# ESSENTIALS OF
# HUMAN DISEASE

## LEONARD V. CROWLEY, MD

Biology Department
Century College
University of Minnesota Medical Center, Fairview
Minneapolis, Minnesota

## JONES AND BARTLETT PUBLISHERS

*Sudbury, Massachusetts*

BOSTON    TORONTO    LONDON    SINGAPORE

## World Headquarters

Jones and Bartlett Publishers
40 Tall Pine Drive
Sudbury, MA 01776
978-443-5000
info@jbpub.com
www.jbpub.com

Jones and Bartlett Publishers
Canada
6339 Ormindale Way
Mississauga, Ontario L5V 1J2
Canada

Jones and Bartlett Publishers
International
Barb House, Barb Mews
London W6 7PA
United Kingdom

Jones and Bartlett's books and products are available through most bookstores and online booksellers. To contact Jones and Bartlett Publishers directly, call 800-832-0034, fax 978-443-8000, or visit our website, www.jbpub.com.

Substantial discounts on bulk quantities of Jones and Bartlett's publications are available to corporations, professional associations, and other qualified organizations. For details and specific discount information, contact the special sales department at Jones and Bartlett via the above contact information or send an email to specialsales@jbpub.com.

The author, editor, and publisher have made every effort to provide accurate information. However, they are not responsible for errors, omissions, or for any outcomes related to the use of the contents of this book and take no responsibility for the use of the products and procedures described. Treatments and side effects described in this book may not be applicable to all people; likewise, some people may require a dose or experience a side effect that is not described herein. Drugs and medical devices are discussed that may have limited availability controlled by the Food and Drug Administration (FDA) for use only in a research study or clinical trial. Research, clinical practice, and government regulations often change the accepted standard in this field. When consideration is being given to use of any drug in the clinical setting, the health care provider or reader is responsible for determining FDA status of the drug, reading the package insert, and reviewing prescribing information for the most up-to-date recommendations on dose, precautions, and contraindications, and determining the appropriate usage for the product. This is especially important in the case of drugs that are new or seldom used.

## Production Credits

Chief Executive Officer: Clayton Jones
Chief Operating Officer: Don W. Jones, Jr.
President, Higher Education and Professional Publishing: Robert W. Holland, Jr.
V.P., Design and Production: Anne Spencer
V.P., Sales and Marketing: William J. Kane
V.P., Manufacturing and Inventory Control: Therese Connell
Publisher, Higher Education: Cathleen Sether
Acquisitions Editor: Shoshanna Goldberg

Senior Associate Editor: Amy L. Bloom
Production Manager: Julie Champagne Bolduc
Associate Production Editor: Jessica Steele Newfell
Associate Marketing Manager: Jody Sullivan
Composition: Glyph International
Cover Design: Kristin E. Parker
Cover Image: Courtesy of Leonard V. Crowley
Printing and Binding: Courier Kendallville
Cover Printing: Courier Kendallville

### Library of Congress Cataloging-in-Publication Data

Crowley, Leonard V.
  Essentials of human disease / Leonard V. Crowley.
    p. ; cm.
  Includes bibliographical references and index.
  ISBN-13: 978-0-7637-6590-3 (pbk. : alk. paper)
  ISBN-10: 0-7637-6590-2 (pbk. : alk. paper)
 1. Physiology, Pathological—Textbooks. I. Title.
  [DNLM: 1. Disease—Programmed Instruction. 2. Pathology—Programmed Instruction. QZ 18.2 C953e 2011]
 RB112.C757 2011
  616.07—dc22

          2009042690

6048
Printed in the United States of America
13 12 11 10 09   10 9 8 7 6 5 4 3 2 1

# Dedication

Dedicated to my wife, who was very helpful and understanding, and also to the many students to whom I have taught human disease concepts. They have been my colleagues as well as my students, and I have enjoyed my association with them.

# Brief Contents

# Contents

# Chapter 9
## Blood Coagulation Abnormalities and Circulatory Disturbances  155

# Chapter 10
## The Cardiovascular System  176

# Chapter 22
## The Musculoskeletal System  491

# Preface

## Purpose and Scope of the Book

*Essentials of Human Disease* is a consolidated and modified version of the very successful *Introduction to Human Disease*, now in its 8th edition. The book is designed to appeal to allied health students who have limited time to master basic disease concepts. Despite time limitations, they want to learn the essential structural and functional characteristics of the common and important diseases, as well as the principles of diagnosis and treatment, and they want the material presented in a user-friendly non-intimidating manner. In order to accomplish these objectives, some diseases considered in *Introduction to Human Disease* had to be eliminated or reduced in content. On the other hand, other items of interest were added to appeal to students, and the format was modified in order to encourage the students to take an active role in the learning process.

Most students have had some previous exposure to anatomy and physiology, and they are often pleasantly surprised to find that the basic concepts relating to human disease are quite straightforward, easy to understand, and extremely interesting. Every organ system has key structural features and physiologic functions, which are reviewed at the beginning of each chapter. All is well when the systems function properly, and when systems do *not* function as they should, students can usually grasp that disease may be the end result. Moreover, when the student understands the anatomic and physiologic changes associated with a given disease, it is not difficult to deduce the clinical manifestations of the disease, and to understand how treatment favorably influences the course and outcome of the disease.

Many students derive tremendous satisfaction from watching their knowledge base relating to human disease grow by leaps and bounds as they proceed through the course, and many students who have taken a human disease course have gone on to careers in biology, medicine, nursing, and other health fields.

Each chapter in the book begins with learning objectives, followed by a brief review of the anatomy and physiology of the organ system discussed in the chapter, which leads into a systematic survey of the pathology, pathophysiology, clinical manifestations, and principles of treatment of the diseases covered. Each chapter ends with a chapter summary, questions for review, student exercises, and an annotated bibliography that summarizes the concepts in the articles cited.

Features that will facilitate learning include the following:

1. Definitions of key terms in bold type in the text are included in the margin of the page where the term appears, as well as in the glossary at the end of the book.
2. Tables are used liberally to reinforce and summarize key material in the text, such as essential features of bacterial, fungal, and parasitic diseases, characteristics of the various types of congenital heart disease, and principles of diagnosis and treatment of heart attacks.
3. Chapters dealing with similar or related subjects are consolidated, and a separate chapter on nutrition and disease has been included.
4. "A Closer Look" boxes have been included in some chapters. These boxes discuss important physicians and scientists who contributed to the diagnosis or treatment of specific diseases, and add interesting insights into the diseases and the persons involved.
5. *Interactive Activities* are included at the end of each chapter. They consist of multiple-choice, matching, true or false, and fill-in-the-blank questions. *Critical Thinking* questions ask a "real world" question about a disease-related subject as would be proposed by a fellow student, parent, or friend. This format requires students to evaluate their knowledge of the subject and then come up with an appropriate answer to the question. The answers to the odd-numbered questions are provided at the back of the book. (Instructors may obtain electronic access to all answers.) The questions and answers can serve as a focus for classroom discussion.

## Organization

The book is organized into two main sections. The first section, comprising the first 9 chapters, deals with general concepts and diseases affecting the body as a whole. The second section, which includes the remaining 13 chapters, considers the various organ systems and their diseases.

In the first section, Chapter 1 discusses manifestations of disease, classification, diagnosis, and principles of treatment. Chapter 2 considers the organization and basic function of cells and tissues, genes, chromosomes, cell division, and chromosome analysis, as well as the HLA system and its relation to disease. Chapters 3 and 4 consider the body's defenses, the inflammatory reaction, the immune system, and their disorders. Chapters 5 and 6 are concerned with the various pathogenic microorganisms, fungi, parasites, and the diseases they cause. Chapter 7 considers congenital and hereditary diseases, and Chapter 8 deals with tumors. Chapter 9 describes coagulation of the blood and the conditions in which the blood does not clot normally, as well as the conditions in which the blood clots too readily and its complications—thrombosis and embolism.

In the second section, the individual organ systems are considered in a systematic manner, with emphasis on the more common and important diseases. Basic pathophysiology, pathology, and principles of diagnosis and treatment are discussed. Chapter 10 describes diseases of the cardiovascular system and related items, including the acute coronary syndrome classification of coronary heart disease. Diseases of the hematopoietic and lymphatic systems are considered together in Chapter 11, followed by diseases of the respiratory system in Chapter 12. Chapters 13 and 14 are best considered as a unit: diseases of the breast, female reproductive system, prenatal development, and diseases associated with pregnancy. Chapter 15 considers kidney diseases and the closely associated diseases of the male reproductive system, which are best considered as a unit. Chapter 16 describes derangements of the liver, biliary system, and pancreas, including diabetes mellitus. Gastrointestinal tract diseases follow in Chapter 17, including sections on eating disorders and their treatment, and Chapter 18 deals with nutrition and disease. Chapter 19 departs from the organ system approach and considers disturbances in fluid, electrolyte, and acid–base balance, which follows the discussion in earlier chapters of the diseases in which these conditions occur. The final three chapters deal, respectively, with diseases of the endocrine glands, nervous system, and musculoskeletal system.

## Study Aids and Special Features

Various learning and study aids are included to enhance the usefulness of the book. Learning objectives, review questions, and chapter summaries are provided for each chapter. Literature for further study is listed at the end of each chapter, and a listing of general references is included at the end of the book. These additional resources should prove useful to students who wish to pursue a subject in greater detail. A glossary with a pronunciation guide is appended to the end of the text. This may prove useful to students who have not had a course in medical terminology, and can serve as a convenient reference for other students who wish to have a quick review of a particular term. Words appearing in the glossary are set in boldface type in the text.

## Additional Resources

### Companion Web Site

The Web site to accompany *Essentials of Human Disease* (http://health.jbpub.com/humandisease/essentials) offers the following resources to enhance learning and comprehension:

**For Students:** Anatomy and Physiology Review, Chapter Outlines, Web Links, Practice Quizzes, Interactive Glossary, Flashcards, and Crosswords

**For Instructors:** PowerPoint Presentations, Lecture Outlines, TestBank, and Answers to Interactive Activities

### Instructor's Media CD-ROM

The **Instructor's Media CD-ROM** includes PowerPoint Presentations and an extensive PowerPoint Image and Table Bank.

For more information about these resources, please contact your sales representative.

## Acknowledgments

Many people helped with the initial edition of *Introduction to Human Disease*, on which the *Essentials of Human Disease* is based. Several colleagues with whom I practiced at hospitals in Minneapolis and St. Paul made helpful suggestions, as did colleagues in the Department of Laboratory Medicine and Pathology, and the Department of Family Practice and Community Health at the University of Minnesota, College of Medicine. Staff members at the West Side Community Health Center in St. Paul were also very helpful, and some of the case studies used in the book were based on these clinical contacts.

Judie Coulter, the senior departmental secretary in the Biology Department at Century College, provided invaluable assistance in converting the 8th edition of *Introduction to Human Disease* to the new *Essentials* book, by organizing the book chapters and preparing the book for publication. It would have been very difficult to accomplish the task without her help.

# General Concepts of Disease: Principles of Diagnosis

## LEARNING OBJECTIVES

1. Define the common terms used to describe disease, such as *lesions*, *organic* and *functional disease*, *symptomatic* and *asymptomatic disease*, *etiology*, and *pathogenesis*.

2. List the major categories of human disease.

3. Explain the approach that a practitioner uses to make a diagnosis and decide on a patient's treatment.

4. Describe the various types of diagnostic tests and procedures that can help the practitioner in making a diagnosis and deciding on proper treatment.

## Characteristics of Disease

Any disturbance of structure or function of the body may be regarded as **disease**. A disease is often associated with well-defined, characteristic structural changes, called **lesions**, that are present in various organs and tissues. One can recognize lesions by examining the diseased tissue with the naked eye, which is called a gross examination, or with the aid of a microscope, which is called a histologic examination. Sometimes histologic examinations are supplemented by specialized studies that evaluate the properties of the cell membranes and the proteins within the cells. A disease associated with structural changes is called an **organic disease**. In contrast, a functional disease is one in which no morphologic abnormalities (*morphe* = structure or shape) can be identified even though body functions may be profoundly disturbed. However, as we develop new methods for studying cells, we can sometimes identify previously unrecognized abnormalities that disturb cell functions. Consequently, many of the traditional distinctions between organic and functional disease are no longer as sharply defined as in the past.

**Pathology** is the study of disease, and a pathologist is a physician who specializes in diagnosing and classifying diseases primarily by examining the morphology of cells and tissues. A clinician is any physician or other health practitioner who cares for patients.

A disease may cause various subjective manifestations, such as weakness or pain, in an affected individual: These are called symptoms. A disease may also produce objective manifestations, detectable by the clinician, that are called signs or physical findings. In many diseases, the quantity of blood cells in the circulation may change, and so may the biochemical constituents in the body fluids. These alterations are reflected as abnormal laboratory test results.

A disease that causes the affected individual no discomfort or disability is called an asymptomatic disease or illness. A disease is often asymptomatic in its early stages. If the disease is not treated, however, it may progress to the stage where it causes subjective symptoms and abnormal physical findings. Therefore, the distinction between asymptomatic and symptomatic disease is one of degree, depending primarily on the extent of the disease.

The term **etiology** means cause. A disease of unknown etiology is one for which the cause is not yet known. Unfortunately, many diseases fall into this category. If the cause of a disease is known, the agent responsible is called the etiologic agent. The term **pathogenesis** refers to the manner by which a disease develops, and a **pathogen** is any microorganism, such as a bacterium or virus, that can cause disease.

**disease**
Any disturbance of the structure or function of the body.

**lesion** (lē′shun) Any structural abnormality or pathologic change.

**organic disease**
A disease associated with structural changes in the affected tissue or organ.

**pathology** The study of the structural and functional changes in the body caused by disease.

**etiology** (ē-tē-ol′ō-jē) The cause, especially the cause of a disease.

**pathogenesis** (path-ō-jen′e-sis) Manner in which a disease develops.

**pathogen** (path-ō-jen′) A disease-causing bacterium or other harmful organism.

# Classifications of Disease

Diseases tend to fall into several large categories, although the diseases in a specific category are not necessarily closely related. Rather, the lesions produced by the various diseases in a category are morphologically similar or have a similar pathogenesis. Diseases are conveniently classified in the following large groups:

1. Congenital and hereditary diseases
2. Inflammatory diseases
3. Degenerative diseases
4. Metabolic diseases
5. Neoplastic diseases

## Congenital and Hereditary Diseases

Congenital and hereditary diseases are the result of developmental disturbances. They may be caused by genetic abnormalities, abnormalities in the numbers and distribution of chromosomes, intrauterine injury as a result of various agents, or an interaction of genetic and environmental factors. Hemophilia, the well-known hereditary disease in which blood does not clot properly, and congenital heart disease induced by the German measles virus are examples of diseases in this category.

## Inflammatory Diseases

Inflammatory diseases are those in which the body reacts to an injurious agent by means of inflammation. Many of the diseases characterized by inflammation, such as a sore throat or pneumonia, are caused by bacteria or other microbiologic agents. Others, such as "hay fever," are a manifestation of an allergic reaction or a hypersensitivity state in the patient. Some diseases in this category appear to be caused by antibodies formed against the patient's own tissues, as occurs in some uncommon diseases classified as autoimmune diseases. The etiology of still other inflammatory diseases has not been determined.

## Degenerative Diseases

In degenerative diseases, the primary abnormality is degeneration of various parts of the body. In some cases, this may be a manifestation of the aging process. In many cases, however, the degenerative lesions are more advanced or occur sooner than would be expected if they were age related, and they are distinctly abnormal. Certain types of arthritis and "hardening of the arteries" (arteriosclerosis) are common examples of degenerative diseases.

## Metabolic Diseases

The chief abnormality seen in metabolic diseases is a disturbance in some important metabolic process in the body. For example, the cells may not be utilizing glucose normally, or the thyroid gland may not properly regulate the rate of cell metabolism. Diabetes, disturbances of endocrine glands, and disturbances of fluid and electrolyte balance are common examples of metabolic diseases.

## Neoplastic Diseases

Neoplastic diseases are characterized by abnormal cell growth that leads to the formation of various types of benign and malignant tumors.

# Health and Disease: A Continuum

Health and disease may be considered two extremes of a continuum. At one extreme is severe, life-threatening, disabling illness with its corresponding major effect on the physical and emotional well-being of the patient. At the other extreme is ideal good health, which may be defined as a state of complete physical and mental well-being. The healthy person is emotionally and physically capable of leading a full, happy, and productive life that is free of anxiety, turmoil, and physical disabilities that limit activities. Between these two extremes are many gradations of health and disease, ranging from mild or short-term illness that limits activities to some extent through moderate good health that falls short of the ideal state. The midpoint in this continuum may be considered a "neutral" position in which one is neither ill nor in ideal good health. In this continuum, most of us are somewhere between mid-position and the ideal state.

The goal of traditional medicine is to cure or ameliorate disease. This is accomplished by various means, ranging from administering an antibiotic to cure an infection to very complex "high-technology" treatments such as kidney transplants and heart surgery. The advances of modern medicine have done much to relieve suffering and advance human welfare, but modern medicine does not guarantee good health. Health is more than an absence of disease; it is a condition in which body and mind function efficiently and harmoniously as an integrated unit. Consequently, we must take an active part in achieving good health by assuming some responsibility for our own physical and emotional well-being. This means practicing such commonsense measures as eating properly, exercising moderately, and avoiding harmful excesses such as overeating, smoking, heavy drinking, or using drugs, which can disrupt physical or emotional well-being. Taking responsibility for one's health also requires using one's mind constructively, expressing emotions, and feeling good about oneself. Positive mental attitudes are essential for good health because negative feelings may be reflected in disturbed bodily functions that are manifested as disease.

# Principles of Diagnosis

The determination of the nature and cause of a patient's illness by a physician or other health practitioner is called a **diagnosis**. It is based on the practitioner's evaluation of the patient's subjective symptoms, the physical findings, and the results of various laboratory tests, together with other appropriate diagnostic procedures. When the practitioner has reached a diagnosis, he or she can then offer a **prognosis**: an opinion concerning the eventual outcome of the disease. Then a course of treatment is instituted.

**diagnosis** The determination of the nature and cause of a patient's illness.

**prognosis** The probable outcome of a disease or a disorder; the outlook for recovery.

## The History

The clinical *history* is a very important part of the evaluation. It consists of several parts:

1. The history of the patient's current illness
2. The past medical history
3. The family history
4. The social history
5. The review of systems

The history of the present illness elicits details concerning the severity, time of onset, and character of the patient's symptoms. Many diseases have characteristic symptoms. The patient's description of the oppressive substernal pain of a heart attack or the pain and urinary disturbances associated with a bladder infection, for example, may provide very helpful information that suggests the correct diagnosis. The past medical history provides details of the patient's general health and previous illnesses. These data may shed light on the patient's current problems as well. The family history provides information about the health of the patient's parents and other family members. Some diseases, such as diabetes and some types of heart disease, tend to run in families. The social history deals with the patient's occupation, habits, alcohol and tobacco use, and similar data. This information may also relate to the patient's general health and current problems. The review of systems inquires as to the presence of symptoms other than those disclosed in the history of the present illness; such symptoms might suggest disease affecting other parts of the body. For example, the practitioner inquires about such symptoms as pain or burning on urination, which suggest an abnormality of the urinary tract, and coughing, shortness of breath, or chest pain, which may indicate disease of the respiratory system. In this way, possible dysfunctions of other organ systems are evaluated by systematic inquiry.

## The Physical Examination

The physical examination is a systematic examination of the patient. The practitioner places particular emphasis on the part of the body affected by the illness, such as the ears, throat, chest, and lungs in the case of a respiratory infection. Any abnormalities detected on the physical examination are correlated with the clinical history. At this point, the practitioner begins to consider the various diseases or conditions that would fit with the clinical findings. Sometimes, more than one possible diagnosis needs to be considered. In a differential diagnosis the practitioner considers a number of diseases that are characterized by the patient's symptoms. For example, if a patient complains of shortness of breath and abnormalities are detected when the lungs are examined with a stethoscope, the practitioner may consider both chronic lung disease and chronic heart failure in the differential diagnosis.

Often the practitioner can narrow the list of diagnostic possibilities and arrive at a correct diagnosis by using selected laboratory tests or other specialized diagnostic procedures. In difficult cases, the clinician may also wish to obtain the opinion of a medical consultant, who is a physician with special training and experience in the type of medical problem presented by the patient.

## Treatment

After the diagnosis has been established, a course of treatment is initiated. There are two different types of treatment: specific treatment and symptomatic treatment.

A specific treatment is one that exerts a highly specific and favorable effect on the basic cause of the disease. For example, an antibiotic may be given to a patient who has an infection that is responsive to the antibiotic, or insulin may be given to a patient with diabetes. Symptomatic treatment, as the name implies, makes the patient more comfortable by alleviating symptoms but does not influence the course of the underlying disease. Examples are the treatment of fever, pain, and cough by means of appropriate medications. Unfortunately, there are no specific treatments for some diseases. Consequently, the clinician must be content with treating the manifestations of the disease without being able to influence its ultimate course.

When dealing with patients who have long-standing chronic disease such as chronic heart, kidney, or lung disease, or some types of cancer, the physician may be assisted by a disease management team composed of a group of persons with special skills that are useful in the care and treatment of patients with these diseases. The management team may include persons who can explain to patients the nature of their disease, the goals of treatment, and how patients can contribute to their own care. Other health-care team members such as dieticians, nurse clinicians, physician's assistants, respiratory therapists, physiotherapists, and pharmacists can bring their own special skills to help physicians care for patients with chronic illnesses who require long-term care and who have special needs. Often the team approach to management of patients with chronic diseases reduces the long-term costs of medical care, improves the patient's satisfaction with the quality of his or her medical care, and contributes to a more favorable response to treatment.

# Screening Tests for Disease

## Purpose and Requirements for Effective Screening

Many diseases that respond to treatment are asymptomatic initially. If untreated, however, the disease often progresses slowly, causing gradual but progressive organ damage until eventually the person is seriously ill with far advanced organ damage caused by the disease. Unfortunately, treatment of late-stage disease is often much less effective and may not be able to restore the function of the organs that have been damaged. Had the disease been identified and treated in its early asymptomatic stage, the disease-related organ damage could have been prevented or minimized, and the affected person would have been spared the discomfort, disability, and shortened survival associated with late-stage disease.

A successful screening program should fulfill the following requirements:

1. A significant number of persons must be at risk for the disease in the group being screened.
2. A relatively inexpensive noninvasive test must be available to screen for the disease that does not yield an excessively high number of false-positive or false-negative results.
3. Early identification and treatment of the disease will favorably influence the health or welfare of the person with the disease.

## Groups Suitable for Screening

Screening tests should target a group of persons in whom there is a relatively high frequency of disease, and tests should also target the age group in whom the disease is likely to be present. If the disease, for example, has its onset in middle age, then screening adolescents and children in the target group would not be productive.

## Suitable Screening Tests

Screening a group of persons for a disease in its early asymptomatic stage requires some type of test that can identify some characteristic manifestation of the disease, such as high blood sugar in the case of diabetes, or the presence of blood in the stool in the case of a colon tumor. A test used for screening should be reasonably inexpensive and should have few false-positive results (test is positive when no disease is present) and few false-negative results (test is negative when disease is present). If the test produced a large number of false-positive results in the group being screened, many persons with false-positive test results would have to undergo more extensive and sometimes invasive testing, as well as a comprehensive medical evaluation, only to find that the test result was a "false alarm" and that they did not have the disease. On the other hand, less sensitive screening tests would yield an excess of false-negative tests, and many persons who actually had the disease would not be detected.

## Benefits of Screening

Screening test results should provide some benefit to the person being screened. Generally, there is no point in screening for a disease if no treatment is available to arrest the progression of the disease.

Examples of widely used cost-effective screening tests for disease include urine tests to detect glucose in the urine as a screening test for diabetes, tests to detect blood in the stools to screen for colon tumors, Papanicolaou smears (Pap tests) to screen for abnormalities in the epithelium of the uterine cervix that predispose to cancer, and breast x-ray examinations (mammograms) to screen for very early breast cancer at a stage when it can be treated most effectively.

## Screening for Genetic Disease

Screening tests can also be used to screen for carriers of some genetic diseases that are transmitted from parent to child as either dominant or recessive traits. When many persons in a population carry a recessive gene that can be detected by relatively simple screening tests, identifying carriers allows the affected persons to make decisions regarding future childbearing or management of a future pregnancy. One high-incidence recessive gene for which screening is available is the sickle hemoglobin gene, which occurs in about 8 percent of the black population. A child born to two carriers of the sickle hemoglobin gene who receives the sickle hemoglobin gene from each parent will develop a severe anemia called sickle cell anemia. The sickle hemoglobin gene and its clinical manifestations are considered in Chapter 11. Other examples of genetic diseases for which screening is available are described in Chapter 7.

# Diagnostic Tests and Procedures

A wide array of diagnostic tests and procedures are available to help the practitioner diagnose and treat the patient properly. They fall into two classifications: invasive procedures and noninvasive procedures. Invasive procedures are so-named because the patient's body is actually "invaded" in some way in order to obtain diagnostic information. Such procedures involve introducing needles, catheters, or other instruments into the patient's body. Noninvasive procedures are those that entail no risk or minimal risk or discomfort to the patient, such as a chest x-ray or an examination of the urine.

Many diagnostic procedures entail some degree of risk or discomfort to the patient. The risk is greater with invasive procedures, but even some noninvasive procedures are not completely harmless. A chest x-ray, for example, exposes the patient to radiation. Even a relatively simple procedure such as the collection of a blood sample for a laboratory test may be complicated by bleeding around the vein or by formation of a blood clot in the vein at the site of puncture. Therefore, with any diagnostic procedure, the practitioner must balance the possible disadvantages to the patient against the benefits that may be derived from the information obtained by the procedure. Patients also must be fully informed about the possible risks and benefits so that they can make informed decisions as to whether to consent to the procedure. It would be unwise to perform a potentially risky diagnostic procedure if the information gained would not contribute significantly to the diagnosis or would not greatly influence the course of treatment. The physician would be much more likely to employ a diagnostic procedure that could provide much useful information at little or no risk to the patient.

Diagnostic tests and procedures can be classified in several major categories:

1. Clinical laboratory tests
2. Tests that measure the electrical activity of the body
3. Tests using radioisotopes
4. Endoscopy
5. Ultrasound procedures
6. X-ray examinations
7. Magnetic resonance imaging (MRI)
8. Cytologic and histologic examination of cells and tissues removed from the patient

## Clinical Laboratory Tests

Clinical laboratory tests have many uses. They can be used to determine the concentration of various constituents in the blood and urine, which are frequently altered by disease. For example, the concentration of a substance in the blood called urea is elevated if the kidneys are not functioning properly, because this constituent is normally excreted by the kidneys. The concentrations of hemoglobin and the quantity of red cells are reduced in patients with anemia. One can also determine the level of enzymes in the blood. Sometimes the enzyme level is elevated because (1) enzymes are leaking from diseased or injured organs, (2) enzyme synthesis is increased as a result of disease, or (3) excretion of enzymes is impaired because disease has caused blockage of normal excretory pathways.

Clinical laboratory tests are also used to evaluate the functions of organs. Clearance tests measure the rate at which a substance such as urea or creatinine is removed from blood and excreted in the urine. This provides a measure of renal (kidney) function. Pulmonary function tests measure the rate at which air moves in and out of the lungs. Determinations of the concentration of oxygen and carbon dioxide in the blood also can indicate how well the lungs are working. A simple device is available that can be applied to the finger that can calculate rapidly the amount of oxygen carried by hemoglobin as another measure of pulmonary function. Tests that measure the uptake and excretion of various substances by the liver are used as a measure of liver function. Microbiologic tests detect the presence of disease-producing organisms in urine, blood, and feces. Other tests can determine the responsiveness of the organisms to antibiotics. Serologic tests detect and measure the presence of antibodies as an indication of response to infectious agents.

## Tests of Electrical Activity

Several different tests measure the electrical impulses associated with various bodily functions and activities. These include the electrocardiogram (ECG), the electroencephalogram (EEG), and the electromyogram (EMG). The most widely used of these tests is the ECG. Electrodes attached to the arms, legs, and chest are used to measure the serial changes in the electrical activity of the heart during the various phases of the cardiac cycle. The ECG also identifies disturbances in the heart rate or rhythm and identifies abnormal conduction of impulses through the heart. Heart muscle injury, such as occurs after a heart attack, can also be recognized by means of characteristic abnormalities in the cardiogram. The EEG measures the electrical activity of the brain,

often called brain waves, by means of small electrodes attached to different areas in the scalp. Brain tumors, strokes, and many other abnormalities of cerebral structure or function may cause altered brain wave patterns that are detected by this examination. The EMG measures the electrical activity of skeletal muscle during contraction and at rest. Abnormal electrical activity is often encountered in various inflammatory or degenerative diseases involving the skeletal muscles.

## Radioisotope Studies

The function of various organs can be evaluated by administering a substance labeled with a radioactive material called a radioisotope. Specially designed radiation detectors then measure the uptake and excretion of the labeled substance. For example, the ability of the thyroid gland to concentrate and utilize radioactive iodine is used to measure thyroid function and can also be used to detect tumors within the thyroid gland. Another procedure can be used to detect the presence of blood clots in the lung that impede blood flow to parts of the lung. Phosphorus-containing isotopes are concentrated in the skeletal system. If there are deposits of tumor in bone, the isotopes are concentrated around the tumor deposits and can be easily identified ( Figure 1-1 ). Radioactive materials injected intravenously can also be used to evaluate blood flow to heart muscle and to identify areas of damaged heart muscle.

## Endoscopy and Laparoscopy

An **endoscopy**, or endoscopic examination (*endo* = within + *skopeo* = examine), is an examination of the interior of the body by means of various types of rigid or flexible tubular instruments that are named according to the part of the body they are designed to examine. These instruments have a system of lenses for viewing and a light source to illuminate the region being examined. An esophagoscope, for example, is used to examine the interior of the esophagus, a gastroscope to examine the stomach, and a bronchoscope to examine the trachea and major bronchi. An instrument for viewing the interior of the bladder is called a cystoscope. A sigmoidoscope is a rigid tube used to examine the rectum and the sigmoid colon, and a colonoscope is a flexible tube that can be used to examine the entire length of the colon.

An instrument called a **laparoscope** is used to visualize the abdominal and pelvic organs, and the procedure is called laparoscopy, which can be used not only to examine abdominal and pelvic organs, but also to perform various surgical procedures, such as removal

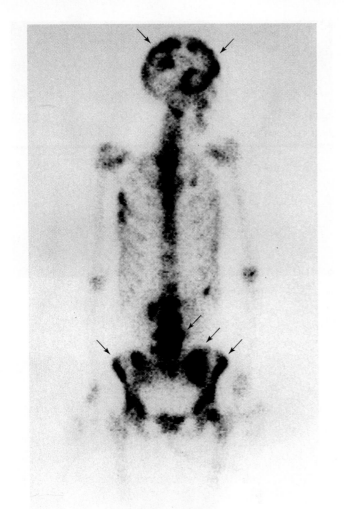

Radioisotope bone scan of head, chest, and pelvis. Dark areas (*arrows*) indicate the concentration of radioisotope around tumor deposits in bone.

of the gallbladder (cholecystectomy), appendix (appendectomy), ovary (oophorectomy), and other surgical procedures that formerly required much larger abdominal incisions. To perform a laparoscopic procedure the peritoneal cavity is inflated first with carbon dioxide that separates the organs within the peritoneal cavity so that they can be visualized more easily. Then the laparoscope is inserted through a small incision in the abdominal wall, often in or near the umbilicus. If a surgical procedure is to be performed such as an appendectomy (removing the appendix) or cholecystectomy (removing the gallbladder), one or two additional small incisions are needed to insert the instruments used to perform the surgical procedure and remove the organ from the abdominal cavity.

## Ultrasound

Ultrasound is a technique for mapping the echoes produced by high-frequency sound waves transmitted into the body. Echoes are reflected wherever there is a change in the density of the tissue. The reflected waves are recorded on sensitive detectors, and images are produced. This method is widely used to study the uterus during pregnancy because it does not require the use of potentially harmful radiation and poses no risk to the fetus ( Figure 1-2 ). The technique can be used to determine the position of the placenta and the fetus within the uterus; it can also identify some fetal abnormalities and detect twin pregnancies. Ultrasound is also used to study the structure and function of the heart valves.

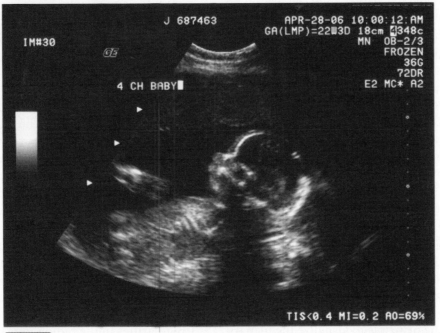

Ultrasound examination of a 22-week-old fetus. (Image courtesy of Belinda Thresher.)

The procedure can detect valve abnormalities and identify blood clots that sometimes form on the heart valves in association with infection of the valve (described in Chapter 10). Ultrasound can determine the thickness of the ventricular walls and septum and the size of the ventricular chambers during the contraction and relaxation of the heart (systole and diastole). Ultrasound can identify gallstones in the gallbladder and abnormalities in the prostate suspicious for prostate cancer. The technique has many other applications in medicine.

## X-Ray Examination

X-ray examinations are conducted in many ways, but the basic principle is the same for all types of x-ray studies. X-rays are passed through the part of the body to be examined, and the rays leaving the body expose an x-ray film. The extent to which the rays are absorbed by the tissues as they pass through the body depends on the density of the tissues. Tissues of low density, such as the air-filled lungs, transmit most of the rays, and thus, the film exposed to x-rays passing through them appears black. Tissues of high density, such as bone, absorb most of the rays; the film remains unexposed and appears white. Tissues of intermediate densities appear as varying shades of gray. The x-ray image produced on the film is called a radiograph or **roentgenogram**. The same basic principle is used to obtain x-ray films of the breast. This procedure is called a **mammogram**. The applications and limitations of the mammogram procedure are considered in Chapter 13 in the section on diseases of the breast.

**roentgenogram**
(rent′gen-ō-gram)
A photograph taken with x-rays.

**mammogram** (mam′ō-gram) An x-ray of the breast, used to detect tumors and other abnormalities within the breast.

Although the linings of internal organs such as the intestinal tract, urinary tract, bronchi, fallopian tubes, and biliary tract have little contrast, they can be examined by administering a dense radiopaque substance called contrast medium. It coats and adheres to the lining of the structure being examined and enhances its visibility. To examine the interior of the gastrointestinal tract, for example, one gives the patient a suspension of barium sulfate to swallow or administers it as an enema. The opaque barium coats the lining of the intestinal tract, and an abnormality in the lining shows on the film as an irregularity in the column of barium ( Figure 1-3 ). The lining of the bronchi can be visualized by instilling a radiopaque oil into the bronchi. The oil forms a thin film on the bronchial mucosa and delineates the contours of the bronchi. This procedure is called a bronchogram ( Figure 1-4 ).

One uses the same principle to visualize the urinary tract. A radiopaque substance is injected into a vein and

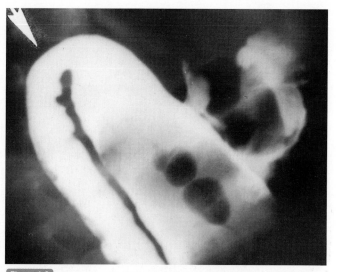

Figure 1-3    X-ray film after injection of radiopaque barium sulfate suspension into colon (barium enema), illustrating narrowed area (*arrow*) that impedes passage of bowel contents.

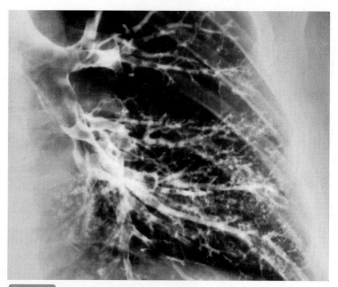

Figure 1-4    Bronchogram illustrating normal branching of bronchi and bronchioles that are normal in caliber and appearance.

is excreted in the urine as the blood flows through the kidney, outlining the contour of the urinary tract. This is called an intravenous pyelogram (IVP) ( Figure 1-5 ). Another method is to introduce the dye directly into both ureters through tubes that are inserted into both ureters by means of a cystoscope introduced into the bladder. This procedure is called a retrograde pyelogram. To visualize the gallbladder, the patient ingests tablets of radiopaque material that is absorbed into the circulation, excreted by the liver in the bile, and concentrated in the gallbladder. Gallstones can be identified because they occupy space in the gallbladder and cause irregularities in the radiopaque material concentrated there ( Figure 1-6 ).

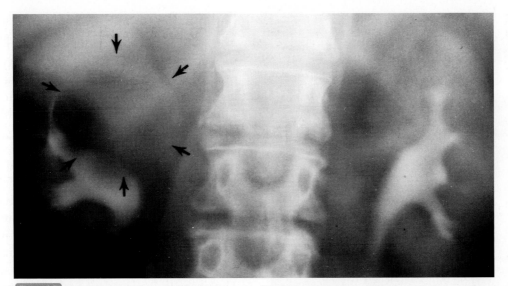

**Figure 1-5** Intravenous pyelogram (IVP). *Arrows* outline filling defect caused by a large cyst in the kidney that distorts the renal pelvis and calyces. The opposite kidney appears normal.

**A**

**B**

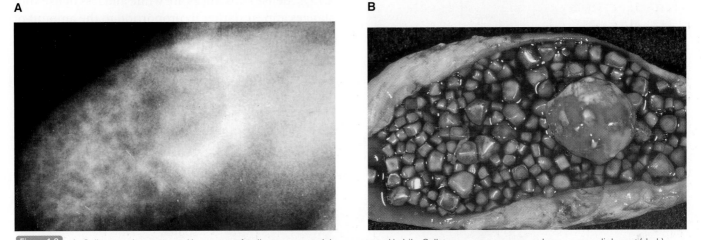

**Figure 1-6** **A,** Gallstones demonstrated by means of radiopaque material concentrated in bile. Gallstones occupy space and appear as radiolucent (dark) areas within radiopaque (white) bile. Note the large radiolucent area, indicating a large gallstone, surrounded by smaller radiolucent areas, representing multiple smaller stones. **B,** Opened gallbladder removed surgically from the same patient. Compare appearance and location of stones with x-ray appearance.

One can also use contrast material to study the flow of blood in large arteries and to identify areas of narrowing or obstruction. This procedure is called an **arteriogram** or **angiogram** (*angio* = blood vessel). A small flexible catheter is inserted into a large artery in the arm or leg and advanced into the aorta until it is positioned at the opening of the artery that is to be examined. Radiopaque material is then injected through the catheter. It mixes with the blood, and its flow through the vessel is followed by means of a series of x-ray films. If the vessel is narrowed by disease, the film will show areas in which the column of opaque material is narrowed. A complete obstruction of the vessel appears as an interruption of the column. Arteriography is often used to detect narrowing or obstruction of the coronary arteries or of the carotid arteries in the neck, which carry blood to the brain

(**Figure 1-7**). Obstruction of the pulmonary arteries by blood clots also can be identified by arteriography. In this case, the catheter used to inject the radiopaque material is inserted into a large vein in the arm, threaded up the vein and through the right side of the heart, and positioned in the pulmonary artery.

This same basic method can be used to study the flow of blood through the heart and can detect abnormal communications between cardiac chambers. This type of study is called **cardiac catheterization.**

**arteriogram**
(är-tēr´ē-ō-gram) An x-ray technique for studying the caliber of blood vessels by injection of radiopaque material into the vessel.

**angiogram**
(an´jē-ō-gram) Same as *arteriogram*.

**cardiac catheterization**
A specialized technique to determine the blood flow through the chambers of the heart, and to detect abnormal communications between cardiac chambers.

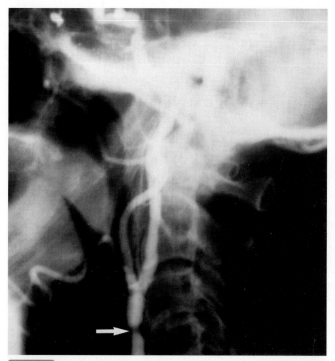

**Figure 1-7** Narrowing of carotid artery in neck (*arrow*) demonstrated by carotid angiogram.

## Computed Tomographic Scans

A **computed tomographic scan** (**CT scan**) is performed by a highly sophisticated x-ray machine that produces images of the body in cross section by rotating the x-ray tube around the patient at various levels. The x-ray tube is mounted on a movable frame opposite an array of sensitive radiation detectors that encircle the patient. As the x-ray tube moves around the patient, the radiation detectors record the amount of radiation passing through the body (Figure 1-8). In computerized scanning, the amount of radiation absorbed is not read directly on an x-ray film. Instead, the data from the radiation detectors are fed into a computer, which reconstructs the data into an image that reproduces the patient's anatomy as a cross-section picture. The image is displayed on a television monitor and can be recorded on film (Figure 1-9). As with conventional x-rays, dense substances are white and less dense substances appear darker in proportion to the amount of

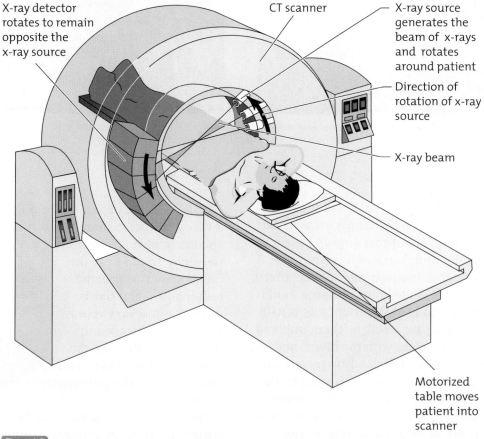

X-ray detector rotates to remain opposite the x-ray source

CT scanner

X-ray source generates the beam of x-rays and rotates around patient

Direction of rotation of x-ray source

X-ray beam

Motorized table moves patient into scanner

**Figure 1-8** Computed tomographic (CT) scan. The patient lies on a table that is gradually advanced into the scanner. X-ray tube mounted in scanner rotates around patient, and radiation detectors also rotate so that detectors remain opposite the x-ray source. Data from radiation detectors generate computer-reconstructed images of the patient's body at multiple levels.

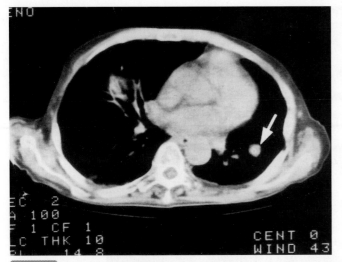

Figure 1-9 CT scan of chest. Mediastinum and heart appear white in the center of scan, with less dense lungs on either side. The *arrow* indicates a lung tumor, which appears as a white nodule in the lung.

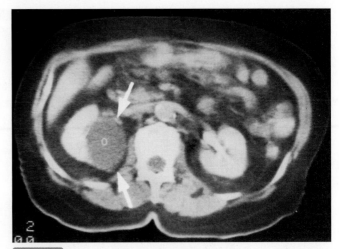

Figure 1-10 CT views of the abdomen at the level of kidneys, illustrating a fluid-filled cyst in the kidney (*arrow*). The cyst appears less dense than surrounding renal tissue. The opposite kidney (*right side of photograph*) appears normal.

radiation they transmit. The individual organs appear sharply separated from one another because the various parts of the body are separated by planes of fat, which have very low density. These separations increase contrast between adjacent organs. Abnormalities of internal organs that cannot be identified by means of standard x-ray examinations can often be discovered with CT scans. (Figure 1-10) shows a renal cyst located by CT scan.

CT delivers a much greater dose of radiation than a standard x-ray examination, such as a chest x-ray, and some physicians are concerned that repeated CT examinations may deliver a significant and possibly excessive amount of radiation to the patient. Ultrasound examination, which sometimes can provide the same information without any radiation exposure, is recommended whenever it can substitute for CT to provide comparable diagnostic information.

## Magnetic Resonance Imaging

Magnetic resonance imaging (MRI) produces computer-constructed images of various organs and tissues somewhat like CT scans. The device consists of a strong magnet capable of developing a powerful magnetic field, coils that can transmit and receive radio frequency waves, and a computer, which receives impulses from the scanner and forms them into images that can be interpreted. The MRI scanner with the enclosed magnet and coils appears similar to a CT scanner. The patient lies on a table that is gradually moved into the scanner, as is done in CT scans. The principle of MRI, however, is quite different from that of CT scanning, which uses ionizing radiation to construct images based on the density of tissues. In contrast, the computer-generated images obtained by MRI scans depend on the response of hydrogen protons (positively charged particles in the nucleus around which electrons rotate) contained within water molecules when they are placed in a strong magnetic field. Body tissues, which have a high water content, are a rich source of protons capable of excitation. The intensity of the signals produced is related to the varying water content of body tissues. Because an MRI does not use ionizing radiation, the patient does not receive radiation exposure. An MRI does expose the patient to strong magnetic fields and radio waves, but this appears relatively safe, on the basis of current knowledge.

**computed tomographic (CT) scan**

(tō-mō-graf′ik) An x-ray technique producing detailed cross-sectional images of the body by means of x-ray tube and detectors connected to a computer. Sometimes called a CAT scan.

## Applications

An MRI detects many of the same types of abnormalities detected by a CT, and a CT is superior to an MRI for many applications. An MRI, however, offers distinct advantages over CT in special situations, as, for example, when attempting to detect abnormalities in tissues surrounded by bone, such as lesions in the spinal cord, orbits, or near the base of the skull (Figure 1-11). In these locations, bone interferes with scanning because of its density, but it does not produce an image in MRI because the water content of bone is low. MRI also provides a sharp contrast between gray and white matter within the brain and spinal cord, which differ in their water content. For this reason, the technique is useful for demonstrating areas where myelin sheaths of nerve fibers have been damaged, as in a neurologic disease called multiple sclerosis (described in Chapter 21, The Nervous System).

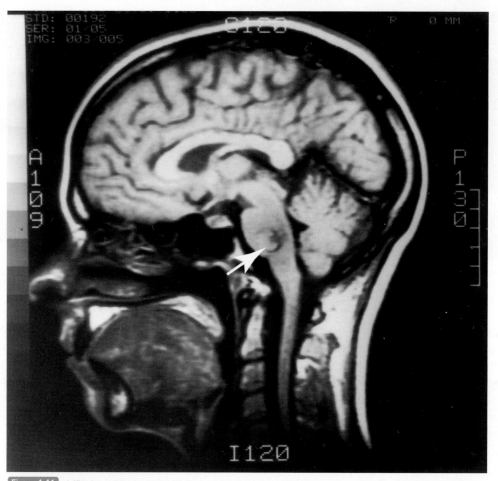

**Figure 1-11** MRI view of the brain, which is clearly visible because skull bones are not visualized by MRI. The white line surrounding the brain represents scalp tissue. The *arrow* indicates a malformation composed of blood vessels within the brain stem.

## Cytologic and Histologic Examinations

Cells covering the surfaces of the body are continually cast off and replaced by new cells. Abnormal cells can often be identified in the fluids or secretions that come in contact with the epithelial surface. This type of examination is called a Papanicolaou smear, or simply **Pap smear**, after the physician who developed the procedure.

It is widely used as a screening test for recognizing early cancer of the uterus and can be used to detect cancers in other locations as well. The Pap smear is discussed in the section on neoplasms in Chapter 11.

Diseased tissues have abnormal structural and cellular patterns that can be recognized by the pathologist. Consequently, it is often possible to

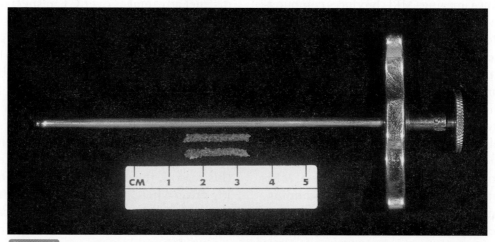

**Figure 1-12** Two samples of bone marrow (adjacent to scale) obtained from pelvic bone by means of a specially designed needle, shown in the upper part of the photograph.

determine the cause of a patient's disease by histologic examination of a small sample of tissue removed from the affected tissue or organ. This procedure is called a **biopsy**. Samples of tissue can be obtained from any part of the body. Gastroscopes, bronchoscopes, and other instruments used for endoscopic examination, for example, are constructed so that specimens for biopsy can be obtained while the internal organs are being examined. Biopsy specimens can also be taken directly from internal organs such as the liver or kidney by inserting a thin needle through the skin directly into the organ. Samples of bone marrow are obtained in this way, and bone-marrow biopsy is often performed to diagnose blood disease ( Figure 1-12 ).

**Pap smear** A study of cells from various sources, commonly used as a screening test for cancer.

**biopsy** (bī′op-sē) Removal of a small sample of tissue for examination and diagnosis by a pathologist.

## A Closer Look

*In the late nineteenth century a Canadian physician completely revolutionized medical education and medical practice in the United States and moved American medicine into the twentieth century.*

His name was William Osler. He was born in Ontario, Canada, in 1849. He received his MD from McGill University in Montreal, followed by postgraduate studies in London, Berlin, and Vienna. In 1874 he returned as professor to McGill University, where he taught medicine, anatomy, physiology, and pathology. In 1888, he was recruited as physician-in-chief at a soon-to-open Johns Hopkins Hospital, and professor of medicine at a planned Johns Hopkins medical school in Baltimore, Maryland. Osler revolutionized the medical curriculum, shifting emphasis from didactic lectures to clinical instruction of medical students in the hospital wards, where the students learned by doing: obtaining a clinical history from the patient, performing a physical examination, and formulating diagnostic possibilities and prognoses under the watchful eye of the physician–instructor. He was soon recognized as a superb clinician, teacher, and clinical investigator who treated students as colleagues. He wrote one of the first textbooks of medicine, *The Principles and Practice of Medicine*, which remained the standard medical textbook for the next 40 years. In 1905, Osler left Baltimore to accept a very prestigious appointment at Oxford University in England as Regius Professor of Medicine, where he continued until his death in 1919.

# CHAPTER REVIEW

## Summary

Disease is a disturbance of the structure or function of the body that produces various manifestations consisting of symptoms and signs, and is associated with abnormal laboratory test results. Symptoms are what the patient tells the physician or health practitioner about how the disease is affecting the patient, such as causing a headache, sore throat, burning on urination, or chest pain. Signs are objective manifestations that the practitioner can identify by examining the patient, such as identifying a skin rash, a throat inflammation, or enlarged tender lymph nodes in the neck. Often the practitioner will perform various laboratory tests to obtain further information about the disease, such as performing a urinalysis or urine culture if a urinary tract infection is suspected, or a chest x-ray if pneumonia is suspected. Many different types of tests are described, each having specific applications and limitations as described in the chapter. The clinician's task is to determine the nature of the disease (make a diagnosis), estimate the probable outcome of the disease (prognosis), and then treat the patient (symptomatic and specific treatment).

Often, screening tests are used to identify persons in a population who have a higher-than-normal risk of a specific disease, or who have an early asymptomatic disease that can be treated successfully before the disease can cause significant organ damage. Screening requires (1) a "screenable population" (significant frequency of disease in the population selected for screening), (2) a reliable cost-effective test to identify the disease that can be performed without risk to the patient, and (3) evidence that early detection of the disease will favorably influence outcome.

## Questions for Review

1. What are the five major categories of disease?
2. What are the definitions of the following terms: *etiology*, *symptom of disease*, *sign of disease*, *diagnosis*, and *prognosis*?
3. How does an organic disease differ from a functional disease?
4. What principal factors does the physician evaluate in arriving at a diagnosis?
5. What is the difference between specific and symptomatic treatment?
6. What are the major categories of diagnostic tests and procedures that can help the practitioner make a diagnosis? Give some examples.
7. What is the difference between an invasive and a noninvasive procedure?
8. What are the basic concepts on which the following procedures are based: Pap smear, x-ray examinations, ultrasound, electrocardiogram, and CT scans?

## Supplementary Reading

Guttmacher, A. E., Collins, F. S., and Carmona, R. H. 2004. The family history: More important than ever. *New England Journal of Medicine* 351:2333–35.

We do patients a disservice if we fail to realize the value of the family history in pinpointing some of the more common diseases that have a hereditary or genetic component. Patients are encouraged to bring their family history to their health-care provider for further discussion, evaluation, and use.

Khoury, M. J., McCabe, L., and McCabe, E. R. B. 2003. Population screening in the age of genomic medicine. *New England Journal of Medicine* 348:50–58.

Newborn infants are routinely screened for several inherited diseases so that early diagnosis can allow prompt treatment, thereby preventing the long-term adverse effects caused by the disease. Screening of adults for selected diseases can also provide benefits to the affected persons.

McNutt, R. A. 2004. Shared medical decision making: Problems, process, progress. *Journal of the American Medical Association* 292:2516–18.

Decisions about options for treatment of a disease should be a joint effort on the part of both the physician and the patient, and the patient needs to understand that every decision is influenced by uncertainty and risk. The physician can explain the possible risks and benefits of various methods of treatment, but the patient must make the final decision.

Paltiel, A. D., Weinstein, M. C., Kimmel, A. D., et al. 2005. Expanded screening for HIV in the United States—an analysis of cost effectiveness. *New England Journal of Medicine* 352:586–95.

One-time screening for HIV antibodies in high-risk groups allowed earlier detection of the infection and improved survival time among high-risk populations. Routine HIV screening every 3–5 years among high-risk groups is cost effective.

Pratt, D. S., and Kaplan, M. M. 2000. Evaluation of abnormal liver enzyme tests in asymptomatic patients. *New England Journal of Medicine* 342:1266–71.

Automated routine laboratory testing is often part of an annual medical examination and may reveal unsuspected liver or biliary tract disease, which can be influenced favorably by early recognition and treatment.

Zuckerman, S., Lahad, A., Shmueli, A., et al. 2007. Carrier screening for Gaucher's disease. Lessons for low-penetrance treatable diseases. *Journal of the American Medical Association* 298:1281–90.

A screening program in Israel was instituted to detect asymptomatic carriers of a Gaucher disease gene mutation, which occurs in about 6 percent of the Ashkenazi Jewish population, in order to identify couples at risk of conceiving a child with the disease. The screening was controversial because carriers are asymptomatic and many affected children have relatively mild disease. Screening provided couples with knowledge of their carrier state, and did reduce the number of pregnancies terminated because the fetus was affected, but was less cost-effective than the screening program to detect carriers of the gene mutation responsible for Tay-Sachs disease, which is a more severe, progressive, and rapidly fatal disease in affected infants.

# Interactive Activities

## Multiple Choice

Select the correct answer.

1. Which of the following statements regarding identification of inherited disease in newborn infants by screening tests is INCORRECT?
   A. Screening is unlikely to be useful because most inherited diseases do not respond to treatment.
   B. Long-term harmful effects of inherited diseases can often be prevented by early identification and treatment.
   C. Identification of a hereditary disease in a newborn may allow the parents to make an informed decision regarding future pregnancies based on the nature of the inherited disease and its prognosis.

2. A government agency proposes a pilot program to screen a population for a disease by means of a blood test. The characteristics of the disease and the screening test are listed. Which of these statements indicates that the proposed screening test is unlikely to be worthwhile?
   A. The disease occurs with moderate frequency in the population (about 1 per 1000).
   B. The disease progresses very slowly in affected persons.
   C. No specific method of treatment is available at the present time.
   D. The test is relatively inexpensive (about $15.00).
   E. The test is quite specific and produces very few false-positive and false-negative results.

3. A patient has a chronic cough, fever, and a purulent (pus-filled) sputum. A lung infection (pneumonia) is suspected. Which of the listed diagnostic tests is LEAST LIKELY to provide useful information?
   A. White blood cell count and differential count
   B. Chest x-ray
   C. Culture of sputum for disease-producing microorganisms
   D. Urinalysis
   E. Computed tomographic (CT) scan

4. The opinion of a physician or other health-care practitioner concerning the probable outcome of the disease is called
   A. Diagnosis          C. Prognosis
   B. Etiology           D. Pathology

5. A young woman has a skin rash caused by an allergic reaction to an antibiotic. The patient's condition would be interpreted as
   A. An infection
   B. An inflammation
   C. A degenerative disease
   D. A metabolic disease

## Critical Thinking

1. The frequency of the sickle cell hemoglobin gene in the African American population is about 8 percent. Two African Americans plan to marry and raise a family. The woman suggests that they both have a screening test for the sickle-cell hemoglobin gene before they marry, and the man asks what you think about the idea. What would you tell him? Explain your reasons.

2. A computed tomographic (CT) scan of the chest and abdomen can provide information about the structure of internal organs that could not be obtained by a routine medical history, physical examination, and a panel of basic laboratory tests. A young couple in good health would like to have an annual CT of the chest and abdomen. They believe it will be able to detect an early stage of an unsuspected organ disease that could be identified and treated early when the treatment would be most effective. They ask for your opinion. What would you tell them? Explain your answer.

# 2

# Genes, Chromosomes, Cells, and Tissues: Their Structure and Function in Health and Disease

## LEARNING OBJECTIVES

1. Describe how cells are organized to form tissues.
2. Describe how tissues are organized to form organ systems.
3. Describe how cells utilize the genetic code within DNA chains to convey genetic nformation to daughter cells during cell division.
4. Explain the process by which the DNA in the nucleus directs the synthesis of enzymes and other proteins in the cytoplasm.
5. Explain how an aging cell becomes increasingly vulnerable to injury.
6. Illustrate how materials move in and out of cells. List five processes by which cells adapt to changing conditions.
7. Describe how chromosomes are studied. Describe how a karyotype is determined.
8. Compare mitosis and meiosis.
9. Compare spermatogenesis and oogenesis. Explain the implications of abnormal chromosome separations in the course of meiosis in older women.
10. Describe the inheritance pattern of genes and define dominant, recessive, codominant, and sex-linked inheritance.

## Organization of Cells

The cell is the basic structural and functional unit of the body. Tissues are groups of similar cells arranged to perform a specific function. Tissues in turn are grouped together in different proportions to form organs, and groups of organs functioning together form organ systems. Finally, the various organ systems are integrated to form a functioning organism. Dysfunction at any of these levels of organization can cause disease.

# The Cell

Cells having different functions differ somewhat in structure, but all have certain features in common ( Figure 2-1 ). Each cell consists of a nucleus surrounded by the cytoplasm. The nucleus, which contains the genetic information stored in the cell, directs the metabolic functions of the cell, and structures in the cytoplasm carry out these directions. Within the cytoplasm are numerous small structures called **organelles**, which play an important part in the functions of the cell. The cytoplasm also contains filaments of structural protein that form the framework (cytoskeleton) of the cell. Some cells also contain filaments of contractile protein. The cytoplasm, nucleus, and organelles are surrounded by membranes composed of lipid and protein molecules, which separate these structures from one another.

## The Nucleus

The nucleus contains two different types of nucleic acid combined with protein. **Deoxyribonucleic acid (DNA)** is contained in the chromosomes, which are long and thin in the nondividing cell and cannot be identified as distinct structures. Instead, they appear as a network of granules called nuclear chromatin. **Ribonucleic acid (RNA)** is contained in spherical intranuclear structures called nucleoli (singular; nucleolus). The nucleus is separated from the cytoplasm by a double-layered nuclear membrane. Small pores in the nuclear membrane permit the nucleus and cytoplasm to communicate.

## The Cytoplasm

The cytoplasm of the cell consists of a mass of protoplasm surrounded by a cell membrane, which acts selectively to allow some materials to pass into and out of the cell while it restricts the passage of others. It contains various organelles and may also contain products secreted by the cell, such as glycogen and fat. The most important organelles are the mitochondria, endoplasmic reticulum, Golgi apparatus, lysosomes, centrioles, and the tubules and filaments comprising the cytoskeleton of the cell. Their functions are summarized in Table 2-1 . Figure 2-2 illustrates how lysosomes perform their digestive functions. Some diseases are associated with characteristic abnormalities in cytoplasmic organelles.

**organelle** A small structure present in the cytoplasm of the cell, such as a mitochondrion.

**deoxyribonucleic acid (DNA)** The nucleic acid present in the chromosomes of the nuclei of cells that carries genetic information.

**ribonucleic acid (RNA)** A type of nucleic acid contained in the nucleoli of cells. A component of messenger, transfer, and ribosomal RNA.

**tissue** A group of similar cells joined to perform a specific function.

# Tissues

A **tissue** is a group of similar cells joined together to perform a specific function. Tissues are classified into four major groups:

1. Epithelium
2. Connective and supporting tissues
3. Muscle tissue
4. Nerve tissue

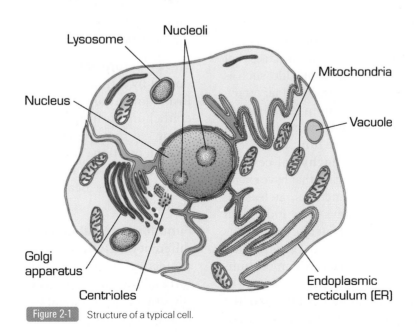

Figure 2-1   Structure of a typical cell.

## Table 2-1 Major Cell Organelles and Their Functions

| Organelle | Function |
| --- | --- |
| Mitochondria | Convert food materials into energy to make adenosine triphosphate (ATP) used to power the chemical reactions in the cell |
| Rough endoplasmic reticulum (RER) | Tubular ribosome-containing channels that synthesize protein to be secreted by cells |
| Smooth endoplasmic reticulum (SER) | Tubular channels containing enzymes that synthesize lipids and some other compounds within the cells |
| Golgi apparatus | Flat sacs located near nucleus attach carbohydrate molecules to the proteins synthesized by RER |
| Lysosomes | Spherical organelles in cytoplasm containing digestive enzymes that break down worn-out cell organelles and material brought into cell by phagocytosis |
| Centrioles | Short cylinders that form the mitotic spindle that separates chromosomes during cell division |
| Cytoskeleton | Protein tubules and filaments that form structural framework of cells and promote cell functions such as motility and phagocytosis |

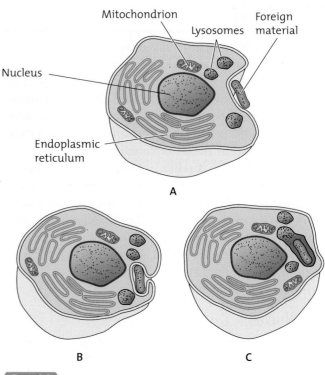

**Figure 2-2** Digestion of engulfed material by lysosomes. **A,** Extensions of cytoplasm from phagocytic cell begin to surround particulate material. **B,** Cytoplasmic extensions engulf material and form a phagocytic vacuole containing the engulfed material. **C,** Lysosome and phagocytic vacuole merge, and enzymes from the lysosome digest the engulfed material.

**parenchymal cell**
(par-en′ki-mul) The functional cell of an organ or tissue.

**parenchyma**
(par-en′ki-muh) The functional cells of an organ, as contrasted with the connective and supporting tissue that forms its framework.

**endothelium**
(en-dō-thē′lē-um) The internal lining of blood vessels and interior of heart.

**mesothelium** (me-sō-thē′li-um) A layer of flat squamous epithelial cells that covers the surfaces of the pleural, pericardial, and peritoneal cavities.

## Epithelium

Epithelium consists of groups of cells closely joined together ( Figure 2-3 ). Epithelial cells cover the exterior of the body and line the interior body surfaces that communicate with the outside, such as the gastrointestinal tract, urinary tract, and vagina. Epithelium forms glands such as the thyroid and pancreas and also makes up the functional cells (often called **parenchymal cells** or **parenchyma**) of organs that have excretory or secretory functions, such as the liver and the kidneys. The individual cells may be flat and platelike (squamous cells), cube-shaped (cuboidal cells), or tall and narrow (columnar cells). Many columnar epithelial cells have become specialized to absorb or secrete, and some contain hairlike processes called cilia. Epithelial cells may be arranged in a single layer (simple epithelium) or may be several layers thick (stratified epithelium).

**Endothelium and Mesothelium** The interiors of the heart, blood vessels, and lymphatic vessels are lined by a layer of simple squamous epithelium called **endothelium** (*endo* = within). A similar type of epithelium lining the pleural, pericardial, and peritoneal cavities is called **mesothelium** (*meso* = middle).

**The Structure of Epithelium** Epithelial cells are supported by a thin basement membrane. The cells are firmly joined to each other, and the deeper layers of epithelium are firmly anchored to the basement membrane, so that the epithelial cells remain relatively fixed in position. There are no blood vessels in epithelium. The cells are nourished by diffusion of material from capillaries located in the underlying connective tissue.

**Functions of Epithelium** Epithelium performs many different functions. All types of epithelium perform a protective function. Stratified squamous epithelium forms the external covering of the body and also lines the oral cavity, esophagus, and vagina. The top layer of skin cells also accumulates a fibrous protein called

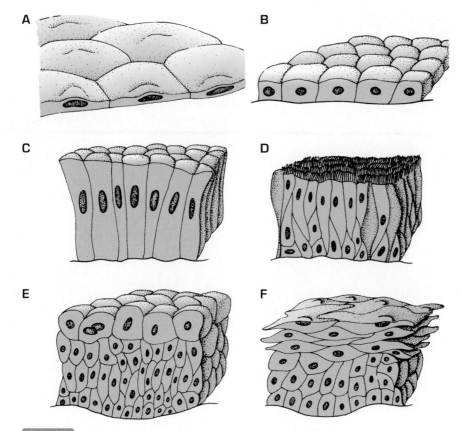

**Figure 2-3** Common types of epithelia. **A,** Simple squamous. **B,** Cuboidal. **C,** Columnar. **D,** Pseudostratified columnar (ciliated). **E,** Transitional. **F,** Stratified squamous.

**keratin** to provide additional protection ( **Figure 2-4** ). Columnar epithelium, such as that lining the intestinal tract, is specialized to absorb and secrete. Other types of epithelium form glands that secrete mucus, sweat, oil, enzymes, hormones, or other products.

## Connective and Supporting Tissues

Connective and supporting tissues consist of relatively small numbers of cells incorporated in a large amount of extracellular material called **matrix** in which are embedded various types of fibers. The proportions of cells, fibers, and matrix vary greatly in different types of connective tissue. Connective tissue fibers are of three types. Collagen fibers are long, flexible fibers composed of a protein called collagen. They are strong but do not stretch. Elastic fibers are not as strong as collagen but stretch readily and return to their former shape when the stretching force is released. Reticulin fibers are very similar to collagen but are quite thin and delicate.

Connective and supporting tissues include various types of loose and dense fibrous tissue, elastic tissue, reticular tissue, adipose tissue, cartilage, and bone. Elastic tissue forms membranes that are wrapped around the

walls of blood vessels and are responsible for the characteristic distensibility of large arteries.

Reticular tissue is a special type of connective tissue characterized by a fine meshwork of fibers that form the supporting framework of various organs such as the liver, spleen, and lymph nodes.

Adipose tissue consists of large numbers of fat cells. Fat is a stored form of energy and also functions as padding and insulation.

Cartilage is a type of supporting tissue in which the cells are dispersed in a dense matrix.

Bone is a highly specialized, rigid supporting tissue in which the matrix containing the bone-forming cells is impregnated with calcium salts.

## Muscle Tissue

Muscle cells contain filaments of specialized intracellular contractile proteins called actin and myosin. These are arranged in parallel bundles. During contraction of muscle fibers, actin filaments slide inward on the myosin filaments, somewhat like pistons, causing the

**keratin**
An insoluble sulfur-containing protein that is the principal constituent of the hair and nails.

**matrix** (mā′trix) Material in which connective-tissue cells are embedded.

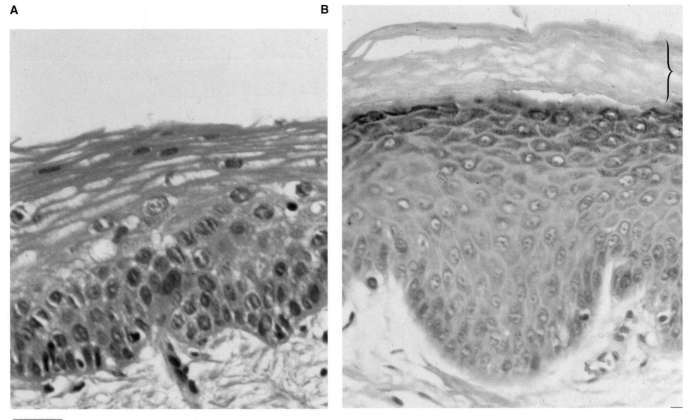

**Figure 2-4** **A,** Nonkeratinized stratified squamous epithelium. **B,** Keratinized stratified squamous epithelium. The keratin layer (bracket) forms a dense acellular covering that protects the underlying epithelial cells (original magnification × 400).

fibers to shorten. There are three types of muscle fibers. Smooth muscle is located primarily in the walls of hollow internal organs such as the gastrointestinal tract, biliary tract, and reproductive tract and is also present in the walls of the blood vessels. Smooth muscle functions automatically and is not under conscious control. Striated muscle moves the skeleton and is under voluntary control. Cardiac muscle is found only in the heart. It resembles striated muscle but has some features common to both smooth and voluntary muscle.

## Nerve Tissue

Nerve tissue is composed of nerve cells called **neurons**, which transmit nerve impulses and supporting cells called **neuroglia**. Neuroglial cells are more numerous than neurons and perform various functions to assist neurons.

## Organs and Organ Systems

An organ is a group of different tissues that is integrated to perform a specific function. Generally, one tissue performs the primary function characteristic of the organ, and the other tissues perform a supporting function, such as providing the vascular and connective-tissue framework for the organ. The functional cells of an organ are often called **parenchymal cells.** The supporting framework of the organ is called the **stroma.** An organ system is a group of organs that is organized to perform complementary functions, such as the reproductive system, the respiratory system, and the digestive system. Finally, the various organ systems are integrated into a functioning individual.

# Cell Function and the Genetic Code

The chromosomes contain a series of messages called the **genetic code**. It is this code that regulates the various functions of the cell. The genetic code is contained within the structure of DNA and is transmitted to each newly formed cell in cell division.

## The Structure of DNA

The chromosomes are composed of DNA combined with protein. The basic structural unit of DNA, called a nucleotide, consists of a phosphate group linked to

**neuron**
(nū′ron) A nerve cell, including the nerve cell body and its processes.

**neuroglia**
(noo-rog′-lē-ah) Supporting cells of tissue of the nervous system.

**stroma** (strō′muh) The tissue that forms the framework of an organ.

**genetic code** (jen-et′ik kōd) The information carried by the codons of DNA molecules in chromosomes.

a five-carbon sugar, deoxyribose, which in turn is joined to a nitrogen-containing compound called a base (Figure 2-5A). There are two different types of DNA bases: a purine base, which contains a fused double ring of carbon and nitrogen atoms, and a pyrimidine base, which contains only a single ring. There are four different bases in DNA: the purine bases adenine and guanine and the pyrimidine bases thymine and cytosine. Consequently, there are four different nucleotides in DNA, each containing a different base (Figure 2-5B). A DNA molecule consists of two strands of DNA that are held together by weak chemical attractions between the bases of the adjacent chains. The DNA chains are twisted into a double spiral somewhat like a spiral staircase, with the sugar and phosphate groups forming the two railings and the complementary base pairs forming the steps (Figure 2-6A, Figure 2-6B, and Figure 2-6C).

## Duplication (Replication) of DNA

As a cell prepares to divide, the double strands of DNA duplicate themselves. The two chains separate, and each chain serves as the model for the synthesis of a new chain (Figure 2-6C). The process of duplication forms two double strands, each containing one of the

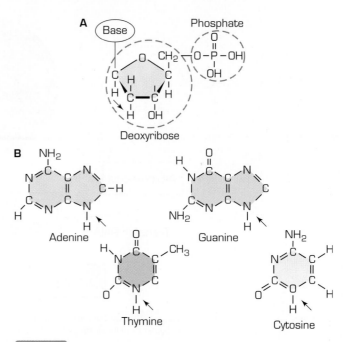

**Figure 2-5** General structure of DNA nucleotide. **A,** Deoxyribose is identical to ribose except for the absence of an oxygen atom (site of missing oxygen indicated by *arrow*). **B,** Structure of the bases. The *arrows* indicate sites at which bases are joined to deoxyribose.

original strands plus a newly formed strand. In this way, each of the two daughter cells produced by cell division

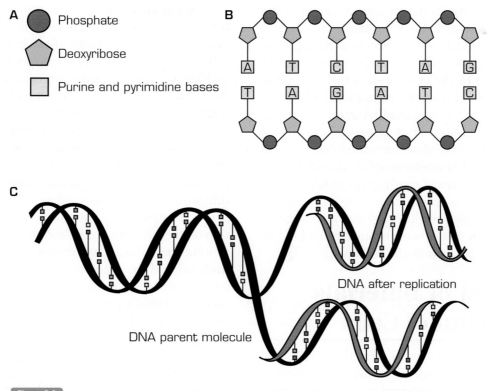

**Figure 2-6** **A,** Components entering into the formation of a DNA molecule. **B,** Structure of double-stranded DNA. **C,** Duplication (replication) of a DNA molecule.

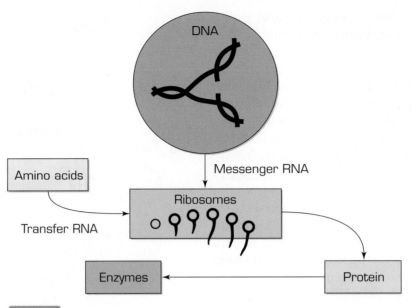

Figure 2-7    Role of messenger RNA and transfer RNA in the synthesis of enzymes and other proteins by ribosomes in the cytoplasm.

receives an exact duplicate of the genetic information possessed by the chromosomes of the parent cell.

## The Genetic Code

The DNA in the nucleus "tells the cell what to do" by directing the synthesis of enzymes and other proteins by the ribosomes located in the cytoplasm. The "instructions" are carried by messenger RNA (mRNA), so named because it carries the message encoded in the DNA to the ribosomes in the cytoplasm.

The mRNA strand leaves the nucleus through the pores in the nuclear membrane and becomes attached to the ribosomes in the cytoplasm, which are small nucleoprotein particles where enzymes and other proteins are constructed from individual amino acids. The combination of amino acids required to assemble a protein is determined by the information contained in the mRNA strand. The amino acids are transported to the ribosomes by means of another type of RNA called transfer RNA (tRNA), so named because it "picks up" the required amino acids from the cytoplasm and transfers them to the ribosomes where they are assembled in proper order, as specified by the mRNA ( Figure 2-7 ).

# Movement of Materials Into and Out of Cells

In order for the cell to function properly, oxygen and nutrients must enter the cell, and waste products must be eliminated. Materials entering and leaving the cell must cross the cell membrane, which limits the passage of some molecules and is freely permeable to others. Materials cross the cell membrane in three ways:

1. Diffusion and osmosis
2. Active transport
3. Phagocytosis and pinocytosis

## Diffusion and Osmosis

Diffusion is the movement of dissolved particles (solute) from a more concentrated to a more dilute solution. Osmosis is the movement of water molecules from a dilute solution to a more concentrated solution ( Figure 2-8 ). Both are passive processes that do not require the cell to expend energy. If the membrane is freely permeable to both water and solute particles (Figure 2-8A and 2-8B), the solute particles diffuse from the higher solute concentration on the right side of the membrane into the lower solute concentration on the left side. At the same time, water molecules diffuse in the opposite direction, from the more dilute solution on the right side of the membrane into the more concentrated solution on the left side. At equilibrium, the concentrations of solute particles and water molecules are the same on both sides of the membrane. Solute and water molecules continue to move in both directions across the membrane after equilibrium is attained, but the movements are equal in both directions, which does not change in the equilibrium volume and concentration of the solutions on the two sides of the membrane.

The situation is quite different if the membrane is not permeable to the solute particles in the solution on one side of the membrane (Figure 2-8C, 2-8D). Water

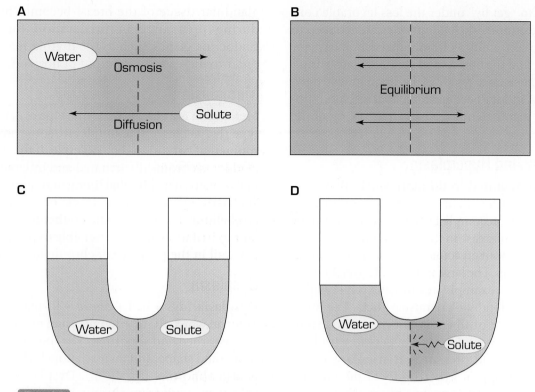

**Figure 2-8** **A,** Processes of osmosis and diffusion across a porous membrane indicated by *dashed line.* **B,** At equilibrium, the concentrations of water and solute molecules are equal on both sides of the membrane. **C,** The left compartment of U tube contains water. The right compartment contains solute impermeable to membrane. **D,** Water molecules diffuse freely across the membrane, but solute molecules are unable to diffuse. The volume of solute increased by diffusion of water molecules into the solute. The volume of water in the left limb of the U tube falls as water moves into the solute in the right limb of the U tube.

molecules move by osmosis from the left side of the membrane into the more concentrated solution on the right side (containing fewer water molecules). Because diffusion of solute is restricted by the membrane but movement of water molecules across the membrane is not, the volume of the solution on the right side of the membrane increases, and its solute concentration falls as the water molecules move by osmosis across the membrane. Eventually, the solutions on both sides of the membrane have the same concentration of water molecules, but their volumes are quite different.

## Active Transport

Active transport is the transfer of a substance across the cell membrane from a region of *low concentration* to one of *higher concentration.* The process requires the cell to expend energy because the substance must move against a concentration gradient. Many metabolic processes depend on active transport of ions or molecules.

## Phagocytosis and Pinocytosis

Phagocytosis is the ingestion of particles that are too large to pass across the cell membrane. The cytoplasm flows around the particle, and the cytoplasmic processes fuse, engulfing the particle within a vacuole in the cytoplasm of the cell. A similar process called pinocytosis consists of the ingestion of fluid rather than solid material.

# Adaptations of Cells to Changing Conditions

Cells respond to changing conditions in various ways. Common adaptive mechanisms are:

1. Atrophy
2. Hypertrophy and hyperplasia
3. Metaplasia
4. Dysplasia
5. Increased enzyme synthesis

In many instances, the adaptation enables the cells to function more efficiently. Sometimes, however, the adaptive change may be detrimental to the cell, as occurs in dysplasia.

## Atrophy

Atrophy is a reduction in the size of cells in response to diminished function, inadequate hormonal stimulation, or reduced blood supply. The cell decreases in size in order to "get by" under the less favorable conditions. For example, skeletal muscles are reduced in size when an extremity is immobilized in a cast for long periods, and the breasts and genital organs shrink after menopause as a result of inadequate estrogen stimulation. A kidney becomes smaller if its blood supply becomes insufficient because of narrowing of the renal artery.

## Hypertrophy and Hyperplasia

If cells are required to do more work, they may increase either their size or their number in order to accomplish their task. *Hypertrophy* is an increase in the size of individual cells without an actual increase in their numbers. The large muscles of a weight lifter, for example, result from hypertrophy of individual muscle fibers. The number of fibers is not increased. Similarly, the heart of a person with high blood pressure often enlarges as a result of hypertrophy of the individual cardiac muscle fibers. This occurs because the heart must work harder in order to pump blood at a higher than normal pressure. **Hyperplasia** is an increase in the size of a tissue or organ caused by an increase in the number of cells. Hyperplasia occurs in response to increased demand. For example, the glandular tissue of the breast becomes hyperplastic during pregnancy in preparation for lactation. Endocrine glands such as the thyroid may enlarge in order to increase their output of hormones.

## Metaplasia

**Metaplasia** is a change from one type of cell to another type that is better able to tolerate some adverse environmental condition. For example, if the lining of the bladder is chronically irritated and inflamed, the normal transitional epithelial lining may assume the characteristic structure of a thick layer of squamous epithelium. The metaplastic epithelium is more resistant to irritation and is better able to protect the bladder wall in the presence of chronic infection.

## Dysplasia

**Dysplasia** (*dys* = bad + *plasia* = formation) is a condition in which the development and maturation of cells are disturbed and abnormal. The individual cells vary in size and shape, and their relationship to one another is also abnormal ( Figure 2-9 ). Dysplasia of epithelial cells may result from chronic irritation or inflammation. In some cases, dysplasia may progress to formation of a tumor; this is called **neoplasia**. The epithelium covering the uterine cervix is a common site of dysplasia, and cervical epithelial dysplasia sometimes progresses to cervical cancer. This subject is discussed in Chapter 13.

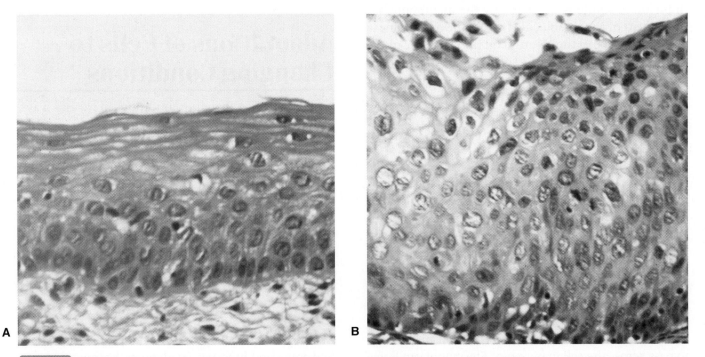

Figure 2-9 Comparison of normal, nonkeratinized stratified squamous epithelium. **A,** With dysplastic epithelium. **B,** Note the variation in nuclear size, polarity, and staining reaction (original magnification × 400).

## Increased Enzyme Synthesis

Increased synthesis of enzymes is another adaptive change that occurs in cells. Sometimes cells are called on to inactivate or detoxify drugs or chemicals by means of the enzymes present in the smooth endoplasmic reticulum (SER). If increased demands are placed on the cells, they respond by synthesizing more SER enzymes so that drugs or chemicals can be processed more efficiently. After the cells increase their ability to handle such chemicals or drugs, they can rapidly eliminate other substances that are handled by means of the same enzyme systems. A person accustomed to heavy consumption of alcohol, for example, is able to metabolize the alcohol more efficiently because of this adaptive change. Such an individual may also metabolize and eliminate other drugs at a greatly accelerated rate. Consequently, if a physician administers a medication that is metabolized by the same enzyme systems, the usual therapeutic doses of the medications may be ineffective.

# Cell Injury, Cell Death, and Cell Necrosis

## Cell Injury

An injured cell may exhibit various morphologic abnormalities. The two most common changes are cell swelling and fatty change.

**Cell Swelling**  A normally functioning cell actively transports potassium into the cell and moves sodium out. This process requires the cell to expend energy. If the cell is injured and unable to function normally, the transport mechanism begins to fail. Sodium diffuses into the cell, and water moves into the cell along with the sodium, causing the cell to swell. If the swelling continues, fluid-filled vacuoles may accumulate within the cell, and eventually, it may rupture.

**Fatty Change**  If the enzyme systems that metabolize fat are impaired, leading to accumulation of fat droplets within the cytoplasm, fatty change may occur. This condition is a common manifestation of liver cell injury because liver cells are actively involved in fat metabolism.

## Cell Death and Cell Necrosis

A cell dies if it has been irreparably damaged. Several hours after the cell dies, various structural changes begin to take place within the nucleus and cytoplasm. Lysosomal enzymes are released and begin to digest the cell. The nucleus shrinks and either dissolves or breaks into fragments. These structural changes are termed cell **necrosis**. All necrotic cells are dead, but a dead cell is not necessarily necrotic because the structural changes that characterize cell death take several hours to develop. Necrotic cells are easily recognized on histologic examination because they appear quite different from normal cells in both their structural and their staining characteristics ( Figure 2-10 ).

**necrosis** (nek-rōsis) Structural changes associated with cell death.

## Programmed Cell Death

Not all cell death results from cell injury. All normal cells have a predetermined life span and are programmed to die after a specific period of time. The number of functional cells in all our body tissues is determined by a balance between proliferation of new cells and death of older "worn-out" cells. The older cells die because they are genetically programmed to "shut down" when they have reached the end of their predetermined life span. The rates of cell proliferation and cell death vary in different body tissues. Sometimes cells may continue to proliferate instead of dying as they should. Excessive numbers of cells may accumulate in organs or tissues, which disrupts their functions and leads to disease.

# Aging and the Cell

All organisms grow old and eventually die, and each species has a predetermined life span. Although human life expectancy has increased over the years, the increase is chiefly because early deaths from infectious diseases, accidents, and other conditions have been greatly reduced. The causes of aging are not well understood but appear to reside in the cell. Although each type of cell has a definite life span, under normal circumstances cell longevity is also influenced by environmental factors.

Many investigators believe that aging of cells is genetically programmed and is an inherent property of the cell itself. Examples can be seen in the graying of the hair, which is the result of an eventual failure of the hair cells to produce pigment, and in menopause, which is a predetermined failure of reproductive function. Aging changes in the brain appear to be caused by the wearing out and eventual death of neurons, which are not capable of cell division. The common type of arthritis seen in older persons begins as an aging change in the cartilage covering the ends of the bones.

As a cell ages, many of its enzyme systems become less active, and the cell becomes less efficient in carrying out its functions. The cell also becomes more

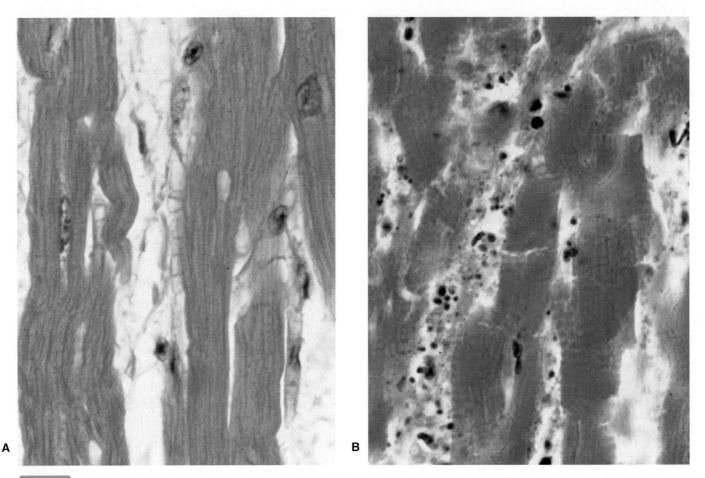

**Figure 2-10** Comparison of normal cardiac muscle fibers. **A,** With necrotic fibers. **B,** Note the fragmentation of fibers, the loss of nuclear staining, and the fragmented bits of nuclear debris (original magnification × 400).

susceptible to harmful environmental influences that may shorten its life. For example, the life span of a red cell is 4 months, and therefore the red cells circulating in the bloodstream vary greatly in age, ranging from newly produced cells to those nearing the end of their life span. Each red cell contains enzyme systems that generate its energy, enable it to perform its varied metabolic functions, and maintain the hemoglobin in a condition suitable for transporting oxygen. As the red cell ages and its enzyme systems gradually decline, the cell is less able to protect itself from injury than is a young, "vigorous" cell. If the red cells are exposed to harmful drugs or antibodies that damage the cell membranes, it is the older cells that bear the brunt of the damage and die. The younger cells are able to survive and continue to function.

An example of aging change in cells that affects the organism as a whole can be seen in the lymphocytes of which our immune system is composed. These cells help eliminate pathogenic organisms and also eliminate any of our own cells that become abnormal and have the potential of forming tumors. The cells of the immune system become less efficient as they age. Consequently, the aging individual becomes more susceptible to various infectious diseases, which can shorten the life span. The aging immune system also becomes less able to eliminate abnormal cells that arise sporadically within the body. This may predispose to the formation of malignant tumors, which occur with increasing frequency in older persons.

Aging of cells may also be caused by damage to cellular DNA, RNA, and cytoplasmic organelles that occurs at a pace more rapid than the cell's ability to repair itself. According to this concept, these components become damaged by radiation or other environmental factors or by accumulation of metabolic products within cells. Eventually, the cells begin to malfunction. Some cells can repair the damage and continue to function. Others cannot and die. The more efficient the repair process within the cell, the more likely the cell is to survive.

In summary, cells have a finite life span. However, the less they are exposed to harmful environmental influences and the more efficient they are in repairing their own malfunctions, the greater their chances for survival to a "ripe old age."

# Chromosomes

The activities of cells are controlled by the chromosomes present in the nucleus. In the somatic cells (cells other than those giving rise to eggs and sperm), chromosomes exist in pairs. One member of each pair is derived from the male parent and one member from the female parent. Except for the sex chromosomes, both members of the pair are similar in size, shape, and appearance and are called **homologous chromosomes**. In human beings, the normal chromosome component is 22 pairs of **autosomes** (the general term for chromosomes other than the sex chromosomes) and one pair of sex chromosomes.

As described previously, the chromosomes are composed of double coils of deoxyribonucleic acid (DNA) combined with protein. The genes, which are the basic units of inheritance, are segments of the DNA chains that determine some property of the cell. Genes are sometimes described as being arranged along the chromosome like beads on a string.

The sum total of all the genes contained in a cell's chromosomes is called its **genome** and is the same in all cells; however, not all genes are expressed (active) in all cells, and not all genes are active all the time. Some genes code for specific enzymes or other proteins that the cell needs in order to function, and others act as regulators to control the activities of neighboring genes. An enzyme or other protein specified by a gene, which is transcribed into messenger RNA and translated through transfer RNA and cytoplasmic ribosomes into protein, is called the **gene product**.

The genes that are expressed in a given cell determine both its structure and its functions, which is why a liver cell, for example, has a different structure from that of a blood cell and functions differently as well.

## Sex Chromosomes

Genetic sex is determined by the composition of X and Y chromosomes. The cells of a normal female contain two X chromosomes, and those of a normal male contain one X and one Y chromosome. The small Y chromosome consists almost entirely of genes concerned with male sexual differentiation. In contrast, the large X chromosome contains a large number of genes that direct many important cell activities.

### X Chromosome Inactivation: The Lyon Hypothesis

Because the cells of the female contain two X chromosomes, they would be expected to contain much more genetic material than those of the male, whose cells contain only one X chromosome. Female cells, however, function as though they contained only genetic material equivalent to that of a single X chromosome. The reason for this paradoxical behavior is that one of the X chromosomes is inactivated and nonfunctional. In the female, the genetic activity of both X chromosomes is only essential during the first week of embryonic development. Thereafter, one of the X chromosomes in each of the developing cells is inactivated. With only rare exceptions, the inactivation occurs in a random manner, as illustrated in ( Figure 2-11 ). After the initial inactivation of an X chromosome has occurred, the same paternal- or maternal-derived X chromosome will also be inactivated in all descendants of the precursor cell. The inactivated X chromosome appears as a small, dense mass of chromatin attached to the nuclear membrane of somatic cells. This structure can be identified in the cells of a normal female and is called a sex chromatin body or **Barr body** after the man who first described it ( Figure 2-12A ).

Because the X chromosome inactivation is random, the inactivated X is of paternal origin in some cells and of maternal origin in others, and the percentages of inactivated paternal- and maternal-derived X chromosomes are not necessarily equal. Consequently, the genes on the X chromosome that function in a woman's cell will depend on which X chromosome is active in the cell, as the other X chromosome is inactivated and nonfunctional. According to this concept, called the Lyon hypothesis after the woman who first described it, a female is composed of a mixture of two types of cells with respect to the active X chromosome. This hypothesis has explained some of the peculiarities of the behavior of genes carried on the X chromosome in males and females, as described in later sections dealing with X-linked genetic diseases.

### Identification of Sex Chromosomes in Intact Cells

An inactivated X chromosome in an intact cell of a normal female can be identified as a sex chromatin body attached to the nuclear membrane of the cell (Figure 2-12A). It is also possible to identify the Y chromosome in the cells of a normal male. The Y chromosome stains intensely with certain fluorescent dyes as a bright fluorescent spot within the nucleus of the intact cell when a suitably stained preparation is examined microscopically under ultraviolet light ( Figure 2-12B ).

A combination of staining and ultraviolet light makes it possible to determine the X and Y chromosome

**homologous chromosomes** A matched pair of chromosomes, one derived from each parent.

**autosome** (aw´tō-sōm) A chromosome other than a sex chromosome.

**genome** (jee´nō-m) The total of all the genes contained in a cell's chromosomes.

**gene product** A protein or enzyme specified (coded) by a gene.

**Barr body** The inactivated X chromosome that is applied to the nuclear membrane in the female. Sex chromatin body.

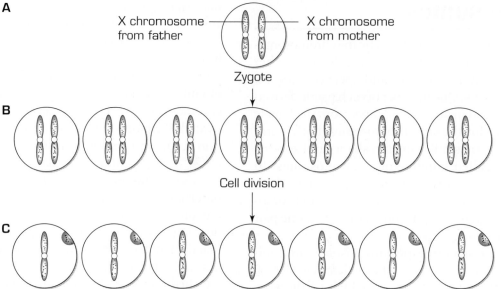

**A**

X chromosome from father ——— ——— X chromosome from mother

Zygote

**B**

Cell division

**C**

Random inactivation of one X chromosome

**Figure 2-11** Concept of random inactivation of X chromosome. **A,** Fertilized egg (zygote) contains two functionally active X chromosomes, and both are necessary during early development. **B,** Cell divisions of the zygote give rise to many daughter cells, each containing two active X chromosomes. **C,** One of the X chromosomes in each cell (either the X chromosome derived from the mother or from the father) is inactivated in a random manner, giving rise to two cell populations with respect to the X chromosome. The descendants of each of these cells also contain the same inactivated X chromosome.

**mitosis** The type of cell division of most cells in which chromosomes are duplicated in the daughter cells and are identical with those in the parent cell. The characteristic cell division found in all cells in the body except for the gametes.

**meiosis** (mi-o′sis) A special type of cell division occurring in *gametes* (ova and sperm), in which the number of chromosomes is reduced by one-half in the ovum and sperm.

**gametogenesis** The development of mature eggs and sperm from precursor cells.

**daughter cell** A cell resulting from division of a single cell (called the *parent cell*).

composition of intact cells. The cells of the normal male possess the fluorescent spot but lack the sex chromatin body, and the cells of the normal female contain the sex chromatin body but lack the fluorescent spot. Cells for examination are usually obtained by scraping the mucosa of the cheek gently with a tongue depressor and preparing slides from this material. However, cells obtained from any convenient site may be used for examination.

# Cell Division

There are two types of cell division: **Mitosis** is characteristic of somatic cells. **Meiosis** is a specialized type of cell division that occurs during the development of the eggs (ova) and sperm, a process called **gametogenesis**. In mitosis, each of the two new cells (called the **daughter cells**) resulting from the cell division receives the same number of chromosomes that were present in the precursor cell (called the **parent cell**). In meiosis, the number of chromosomes is reduced so

**A**

**B**

**Figure 2-12** **A,** Characteristic appearance of sex chromatin body (Barr body) in the nucleus of a squamous epithelial cell. **B,** Fluorescent Y chromosome (*arrow*) in nucleus of intact cell.

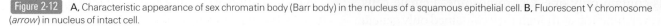

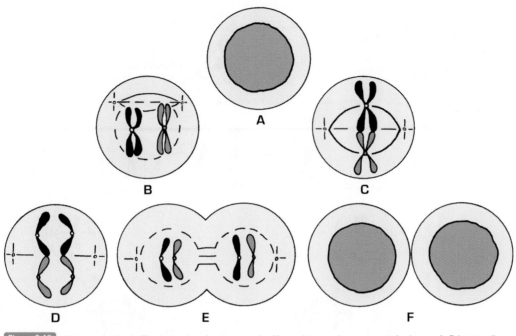

**Figure 2-13** Stages of mitosis. The behavior of only one pair of homologous chromosomes is shown. **A,** Prior to cell division. **B,** Prophase. **C,** Metaphase. **D,** Anaphase. **E,** Telophase. **F,** Daughter cells resulting from mitosis, each identical to the parent cell.

that the daughter cells receive only half of the chromosomes possessed by the parent cell.

## Mitosis

Mitosis is characteristic of somatic cells, but not all mature cells are able to divide. Some mature cells, such as cardiac muscle cells and nerve cells, do not divide. Others, such as connective tissue cells and liver cells, divide as needed to replace lost or damaged cells or to heal an injury. Yet others divide continually, such as those lining the testicular tubules that produce sperm cells and those in the bone marrow that continually replace the circulating cells in the bloodstream. Regardless of the frequency of cell division, the rate of cell division is controlled closely to match the body's needs, and excess cells are not normally produced.

Many factors regulate cell growth and cell division. Normal cells divide often enough to accomplish their functions and replenish cell losses from injury or normal aging but restrain excessive proliferation. Moreover, normal cells cannot continue to divide indefinitely. They are programmed to undergo a limited number of cell divisions, and then they die.

Before a cell begins mitosis, its DNA chains are duplicated to form new chromosome material. Each chromosome and its newly duplicated counterpart lie side by side. The two members of the pair are called **chromatids**. When the chromosomes shorten in the course of cell division, each chromosome can be seen to actually consist of two separate chromosomes that are still partially joined where the spindle fibers attach. The term *chromatids* is applied to the still-joined chromosomes at this stage. Mitosis is the process by which chromatids separate. As soon as they separate, they are again called chromosomes.

Mitosis is divided into four stages ( Figure 2-13 ): prophase, metaphase, anaphase, and telophase.

**Prophase** Each chromosome thickens and shortens. The centrioles migrate to opposite poles of the cell and form the mitotic spindle, which consists of small fibers radiating in all directions from the centrioles. Some of these spindle fibers attach to the chromatids. The nuclear membrane breaks down toward the end of prophase.

**Metaphase** The chromosomes line up in the center of the cell. At this stage, the chromatids are partially separated but still remain joined at a constricted area called the centromere, which is the site where the spindle fibers are attached.

**Anaphase** The chromatids constituting each chromosome separate to form individual chromosomes, which are pulled to opposite poles of the cell by the spindle fibers.

**Telophase** The nuclear membranes of the two daughter cells reform, and the cytoplasm divides,

**chromatid**
(krō′mä-tid) One of two newly formed chromosomes held together by the centromere.

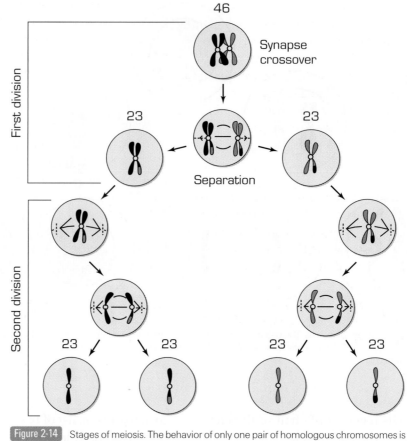

**Figure 2-14** Stages of meiosis. The behavior of only one pair of homologous chromosomes is indicated. In the first meiotic division, each daughter cell receives only one member of each homologous pair, and the chromosomes are not exact duplicates of those in the parent cell. The second meiotic division is like a mitotic division, but each cell contains only 23 chromosomes.

forming two daughter cells. Each is an exact duplicate of the parent cell.

## Meiosis

Meiotic cell division reduces the number of chromosomes by half and also leads to some intermixing of genetic material between homologous chromosomes. The process entails two separate divisions called the first and second meiotic divisions ( Figure 2-14 ).

**First Meiotic Division** As in mitosis, each chromosome duplicates itself before beginning cell division, forming two chromatids. During *prophase*, each homologous pair of chromosomes comes to lie side by side over their entire length. This association is called a **synapse**. At this stage, there is frequently some interchange of segments between homologous chromosomes, which is called a **crossover**. The pairing of homologous chromosomes and the interchange of genetic material during prophase are the characteristic features of meiosis. In the female, the two X chromosomes synapse in the same way as autosomes, but in the male, the X and Y chromosomes synapse end to end and do not exchange segments.

In *metaphase*, the paired chromosomes become arranged in a plane within the middle of the cell. During *anaphase*, the homologous chromosomes separate and move to opposite poles of the cell. Each chromosome consists of two chromatids, but they do not separate at this stage. In *telophase*, two new daughter cells are formed. Each daughter cell contains only one member of each homologous pair of chromosomes; consequently, the chromosomes in each daughter cell are reduced by half. The chromosomes in the daughter cells are also somewhat different from those in the parent cell because of the interchange of genetic material during synapse.

**Second Meiotic Division** The second meiotic division is similar to a mitotic division. The two chromatids composing each chromosome separate, and two new daughter cells are formed, each containing half of the normal number of chromosomes.

**synapse**
(sin′aps) Pairing of homologous chromosomes in meiosis.

**crossover** Interchange of genetic material between homologous chromosomes during synapse and meiosis.

# Gametogenesis

The testes and ovaries, called **gonads**, contain precursor cells called **germ cells**, which are capable of developing into mature sperm or ova. The mature germ cells are called **gametes**, and the process by which they are formed is gametogenesis. The development of sperm (spermatogenesis) and of ova (oogenesis) is similar in many respects ( Figure 2-15 ).

## Spermatogenesis

The precursor cells in the testicular tubules are called spermatogonia (singular term; spermatogonium). Each contains a full complement of 46 chromosomes. Spermatogonia divide by mitosis to form primary spermatocytes, which, like the precursor cells, contain 46 chromosomes. The primary spermatocytes then divide by meiosis. In the first meiotic division, each primary spermatocyte forms two secondary spermatocytes, each containing 23 chromosomes. Each secondary sperma-

tocyte completes the second meiotic division and forms two **spermatids**, also containing 23 chromosomes, and the spermatids mature into sperm. The entire process of spermatogenesis takes about 2 months, and sperm are being produced continually.

## Oogenesis

The precursors of the ova are called oogonia (singular term; oogonium). Each contains 46 chromosomes. Oogonia divide repeatedly in the fetal ovaries before birth, forming primary oocytes, which contain 46 chromosomes. The oocytes then become surrounded by a single layer of cells called **granulosa cells** or follicular cells, forming structures called primary follicles ( Figure 2-16 ). The primary oocytes in the follicles begin the prophase of the first meiotic division

**gonad**
(gō′nad)
A general term referring to either the ovary or the testis.

**germ cell** A precursor cell capable of developing in mature sperm or ovum.

**gametes** Reproductive cells, eggs, and sperm, each containing 23 chromosomes, which unite during fertilization to form a zygote containing 46 chromosomes.

**spermatids** Germ cells in a late stage of sperm development just before complete maturation to mature sperm.

**granulosa cells** (gran-u-lō′suh) Cells lining the ovarian follicles.

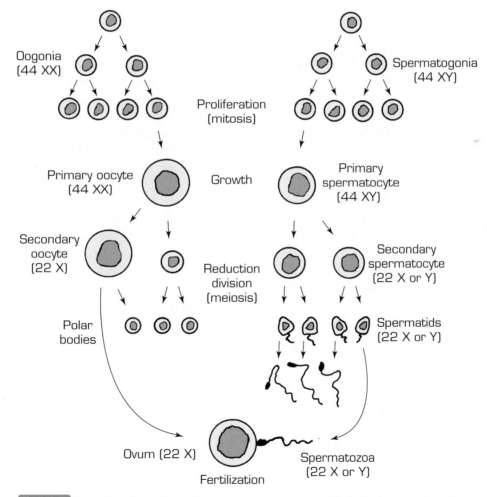

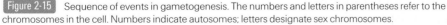

Figure 2-15 Sequence of events in gametogenesis. The numbers and letters in parentheses refer to the chromosomes in the cell. Numbers indicate autosomes; letters designate sex chromosomes.

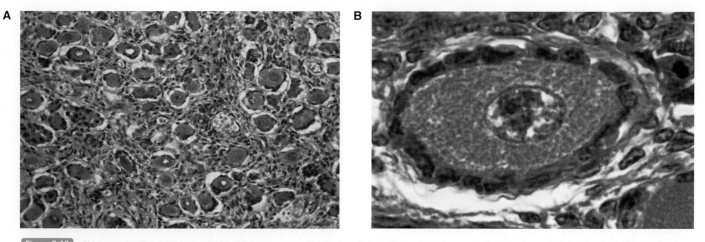

**Figure 2-16** **A,** Low-magnification photomicrograph of the ovary of a newborn infant, illustrating a large number of primary follicles distributed throughout the ovary (original magnification × 100). **B,** High-magnification photomicrograph illustrating a primary follicle composed of a central oocyte surrounded by a collar of granulose cells (original magnification × 400).

during fetal life but do not carry the division through to completion. A very large number of primary follicles are formed, but many of them degenerate during infancy and childhood. However, about a half million of the primary follicles persist into adolescence, and the loss continues throughout the woman's reproductive years. During each reproductive cycle, several oocytes begin to mature; however, usually only one is ovulated, and the others degenerate. Nevertheless, there is still a great excess of oocytes. Even if one egg were released over a reproductive span of 40 years, only 480 eggs would be ovulated, and only a few, if any, would ever be fertilized. At menopause, only a few thousand oocytes remain, and the decline continues until eventually there are no oocytes left in the ovaries of a postmenopausal woman.

The ovaries with their contained primary follicles remain inactive until puberty. Then cyclic ovulation begins under the influence of the pituitary gonadotropic hormones. During each menstrual cycle, a number of primary follicles begin to grow, but normally only one follicle comes to full maturity and is ovulated. When the oocyte is discharged, it completes its first meiotic division and gives rise to two daughter cells, which are unequal in size. One daughter cell, which receives half of the chromosomes (one member of each homologous pair) and almost all of the cytoplasm, is called a secondary oocyte (23 chromosomes). The other daughter cell, which receives the remaining 23 chromosomes but almost none of the cytoplasm, is called the first **polar body** and is discarded. The newly formed secondary oocyte promptly begins its second meiotic division, which will lead to the formation of the mature ovum and a second polar body, each containing 23

**polar body**
Structure extruded during the meiosis of the oocyte. Contains discarded chromosomes and a small amount of cytoplasm.

chromosomes. The meiotic division is not completed, however, unless the ovum is fertilized.

## Comparison of Spermatogenesis and Oogenesis

Spermatogenesis and oogenesis have many similarities, but there are two major differences.

First, four spermatozoa are produced from each precursor cell in spermatogenesis, but only one ovum is formed from each precursor cell in oogenesis. The other three "daughter cells" derived from the meiotic divisions are discarded as polar bodies.

Second, spermatogenesis occurs continually and is carried through to completion in about 2 months. Consequently, seminal fluid always contains relatively "fresh" sperm. In contrast, the oocytes are not produced continually. All of the oocytes present in the ovary were formed before birth and have remained in a prolonged prophase of the first meiotic division from fetal life until they are ovulated. This may be why congenital abnormalities that result from abnormal separation of chromosomes in the course of gametogenesis are more frequent in older women. The ova released late in a woman's reproductive life have been held in prophase for as long as 45 years before they finally resume meiosis at the time of ovulation. These ova have been exposed for many years to potentially harmful radiation, chemicals, or other injurious agents, and this predisposes them to abnormal separation of chromosomes when cell division is resumed. If the chromosomes do not separate normally in meiosis, an ovum may end up with either an excess or a deficiency of chromosomes. If the abnormal ovum is fertilized, a fetus that has an abnormal number of chromosomes may be conceived. This subject is considered in Chapter 7.

# Chromosome Analysis

The chromosome composition of the human cell can be studied with great accuracy by culturing cells in a suitable medium. The presence of abnormalities in chromosome number or structure also can be detected in this way. Usually, human blood is used as a source of cells for these studies; the blood lymphocytes can be induced to undergo mitotic division. Certain chemicals are added to stop the mitotic division after the chromosomes have become separate and distinct, and consequently, many cells arrested in mitosis accumulate in the culture medium. Additional methods are employed to cause swelling of the cells, which are then prepared, and the chromosomes can be examined. Figure 2-17 illustrates the appearance of a swollen cell arrested in mitosis with the chromosomes well separated. A normal dividing cell arrested in mitosis contains 46 chromosomes, each consisting of two chromatids joined at their centromeres. Chromosomes are classified according to their size, the location of the centromere, the relative lengths of the chromatids that extend outward from the centromere (called the arms of the chromosome), and the pattern of light and dark bands along the chromosome.

Each chromosome has its own unique structure. The individual chromosomes are arranged in a standard pattern called a **karyotype**. Figure 2-18 illustrates the karyotype of a female, as indicated by the paired X chromosomes, with Y chromosome absent. The karyotype illustrated is not normal; there is an extra chromosome 21.

# Genes and Inheritance

A gene is a section of the DNA chain that determines some property of the cell. Each gene occupies a specific site on the chromosome; this site is called the **locus** of the gene. Chromosomes exist in pairs except in the ova and sperm. Consequently, genes are also paired, and the members of each pair are located at corresponding gene loci on homologous chromosomes. Alternate forms of a gene that can occupy the same locus are called **alleles**, and any one chromosome can carry only one allele at a given locus. An individual is homozygous for a gene if both alleles are the same and heterozygous if the alleles are different.

Genes are responsible for inherited traits, but the effects that they produce (called the expression of the gene) vary with different genes. A **recessive gene** is one that produces an effect only in the homozygous state. A **dominant gene** expresses itself in either the heterozygous or the homozygous state. Sometimes both alleles of a pair are expressed. Such alleles are called codominant. For example, each of the alleles that direct hemoglobin synthesis induces the formation of a specific type of hemoglobin in the red blood cells. If two different alleles are present, two different types of hemoglobin are produced.

**karyotype** (kār′-ē-ō-é-type) An arrangement of chromosomes from a single cell arranged in pairs in descending order according to size of the chromosomes and the positions of the centromeres.

**locus** The position of a gene on a chromosome. Different forms (*alleles*) of the same gene are always found at the same locus on a chromosome.

**allele** (äh′lēl) One of several related genes that may occupy the same locus on a homologous chromosome.

**recessive gene** A gene that expresses a trait only when present in the homozygous state.

**dominant gene** A gene that expresses a trait in the heterozygous state.

**A**

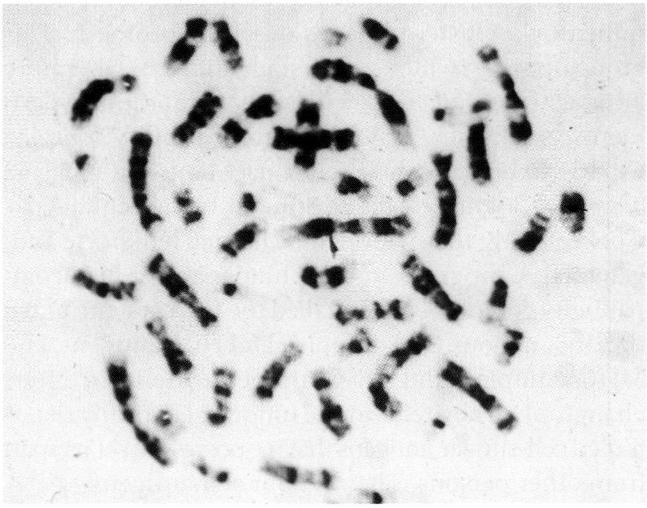

**B**

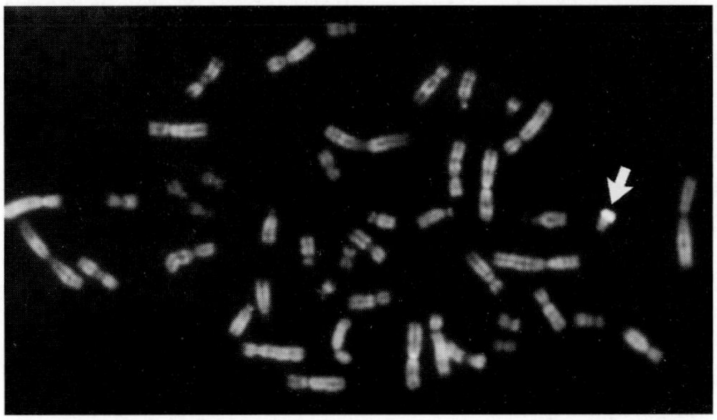

Figure 2-17  The appearance of chromosomes from a single cell arrested in mitosis, illustrating the banded pattern that facilitates the identification of individual chromosomes. The two chromatids composing each chromosome lie side by side. **A,** Giemsa stain (photograph-courtesy of Dr. Jorge Yunis). **B,** Fluorescent stain. The *arrow* indicates an intensely stained Y chromosome (photograph courtesy of Patricia Crowley-Larsen).

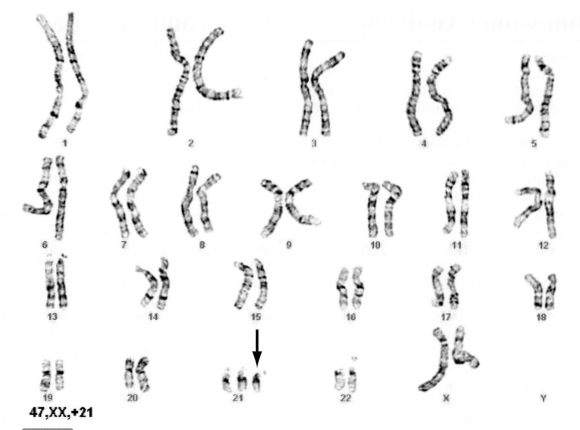

47,XX,+21

**Figure 2-18** Karyotype of a female. Karyotype is not normal. There is an extra chromosome 21(*arrow*). (Karyotype courtesy of Patricia Crowley-Larsen.)

Genes carried on sex chromosomes are called **sex-linked genes**, and the effects that they produce are called sex-linked traits. The small Y chromosome carries few genes other than those that direct male sex differentiation, but the much larger X chromosome carries many genes in addition to those concerned with sexual development. For practical purposes, only X-linked traits are recognized, and most are recessive. The female carrier of a recessive X-linked trait is normal because the effect of the defective allele on one X chromosome is offset by the normal allele on the other X chromosome. The male, however, possesses only one X chromosome. Consequently, he can be neither heterozygous nor homozygous for X-linked genes and is called **hemizygous** (*hemi* = half) for genes carried on the X chromosome. If the male receives an X chromosome containing a defective gene, the normal offsetting allele possessed by the female carrier is lacking, and the defective X-linked gene functions like a dominant gene when paired with the Y chromosome.

# Genes of the Histocompatibility (HLA) Complex

Successful transplantation of organs from one person to another requires that the antigens present on the cells of the organ donor resemble as closely as possible those of the recipient. The antigens present on cells are determined by a cluster of genes on chromosome 6. This group of genes, which was first identified in laboratory animals in connection with transplantation experiments, is called the **major histocompatibility complex** (MHC). In humans, these cell-surface proteins (antigens) were first identified on peripheral blood leukocytes. Consequently, they were named **human leukocyte antigens** (HLA antigens), and the human major histocompatibility complex is often called the HLA system. Often the designations HLA complex and HLA antigens, and MHC complex and MHC antigens, are used interchangeably. They refer to the unique genetically determined cell-surface antigens that we possess to set us apart from other persons. They are our **self-antigens**.

Although the HLA surface proteins are often called HLA antigens, their antigenicity actually depends on whether they are one's own proteins or the HLA proteins of another person. The HLA proteins on a person's own cells (self-antigens) are unique for the person possessing them and are recognized by the immune system as being part of that person, not as being foreign; they are, however, foreign proteins (non–self-antigens) in another person in whom they are antigenic and incite an immune response.

Originally, MHC proteins were considered of interest only with respect to organ transplantation because transplantation of cells containing MHC proteins different from those of the transplant recipient was followed by rejection of the transplant unless the immune system was suppressed. However, we know now that they have a much larger role, in that they also take part in generating immune responses to foreign antigens of all types. The HLA complex consists of four separate but closely linked gene loci designated HLA-A, HLA-B, HLA-C, and HLA-D, and there are additional subdivisions within the HLA-D locus. Each locus has an equally large number of alleles. Over 50 different alleles, for example, have been identified at the HLA-B locus alone, and many alleles are identified at other HLA gene loci as well. Each allele is designated by a specific letter to designate the locus and a number to indicate the allele, such as HLA-B27. A set of HLA genes on one chromosome is called a haplotype and is transmitted as a unit. Because chromosomes are paired, each person has two haplotypes, each consisting of four HLA genes. The two haplotypes together determine a total of eight HLA proteins on the cell. Because of the large number of alleles in the HLA system, the chances of two persons who are not identical twins having the same HLA proteins on their cells is very remote. When performing HLA typing of proposed donors for an organ transplant one attempts to match the major antigens of the donor as closely as possible with those of the recipient. It is impossible to get a perfect match because of the huge number of HLA alleles, but the more closely the HLA antigens match, the better the chances that the graft will survive.

Figure 2-19 illustrates the inheritance of HLA haplotypes, as shown in the illustration of the haplotypes of the first four children. In this example, each child receives one of two possible haplotypes from each parent. Consequently, a child has only one haplotype in common with each parent. Because of the way in which chromosomes are transmitted from parent to child, a child can have any one of four different haplotypes. Each of the first four children has a different combination of HLA haplotypes. The fifth child, however, has the same haplotypes as the second child, indicating that organ transplantation between these two children would have a better chance for success than would transplantation between individuals having different haplotypes.

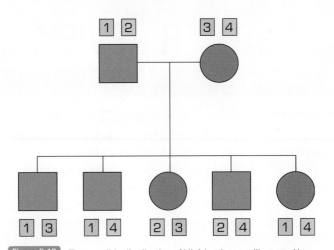

**Figure 2-19** The possible distribution of HLA haplotypes illustrated in a family of five children. Each haplotype consists of four separate linked HLA genes and is arbitrarily designated by an Arabic numeral. The four possible combinations of haplotypes are illustrated in the first four children. In this example, the haplotype of the fifth child is the same as that of the second child.

# Genes and Recombinant DNA Technology (Genetic Engineering)

Genes direct the synthesis of gene products—that is, enzymes or other proteins that play a role in the activities of the cells that make the proteins. Cells make many important biologic products, such as insulin, growth hormone, proteins that regulate the immune responses, and proteins that activate the body's clot-dissolving mechanisms. Many of these proteins are used in clinical medicine: insulin to treat diabetes; growth hormone, which allows a child with a growth hormone deficiency to grow normally; and proteins to unplug blocked coronary arteries of patients with heart attacks. Recent advances in DNA technology have led to the development of methods for large-scale production of these and many other important biologic products. The technology that paved the way for these advances has been called either recombinant DNA technology (because genes from two different sources are being recombined in a single organism) or genetic engineering (because genes are being manipulated).

Whatever name one uses for it, the process requires the insertion of a gene that encodes a desired product, such as insulin, into a bacterium or yeast. After the gene has been inserted, the microorganism contains not only its own genes, but also the new gene, which directs the synthesis of the desired protein. The microorganism–foreign gene combination divides repeatedly to produce large quantities of the desired protein that can be purified and used for various purposes.

# CHAPTER REVIEW

## Summary

The cell is the basic structural and function unit of the body. All cells have similar features (nucleus, cytoplasm, organelles) but many cells are specialized to perform specific functions. The nucleus contains the genetic material (23 pairs of chromosomes = the geonome) that directs the functions of the cell (via messenger RNA). The cytoplasm contains the various organelles that carry out the functions specified by DNA. Groups of similar cells form tissues. Tissues are organized to form organs, and groups of organs form organ systems.

Epithelium covers the exterior of the body, lines the interior of organs such as the respiratory and GI tract, lines body cavities, forms glands, and forms the functional cells of organs that have excretory or secretory functions (such as the liver and kidneys). Epithelium is classified on the basis of its structure as simple or stratified, and by the characteristics of the epithelial cells. Connective tissue connects and supports. Muscle contracts, and nerve tissue conducts.

Materials move in and out of cells across cell membranes by active transport, phagocytosis, and pinocytosis (active processes that require the cell to expend energy), and by diffusion and osmosis (passive non-energy–requiring processes).

Cells adapt to changing conditions (atrophy, hypertrophy, hyperplasia, metaplasia, dysplasia, and increased enzyme synthesis). Injured cells exhibit structural and functional abnormalities; swelling, fatty change, necrosis. Normal cells don't last forever. They have a predetermined life span, and they wear out. However, some tumor cells can proliferate indefinitely. They are "immortal."

Chromosomes occur in pairs: 22 matched pairs of homologous chromosomes called autosomes (non-sex chromosomes) and one pair of sex chromosomes (XX = females; XY = males). One member of each chromosome pair comes from each parent. Genes occupy specific sites on chromosomes called gene loci. There are paired gene loci on the paired chromosomes. At any gene locus, any one of several related genes can occupy the locus. These alternative forms of genes are called alleles or allelic genes. A person is homozygous for a gene if both gene loci possess the same allelic gene, and is heterozygous if the alleles are different.

There are two types of cell division; mitosis characteristic of somatic cells and meiosis in germ cells. Each cell has already duplicated its DNA before it ever starts to divide. Mitosis is simply a separation of already duplicated chromosomes. Each precursor (parent) cell produces two daughter cells, each identical to the parent cell. In contrast, meiosis involves two separate cell divisions. In the first division, there is some intermixing of genetic material between homologous chromosomes (synapse), followed by chromosome separation, giving rise to two daughter cells, each containing only 23 chromosomes. The second meiotic division is just like mitosis, but there are only 23 chromosomes (each composed of two chromatids) in each of the two daughter cells. The chromatids separate and are distributed to the two daughter cells during the second meiotic division. In spermatogenesis, four sperm are formed from each precursor cell. In oogenesis only one ovum is formed; the other three products of the meiosis are discarded as polar bodies.

The HLA (MHC) system is important. It is a system of interconnected (linked) genes located at gene loci on one pair of homologous chromosomes that determine specific proteins (self-antigens) called HLA or MHC proteins on the surface of cells. The HLA genes are transmitted in sets called haplotypes, one set provided by each parent. There are multiple possible alleles at each gene locus, and there are so many possible gene combinations that each individual has a unique set of HLA antigens (except identical twins possessing identical genes). Certain HLA types appear to be associated with increased susceptibility to certain diseases.

## Questions for Review

1. How does the nucleus direct the activities of the cell? What is the genetic code, and what is its role in directing the functions of the cell?
2. How is epithelium classified, and what are its functions? What are mesothelium and endothelium?
3. What is the difference between atrophy and hypertrophy, between metaplasia and dysplasia, and between cell death and cell necrosis?
4. What factors cause a cell to age?

5. What is meant by the following terms: *homologous chromosomes*, *autosomes*, *sex chromosome*, *Barr body*, *gene*, *gametogenesis*, and *centrosome*?
6. How does the process of mitosis compare with meiosis?
7. What are the differences between spermatogenesis and oogenesis?
8. What is a chromosome karyotype?
9. What is the MHC? What is its function?
10. What is a haplotype? How are haplotypes inherited by children from their parents?

# Interactive Activities

## Matching

Match the organelle with its function.

| Organelle | Function |
|---|---|
| 1. Cytoskeleton | A. Convert food materials into energy to make adenosine triphosphate (ATP) used to power the chemical reactions in the cell |
| 2. Rough endoplasmic reticulum (RER) | B. Tubular ribosome-containing channels that synthesize protein to be secreted by cells |
| 3. Lysosomes | C. Tubular channels containing enzymes that synthesize lipids and some other compounds within the cells |
| 4. Golgi apparatus | D. Flat sacs located near the nucleus attach carbohydrate molecules to the proteins synthesized by RER |
| 5. Smooth endoplasmic reticulum | E. Spherical organelles in cytoplasm containing digestive enzymes that break down worn out cell organelles and material brought into cells by phagocytosis |
| 6. Centrioles | F. Short cylinders that form the mitotic spindle that separates chromosomes during cell division |
| 7. Mitochondria | G. Protein tubules and filaments that form structural framework of cells and promote cell functions such as motility and phagocytosis |

## True or False

Indicate whether the following statements are true or false by writing T or F at the end of the statement.
1. Chromosomes normally exist in pairs called homologous chromosomes._____
2. Genes exist in pairs and the members of each pair are located at corresponding sites (gene loci) on homologous chromosomes._____

3. Certain HLA types appear to predispose to specific diseases._____
4. An individual is heterozygous for a gene if the genes at corresponding sites (gene loci) are the same, and homozygous for the gene if the genes are different._____
5. A dominant gene expresses itself in either the homozygous or heterozygous state._____
6. A defective X-linked gene functions as a dominant gene in females as well as males._____

## Critical Thinking

1. Charles Brown is a weight lifter and has large back, neck, and arm muscles. He believes that his muscles are larger because his high-protein diet is causing him to develop more muscle fibers. He believes that increasing his protein intake will form even more muscle fibers, and asks your opinion. What would you tell him?
2. James Smith has chronic kidney disease and will need a kidney transplant. His younger brother Andrew has the same HLA type that James has and wants to know whether this guarantees that the transplanted kidney will survive if he donates his kidney. What would you tell Andrew?
3. Sally Smith's brother has hemophilia, which is a genetically transmitted disease caused by an abnormal gene carried on the X chromosome. Sally wants to know whether she also carries the gene, which she could transmit to her children. What would you tell Sally? Be prepared to explain your answer to her.

# 3

# Inflammation and Repair

1. List the characteristics and clinical manifestations of an acute inflammation. Differentiate inflammations on the basis of their component of fluid and inflammatory cells (serous, purulent, fibrinous, and hemorrhagic inflammations).

2. Describe the possible outcomes of an inflammatory reaction.

3. Name the chemical mediators of inflammation. Explain how they interact to intensify the inflammatory process.

4. Describe the harmful effects of inflammation. Explain why it is sometimes necessary to suppress the inflammatory process.

5. Compare inflammation and infection. Name some of the terms used to describe infections.

## The Inflammatory Reaction

The inflammatory reaction is a nonspecific response to any agent that causes cell injury. The agent may be physical (such as heat or cold), chemical (such as a concentrated acid or alkali or another caustic chemical), or microbiologic (such as a bacterium or virus). The inflammatory reaction is characterized by both local and systemic effects, as indicated diagrammatically in Figure 3-1.

Local effects consist of dilatation (expansion) of blood vessels and increased vascular permeability.

Leukocytes (white blood cells) are attracted to the site of injury. They adhere to the endothelium of the small blood vessels, force their way through the walls, and migrate to the area of tissue damage ( Figure 3-2 ). The characteristic signs of inflammation are heat, redness, tenderness, swelling, and pain. The increased warmth and redness of the inflamed tissues are caused by dilatation of capillaries and slowing of blood flow through the vessels. Swelling occurs because the extravasation (leakage) of plasma from the dilated and more permeable vessels causes the volume of fluid in the inflamed

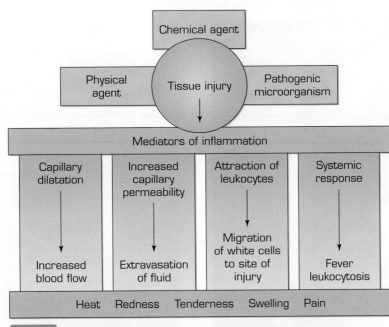

**Figure 3-1** Local and systemic effects of tissue injury caused by various injurious agents.

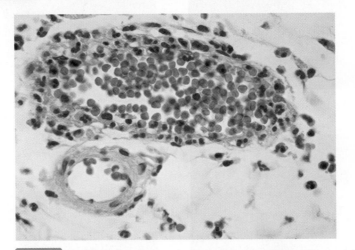

**Figure 3-2** Photomicrograph illustrating leukocytes adherent to capillary endothelium and migrating through wall to site of tissue injury (original magnification × 160).

tissue to increase ( Figure 3-3 ). The tenderness and pain are secondary to irritation of sensory nerve endings at the site of the inflammatory process.

The polymorphonuclear leukocyte is the most important cell in the acute inflammatory response. It is an actively phagocytic cell that is attracted to the area by the cell injury. Mononuclear cells (monocytes, macrophages) appear later in the inflammation reaction. One of their major functions is to clean up the debris produced by the inflammatory process. These cells are also active in chronic inflammatory reactions.

The fluid mixture of protein, leukocytes, and debris that forms during the inflammatory process is called **exudate**. Its proportions of protein and inflammatory cells vary in different exudates, and the appearance of the exudate will also vary. It is convenient to describe an exudate as serous, purulent, fibrinous, or hemorrhagic based on its appearance. If the exudate consists primarily of fluid containing very little protein, the term *serous exudate* is used. If a large amount of serous fluid accumulates in injured tissues—as, for example, after a severe burn of the skin—blisters may form ( Figure 3-4 ). An exudate consisting largely of inflammatory cells is called a *purulent exudate*, and the creamy yellow exudate is called pus. The term *fibrinous exudate* is used if the fluid in the exudate is rich in a blood protein called fibrinogen, which coagulates and forms fibrin, producing a sticky film on the surface of the inflamed tissue ( Figure 3-5 ). (The proteins concerned in the coagulation of the blood are considered in Chapter 9.) A *hemorrhagic exudate* occurs when the inflammatory process had ruptured many small capillaries, allowing red blood cells to escape into the tissues so that the exudate appears bloody.

**exudate**
(ex′yū-dāt)
The fluid, leukocytes, and debris that accumulate as a result of an inflammation.

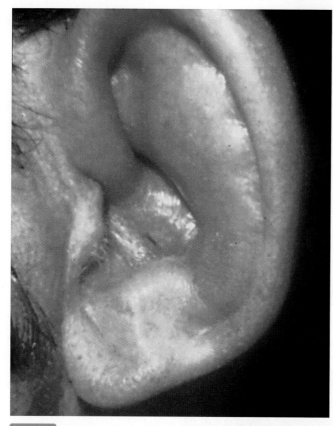

Figure 3-3 Marked swelling of ear caused by acute inflammation.

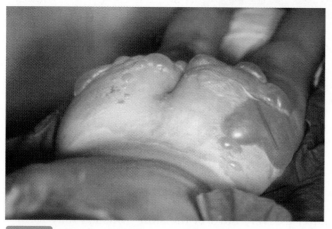

Figure 3-4 Extensive burn with marked leakage (extravasation) of fluid into the burned area leading to formation of large blisters.

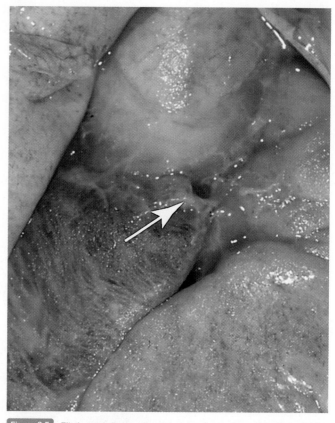

Figure 3-5 Fibrinous inflammation involving the surface of the heart (epicardium) and pericardium. The pericardial sac has been opened to expose the surface of the heart, which appears rough because fibrin has accumulated on the epicardium. The *arrow* indicates a large aggregate of fibrin adjacent to the right atrial appendage.

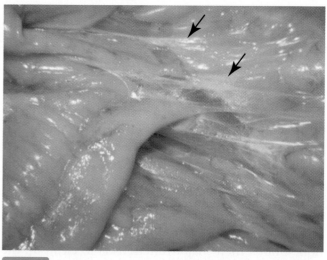

Figure 3-6 Multiple fibrous adhesions (*arrows*) between loops of small intestine resulting from previous abdominal inflammation.

If a fibrinous exudate involves two surfaces in close proximity, such as adjacent loops of small intestine, the surfaces may stick together. This type of inflammation often heals by ingrowth of fibrous tissue, which binds the adjacent surfaces together by means of fibrous bands called **adhesions** ( Figure 3-6 ).

If the inflammatory process is severe, systemic effects become evident. The individual feels ill, and the temperature is elevated. The bone marrow accelerates its production of leukocytes so that the number of leukocytes circulating in the bloodstream increases.

The outcome of an inflammation depends on how much tissue damage has resulted from the inflammation. If the inflammation is mild, it soon subsides, and the tissues return to normal. This process is called resolution.

**adhesions**
(ad-hē′shuns) Bands of fibrous tissue that form subsequent to an inflammation, and bind adjacent tissues together.

If the inflammatory process is more severe, tissue is destroyed to some extent and must be repaired ( Figure 3-7 ). During healing, damaged cells are replaced, and the framework of the injured tissue is repaired as an ingrowth of cells produces connective-tissue fibers and new blood vessels. Scar tissue replaces large areas of tissue destruction ( Figure 3-8 ). Sometimes, the scarring subsequent to a severe inflammation is so severe that function is seriously disturbed ( Figure 3-9 ).

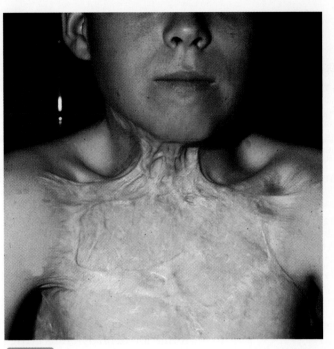

Figure 3-9    Marked scarring after the healing of a severe burn, which has restricted motion of neck and arms. Skin grafting was required to improve function.

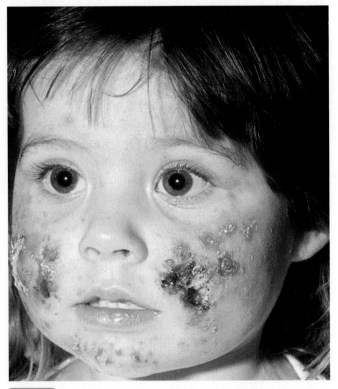

Figure 3-7    Acute inflammation of face with superficial necrosis of skin. Crusts of dried exudate (scabs) have formed on skin surface.

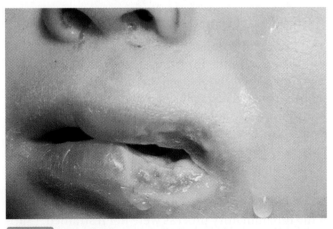

Figure 3-8    Extensive tissue destruction of lower lip, which is covered with inflammatory exudate. Child chewed an electric light cord, exposing bare wire, and sustained a severe electrical burn of lip.

## Chemical Mediators of Inflammation

The inflammatory reaction is a nonspecific, stereotyped response to tissue injury and is much the same no matter what caused the injury. For example, an injury caused by dropping a book on your foot produces the same type of inflammatory response as does a severe sunburn in the same region. The reason is because *the inflammatory response is not directly caused by the tissue injury*. It is caused by chemical agents called *mediators of inflammation* that are formed and released when the tissue is damaged. Some mediators are derived from cells, and others are formed from proteins in the blood plasma that accumulate in the injured area.

**Cell-Derived Mediators**  **Mast cells**, a major source of cell-derived mediators, are specialized cells that are widely distributed throughout the connective tissues of the body. Their cytoplasm is filled with granules containing histamine and other chemicals. If tissue is injured, the mast cells discharge their granules, liberating the chemicals to initiate the inflammatory process. Histamine is a potent **vasodilator** (*vas* = blood vessel + *dilate* = expand) and also greatly increases vascular permeability. *Blood platelets* also contain histamine and another mediator called **serotonin**, which are released when platelets adhere to collagen fragments at the site of tissue injury. Other important cell-derived mediators are a group called **prostaglandins** (so named because compounds of this type were first isolated from the prostate gland) and a group of similar compounds called leukotrienes. These biologically active compounds are synthesized by cells from arachidonic acid present in cell membranes in response to stimuli that induce inflammation, and they function as mediators that intensify the inflammatory process.

### Mediators from Blood Plasma

Blood plasma contains various protein substances that circulate as inactive compounds and leak from the permeable capillaries into the area of tissue damage where they become transformed (activated) by a complex process into chemical mediators. One important group of mediators formed in this way is called **bradykinins** (or simply kinins). The series of reactions that leads to the formation of bradykinins is triggered by one of the proteins concerned with blood coagulation, which is activated by the tissue injury.

Mediators of inflammation are also formed from another group of blood proteins called **complement**. Complement consists of a group of proteins that interact in a regular sequence to yield a series of by-products, some of which function as mediators of inflammation. Complement is activated when an antigen combines with an antibody but may also be activated in other ways that do not require an antigen–antibody interaction. The various functions of the complement system are considered in connection with the immune system (see Chapter 4). ( Figure 3-10 ) illustrates how the various mediators interact. The release of mediators from any source not only initiates the inflammatory process, but also induces release of more mediators from other sources, setting off a "chain reaction" that intensifies the inflammatory process.

### The Role of Lysosomal Enzymes in the Inflammatory Process

The cytoplasm of phagocytic neutrophils and monocytes that are attracted to the site of inflammation by chemical mediators contains granules called lysosomes (*lysis* = dissolving + *soma* = body). Lysosomes contain potent enzymes that are capable of digesting the material brought into the cytoplasm of the cells by phagocytosis. During phagocytosis, bacteria or other foreign materials become enclosed within vacuoles in the cell

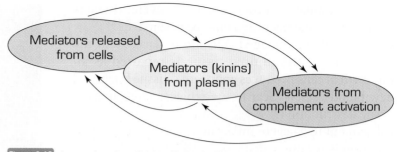

**Figure 3-10** Interaction of mediators of inflammation. Activation of mediators from any source also leads to the formation of mediators from other sources, which intensifies the inflammatory reaction.

cytoplasm, and the lysosomes dissolve the material by discharging their enzymes into the vacuoles, as described in Chapter 2 (Figure 2-2).

In the course of any inflammatory reaction, many neutrophils and monocytes are damaged or destroyed, and their lysosomal enzymes are released. Some lysosomal enzymes also escape from intact leukocytes during phagocytosis. Much of the tissue injury in an area of inflammation is a result of the destructive effect of the lysosomal enzymes released from leukocytes. The tissue injury in turn generates more mediators, and this induces further inflammatory changes.

### Inflammation Caused by Antigen–Antibody Interaction

Antibodies are one of the body's defense mechanisms. This is discussed in Chapter 4. When antigen and antibody interact, an intense inflammatory reaction with marked tissue necrosis often follows. The interaction of antigen and antibody activates complement, and the mediators generated from complement activation induce the inflammatory reaction. Large numbers of leukocytes are attracted to the site, and the release of potent lysosomal enzymes from the leukocytes is the chief cause of the tissue damage.

### Harmful Effects of Inflammation

The tissue injury that results from an inflammation is due in part to the injurious agent and in part to the inflammatory reaction itself. In most cases, the inflammatory process is self-limited and subsides when the harmful agent has been eliminated. At times, however, an inflammatory process may persist and cause extensive, progressive tissue injury. If this occurs, it is sometimes necessary to suppress the inflammatory process by administering adrenal corticosteroid hormones to reduce the tissue damage that would result if the inflammatory process were not restrained. (Suppression of the immune response is considered in Chapter 4.)

# Infection

## Terminology of Infection

The term **infection** is used to denote an inflammatory process caused by disease-producing organisms. A number of different terms are used to refer to infections in various sites. Generally, the ending *-itis* is appended to the name of the tissue or organ in order to indicate an infection or inflammatory process. For example, the terms appendicitis (Figure 3-11), hepatitis, colitis, and pneumonitis refer to inflammation of the appendix, liver, colon, and lung, respectively. An acute spreading infection at any site is called **cellulitis** (Figure 3-12). Usually, this term is used to refer to an acute infection of the skin and deeper tissues. The term **abscess** is used when an infection is associated with breakdown of the tissues and the formation of a localized mass of pus (Figure 3-13). If a localized infection spreads into the lymphatic channels draining the site of inflammation,

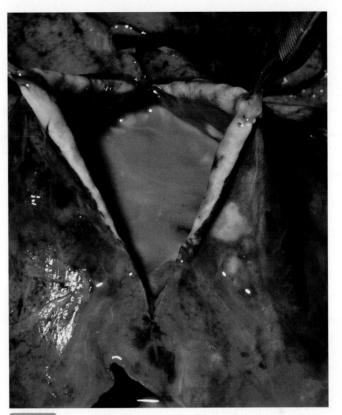

Figure 3-13   Lung abscess. The pleural surface has been incised to expose a large abscess cavity filled with pus.

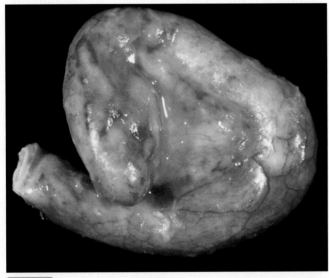

Figure 3-11   Acute appendicitis. Marked inflammatory exudate on the surface of the appendix.

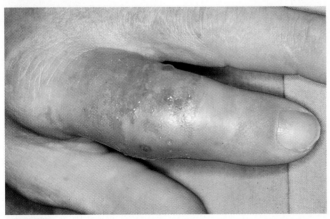

Figure 3-12   Acute infection (cellulitis) of the finger.

the term **lymphangitis** is used. **Lymphadenitis** refers to infection in the regional lymph nodes draining the primary site of infection. The term **septicemia** is used to refer to an overwhelming infection in which pathogenic bacteria gain access to the bloodstream.

## Factors Influencing the Outcome of an Infection

In any infection, the invading organism is pitted against the defenses of the body. Bacteria and other microbiologic agents vary in their ability to cause disease. Many are not harmful to humans. Others, capable of causing human disease, are called **pathogenic** (*pathos* = *disease* + *genic* = producing) organisms. The term **virulence** refers to the ease with which a pathogenic organism can overcome the defenses of the body. A highly virulent organism is one that is likely to produce progressive disease in the majority of susceptible individuals. In contrast, an organism of low virulence is capable of only

**infection** Inflammation caused by a disease-producing organism.

**cellulitis** (sell-ū-lie′tis) An acute spreading inflammation affecting the skin or deeper tissues.

**abscess** (ab′sess) A localized accumulation of pus in tissues.

**lymphangitis** (limf′an-ji′tis) An inflammation of lymph vessels draining a site of infection.

**lymphadenitis** (limf-a-den-ī′tis) An inflammation of lymph nodes draining a site of infection.

**septicemia** (sep-ti-sē′mē-yuh) An infection in which large numbers of pathogenic bacteria are present in the bloodstream.

**pathogenic** (path-ō-jen′ik) Capable of producing disease.

**virulence** (vir′u-lenz) The ability of an organism to cause disease.

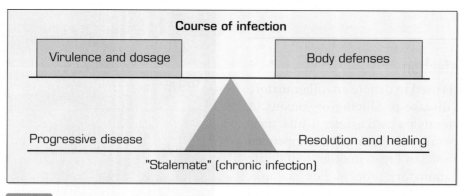

**Figure 3-14** Factors influencing the outcome of an infection.

producing disease in a highly susceptible individual under favorable circumstances.

The outcome of any infection depends on two factors: the virulence of the organism combined with the numbers ("dosage") of the invading organisms and the resistance of the infected individual (often called the **host**). These may be considered balanced against one another, as indicated diagrammatically in (Figure 3-14). When large numbers of organisms of high virulence are introduced into the body, especially when host resistance is lowered, the balance is tipped in favor of the invader, and progressive or fatal disease develops. When the virulence or dosage of the organism is low or the body's resistance is high, the balance is tipped in favor of the host. The infection is then overcome, and healing occurs.

**host** Individual infected with a disease-producing organism.

## Chronic Infection

Sometimes the organism and host are evenly matched. Neither can gain the advantage; the result is a stalemate. Clinically, this results in a *chronic infection*, characterized by a relatively quiet, smoldering inflammation that is usually associated with vigorous attempts at healing on the part of the host. The balance between the host and the invader is precarious. The infection may flare up at times when the pathogen obtains a temporary advantage, or it may become quiescent at other times when the defenses of the host gain the upper hand. Lymphocytes, plasma cells, and monocytes are the predominant cells in chronic inflammatory processes.

# CHAPTER REVIEW

## Summary

The inflammatory reaction is a nonspecific stereotyped response to cell injury. The reason that the response is always the same is because any tissue injury triggers the release of the same type of mediators of inflammation. Mediators come from mast cells (mostly histamine), platelets (serotonin), and other injured cells (prostaglandins, leukotrienes); they also come from blood plasma (bradykinins), and from activation of blood proteins called complement. Lysosomes (packs of digestive enzymes in the cytoplasm of white cells) release their digestive enzymes when white cells degenerate at the site of inflammation, and the released lysosomal enzymes cause further tissue injury. Sometimes the tissue injury caused by the inflammation is so marked that it is necessary to suppress the inflammatory process by means of corticosteroids (such as cortisone) or nonsteroidal anti-inflammatory drugs (such as aspirin or ibuprofen).

*Inflammation* is a general term. If the inflammation is caused by a pathogenic microorganism, we use the term *infection*. Various terms are used to describe an infection: cellulitis (localized infection in the tissues); lymphangitis (infection spreading into lymphatic channels draining the site of infection, with red streaks running up the arm; lymphadenitis (regional lymph nodes involved); abscess (necrosis of tissue with a pocket of pus); and septicemia (bloodstream infection). The outcome of an infection depends on whether the pathogen or body defenses win, or whether they are evenly matched and a chronic infection results.

## Questions for Review

1. What is the inflammatory reaction? What are its clinical manifestations?
2. What factors influence the outcome of an infection?
3. What are mediators of inflammation? How do they function?

4. What is meant by the following terms: *chronic infection*, *pathogenic*, and *complement*?

## Supplementary Reading

Charo, I. F., and Ransohoff, R. M. 2006. The many roles of chemokines and chemokine receptors in inflammation. *New England Journal of Medicine* 354:610–21.

> Chemokines are cytokines that attract leukocytes to the site of inflammation. They also play a role in directing monocytes throughout the body.

Gabray, C., and Kushner, I. 1999. Acute phase proteins and other systemic responses to inflammation. *New England Journal of Medicine* 340:448–54.

> Inflammation is associated with the formation of protein products by liver cells and other tissues that affect the inflammatory response, including C reactive protein (named from its formation in response to the capsule of the pneumococcus, which causes a pulmonary infection) as well as components of complement. Although they have been called acute-phase reactants, they are produced in response to chronic as well as acute inflammation. They also function as markers of inflammation, which can be used to monitor the body's response to inflammation.

Hansson, G. K. 2005. Inflammation, coronary atherosclerosis, and coronary artery disease. *New England Journal of Medicine* 352:1685–95.

> Inflammation plays a role in coronary artery disease (considered in Chapter 10) and other manifestations of vascular disease.

Peters-Golden, M., and Henderson, W. R. 2007. Leukotrienes. *New England Journal of Medicine* 357:1841–54.

> Leukotrienes are made by leukocytes from arachadonic acid, which is a component of cell membranes. They are synthesized in response to many infectious agents, and they enhance the capacity of neutrophils and macrophages to ingest and kill microbes, and also to produce mediators of inflammation that intensify the inflammatory response.

Rhen, T., and Cidlowski, J. A. 2005. Anti-inflammatory action of glucocorticoids—new mechanisms for old drugs. *New England Journal of Medicine* 353:1711–23.

> Inflammation is a response to injury, tissue necrosis, or infection. Infectious microorganisms can activate complement directly without requiring an antigen–antibody interaction to activate complement. Glucocorticoids suppress the inflammatory response by various mechanisms, but also produce undesirable side effects.

Weiss, G., and Goodnough, W. G. 2005. Anemia of chronic disease. *New England Journal of Medicine* 352:1011–23.

> Cytokines released as a result of inflammation impair iron uptake and hemoglobin synthesis, which leads to anemia in many persons with chronic infections.

## Interactive Activities

### Matching

Match the term with its definition.

| Term | Definition |
|------|-----------|
| 1. Exudate | A. A disease-producing organism |
| 2. Infection | B. Inflammation of a lymph node |
| 3. Mediators of inflammation | C. Products released from cells and from blood proteins that are responsible for the features of an inflammatory reaction |
| 4. Leukocytes | D. An inflammation caused by a pathogenic microorganism |
| 5. Pathogen | E. White blood cells |
| 6. Lysosomes | F. Ingestion of material by neutrophils and monocytes |
| 7. Lymphadenitis | G. Spherical structures in the cytoplasm containing potent digestive enzymes |
| 8. Septicemia | H. Fluid and leukocytes accumulate at the site of tissue injury |
| 9. Antibodies | I. Proteins made by plasma cells |
| 10. Phagocytosis | J. Pathogenic microorganisms circulating in the bloodstream |

### True or False

Indicate whether the following statements are true or false by writing T or F at the end of the statement.

1. Mediators of inflammation are produced primarily by neutrophils.____
2. The plasma cell is the most important cell in the acute inflammatory reaction.____
3. Extensive destruction of tissue caused by inflammation is often followed by scarring.____
4. The inflammatory reaction concentrates leukocytes and antibodies at the site of the inflammation.____
5. Activation of blood proteins called complement generates mediators of inflammation.____

### Critical Thinking

1. While working in his garden Ambrose Torson cut his hand on the sharp edge of a garden rake. He washed the wound with soap and water and applied an adhesive bandage. The next day the wound was swollen and he didn't feel well; he also noted some red streaks extending from the wound toward his wrist, and some enlarged tender lymph nodes in his axilla (arm pit). He told his next door neighbor Mary, who is an emergency room nurse at a local hospital, about his problem. She told him what was happening and what he should do. What do you think she told him?

# Immunity, Hypersensitivity, Allergy, and Autoimmune Diseases

## LEARNING OBJECTIVES

1. List the basic features of cell-mediated and humoral immunity. Explain the role of lymphocytes in the immune response.

2. Compare immunity and hypersensitivity. Explain why it is sometimes necessary to suppress the immune response, and describe how this is accomplished.

3. List the five classes of antibodies, and explain how they differ from one another.

4. Describe the pathogenesis of allergic manifestations and the role of IgA in allergy. Compare the methods of treatment.

5. Summarize the theories concerning the pathogenesis of autoimmune disease, the clinical manifestations, and the methods of treatment.

## The Body's Defense Mechanisms

The body has two separate defense mechanisms for dealing with pathogenic microorganisms and other potentially harmful substances. One mechanism consists of the inflammatory reaction, which is a nonspecific response to any harmful agent and includes phagocytosis of the material by neutrophils and macrophages. The second, which depends on the immune system, consists of the development of an acquired immunity. The two mechanisms complement one another and function together to protect an individual from disease.

Acquired immunity, which develops after contact with a pathogenic microorganism, is only one manifestation of a person's capacity to react to a large number of foreign antigens. There are two different types of acquired immunity: humoral immunity (also called

Figure 4-1

antibody-mediated immunity) and cell-mediated immunity. **Humoral immunity** is associated with the production of antibodies that can combine with and eliminate the foreign material, and is the body's major defense against many bacteria and bacterial toxins. **Cell-mediated immunity** is characterized by the formation of a population of lymphocytes that can attack and destroy the foreign material. It is the main defense against viruses, fungi, parasites, and some bacteria. Cell-mediated immunity is the mechanism by which the body rejects transplanted organs and eliminates the abnormal cells that sometimes arise spontaneously in cell division.

Acquired immunity is often associated with a stage of altered reactivity to bacterial products or foreign material, leading to an intense inflammatory reaction at the site of contact with the foreign antigen. This increased responsiveness is called **hypersensitivity**. For example, contact with the tubercle bacillus leads to cell-mediated immunity and is also associated with the development of tissue hypersensitivity to antigens of the tubercle bacillus. An individual who displays hypersensitivity to an organism or its products usually possesses some degree of immunity as well.

Normally, a person develops an immune response not against cell proteins in his or her own cells and tissues (called self-antigens) but only against foreign antigens (called non–self-antigens) because the body has developed a tolerance to the self-antigens present within it. Any lymphocytes that are inadvertently programmed in the course of prenatal development to react against self-antigens are destroyed or inactivated or their functions are suppressed.

However, there are some diseases that result when our own immune system attacks us, producing groups of destructive lymphocytes and injurious antibodies directed against our own cells and tissues, which may cause considerable organ damage. Antibodies directed against us are called **autoantibodies** (*auto* = self), and the diseases resulting from tissue damage caused by our own immune system are called **autoimmune diseases**.

**humoral immunity** Immunity associated with formation of antibodies produced by plasma cells.

**cell-mediated immunity** Immunity associated with population of sensitized lymphocytes.

**hypersensitivity** A state of abnormal reactivity to a foreign material.

**autoantibody** (aw′tō-an′ti-bod-ē) An antibody formed against one's own cells or tissue components.

**autoimmune disease** A disease associated with formation of cell-mediated or humoral immunity against the subject's own cells or tissue components.

**lymphokine** (limf′ō-kin) A soluble substance liberated by lymphocytes.

**monokine** A cytokine secreted by monocytes and macrophages.

**cytokine** A general term for any protein secreted by cells that functions as an intercellular messenger and influences cells of the immune system. Cytokines are secreted by macrophages and monocytes (monokines), lymphocytes (lymphokines), and other cells.

**interferon** (in-tur-fēr′on) A broad-spectrum antiviral agent manufactured by various cells in the body.

**interleukin** A general term for a cytokine liberated by lymphocytes that causes a response in other cells.

# Immunity

## The Role of Lymphocytes in Acquired Immunity

The important cells of the immune system are the lymphocytes ( Figure 4-1 ), which respond to foreign antigens and the macrophages and related cells that process the antigen and "present" it to the lymphocytes.

The various cells of the immune system communicate with one another and produce many of their effects by secreting soluble protein (peptide) chemical messengers. Those secreted by lymphocytes are called **lymphokines**, and those secreted by monocytes are called **monokines**. The general term **cytokines** is used to designate any chemical messengers that take part in any function of the immune system, and some cytokines have specific names. Those that act by interfering with the multiplication of viruses within cells are called **interferons**. Those that send regulatory signals between cells of the immune system are called **interleukins**. Cytokines that can destroy foreign or abnormal cells are called **tumor necrosis factors**, so named because they can destroy tumor cells, although their destructive functions are not restricted to tumor cells.

## Development of the Lymphatic System

**Development of Immune Competence** The precursor cells of the lymphocytes are formed initially from stem cells in the bone marrow, and they eventually develop into either of two groups of lymphocytes,

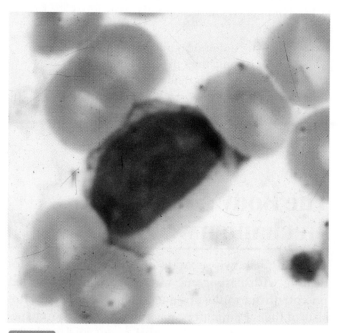

Figure 4-1 Structure of mature lymphocyte in the peripheral blood (original magnification × 1000).

depending on where they undergo further development and "learn" their functions, a process called developing immune competence. In the fetus, some of these precursor cells migrate from the marrow into the thymus, where they undergo further maturation and develop into cells that are destined to form a specific type of lymphocyte called T (thymus-dependent) **lymphocytes**. Other lymphoid cells remain within the bone marrow, where they differentiate and develop into cells destined to form a second specific type of lymphocyte called **B** (bone-marrow) **lymphocytes**.

The programming process by which lymphocytes acquire immune competence involves a rearrangement of genes within the developing T and B lymphocytes. Each programmed lymphocyte develops antigen receptors on its cell membrane that enable the lymphocyte to "recognize" and respond to a specific antigen. The antigen receptors of B lymphocytes are immunoglobulin (antibody) molecules, each a copy of the antibody that the B lymphocyte will eventually produce when stimulated by the appropriate antigen. T lymphocytes develop somewhat different types of receptors, but they serve the same functions as those on B cells. When the programming process has been completed, many millions of different T and B cells have formed, each programmed to recognize and respond to a different antigen. Although a single lymphocyte can respond to only a single antigen, there is such an enormous population of lymphocytes that some member of the "immunologic response team" can respond to any antigen the individual may ever encounter.

**Migration and Circulation of Lymphocytes** Before birth, the precursor cells of both T and B lymphocytes migrate into the spleen, lymph nodes, and other sites. Here they proliferate to form the masses of mature lymphocytes that populate the various lymphoid organs.

T lymphocytes are usually classified into two major groups based on the type of protein molecules, called CD (cluster of differentiation) antigens, on their cell membranes. Lymphocytes containing CD4 antigens are usually called T4 lymphocytes, and those with CD8 antigens are called T8 lymphocytes. As is described later, each group of T lymphocytes has different functions and responds somewhat differently when stimulated by an antigen.

Lymphocytes vary in their life span. Some have only a short survival time, but others live for many years. Lymphocytes do not remain localized within lymphoid organs. They continually move back and forth between the bloodstream and the various lymphoid tissues. T and B lymphocytes are both present in the circulation and can be distinguished by special techniques.

About two-thirds of the circulating lymphocytes are T lymphocytes, and most of the rest are B lymphocytes. From about 10 to 15 percent of the circulating lymphocytes, however, have neither T nor B cell receptors. These cells are called **natural killer cells** or, simply, **NK cells**. Their major targets are virus-infected cells and cancer cells, which they can attack and destroy by secreting destructive lymphokines, even though they have not been previously exposed to the foreign antigens that they are attacking. Furthermore, NK cells can destroy the target cells as soon as they are encountered, in contrast to T and B cells, which need time to become activated and function effectively. Although NK cells are not actually part of either the cell-mediated or the humoral immune-defense systems, their functions are to some extent regulated by the immune system.

## Response of Lymphocytes to Foreign Antigens

Entry of a foreign antigen into the body triggers a chain of events that involves interactions between T and B lymphocytes and macrophages or similar antigen-processing cells. Macrophages are monocytes that have left the bloodstream and taken up permanent residence in the tissues throughout the body where they phagocytose and process antigens. Another important group of widely distributed antigen-processing cells are called dendritic cells, named from their long cytoplasmic processes that resemble the dendrites of a nerve cell. T and B lymphocytes respond differently to foreign antigens. T lymphocytes can only respond to processed antigens, but B lymphocytes can process intact antigens and display the fragments on their cell membranes.

Figure 4-2 illustrates the interaction of antigen processing cells with T and B cells to generate an immune response. The initial contact with a foreign antigen is followed by a lag phase of a week or more before an immune response is demonstrated. This lag corresponds to the time required for processing the antigen and for the lymphocytes to respond. After the body's immune mechanisms have reacted to a foreign antigen, however, some of the lymphoid cells retain a "memory" of the antigen that induced sensitization. They pass this information to succeeding generations of lymphocytes. Consequently, any later contact with the same antigen provokes a renewed proliferation of sensitized lymphocytes or antibody-forming plasma cells.

**tumor necrosis factor** A cytokine that can destroy foreign or abnormal cells.

**lymphocyte** (limf'ō-sit) A mononuclear blood cell produced in lymphoid tissue that takes part in cell-mediated and humoral immunity.

**T lymphocyte** A type of lymphocyte associated with cell-mediated immunity.

**B lymphocyte** A lymphocyte that differentiates into plasma cells and is associated with humoral immunity.

**natural killer cells** Lymphocytes capable of destroying foreign or abnormal cells, although they have not had any prior antigenic contact with the cells.

**NK cells** An abbreviation for natural killer cells.

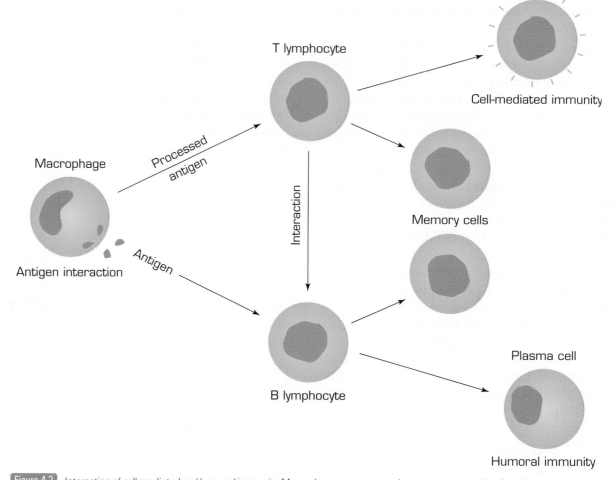

**Activated T lymphocyte**

**T lymphocyte**

**Cell-mediated immunity**

**Macrophage**

*Processed antigen*

*Interaction*

**Memory cells**

**Antigen interaction**

*Antigen*

**Plasma cell**

**B lymphocyte**

**Humoral immunity**

**Figure 4-2**  Interaction of cell-mediated and humoral immunity. Macrophage processes and presents processed antigen fragments to T lymphocyte; B lymphocyte processes intact antigen and displays fragments of the same antigen on its cell membrane. T lymphocyte, which has responded to the same antigen, stimulates the B lymphocyte to proliferate, mature into plasma cells, and make antibodies.

**Role of Major Histocompatibility Proteins in Displaying Processed Antigen**  The major histocompatibility complex (MHC) proteins play an essential role in "presenting" processed antigen to the responding cells of the immune system in order to generate an immune response. The MHC proteins are carbohydrate–protein (glycoprotein) molecules on the surface of cells that distinguish the cells of one person from those of another, as described in Chapter 2. There are two major classes of MHC proteins: MHC Class I proteins are present on all nucleated cells; MHC Class II proteins are restricted to B lymphocytes, macrophages and related antigen-processing cells, and some activated T lymphocytes. The main function of the MHC proteins is to serve as a carrier for the processed foreign antigen fragments on the surface of cells, to which the immune system can respond.

**T-Lymphocyte Response to Antigen**  T lymphocytes are unable to respond to a foreign antigen until a macrophage or similar macrophagelike antigen-processing cell has phagocytosed the antigen, digested it, and displayed on its cell membrane the antigen fragments combined with its own MHC Class II proteins. In response to the displayed antigen-MHC Class II proteins, the T lymphocyte having the corresponding antigen receptors responds by proliferating and forms a group (clone) of identical T cells. The macrophages are also activated when they process and present antigen to T cells, and they secrete a cytokine that stimulates the T cells to proliferate.

**B-Lymphocyte Response to Antigen**  B lymphocytes have immunoglobulin molecules on their cell membranes that function as antigen receptors, and they can bind entire antigen molecules to their receptors. Then the bound antigen is transported across the cell membrane into the cell, where it is processed into fragments within the cytoplasm of the B lymphocyte. Finally, the processed fragments are displayed on the cell membrane along with the B lymphocyte's own MHC Class II proteins. The T lymphocytes that have also responded to the same antigen are activated by the displayed antigen–MHC protein complex on the B lymphocytes, and they perform a "helper cell" function by secreting lymphokines that induce the B cells to proliferate, mature into plasma cells, and produce antibodies. Figure 4-2 summarizes the interaction of T and B lymphocytes and antigen-processing cells concerned with generating an immune response to a foreign antigen.

**Major Functions of T-Lymphocyte Populations** Two major groups of T cells are recognized: regulator T cells and effector T cells. Their activities are coordinated, and they function together to regulate the immune response and also to act against foreign antigens. The regulator cells are T4 (CD4+) cells. One group functions as helper T cells to promote the immune response by secreting cytokines that activate effector T cells and B cells. Loss or destruction of these cells inhibits the immune response and greatly increases susceptibility to infection. The devastating effect of helper T-cell loss on the immune system is illustrated by the acquired immune deficiency syndrome (AIDS, described in Chapter 6) that is caused by a virus that attacks and destroys helper T lymphocytes. Another group of regulator T4 cells function as suppressor T cells to prevent excessive immune system stimulation by producing inhibitory cytokines.

There are two types of effector T cells: cytotoxic T cells, which are T8 (CD8+) cells, and delayed hypersensitivity T cells, which are T4 (CD4+) cells. Cytotoxic T cells attack and destroy body cells infected with viruses or intracellular bacteria. The infected cells are marked for destruction because some of the viral or bacterial antigens are broken down within the infected cells and transported to the cell surface combined with MHC Class I proteins (present on all nucleated cells). The cytotoxic T cells respond to the foreign antigen–MHC complex by proliferating and secreting cytokines that destroy the infected cells. Cytotoxic T cells can also attack cancer cells, which display antigens different from normal cell antigens combined with MHC Class I proteins, and they are also responsible for the rejection of transplanted organs, which also contain foreign antigens.

Delayed hypersensitivity cells, also called sensitized T cells, are produced by a subgroup of helper T cells. The delayed hypersensitivity T cells respond to foreign antigens processed by macrophages or similar cells by accumulating at the site of the antigenic material, where they secrete a variety of lymphokines that attract macrophages, activate them, and stimulate them to secrete additional cytokines, including interferon and tumor necrosis factor. Some of the lymphokines also stimulate cytotoxic T cells and NK cells, both of which also secrete destructive cytokines. In this way, the delayed hypersensitivity reaction generates an intense inflammatory response directed against the antigens that stimulated the response.

In addition to regulator and effector T cells, a population of long-lived memory cells is also generated that can initiate a rapid cell-mediated immune response on later contact with the same antigen. Table 4-1 summarizes the classification and functions of the immune system cells.

## Table 4-1    Classification and Functions of Immune System Cells

| Cell Function | Cell Type | Action of Cell |
|---|---|---|
| Antigen processing | Macrophages, B lymphocytes, dendritic cells | Process antigen and present to lymphocytes |
| Regulate immune response | Regulator T cells (CD4+) | Cytokines regulate immune system activity |
| Promote cytotoxic immune response | Cytotoxic T cells (CD8+) | Produce cytokines that destroy foreign or abnormal cells displaying antigen fragments combined with MHC Class I antigens |
| Promote delayed hypersensitivity response | Delayed hypersensitivity T cells (CD4+) | Respond to antigen processing cells presenting foreign antigen fragments combined with MHC Class II antigens; produce cytokines that activate and stimulate macrophages, cytotoxic T cells, and NK cells |
| Destroy virus-infected cells and cancer cells | NK cells | Cytokine-mediated cell destruction; no previous contact with antigen required |
| Produce antibodies | Plasma cells | Antigen processed by B lymphocytes and presented to responding T cells stimulates B lymphocytes to mature into plasma cells and make antibodies |

**Relation of MHC Proteins to Effector T-Cell Responses** The two types of effector T cells are restricted in their ability to respond to processed antigens complexed and presented with MHC proteins. Cytotoxic T cells, which are T8 (CD8+) cells, can respond only to antigens complexed with MHC Class I proteins displayed on infected host cells, indicating to the immune system that some of the body's own cells have been infected and should be destroyed. In contrast, delayed hypersensitivity cells, which are T4 (CD4+) cells, can respond only to processed antigen displayed on macrophages or related cells along with MHC Class II proteins, signaling the immune system cells to become activated in order to deal with the threat. Consequently, the manner in which the processed antigen is displayed determines which type of effector T cell will respond to the complexed antigen. Cytotoxic T cells are "designed" to attack and destroy infected host cells or other antigenically foreign or abnormal cells. Delayed hypersensitivity T cells function by orchestrating an intense inflammatory reaction to any type of foreign antigen, including microorganisms such as the tubercle bacillus that are phagocytosed by macrophages. Activated macrophages, assisted by lymphoid cells, are the cells that play a major role in eliminating the antigenic material.

**Immune-Response Genes** The ability to generate an immune response is under genetic control. Genes called **immune-response genes**, which are closely associated with the HLA complex on chromosome 6, control the immune response by regulating T-cell and B-cell proliferation. In this way, the genes regulate the intensity of the cell-mediated immune reaction and control the synthesis of antibody molecules. As a result, they influence resistance to infection and resistance to tumors. They also influence the likelihood of acquiring an autoimmune disease.

**immune-response genes** Genes on chromosome 6 that control the immune response to specific antigens.

**immunoglobulin** (im′mū-nō-glob′u-lin) An antibody protein.

## The Role of Complement in Immune Responses

Complement functions along with the immune system to destroy or inactivate all types of foreign antigens, including invading microorganisms. Complement can be activated in two ways: the classical pathway, which is triggered by antigen–antibody interactions; and the alternative pathway, in which complement is activated by bacterial cell wall material or by-products generated during the inflammatory reaction. When complement is activated, the complement components interact to accomplish several important functions. Some

components function as mediators of inflammation. Other components coat the surface of invading bacteria, which makes them easier for macrophages and neutrophils to phagocytose. Finally, the interaction of the complement components generates a large molecule called an attack complex, which destroys the target microorganism or abnormal cell by "punching holes" in its cell membrane ( Figure 4-3 ).

# Antibodies (Immunoglobulins)

Antibodies are globulins produced by plasma cells and are usually called **immunoglobulins** to emphasize their role in immunity. There are five different classes of immunoglobulins:

1. Immunoglobulin M (IgM)
2. Immunoglobulin G (IgG)
3. Immunoglobulin A (IgA)
4. Immunoglobulin D (IgD)
5. Immunoglobulin E (IgE)

Although the immunoglobulins differ somewhat from one another in their chemical composition, molecular weight, and size, they all have the same basic structure: two matched pairs of polypeptide (protein) chains joined by chemical bonds ( Figure 4-4 ). One pair is called heavy chains. The second pair is only half as long as the heavy chains and is called light chains.

The arrangement of the Ig chains somewhat resembles the appearance of a fork. The ends of the Ig chains that combine with the antigen can be compared with its prongs. The "prong" end of the immunoglobulin molecule, which is different in each antibody, is called the *variable part* of the molecule. It is this part that imparts specificity to the molecule. Because of its structure, the antibody can react only with the specific antigen that induced its formation. The *constant part* of the chain, which can be compared with the handle of the fork, is the same for each major class of antibody. The "handle" end does not combine with antigen but determines other properties of the antibody, such as the ability to activate complement or fix to the surface of cell membranes.

All Ig molecules have the same basic four-chain unit structure, but some immunoglobulins characteristically aggregate to form clusters of two or five individual units. For example, IgM is usually a cluster of five individual units, and IgA is usually a pair of units. An antibody molecule is not a rigid structure. The junction of its constant and variable parts is quite flexible and is called the hinge region. This feature allows the

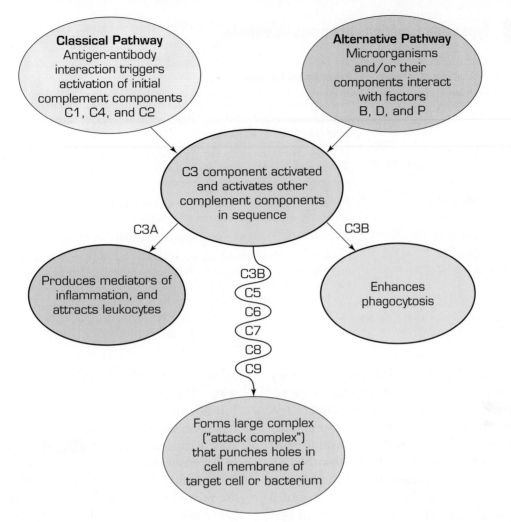

**Figure 4-3** Components and pathways of complement activation that "complement" the body's immune defenses. Individual components named C1 through C9 and factors B, D, and P.

variable end of the Y-shaped molecule to adapt to the configuration of the antigen that it is binding.

IgM, which is present in the blood as a cluster of five individual molecules (a pentamer) joined together, has a star-shaped configuration with the antigen-binding ends projecting outward and the opposite ends of the molecules directed toward the center of the cluster. As a pentamer, IgM forms a very large antibody cluster that is very efficient in combining with large particulate antigens such as fungi; it is often called a macroglobulin because of its large size and high molecular weight. IgG is a much smaller antibody molecule and is the principal type of antibody molecule formed in response to the majority of infectious agents. IgA is produced by

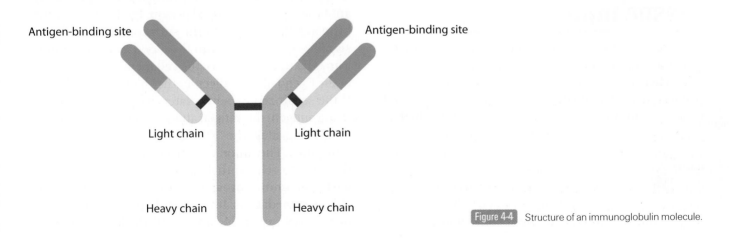

**Figure 4-4** Structure of an immunoglobulin molecule.

## Table 4-2 — Types and Functions of Immunoglobulins

| Immunoglobulin | Usual Type of Secretion | Properties and Functions |
|---|---|---|
| IgM | Pentamer | First Ig formed in response to foreign antigen (primary immune response). Present in bloodstream but not in tissues. Large pentamer antibody cluster very effective for combining with foreign antigen. |
| IgG | Monomer | Most prevalent Ig produced rapidly in large amounts (secondary immune response) to replace IgM. Found in blood and tissues. Crosses placenta to protect fetus until infant immune system can produce antibodies. |
| IgA | Dimer | Present in bloodstream, in secretions produced by mucous membranes (respiratory and GI tract), and breast milk to provide maternal antibody protection to infant. |
| IgD | Monomer | Small amount in bloodstream and on surface of B lymphocytes. Undetermined functions. |
| IgE | Monomer | Present in bloodstream and attaches to mast cells and basophils, which causes allergic response when sensitizing antigen encountered. IgE evolved to protect against parasitic infections common in developing countries, but in developed countries causes allergy problems in susceptible (atopic) persons. |

antibody-forming cells located in the respiratory and gastrointestinal mucosa. It is present in secretions of the respiratory and gastrointestinal tracts. IgA apparently functions by combining with potentially harmful ingested or inhaled antigens, forming antigen–antibody complexes that cannot be absorbed. In this way, IgA prevents the antigens from inducing sensitization. IgD is found on the cell membranes of B lymphocytes, along with the monomeric form of IgM and is present in only minute quantities in the blood. IgE is normally present in only small quantities in the blood of most persons, but its concentration is greatly increased in allergic individuals.

Table 4-2 summarizes the types and functions of the various immunoglobulins.

# Hypersensitivity Reactions: Immune System–Related Tissue Injury

The immune system, while protecting us from foreign antigens that could harm us, may also damage the tissues where the immune response occurs. The desirable effect, which eliminates the foreign antigen, is called **immunity**. The undesirable effect, which is the associated tissue damage, is called **hypersensitivity**. Both are manifestations of the same process. The situation could be compared with the successful efforts of fire fighters in putting out a potentially destructive house fire but

at the same time breaking some windows and causing water damage to the house and furniture.

It is conventional to classify the various types of hypersensitivity reactions based on how the immune system caused the injury (Table 4-3). Four different types of hypersensitivity reactions, usually designated by Roman numerals, are recognized. The first three types are related to antibodies formed in response to antigenic material, and the fourth type is a cell-mediated hypersensitivity reaction. This section deals with the various mechanisms of immunologic injury. Specific examples of immune-mediated organ damage will be considered in connection with the disease of the various organ systems.

## Type I. Immediate Hypersensitivity Reactions: Allergy and Anaphylaxis

Type I hypersensitivity reactions follow contact with foreign antigens that induce formation of specific IgE antibodies in the sensitized person. IgE has the unusual property of attaching to the surface of mast cells and similar cells circulating in the blood called basophils. The IgE attaches itself to the cell membrane by means of the $F_c$ end of the molecule (the "handle of the fork"). If the sensitized person is later exposed to the sensitizing antigen, the antigen attaches to the free antibody-combining sites (the "prongs of the fork") on the IgE molecules. The union of antigen and antibody causes the cells to release their cytoplasmic granules filled with histamine, prostaglandins, and other potent chemical mediators. Immediate hypersensitivity reactions either may be localized, called allergic reactions,

**immunity**
Resistance to disease.

**hypersensitivity** A state of abnormal reactivity to a foreign material.

## Table 4-3  Mechanisms of Immunologic Injury

| Type | Mechanism | Examples |
|------|-----------|----------|
| I: Immediate hypersensitivity | IgE antibodies fix to mast cells and basophils. Later contact with sensitizing antigen triggers mediator release and clinical manifestations. | Localized response: hay fever, food allergy, etc. |
| | | Systemic response: bee sting, or penicillin anaphylaxis, etc. |
| II: Cytotoxic hypersensitivity reactions | Antibody binds to cell or tissue antigen, and complement is activated, which damages cell, causes inflammation, and promotes destruction of antibody-coated cell by phagocytosis. | Autoimmune hemolytic anemia |
| | | Blood transfusion reactions |
| | | Rh hemolytic disease |
| | | Some types of glomerulonephritis |
| III: Immune complex disease | Circulating antigen–antibody complexes form, which activate complement and cause inflammatory reaction. | Some types of glomerulonephritis |
| | | Lupus erythematosus |
| | | Rheumatoid arthritis |
| IV: Delayed (cell-mediated) hypersensitivity | Sensitized (delayed hypersensitivity) T cells release lymphokines that attract macrophages and other inflammatory cells. | Tuberculosis |
| | | Fungus and parasitic infections |
| | | Contact dermatitis |

or may evoke a widespread systemic reaction, called anaphylaxis.

**Allergy** Individuals who develop localized IgE-mediated reactions are predisposed to form specific IgE antibodies (become allergic) to ragweed, other plant pollens, and various other antigens that do not affect most persons. The allergy-prone individual is called an **atopic** person. The sensitizing antigen is called an allergen, and the allergic manifestations are localized to the tissues that are exposed to the allergens—for example, swollen itchy eyes, stuffy nose, and sneezing in a ragweed-sensitive person ( Figure 4-5 ). Because histamine is one of the mediators released from the IgE-coated cells, antihistamine drugs (which block the effects of histamine) often relieve many of the allergic symptoms. A more specific method of treating an allergic individual consists of immunizing the person to the offending allergen by repeated subcutaneous injections of the antigen that induced the allergy, such as an extract of ragweed pollen in a ragweed-sensitive person. This method of treatment, which is called **desensitization**, induces the formation of specific IgA and IgG antibodies against the offending allergen. The IgA and IgG act by combining with the allergen before it can affix to the cell-bound IgE and trigger the release of mediators. In a ragweed-sensitive person, for example, the ragweed-specific IgA present in the secretions of the respiratory tract combines with some of the inhaled ragweed antigen and helps prevent absorption of the allergen. At the same time, the ragweed-specific IgG circulating in the bloodstream combines with much of the absorbed ragweed antigen

before it can interact with the IgE on the surface of the mast cells and basophils. Because less antigen is available to combine with cell-bound IgE and thereby trigger release of mediators, the allergic manifestations are minimized.

**Anaphylaxis** A severe generalized IgE-mediated hypersensitivity reaction may be life threatening and is called **anaphylaxis**. This condition results from an initial exposure to a substance (allergen) that induces the sensitization in a susceptible person. Commonly implicated allergens include penicillin, bee stings, peanuts, latex products, as well as various other sensitizing agents. Once sensitization has occurred, a later exposure to the sensitizing antigen triggers widespread mediator release from IgE-coated mast cells and basophils. This release may lead to a fall in blood pressure with circulatory collapse and is often accompanied by severe respiratory distress caused by a mediator-induced spasm of smooth muscle in the walls of the bronchioles, which restricts air flow into and out of the lungs. Prompt treatment of this immunologic catastrophe with epinephrine and other appropriate agents is essential.

A similar condition called an **anaphylactoid reaction** resembles an anaphylactic reaction but is not caused by IgE and occurs after the first contact with a foreign substance, possibly by stimulating mast cells

**atopic**
(ā-top´ik)
Having a genetic predisposition to certain allergic conditions such as hay fever and asthma.

**desensitization** A method of inducing a diminished response to allergens by inducing the formation of specific IgG and IgA antibodies.

**anaphylaxis** (a-nä-fil-aks´is) A severe generalized IgE-mediated hypersensitivity reaction characterized by marked respiratory distress and fall in blood pressure.

**anaphylactoid reaction**
(a-na-fil-ack´-toyd) A hypersensitivity reaction resembling anaphylaxis but not caused by IgE antibodies.

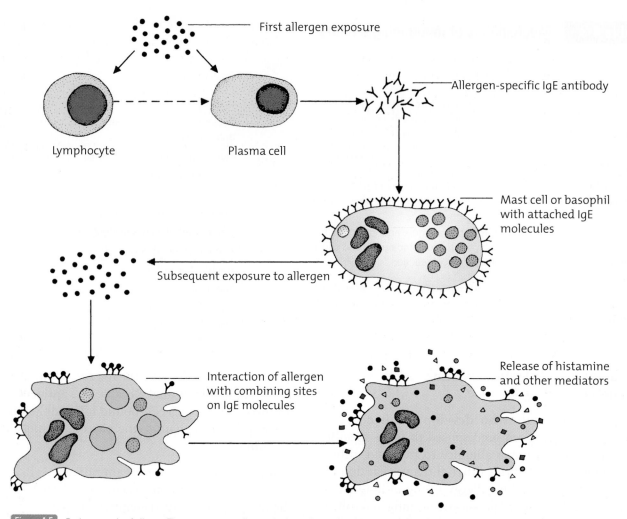

First allergen exposure

Lymphocyte

Plasma cell

Allergen-specific IgE antibody

Mast cell or basophil with attached IgE molecules

Subsequent exposure to allergen

Interaction of allergen with combining sites on IgE molecules

Release of histamine and other mediators

**Figure 4-5** Pathogenesis of allergy. First exposure to allergen induces formation of specific IgE antibody in susceptible individual, which binds to mast cells and basophils by nonantigen receptor end of molecule. Subsequent exposure to allergen leads to an antigen–antibody interaction, liberating histamine and other mediators from mast cells and basophils. These mediators induce allergic manifestations.

directly or by activating complement. Aspirin, other nonsteroidal anti-inflammatory drugs, some antibiotics, and radiopaque iodine-containing contrast material used for x-ray examinations may trigger an anaphylactoid reaction. The treatment is the same as for an anaphylactic reaction.

## Type II. Cytotoxic Hypersensitivity Reactions

In this type of hypersensitivity reaction, antibody formed against a cell or tissue antigen binds to the surface of the target cell or tissue. The antigen–antibody reaction activates complement, and products of complement activation directly or indirectly damage the target. The complement components interact to form a large molecule called an attack complex that directly damages the target cell membrane. Inflammatory cells also are attracted and contribute to the tissue injury by releasing destructive enzymes; they may also destroy the antibody-coated target cells by phagocytosis.

Examples of Type II reactions include transfusion reactions caused by administration of incompatible blood, hemolytic disease of newborn infants caused by Rh incompatibility (Chapter 14), some types of chronic hemolytic anemia associated with autoantibodies directed against red blood cells (Chapter 11), and a type of kidney disease caused by autoantibodies directed against basement membranes of glomerular capillaries (Chapter 15).

## Type III. Tissue Injury Caused by Immune Complexes ("Immune Complex Disease")

In this condition, antigen and antibody form clumps called immune complexes within the circulation that are deposited in the tissues. The antigen–antibody complexes activate complement, and the activated complement components, along with the inflammatory cells that they attract, damage the tissues. Sometimes the immunologic reaction within the tissues is quite severe and leads to thrombosis of blood vessels and considerable tissue necrosis.

An example of organ damage caused by immune complexes is a type of kidney disease called immune complex glomerulonephritis (Chapter 15), in which the complexes are trapped within the glomeruli as the blood flows through the kidneys. Other important diseases in which tissue injury is related to immune complexes include lupus erythematosus, considered in connection with autoimmune disease, and rheumatoid arthritis (Chapter 22).

## Type IV. Delayed (Cell-Mediated) Hypersensitivity Reactions

In delayed hypersensitivity reactions, T lymphocytes rather than antibodies are responsible for the tissue injury. This type of hypersensitivity reaction is commonly encountered in persons who have been infected with the tubercle bacillus and have developed a cell-mediated immune reaction directed against the organism, but some other types of bacteria, as well as fungi and parasites, evoke a similar response. The initial antigenic contact sensitizes the affected individual, and the lymphocytes that generate the cell-mediated immune response are T4 (CD4+) lymphocytes that are called delayed hypersensitivity T cells or, simply, sensitized T cells. After sensitization has occurred, any subsequent contact with the sensitizing antigen induces proliferation of T4 cells that accumulate at the site of antigen contact. The sensitized T cells secrete cytokines that attract and activate macrophages and other lymphocytes, which incites an inflammatory reaction.

Delayed hypersensitivity reactions may also follow skin exposure to poison ivy, as well as various drugs, cosmetics, and chemicals. These agents combine with normal skin proteins to form a complex that induces sensitization. Any later skin contact with the offending agent that induced the initial sensitization provokes an intense cell-mediated inflammatory reaction in the skin, a condition called contact dermatitis.

Unlike immediate hypersensitivity reactions, which are mediated by antibodies, a cell-mediated inflammatory reaction requires from 24 to 48 hours to develop, the delay being the time necessary for sensitized T cells to accumulate at the site and generate an inflammatory reaction. Because this type of reaction takes place in persons who have been infected with the tubercle bacillus, a delayed hypersensitivity reaction is sometimes called tuberculin type hypersensitivity. The commonly used Mantoux skin test to detect infection with the tubercle bacillus is based on the presence or absence of a delayed hypersensitivity reaction to proteins of the tubercle bacillus. If an individual has had a previous contact with the organism, injection of a small test dose of proteins from the tubercle bacillus leads to an inflammatory reaction at the injection site. A positive test, however, only indicates a previous infection with the organism and development of cell-mediated immunity, along with associated hypersensitivity to the tubercle bacillus, but does not necessarily indicate that the person has active tuberculosis.

# Suppression of the Immune Response

## Reasons for Suppression

Cell-mediated and humoral immune responses protect against potentially harmful microorganisms and other foreign substances. These same immunologic mechanisms may at times have undesirable effects:

1. They may be directed against the individual's own cells or tissue components, leading to autoimmune diseases.
2. They are responsible for the rejection of transplanted organs.

## Methods of Suppression

It is sometimes necessary to suppress the immune response to treat certain autoimmune diseases and to perform organ transplants. There are many types of immunosuppressive agents that have found wide application in clinical medicine. The main types of immunosuppressive agents that are commonly used by physicians are as follows:

1. Radiation
2. Immunosuppressive drugs that impede cell division or cell function
3. Adrenal corticosteroid hormones
4. Immunoglobulin preparations

**Radiation and Immunosuppressive Drugs** Radiation destroys normal cells. It exerts its immunosuppressive effect by destroying lymphoid tissue, which plays a key role in both cell-mediated and humoral immunity. There are several types of drugs that can suppress the immune response. Cytotoxic drugs (*cyto* = cell + *toxic* = poisonous) act by suppressing growth and division of lymphocytes. Lymphoid tissue is especially susceptible to the inhibitory effect of these drugs. Antimetabolites, as the name implies, are another group that inhibit important cellular metabolic functions, thereby inhibiting cell proliferation and suppressing the inflammatory reaction. (Cytotoxic drugs and antimetabolites are also used to treat some types of leukemia and malignant tumors, as described in Chapter 8.)

**Corticosteroids** Adrenal corticosteroids act in several ways. They suppress the inflammatory response and impair phagocytosis. They also inhibit protein synthesis, thereby suppressing the growth and division of lymphocytes and inhibiting antibody formation by plasma cells.

## Tissue Grafts and Immunity

An individual will accept a graft of his or her own tissue or that of an identical twin, but not that of another person, because a graft from another person contains HLA antigens foreign to the recipient. The body "recognizes" the foreign antigens in the transplant, which becomes infiltrated by lymphocytes and macrophages and is eventually destroyed. This process is called rejection of the transplanted organ, and it is a manifestation of a cell-mediated immune reaction. Physicians who are treating kidney failure by transplantation can keep a foreign kidney from being rejected by inhibiting the recipient's immunologic defenses, using drugs that suppress the immune response. Transplantation of kidneys and other organs has been successful because it is usually possible to suppress the body's immune responses sufficiently to allow the transplanted organ to survive.

# Autoimmune Diseases

The reasons why an individual forms an autoantibody to his or her own cells or tissue components are not well understood. Unfortunately, after an individual develops an autoimmune disease, it usually "doesn't go away." Although the affected person experiences periods when the disease is in remission or the manifestations are controlled by treatment, the disease persists and often progresses. Three major mechanisms have been postulated to explain the pathogenesis of autoimmune diseases:

1. Alteration of the patient's own self-antigens that causes them to become antigenic and provoke an immune reaction
2. The formation of cross-reacting antibodies against foreign antigens that also attack the patient's own antigens
3. Defective regulation of the immune response by regulator T lymphocytes

The subject's own antigens may be altered by a viral infection or an infection with some other microbiologic agent in such a manner that the immune system no longer recognizes the antigen as a self-antigen, and an immune reaction is generated against the altered antigen ( Figure 4-6A ). Alternatively, some drug or medication ingested by the patient may change the structure of a self-antigen so that it is perceived as foreign and generates an immune response. Cross-reacting antibodies may induce organ damage when an antibody is formed against a foreign antigen, such as an invading bacterium that shares antigenic determinants with some of the subject's own cell or tissue antigens. As a result, the antibody that formed against the antigenic determinants in the foreign antigen cross-reacts with similar antigenic determinants in the subject's own tissues, leading to tissue injury ( Figure 4-6B ).

Defective regulation of the immune system by helper T lymphocytes may lead to autoimmune disease. When lymphocytes are programmed to respond to specific antigens (develop immune competence) in the thymus and bone marrow as the immune system is developing, some lymphocytes are inadvertently programmed

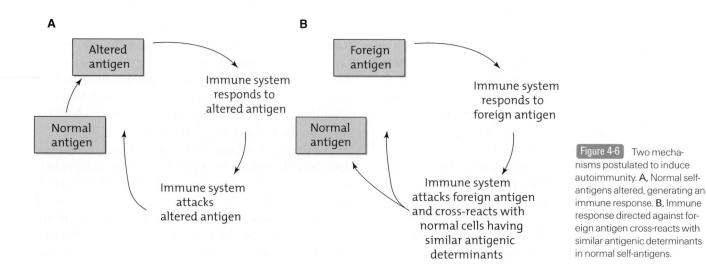

**A**

Altered antigen → Immune system responds to altered antigen

Normal antigen

Immune system attacks altered antigen

**B**

Foreign antigen → Immune system responds to foreign antigen

Normal antigen

Immune system attacks foreign antigen and cross-reacts with normal cells having similar antigenic determinants

Figure 4-6 Two mechanisms postulated to induce autoimmunity. **A,** Normal self-antigens altered, generating an immune response. **B,** Immune response directed against foreign antigen cross-reacts with similar antigenic determinants in normal self-antigens.

to respond to self-antigens. These cell populations are usually destroyed. But some are only suppressed and their "attack" functions are held in check by regulator T lymphocytes. If the regulator function of T cells does not function normally, lymphocytes programmed to recognize self-antigens are no longer held in check. They become activated and attack one's own cells and tissues. Three factors appear to predispose to autoimmune diseases:

1. A genetic component that in part is related to the genes on chromosome 6, which code for our own unique self-antigens.
2. A gender component, as many autoimmune diseases occur much more frequently in women than in men.
3. An infection component in a genetically predisposed individual, as the onset of many autoimmune diseases appears to be associated with a recent infection, often a viral infection. In addition, an infection in a person with a chronic autoimmune disease may cause a flare-up of disease.

## Autoimmune Disease Manifestations and Mechanisms of Tissue Injury

The manifestations of autoimmune disease depend on which cells or tissue components are targeted for attack by the immune system. Some autoimmune diseases attack specific tissues throughout the body, such as bone, cartilage, connective tissue, blood vessels, or skin. Other autoimmune diseases target specific organs, such as individual endocrine glands, kidney, liver, lung, or nervous system. The mechanisms of tissue injury are those described in connection with immune-mediated hypersensitivity reactions and may include humoral mechanisms, cell-mediated mechanisms, or a combination of both. Autoantibody-associated tissue injury results when antibody becomes attached to the cell membrane of the target cells, activating complement and causing complement-mediated destruction of the target, usually assisted by activated macrophages and killer lymphocytes (Type II reaction). Alternatively, antigen and antibody may combine to form immune complexes that are deposited in the tissues and induce a similar type of complement-mediated tissue injury (Type III reaction). Cell-mediated destruction of target tissues is caused by sensitized T lymphocytes that secrete lymphokines, which generate a destructive inflammatory reaction in the target tissue or organ (Type IV reaction).

Not all autoantibodies destroy target tissue. Sometimes they derange the function of the target but do not destroy it. The thyroid gland, for example, may be attacked by two different types of autoantibodies. One type destroys thyroid cells and impairs thyroid function, causing hypothyroidism. Another type stimulates the thyroid cells and makes them hyperfunction, causing hyperthyroidism.

In general, treatment of autoimmune disease is not very satisfactory. Various methods of treatment have been used to minimize inflammation and tissue damage, to suppress the function of the immune system, and to block the destructive effects of cytokines produced by T lymphocytes and macrophages.

Table 4-4 summarizes the features of some of the more important diseases in which autoantibody formation appears to play a role. These diseases are considered in greater detail in subsequent chapters.

## Connective-Tissue (Collagen) Diseases

The fibrous connective tissue that forms the framework of all tissues in the body is called collagen. The term *connective-tissue disease*, or *collagen disease*, is used to describe a group of diseases characterized by necrosis and degeneration of collagen fibers throughout the body. In many instances, autoantibodies directed against antigens present in various cells and tissues can be detected in the serum of affected individuals, and aggregates of antigen combined with antibody (termed *antigen–antibody complexes*) can be identified at the sites of tissue damage. Often, large numbers of lymphocytes and plasma cells accumulate in the affected tissues. These cells are presumed to be responsible for the tissue injury by means of cell-mediated immune reactions and formation of autoantibodies ( Figure 4-7 ). Therefore, the connective-tissue diseases are usually classified as autoimmune diseases.

## Lupus Erythematosus

One of the more common connective-tissue diseases is called lupus erythematosus. This disease is seen most frequently in young women and is characterized by widespread damage to fibrous connective tissue in the skin, articular tissues, heart, serous membranes (pleura and pericardium), and kidneys. Hemolytic anemia, leukopenia, and thrombocytopenia are frequent hematologic manifestations of lupus; these are caused by autoantibodies. Many patients die of renal failure resulting from the severe renal glomerular injury.

Patients with lupus develop a variety of autoantibodies directed against cells and tissues, including antinucleoprotein antibodies and antibodies directed against red cells, white cells, platelets, and plasma proteins. Circulating antigen–autoantibody complexes (immune complexes) form and are deposited in kidney glomeruli, blood vessels, and other tissues. Complement

## Table 4-4 Common Autoimmune Diseases

| | Probable Pathogenesis | Major Clinical Manifestations |
|---|---|---|
| Rheumatic fever | Antistreptococcal antibodies cross-react with antigens in heart muscle, heart valves, and other tissues. | Inflammation of heart and joints |
| Glomerulonephritis | Some cases caused by antibodies formed against glomerular basement membrane; other cases caused by antigen–antibody complexes trapped in glomeruli. | Inflammation of renal glomeruli |
| Rheumatoid arthritis | Antibodies formed against serum gamma globulin. | Systemic disease with inflammation and degeneration of joints |
| Autoimmune blood diseases | Autoantibodies formed against platelets, white cells, or red cells; in some cases, antibody apparently is formed against altered cell antigens, and antibody reacts with both altered and normal cells. | Anemia, leukopenia, or thrombocytopenia, depending on nature of antibody |
| Lupus erythematosus and related collagen diseases | Various antinuclear antibodies cause widespread injury to several organs. | Systemic disease with manifestations in several organs |
| Chronic thyroiditis (Hashimoto disease) | Antithyroid antibody causes injury and inflammatory cell infiltration of thyroid gland. | Hypothyroidism |
| Diffuse toxic goiter (Graves disease) | Autoantibody mimicking thyroid-stimulating hormone (TSH) causes increased output of thyroid hormone. | Hyperthyroidism |
| Diabetes (type 1) | Autoantibodies and activated T lymphocytes destroy pancreatic islet beta cells | Diabetes mellitus caused by insulin deficiency |
| Pernicious anemia | Autoantibodies destroy gastric mucosa cells | Macrocytic anemia and nervous system damage resulting from inadequate absorption of vitamin $B_{12}$ |
| Vasculitis (various types of blood vessel inflammation) | Autoantibody-mediated damage to small, medium, and large blood vessels | Blood vessel damage interferes with blood vessel function and blood supply to tissues |
| Various skin conditions and diseases causing loss of skin pigment or skin blisters | Some autoantibodies damage pigment-producing cells in skin; others attack intercellular connections between skin cells | Pigment cell loss causes areas of skin depigmentation (vitiligo); blisters result from loss of skin intercellular connections |
| Myasthenia gravis | Autoantibodies destroy acetylcholine receptors at muscle–nerve junctions | Muscle weakness resulting from inadequate transmission of impulses from nerves to muscles |

is activated, which generates an inflammatory reaction where the immune complexes are deposited. A characteristic feature of lupus erythematosus is the presence of antinucleoprotein antibodies in the patient's blood, which can be demonstrated by various methods. The original technique consisted of incubating the patient's blood serum with intact white blood cells. The antinucleoprotein antibodies damage many of the leukocytes, causing swelling and loss of structural detail in the cell nuclei. The damaged nuclei are converted into large, homogeneous, spherical "blobs" of blue-staining nuclear debris that becomes surrounded and phagocytized by polymorphonuclear leukocytes.

The phagocytized spherical mass fills the cytoplasm of the cell and displaces the nucleus to the edge of the cell, resulting in the characteristic appearance called an LE cell. This classic method of demonstrating antinucleoprotein antibodies was originally described in 1948 by Hargraves and two associates from the Mayo Clinic and now is primarily of historical interest. The test has been superseded by newer more sensitive techniques, but the method does clearly illustrate the damaging effect of nucleoprotein antibodies on intact cell nuclei ( Figure 4-8 ).

The pathogenesis of lupus is not well understood but appears to be initiated by some event, possibly a

**A**

**B**

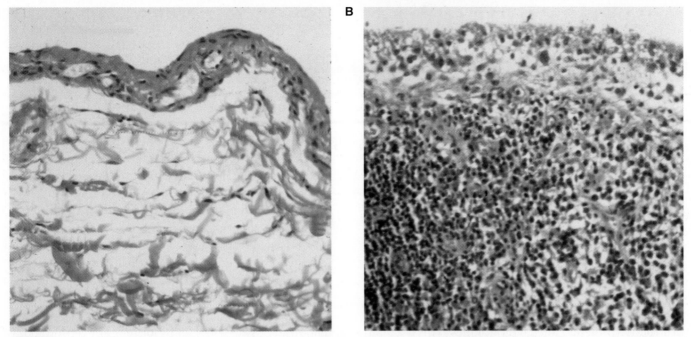

Figure 4-7   Comparison of normal joint lining. **A,** with joint lining in one type of connective tissue disease. **B,** The lining of the affected joint is heavily infiltrated with lymphocytes and plasma cells, and the joint injury is secondary to the inflammatory reaction (original magnification × 400).

viral infection or other antigenic stimulation in a genetically predisposed individual that damages normal MHC antigens so that they are no longer recognized as self-antigens by the immune system. Helper T lymphocytes and B lymphocytes directed against the abnormal self-antigens are activated. The helper T lymphocytes stimulate the B lymphocytes to proliferate. Then the B lymphocytes form the various autoantibodies and generate the antigen–autoantibody complexes that are responsible for the organ damage characteristic of this disease.

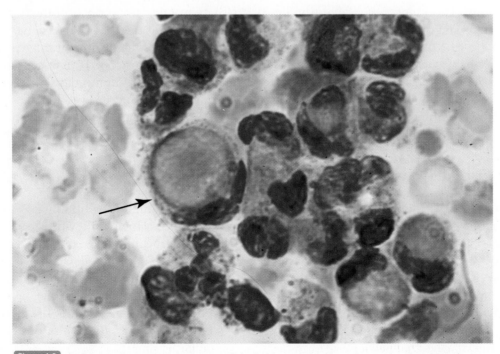

Figure 4-8   Positive test for lupus erythematosus. Spherical mass derived from damaged nucleus (*arrow*) engulfed by neutrophil (original magnification × 1000).

# CHAPTER REVIEW

## Summary

An inflammation caused by a microorganism (infection) differs from other types of inflammation caused by trauma or other types of tissue injury because the pathogen that causes the tissue injury is a foreign substance (non–self-antigen). It is introduced into the body and the body responds by generating an immune response to eliminate the foreign material in addition to giving rise to an inflammation. The immune response may be either cell mediated or antibody mediated (humoral) and sometimes both are generated against the same organism. Cell-mediated immunity is a property of T lymphocytes, which proliferate and accumulate around the foreign material where they secrete destructive proteins called lymphokines. This is a main defense against viruses, fungi, parasites, and some bacteria such as the tubercle bacillus. Humoral immunity is a property of B lymphocytes. When stimulated by foreign material they proliferate and "gear up" to produce large amounts of antibodies that combine with the foreign material. As B lymphocytes proliferate, they become transformed into cells with more cytoplasm that contains lots of ribosomes and rough endoplasmic reticulum. These cells are now called plasma cells and are very efficient "antibody-producing factories." This is our primary defense against most bacteria and bacterial toxins.

There are various classes and types of antibodies (immunoglobulins), and antibody molecules can be compared to a fork. The tines represent the specifity of the antibody, which "spears" the foreign material, and the handle as the class and characteristics of the antibody. IgM is the first antibody formed and is a large structure. IgG (gamma globulin) is formed soon after and becomes the major immunoglobulin. IgA is secreted by B lymphocytes in the mucosa of the GI and respiratory tract, and combines with inhaled or swallowed antigens so that they are not absorbed into the body. IgE is the allergy antibody. IgD is attached to the cell membranes of B lymphocytes, and has some special functions that need not be considered now.

Hypersensitivity reactions are important and the classification system used in your book is generally used. IgE-mediated response triggers localized manifestations (allergy) or more serious systemic reactions to bee stings or penicillin reactions (anaphylaxis). IgG-mediated hypersensitivity responses injure cells by binding to cells and activating complement that causes inflammation and tissue injury; or by forming antigen–antibody aggregates in tissues or in the circulation, which activates complement and induces inflammation.

A delayed hypersensitivity response (tuberculin-type hypersensitivity reaction) is a cell-mediated reaction, not antibody related. Sensitized T lymphocytes accumulate at the site of contact with the foreign material and release lymphokines that attract macrophages and cytotoxic T lymphocytes. These attracted cells secrete cytokines that cause the tissue injury and inflammation. A positive Mantoux test is an example of this type of reaction. As we will see later, much of the tissue necrosis in tuberculosis is the result of a delayed hypersensitivity reaction to products of the tubercle bacillus.

Autoimmune disease occurs when the body develops an immune response to its own antigens (self-antigens), which damages the body's own cells and tissues. The nature of the autoimmune disease is determined by what organ or tissue is being attacked by the antoantibody. Several mechanisms have been proposed to explain why our immune system attacks our own cells.

## Questions for Review

1. What is meant by the following terms: *acquired immunity*, *cell-mediated immunity*, *humoral immunity*, and *hypersensitivity?*
2. What is the role of the lymphocyte in acquired immunity? What is the role of the macrophage?
3. How does the physician manipulate the body's immune reaction to allow kidney transplantation?
4. What is meant by the following terms: *B lymphocyte*, *T lymphocyte*, and *lymphokine?*
5. What are immunoglobulins? What is their basic structure? How do they function?
6. What is meant by the following terms: *light chains*, *macroglobulin*, and *allergy?*
7. What is an autoantibody? What are some of the postulated mechanisms that result in autoantibody formation? What is the effect of autoantibody directed against the patient's own blood cells?

8. What is a connective-tissue disease? What are its manifestations? What is an LE cell?

9. What are antigen–antibody complexes? How do they cause tissue injury?

10. How can the immune response be suppressed? Why is this sometimes necessary?

## Supplementary Reading

Dalakas, M. C. 2004. Intravenous immunoglobulin in autoimmune neuromuscular diseases. *Journal of the American Medical Association* 291:2367–74.

Injections of immunoglobulins are a safe, effective treatment for many autoimmune neuromuscular diseases, although the optimal doses and frequency of administration are still being investigated. The immunoglobulins act by interfering with virtually all of the processes that generate the cytotoxic cells, cytokines, and autoantibodies responsible for autoimmune damage to the target organ or tissue, such as interference with T-cell functions, suppression of cytokines, suppression of autoantibody production by B cells, and interference with its ability to bind to its target.

Delves, P. J., and Roitt, I. M. 2000. The immune system. *New England Journal of Medicine* 343:37–49, and 343:108–17.

A review of current knowledge on this complex system.

Fine, D. M. 2005. Pharmacologic therapy of lupus nephritis. *Journal of the American Medical Association* 293:3053–60.

Sixty percent of adults with lupus develop kidney damage (lupus nephritis) during the course of their disease. The usual treatment method (cyclophosphamide and glucocorticoids) is less desirable in women of child-bearing age, and a regimen substituting a newer drug for cyclophosphamide is a more effective treatment.

Klein, J., and Sato, A. 2000. The HLA system. *New England Journal of Medicine* 343:702–09, and 343:782–86.

A review of current knowledge about our system of self-antigens, how they function, and the abnormalities of genes linked to the HLA complex. The roles of the HLA system in cancer and transplantation are considered.

Rahman, A., and Isenberg, D. A. 2009. Systemic lupus erythematosus. *New England Journal of Medicine* 358:929–39.

Lupus is a serious disease that occurs predominantly in women, and occurs much more frequently in black women than in white women. Antibodies to a common virus infection (Epstein-Barr virus) are almost invariably present, as is EB virus DNA. Most patients have antibodies directed against double-strand DNA, which is characteristic of lupus. Lymphocytes are also activated in the disease. The activity of the disease is related to the antoantibody level in the patient's blood, and many treatment methods are directed toward reducing the autoantibody levels.

## Matching

Match the term with its definition.

| | | | |
|---|---|---|---|
| 1. | Platelets | A. | A disease-producing organism |
| 2. | Infection | B. | Inflammation of a lymph node |
| 3. | Inflammation | C. | Products released from cells and from blood proteins that are responsible for the features of an inflammatory reaction |
| 4. | Leukocytes | D. | A blood protein concerned with blood coagulation |
| 5. | Pathogen | E. | Small structures circulating in the bloodstream that are concerned with blood coagulation |
| 6. | Plasma | F. | Ingestion of material by neutrophils and monocytes |
| 7. | Lymphadenitis | G. | Structures in the cytoplasm containing potent digestive enzymes |
| 8. | Septicemia | H. | An inflammation resulting from tissue injury not caused by a pathogenic microorganism |
| 9. | Antibodies | I. | The cell-free fluid part of the blood |
| 10. | Mediators of inflammation | J. | Pathogenic microorganisms circulating in the bloodstream |
| 11. | Phagocytosis | K. | Proteins made by plasma cells |
| 12. | Fibrinogen | L. | An inflammation caused by a pathogenic microorganism |
| 13. | Lysosomes | M. | White blood cells |
| 14. | Mast cells | N. | A specialized cell in tissues containing histamine and other chemical mediators |

## True or False

Indicate whether the following statements are true or false by writing T or F at the end of the statement.

1. Neutrophils process foreign antigens and present antigen fragments to lymphocytes in order to generate an immune response to the foreign material.

2. Eosinophils produce antibodies that protect us from infections. _____

3. Autoantibodies directed against kidney tissues may damage the kidneys. _____

4. The inflammatory reaction concentrates leukocytes and antibodies at the site of the inflammation. _____

5. Activation of blood proteins called complement generates mediators of inflammation. _____

## Critical Thinking

1. John Reynolds is a 34-year-old employee of a pork processing plant, where he was exposed to aerosolized pig brain tissue. Later he developed progressive inflammatory neuropathy, a neurologic disease. He was told that the condition may have resulted from an occupational exposure to pig brain tissue, but he doesn't understand how such an exposure could cause his problems. What would you tell him?

2. Susan Arnold is a 62-year-old woman who has developed rheumatoid arthritis and is beginning to develop significant joint damage as a result of the disease. Her physician wants to treat her with drugs to suppress her immune system in order to prevent further joint damage. She says that she takes aspirin to relieve her joint pain, and doesn't understand how suppressing her immune system would help her. She is also concerned that suppressing her immune system may make her more susceptible to infection. What would you tell her?

# Pathogenic Microorganisms, Fungi, and Animal Parasites

**5**

1. Explain the characteristics by which bacteria are classified. List and describe the major groups of pathogenic bacteria.

2. Describe the mechanism by which antibiotics inhibit the growth and metabolism of bacteria. Explain the adverse effects of antibiotics.

3. Describe the procedures used in antibiotic sensitivity testing and explain the principles by which the results are interpreted.

4. Explain the mode of action of virus infections and describe how the body's response to viral infection leads to recovery.

5. List the common infections caused by chlamydiae, mycoplasmas, and rickettsiae.

6. Discuss the spectrum of infections caused by fungi. Explain the factors that predispose to systemic infections. Describe the methods used to treat fungus infections.

7. List the common parasitic infections that affect humans.

8. Explain how these infections are acquired.

9. Describe their clinical manifestations, and explain their clinical significance.

# Types of Harmful Microorganisms

The human species coexists with a large number of microorganisms. In most instances, we and our microbiologic associates live in harmony. Of the wide spectrum of organisms found in nature, only a relatively small proportion cause disease in humans. These pathogenic microorganisms are classified into several large groups:

1. Bacteria
2. Chlamydiae
3. Rickettsiae and ehrlichiae
4. Mycoplasmas
5. Viruses
6. Fungi

In addition, humans serve as host to a number of animal parasites capable of causing illness or disability. The various organisms that are injurious to humans vary in their ability to cause disease. A small number of microbiologic agents are extremely virulent. Others are of very low virulence and are capable of causing disease only when the body's normal defenses have already been weakened by a debilitating illness.

# Bacteria

## Classification of Bacteria

Bacteria are classified on the basis of four major characteristics:

1. Shape
2. Gram-stain reaction
3. Biochemical and cultural characteristics
4. Antigenic structure

**Shape**  A bacterium may be spherical (coccus) or rod shaped (bacillus), or it may have a spiral or corkscrew shape. Cocci may grow in clusters (staphylococci), in pairs (diplococci), or in chains (streptococci).

**Gram-Stain Reaction**  In the Gram-stain method, a dried, fixed suspension of bacteria, prepared on a microscope slide, is stained first with a purple dye and then with an iodine solution. Next, the slide is decolorized with alcohol or another solvent; it is then stained with a red dye. Bacteria that resist decolorization and retain the purple stain are called *gram-positive*, whereas those that have been decolorized and accept the red counterstain are termed *gram-negative*. By means of the Gram-stain method, organisms may be characterized as either gram-positive or gram-negative.

**flagella**
(flă-jel'ă) Whip-like processes that propel organisms or sperm.

**spores**  Spherical structures formed within some bacteria that are extremely resistant to heat, disinfectants, and other agents that destroy bacteria. Spores form when conditions are unfavorable for the bacteria, and they can germinate to form actively growing bacteria when conditions are more favorable.

**Biochemical and Cultural Characteristics**  Some bacteria are quite fastidious and can be grown only on enriched media under carefully controlled conditions of temperature and acidity (pH). Other bacteria are hardy and capable of growing on relatively simple culture media under a wide variety of conditions.

Many bacteria grow best in the presence of oxygen (*aerobic organisms*). Some bacteria are able to grow only in the absence of oxygen or under extremely low oxygen tension. These are called *anaerobic* (without oxygen) bacteria. Others grow equally well under either aerobic or anaerobic conditions.

Many bacteria have special structural characteristics. Some bacteria have **flagella**: hairlike processes covering their surface. Flagella give a bacterium its motility; organisms that lack flagella are nonmotile. Some bacteria form **spores**: spherical structures formed within the bacterial cell. Spores can survive under conditions that would kill an actively growing bacterium. They may be considered a dormant, extremely resistant bacterial modification that forms under adverse conditions. Spores can germinate and give rise to actively growing bacteria under favorable conditions.

Most bacteria have distinct biochemical characteristics. Some types of bacteria are capable of fermenting carbohydrates and can bring about many different biochemical reactions under suitable cultural conditions. Each type of bacterium has its own "biochemical profile," which aids in its identification.

**Antigenic Structure**  Each type of bacterium contains a large number of antigens associated with the cell body, the capsule of the bacterium, and the flagella (in the case of motile organisms). The antigenic structure can be determined by special methods, defining a system of antigens unique for each group of bacteria.

**Identification of Bacteria**  The methods of classifying bacteria can be applied to the identification of a specific bacterium. Let us assume, for example, that an organism has been isolated from the blood of a patient with a febrile illness. By means of the Gram-stain reaction, the organism is identified as a gram-negative bacillus. The cultural characteristics indicate that it is not a fastidious organism and is capable of growing on a wide variety of culture media at various temperatures; moreover, it grows well both in the presence of oxygen and under anaerobic conditions. The organism is motile and does not form spores.

At this point, the number of possible organisms consistent with these characteristics has been reduced to relatively few gram-negative bacteria. The number of possibilities is narrowed still further by various biochemical tests indicating that the bacterium does not ferment lactose but is able to ferment glucose and certain other sugars. These and other biochemical tests support the conclusion that the organism is a type of pathogenic bacterium, called *Salmonella*, found in the gastrointestinal tract and capable of causing a typhoid-like febrile illness. The bacterial antigens within the cell body and flagella of the bacteria can be identified to determine the exact type of *Salmonella* responsible for the patient's illness.

Once the organism has been identified, the clinician can begin proper treatment and can institute proper

Table 5-1 **Important Pathogenic Bacteria**

| Type | Gram-Stain Reaction | |
| --- | --- | --- |
| | Gram-Positive | Gram-Negative |
| Cocci | Staphylococci<br>Streptococci<br>Pneumococci | Gonococci<br>Meningococci |
| Bacilli | *Corynebacteria*<br>*Listeria*<br>*Bacilli*<br>*Clostridia* | *Hemophilus*<br>*Gardnerella*<br>*Francisella*<br>*Yersinia*<br>*Brucella*<br>*Legionella*<br>*Salmonella*<br>*Shigella*<br>*Campylobacter*<br>Cholera bacillus<br>Colon bacillus (*Escherichia coli*) and related organisms |
| Spiral organisms | *Treponema pallidum*<br>*Borrelia burgdorferi* | |
| Acid-fast organisms | Tubercle bacillus<br>Leprosy bacillus | |

isolation and control procedures based on the means by which the disease is transmitted.

## Major Classes of Pathogenic Bacteria

The major groups of pathogenic bacteria and their Gram-stain reactions are given in Table 5-1. The diseases caused by these organisms are described in the following section and summarized in Table 5-2.

**Staphylococci**  Staphylococci are normal inhabitants of the skin and nasal cavity and normally are not pathogenic. Some staphylococci, however, are pathogens, and some strains may be extremely virulent. Pathogens usually can be distinguished from nonpathogenic staphylococci by the appearance of their colonies on media containing blood (blood agar plates). Pathogenic staphylococci produce zones of complete hemolysis around the growing colonies ( Figure 5-1 ), in contrast to nonpathogenic staphylococci that do not hemolyze red cells.

Pathogenic staphylococci are a common cause of boils, other skin infections, and postoperative wound infections. Staphylococci may also cause serious pulmonary infections and other types of systemic infections. Staphylococcal infections often pose a serious problem in hospitals because the organisms are widely distributed and many hospitalized patients are

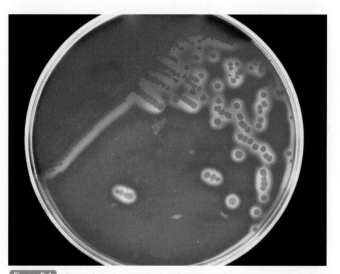

Figure 5-1  Bacteriologic culture plate (blood agar) containing colonies of hemolytic staphylococci. Enzymes produced by the bacteria break down (hemolyze) the blood cells in the culture medium, which cause the clear zones surrounding the colonies.

unusually susceptible to infection. Some strains of staphylococci are highly resistant to antibiotics, and infections caused by antibiotic-resistant staphylococci are extremely difficult to treat.

**Streptococci**  There are many kinds of streptococci, and their pathogenicity varies. These organisms are classified on the basis of their serologic group designated

## Table 5-2  Summary of Major Bacterial Pathogens and the Diseases They Cause

| Cocci | Disease |
|---|---|
| *Staphylococcus aureus* | Various localized and systemic infections |
| *Beta hemolytic streptococcus,* Group A | Pharyngitis, systemic infections, skin and muscle necrosis. |
| | Hypersensitivity response to organism causes rheumatic fever, nephritis. |
| *Beta hemolytic streptococcus,* Group B | Urinary tract and wound infections, systemic infection. |
| | Newborn infection acquired from vaginal organisms in mother. |
| *Streptococci,* other groups | Wound and urinary tract infections. |
| *Streptococcus pneumoniae* (Pneumococcus) | Middle ear and sinus infections. Systemic infection. Lobar pneumonia. Meningitis. |
| *Neisseria gonorrhoeae* (Gonococcus) | Genital tract infections. Bacteremia causing endocarditis, osteomyelitis, septic arthritis. |
| *Neisseria meningitidis* (Meningococcus) | Meningococcal meningitis. |
| **AEROBIC GRAM-POSITIVE RODS** | |
| *Corynebacterium diphtheriae* | Diphtheria. Clinical manifestations caused by toxin production. |
| *Listeria monocytogenes* | Systemic infection. Pregnant women may infect fetus. Persons with impaired immune system very susceptible. |
| **AEROBIC SPORE-FORMING RODS** | |
| *Bacillus anthracis* | Primarily a disease of animals. People infected from contact with wool or animal products. Localized and systemic infection. Potential germ warfare agent. |
| **ANAEROBIC SPORE-FORMING RODS** | |
| *Clostridium perfringens* | Gas gangrene. Muscle necrosis and hemolytic anemia caused by toxin. Gas formation in infected tissues. |
| *Clostridium tetani* | Tetanus ("lockjaw") caused by toxin-induced spasm of voluntary muscles. |
| *Clostridium botulinum* | Botulism. Neuroparalytic toxin produced in improperly processed or canned foods. |
| *Clostridium difficile* | Antibiotic-associated colitis. Loss of normal intestinal flora caused by antibiotics allows overgrowth of *Clostridia.* Toxins produced by *Clostridia* damage bowel mucosa. |
| **GRAM-NEGATIVE RODS** | |
| *Hemophilus influenzae* | Pulmonary infections. Meningitis in susceptible children. |
| *Yersinia pestis* | Plague. Disease of wild rodents transmitted to humans by fleas. Causes systemic infection. Can spread person-to-person if infection spreads to lungs (pneumonic plague). |
| *Brucella* species | Brucellosis. Febrile illness from contact with infected animals or consumption of raw milk from infected animals. |
| *Francisella* species | Tularemia. Febrile illness acquired from flesh of infected animals, usually wild rabbits, or transmitted to humans by bite of infected ticks or deer flies. |
| *Legionella pneumophila* | Legionnaires' disease. Organisms live in water and cause pulmonary infection in persons who inhale aerosolized droplets from showers, air conditioners, or other water sources. No person-to-person spread. |

*(Continued)*

Table 5-2

## Summary of Major Bacterial Pathogens and the Diseases They Cause (cont.)

| Cocci | Disease |
| --- | --- |
| *Salmonella* species | Gastroenteritis and systemic infections. Infection acquired from contaminated food or water sources. |
| *Shigella* species | Dysentery with frequent watery stools. Spread by person-to-person contact, or by contaminated food and water. |
| *Campylobacter* species | Gastroenteritis. May cause systemic infection. Infects many animals. Humans infected from contaminated water, undercooked meat or poultry, or contact with infected animals. |
| *Escherichia coli* | Gastroenteritis, urinary tract, and systemic infections. Some strains (O157:H7) produce toxins that cause hemolytic anemia and kidney damage. |
| SPIRAL ORGANISMS<br>*Treponema pallidum* | Syphilis. Considered in Chapter 8. |
| *Borrelia burgdorferi* | Lyme disease, transmitted from rodents to humans by ticks. Causes febrile illness and arthritis with lesion at site of tick bite. |
| ACID-FAST BACTERIA<br>*Mycobacterium tuberculosis* | Pulmonary tuberculosis. Considered in Chapter 12. |
| *Mycobacterium avium* complex | A normally nonpathogenic organism that may cause an opportunistic infection in AIDS patients. See Case 6-3 in Chapter 6. |

by an uppercase letter, and on the type of hemolysis the organism produces when grown on a solid medium containing blood. Generally, both the letter group and the type of hemolysis are specified when describing a streptococcus.

The serologic classification places the streptococci into major groups based on differences in the carbohydrate antigens present in their cell walls. Most of the streptococci of medical importance are in groups A, B, and D. The classification based on hemolysis describes the organisms as producing either alpha hemolysis, beta hemolysis, or no hemolysis on blood agar plates.

*Alpha hemolytic streptococci* (or simply *alpha streptococci*) produce green discoloration of the blood immediately around the colony and are often called *Streptococcus viridans* because of this growth characteristic (*viridans* = green). These organisms are normal inhabitants of the upper respiratory passages and usually are not pathogenic.

*Beta hemolytic streptococci* (or simply *beta streptococci*) produce a narrow zone of complete hemolysis around the growing colony. One of the most important beta streptococci is called a *group A beta streptococcus*. Many group A beta streptococci are extremely

pathogenic, causing streptococcal sore throat, scarlet fever, serious skin infections, and infections of the uterus after childbirth.

In addition to causing infections in various tissues, some strains of group A beta streptococci are capable of inducing a state of hypersensitivity in susceptible individuals, leading to development of *rheumatic fever* or a type of kidney disease called *glomerulonephritis*. These diseases are considered in greater detail in the sections on the cardiovascular system (Chapter 10) and kidneys (Chapter 15). Fortunately, group A beta streptococci still remain quite sensitive to penicillin and other antibiotics.

Beta streptococci in other groups are also of medical importance. *Group B beta streptococci* may cause urinary tract and wound infections, but they are of greatest importance as a cause of serious infections in newborn infants. They often inhabit (colonize) the rectum and vagina of pregnant women, and the infant may become infected during labor and delivery. Because of the potential hazard of a life-threatening infection in an infant born to a mother colonized by group B beta streptococci, routine rectal and vaginal cultures to detect the organism are recommended for all pregnant women late in pregnancy. Those women who are colonized are treated with intravenous antibiotics during labor to reduce the risk of a serious group B beta streptococcal infection in the infant.

**Pneumococci** Pneumococci (*Streptococcus pneumoniae*) are gram-positive cocci and are classified with the streptococci. They grow in pairs and short chains and have certain biochemical characteristics setting them apart from other streptococci. Pneumococci are a common cause of bacterial pneumonia.

**Gram-Negative Cocci** Most gram-negative cocci are nonpathogenic members of the genus *Neisseria* and are normal inhabitants of the upper respiratory passages. This group has two pathogenic members. The meningococcus (*Neisseria meningitidis*) causes a type of meningitis (inflammation of the membranes surrounding the brain and spinal cord) that frequently occurs in epidemics. The gonococcus (*Neisseria gonorrhoeae*) causes gonorrhea. This disease is transmitted by sexual contact and is discussed in greater detail in Chapter 6.

**Gram-Positive Bacilli** There are several important groups of gram-positive rod-shaped bacteria that can be subdivided on the basis of their oxygen requirements and on their ability to form spores. The two important groups of non–spore-forming aerobic bacteria are *Corynebacteria* and *Listeria*. The two important groups of spore-forming organisms are *Bacilli*, which are aerobic microorganisms, and *Clostridia*, which are anaerobic organisms.

*Aerobic Non–Spore-Forming Gram-Positive Organisms* *Corynebacteria* are a large group of microorganisms. Most are nonpathogenic inhabitants of the skin and other squamous epithelium-lined body surfaces (mucous membranes). However, one member of this group (*Corynebacterium diphtheriae*) causes diphtheria. The organism causes an acute ulcerative inflammation of the throat and produces a potent toxin that can injure heart muscle and nerve tissue.

One important member of the *Listeria* group of microorganisms, called *Listeria monocytogenes*, can cause a very serious infection. The organism is widely distributed in nature: in the soil, on plants, and in the intestinal tract of people and animals. The organism may contaminate dairy products, raw vegetables, and other food products such as soft cheeses, hot dogs, and delicatessen foods. People become infected by eating *Listeria*-contaminated foods, and the persons at greatest risk of serious infections are infants and older people, pregnant women, and persons whose immune system is impaired. *Listeria* infection may be complicated by spread of the organism to the brain and meninges, causing a meningitis or brain abscess. In pregnant women, the organism may also spread through the placenta to infect the unborn infant, leading to intrauterine fetal death or life-threatening infection of the infant.

*Aerobic Spore-Forming Gram-Positive Organisms* Spore-forming aerobes are called *Bacilli*. Only one member of this group is highly pathogenic. This organism is *Bacillus anthracis*, which causes anthrax.

Anthrax is primarily a disease of animals that is rare in the United States, but is a more common animal infection in some other countries. Anthrax spores are highly resistant, can survive for many years in the soil, and can contaminate the hair, wool, or other tissues of animals from countries where anthrax is prevalent. If anthrax spores enter the body of a susceptible animal or person, the spores can germinate to form very large numbers of rapidly growing bacteria, which causes the disease anthrax.

Inhalation of anthrax spores from spore-contaminated wool, yarn, or other animal products causes a severe life-threatening pulmonary and systemic infection with an extremely high mortality. The spores germinate within the pulmonary alveoli, actively proliferate, and produce lethal toxins that cause extensive tissue destruction. Other spores are ingested by macrophages and transported to regional lymph nodes, where they continue to germinate and produce toxins.

Concerns about the use of anthrax spores as a bioterrorism germ warfare agent became a reality in 2001 when a letter containing anthrax spores was mailed to a U.S. senator, processed at a postal facility in Washington, DC, and opened in a senate office building. The spores contaminated the postal facility and senate office building, caused acute inhalation anthrax in five postal workers who worked in the facility where the letter was processed, and also exposed a number of persons who worked in the office building. Persons who may have been exposed to anthrax spores require a prolonged course of antibiotics to prevent development of pulmonary anthrax because antibiotics effective against the germinated form of the anthrax bacillus are not effective against the spore form of the organism, and many spores do not germinate as soon as they are inhaled. Some are ingested by macrophages and transported to the regional lymph nodes, where they may continue to germinate for as long as 2 months after the initial exposure. The long course of antibiotics is required in order to destroy the antibiotic-sensitive vegetative bacteria as they germinate at various times from antibiotic-resistant spores.

*Anaerobic Spore-Forming Gram-Positive Organisms* Anaerobic spore-forming bacilli are called *Clostridia*. These are normal inhabitants of the intestinal tract of animals and humans and are also found in the soil. Members of this group produce potent toxins and cause several important diseases. Some *Clostridia* cause gas gangrene. Some cause tetanus (lockjaw). Some cause botulism, and others cause an intestinal infection.

Gas gangrene, caused by *Clostridium perfringens* and related organisms, develops in dirty, spore-contaminated wounds. These anaerobic organisms germinate and proliferate in dead or devitalized tissues, especially in wounds where considerable necrosis of tissue has taken place. The *Clostridia* produce large amounts of gas by fermenting the necrotic tissues, and they also release powerful toxins that destroy tissues and cause widespread systemic effects.

Another clostridial species, *Clostridium tetani*, produces a potent toxin that causes spasm of voluntary muscles. The common term lockjaw comes from the marked rigidity of the jaw muscles that is a common feature of the disease. Tetanus may be fatal because of respiratory failure resulting from spasm of the muscles concerned with respiration.

*Clostridium botulinum* produces a potent neuroparalytic toxin. Botulism can generally be traced to eating improperly processed or canned foods in which the organism has grown and produced toxin. Botulism is actually a poisoning caused by the ingestion of toxin in food rather than a bacterial infection.

*Clostridium difficile* is the organism responsible for the intestinal infection called antibiotic-associated colitis that sometimes follows use of broad-spectrum antibiotics and is considered in Chapter 17.

**Gram-Negative Bacteria** There are many gram-negative organisms of clinical importance. Several different groups cause important diseases in humans. Members of the genus *Hemophilus* are normal inhabitants of the respiratory tract. One member of this group, *Hemophilus influenzae*, was a common cause of meningitis in infants and young children. Now routine immunization against this organism has greatly reduced the frequency of meningitis and other infections caused by this organism. One member of the genus *Yersinia* is responsible for bubonic plague. A member of the genus *Francisella* produces a somewhat similar illness called tularemia. Members of the genus *Brucella* cause disease in cattle, goats, and hogs that can be transmitted to people from contact with meat or other tissues from infected animals, or from drinking unpasteurized milk from infected cows or goats. In humans, the disease is a febrile illness without any specific features and responds to appropriate antibiotics. *Legionella* causes a serious respiratory illness called Legionnaires' disease.

Other gram-negative organisms of medical importance include a number of closely related organisms that live in the gastrointestinal tract of people and animals. Other members of this group are free-living organisms, widely distributed in nature. Important pathogenic members of the group include *Salmonella*, *Shigella*, *Campylobacter*, and the cholera bacillus (*Vibrio cholerae*). These organisms cause various types of febrile illness and gastroenteritis. The organisms are excreted from the gastrointestinal tract in the feces of infected patients and are transmitted by contaminated food or water.

An organism closely related to *Campylobacter* called *Helicobacter* is of medical importance because it causes chronic inflammation of the stomach lining (chronic gastritis) and stomach ulcers. This organism is considered in connection with the gastrointestinal tract (Chapter 17).

Other members of this large group are of only limited pathogenicity but sometimes produce disease when they are outside of their normal habitat in the gastrointestinal tract. These organisms may cause wound infections, urinary tract infections, and pulmonary infections in susceptible individuals. The best-known enteric bacterium is the colon bacillus (*Escherichia coli*), which is the predominant organism found within the intestinal tract of humans and animals. Some strains of the colon bacillus can produce various toxins that can cause intestinal symptoms ranging from a choleralike diarrhea to a dysentery like acute inflammation of the intestinal tract. One well-known pathogenic strain is designated *E. coli 0157:H7*; the numbers referring to the antigens contained in the bacterial cell and its flagellae. This organism's toxin causes an acute inflammation of the colon characterized by bloody diarrhea and abdominal pain. Sometimes there is also an associated destruction of the patient's red blood cells, with marked anemia and impaired renal function with renal failure. This pathogenic organism is present in the intestinal tract of infected cattle, and people usually become infected by consuming contaminated, incompletely cooked beef or by drinking raw milk.

**Spiral Organisms** The spiral organisms can cause a wide variety of illnesses. The best-known member of this group is *Treponema pallidum*, which causes syphilis, one of the sexually transmitted diseases considered in Chapter 6. Another spiral organism in this group is *Borrelia burgdorferi*, which causes Lyme disease. Transmission to humans is by the bite of an infected tick. Untreated Lyme disease typically progresses through three stages. In the first stage, a roughly circular, localized skin rash appears at the site of the tick bite and is frequently associated with flulike symptoms of fever, chills, and headaches, along with muscular and joint aches and pain. The rash and other manifestations eventually subside, but weeks or months later, many patients develop various neurologic, cardiac, and joint manifestations, which characterize the second stage of the disease. The third stage, which eventually develops in some untreated patients, is characterized by chronic arthritis and various neurologic problems. Diagnosis is usually made by means of various serologic tests, and the disease is usually treated with an antibiotic.

**Acid-Fast Bacteria**  Acid-fast bacteria have a waxy capsule that is stained with difficulty by means of certain red dyes. After the organism has been stained, the stain-impregnated capsule resists decolorization with various acid solvents. This property, attributable to the capsule, is the reason for the term *acid-fast*, used to refer to this type of organism. Acid-fast bacteria cause a special type of chronic inflammatory reaction, called a *chronic granulomatous inflammation*, rather than the polymorphonuclear inflammatory reaction usually seen with bacterial infections.

The best-known acid-fast bacterium is the tubercle bacillus (*Mycobacterium tuberculosis*) responsible for tuberculosis. Mycobacteria other than the tubercle bacillus may at times cause a tuberculosislike disease affecting lungs, lymph nodes, or skin, and some may cause severe systemic infections in immunocompromised persons. (Disseminated infection caused by *Mycobacterium avium complex* in persons with the acquired immune deficiency syndrome is described in Chapter 6.) Another acid-fast bacterium (*Mycobacterium leprae*) causes leprosy.

## Antibiotic Treatment of Bacterial Infections

The discovery of antibiotic compounds and their widespread use to treat various types of infections has been one of the great advances in medicine. Antibiotics are substances that destroy bacteria or inhibit their growth. They are useful clinically because of their ability to injure bacterial cells without producing significant injury to the patient. The bacterial cell is a complex structure containing genetic material, a protein-synthesizing mechanism, numerous enzyme systems concerned with intracellular metabolic functions, a semipermeable cell membrane, and a rigid cell wall. The bacterial genetic material is arranged as a circular DNA molecule that is attached to the cell membrane. Many bacteria also contain smaller circular DNA molecules called **plasmids** that often contain genes coding for various properties useful to bacteria, such as resistance to

**plasmid** (plas´-mid) A small, circular DNA molecule separate from the main bacterial chromosome.

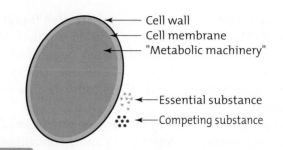

**Figure 5-2**  Various sites of action of antibiotics. Antibiotics may act by disrupting the bacterial cell wall, by disturbing the functions of the cell membrane, or by interfering with the intracellular "metabolic machinery." Some antimicrobial drugs are not directly injurious to the bacterial cell, but compete with essential substances required for bacterial growth and multiplication.

antibiotics and toxin production, but harmful to the persons infected by the bacteria; unfortunately, plasmids possessed by one bacterium can be copied and transferred to other bacteria, which then acquire new growth and survival advantages related to the transferred plasmids. Antimicrobial substances act by interfering with the structure or function of the bacterial cell in one or more of the following ways ( **Figure 5-2** ):

1. Inhibition of cell-wall synthesis
2. Inhibition of cell-membrane function
3. Inhibition of metabolic functions
4. Competitive inhibition

**Inhibition of Cell-Wall Synthesis**  The bacterial cell has a high internal osmotic pressure, and the rigid outer cell wall maintains the shape of the bacterium. In some respects, the function of the cell wall can be compared with a corset or girdle supporting the enclosed cell. Penicillin and several other antibiotics act by inhibiting the synthesis of the bacterial cell wall so that the cell body is exposed. Because of the high osmotic pressure inside the bacterium, the relatively unsupported cell swells and eventually ruptures.

**Inhibition of Cell-Membrane Function**  The cell membrane is a semipermeable membrane surrounding the bacterial protoplasm. It controls the internal composition of the cell by regulating the diffusion of materials into and out of the cell. Some antibiotics act by inhibiting various functions of the cell membrane. Loss of the selective permeability of the cell membrane leads to cell injury and death.

**Inhibition of Metabolic Functions**  Some antibiotics interfere with nucleic acid or protein synthesis by bacteria so that the organisms are unable to carry out essential metabolic functions.

**Competitive Inhibition**  Some antibiotics resemble important compounds required by bacteria for growth and multiplication. The bacteria are unable to distinguish between the essential compound and the antibiotic that resembles it, but the antibiotic cannot be substituted for the required compound in the metabolic process. When the bacteria use the "wrong" compound rather than the "correct" substance, bacterial metabolism is disrupted, leading to inhibition of bacterial growth.

## Antibiotic Sensitivity Tests

In selecting antibiotics to treat a bacterial infection, the practitioner is aided by laboratory tests called antibiotic sensitivity tests. These tests measure, under standardized conditions, the ability of the antibiotic to inhibit the growth of the organism isolated from the patient. One method, called a tube dilution sensitivity test, consists of preparing various dilutions of antibiotics in test tubes and inoculating the tubes with the organism to be tested. The tubes are then incubated for a period of time in order to permit growth of the organism. Finally, determination of the highest dilution of antibiotic that inhibits the growth of the organism indicates the sensitivity of the organism to the drug.

Another method of sensitivity testing consists of inoculating the organism on a bacteriologic plate containing a culture medium. One then places several filter paper disks on the plate, each containing a standardized concentration of a different antibiotic. Next, the plate is incubated to allow the organism to

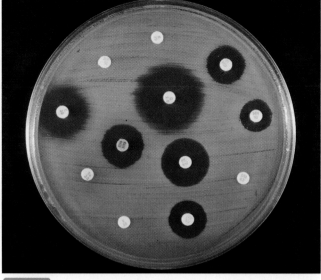

**Figure 5-3** Sensitivity test, illustrating antibiotic-impregnated filter paper disks on surface of culture plate. The clear zone around disk indicates that the antibiotic in the disk has inhibited bacterial growth.

grow. During incubation, the antibiotics in the disks diffuse into the surrounding culture. If the antibiotic inhibits the organism, the organism is unable to grow in the area around the disk, and a circular clear zone free of bacterial growth appears (**Figure 5-3**). The organism is said to be sensitive to the antibiotic. On the other hand, if the growth of the organism is not influenced by the antibiotic, growth will not be inhibited around the disk, and the organism is said to be resistant to the antibiotic.

### A Closer Look

*The discovery of penicillin began with a mold-contaminated microbiologic plate that evolved into a full-scale production effort stimulated by the onset of World War II, and culminated in the widespread availability of a very useful antibiotic.*

Penicillin is the name given to the antibiotic produced by a mold called *Penicillium notatum*. Many investigators and clinicians as far back as the 1800s observed that cultures of bacteria on agar plates were inhibited when molds contaminated the cultures, which set the stage for the observation by Alexander Fleming, an English physician–microbiologist. He was searching for mold-produced products that inhibited bacteria that might be useful for treating infections.

One day, on a culture plate of staphylococci that he was preparing to discard, he observed that a mold had contaminated the culture and inhibited the growth of the adjacent bacteria. He identified the mold and called the mold-produced product *penicillin*. Fleming published his results in 1929 but the observations excited little interest

at the time. Fleming continued his work, assisted by chemists and mold specialists.

In England, the onset of World War II in 1938 accelerated penicillin research and production. Howard Florey, assisted by Ernst Chain and others, formed a large research team to work on the project. Later, from 1941 through 1944, groups in the United States made further progress, culminating in methods for producing large quantities of penicillin, which became available to treat infections caused by penicillin-susceptible microorganisms. In 1945, Fleming, Chain, and Florey shared the Nobel Prize for their work.

The penicillin success story marked a big advance in the ongoing fight against pathogens, and development of other antibiotics followed. However, many organisms have become resistant to antibiotics to which they were previously sensitive, and new antibiotics have been developed to use against the newly resistant organisms. This cycle has been repeated many times. So far, we are ahead of the bacteria, but our supremacy is not guaranteed.

A bacteriology laboratory report that the organism is sensitive to a given antibiotic means that the organism probably can be inhibited by giving the patient the usual therapeutic dose of that drug. A report that the organism is resistant to an antibiotic indicates that a therapeutic dose of antibiotic is unlikely to inhibit the growth of the organism.

It should be emphasized, however, that the sensitivity of an organism to an antibiotic is only one factor influencing a patient's response to an infection. Other factors include the patient's own resistance and the antibiotic's ability to diffuse in sufficient quantities into the site of the infection.

## Adverse Effects of Antibiotics

**Toxicity**  Antibiotics are useful because they are much more toxic to bacteria than they are to the patient. Antibiotics vary in their effects on people, but all are toxic to some degree. Some injure the kidneys; others injure nerve tissue or the blood-forming tissues. Penicillin and other antibiotics that act by interfering with bacterial cell-wall synthesis are relatively nontoxic, probably because the body cells have no structure comparable to the bacterial cell wall. Some antibiotics that interfere with bacterial metabolic functions can at times produce similar derangements in the patient's own metabolic functions. For example, tetracycline is a relatively nontoxic antibiotic, excreted chiefly by the kidneys. If renal function is impaired, very high blood levels of antibiotic may develop after administration of the usual therapeutic doses of the drug; this may cause severe impairment of the patient's own cellular metabolic functions.

**Hypersensitivity**  Some antibiotics induce a marked hypersensitivity that can lead to a fatal reaction if the drug is later administered to a sensitized patient. Penicillin is capable of inducing extremely severe anaphylactic reactions, although the antibiotic itself has a very low toxicity.

**Alteration of Normal Bacterial Flora**  The normal bacterial flora in the oral cavity, the colon, and other locations may be altered by antibiotics. If the normal bacteria are destroyed, there may be overgrowth of resistant bacteria and fungi previously controlled by the normal flora. These resistant organisms may cause infections in susceptible patients.

**Development of Resistant Strains of Bacteria**  Some bacteria that are initially sensitive to antibiotics eventually become resistant. There are two ways in which an organism becomes resistant. It may undergo a spontaneous mutation that conveys resistance, or it may acquire resistance genes transferred by a plasmid from another bacterium.

Spontaneous mutations do not occur frequently in cell division, but many bacteria divide so rapidly that spontaneous mutations can present a problem if the rapidly dividing bacteria are not quickly eliminated by the antibiotic. After a mutation that conveys antibiotic resistance occurs, the mutant organism has an advantage over its antibiotic-sensitive counterpart because it can flourish in the presence of the antibiotic while the antibiotic-sensitive organisms are eliminated.

Plasmid-acquired resistance can be a major problem because the transferred resistance genes may convey resistance to multiple antibiotics, and transfers can take place between bacteria of different types. Now both bacteria possess antibiotic-resistance genes, which they in turn can pass to other bacteria.

There are a number of mechanisms by which resistant bacteria can circumvent an antibiotic's effect. Such mechanisms include (1) developing enzymes to destroy the antibiotic, (2) either changing their cell-wall structure so that the antibiotic is unable to get into the cell or developing mechanisms to expel the antibiotic as soon as it enters the cell and before it can disturb bacterial functions, and (3) changing their intracellular "metabolic machinery" so that the antibiotic is no longer able to disturb bacterial functions.

Widespread use of an antibiotic predisposes to the development of resistant strains. This may complicate the treatment of patients who become infected with antibiotic-resistant organisms. Staphylococci, in particular, have raised this problem because many strains isolated from hospital patients have been found to be highly resistant to a large number of antibiotics. Treatment of gonorrhea also has been complicated by the development of a high degree of penicillin resistance in many strains of gonococci; consequently, prolonged courses of therapy and much larger doses of antibiotic are required to eradicate the infections. Even the pneumococcus is no longer uniformly sensitive to penicillin, as it was in the past. Some strains are resistant to penicillin and other drugs normally used against them. Resistant strains of tubercle bacilli also have developed, hindering treatment of tuberculosis with antituberculosis drugs. On the other hand, some bacteria still remain quite sensitive to antibiotics. For example, group A beta streptococci remain sensitive to penicillin, despite widespread use of penicillin to treat streptococcal infections. *Treponema pallidum*, the organism responsible for syphilis, also has remained quite sensitive to penicillin, even though the drug has been used to treat syphilis for many years.

# Chlamydiae

The chlamydiae are very small, gram-negative, non-motile bacteria that were once thought to be large viruses. They are deficient in certain enzymes, and can live only as parasites inside the cells of the individual that they infect. They are taken into the cells of the host by phagocytosis, where they divide to form large intracytoplasmic clusters of organisms called *inclusion bodies*. These resemble inclusion bodies formed in some viral diseases. Their growth can be inhibited by various antibiotics that inhibit protein synthesis, such as tetracycline and erythromycin. Some strains of chlamydiae are also inhibited by sulfonamide drugs.

Chlamydiae cause several different types of diseases. The most common chlamydial disease affects the genital tract and is transmitted by sexual contact. In the male, it causes an inflammation of the urethra called *nongonococcal urethritis*. In the female, it causes an inflammation of the uterine cervix that may spread to the fallopian tubes and ovaries as well. If a mother has a chlamydial infection of the cervix, infected secretions may get into her infant's eyes during childbirth and cause an inflammation called *inclusion conjunctivitis*. The name is based on the fact that characteristic inclusions can be demonstrated in the infected cells of the infant's conjunctiva. Other chlamydiae cause pulmonary infections.

# Rickettsiae and Ehrlichiae

Rickettsiae are very small intracellular bacteria that can multiply only within the cells of an infected person. Many small animals and dogs are infected. The rickettsiae are transmitted to humans by insect bites, and they multiply in the endothelial cells of small blood vessels, which become swollen and necrotic, leading to thrombosis, rupture, and necrosis. Clinically, a rickettsial infection usually causes a febrile illness, often associated with a skin rash. Typhus and Rocky Mountain spotted fever are the most common rickettsial diseases. These organisms are sensitive to some antibiotics (tetracyclines and chloramphenicol). Similar organisms called *ehrlichiae* (named after a famous immunologist, Paul Ehrlich) are also transmitted by ticks, and infect white blood cells rather than endothelial cells. The infected white cells contain small, compact clusters of organisms that can be identified in blood smears. The disease called *ehrlichiosis* is a febrile illness similar to infections caused by rickettsiae and may be associated with a skin rash. Ehrlichiosis can be treated successfully with a tetracycline antibiotic.

# Mycoplasmas

The mycoplasmas are very small bacteria that are very fragile because they lack a cell wall. One member of this group causes a type of pneumonia called *primary atypical pneumonia*. Mycoplasmas respond to the antibiotics tetracycline and erythromycin.

# Viruses

Viruses are the smallest infectious agents. A typical virus consists of a molecule of nucleic acid (either DNA or RNA), its *genome*, enclosed within a protein shell called a capsid. The capsid is made of subunits called capsomeres that are arranged in a precise geometric fashion around the genome. Many viruses are also covered by an outer lipid envelope acquired from the cytoplasm of the host cell when the virus buds from the infected cell. Projections from the surface of the virus allow the virus to attach to the cell that it will infect. Viruses vary greatly in size. The smallest are only slightly larger than protein molecules, whereas the largest viruses approach the size of a bacterium.

The nucleic acid of the virus genome may be arranged in either a single or a double strand, and the complexity of the viral genome varies. Some viruses have as many as 400 genes within their nucleic acid structure, whereas others have as few as eight. Viruses have few metabolic enzymes and therefore must rely on the cells of the infected person to carry out their activities. When a virus invades the cell, the viral genome directs the metabolic processes of the cell to synthesize more virus particles. In many respects, the virus may be likened to a criminal who takes over a business, forcing it to function for the criminal's benefit rather than for the benefit of the owner ( Figure 5-4 ).

## Classification of Viruses

An older classification of viruses was based on the major clinical features of the viral infection, and viruses were classified on the basis of the portion of the body or organ system in which the viral infection produced the most prominent clinical manifestations. A more modern classification categorizes viruses on the basis of their nucleic acid structure, size, structural configuration, and biologic characteristics. In this classification, several large groups of viruses are recognized, and a large number of viruses are identified in each group. Table 5-3 presents a simplified classification of viruses and the diseases they cause.

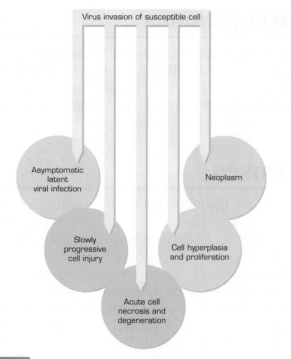

**Figure 5-4** Summary of possible effects of a virus infection on susceptible cells.

| Table 5-3 | Simplified Classification of Common Virus Infections |
|---|---|

| DNA Viruses | Diseases |
|---|---|
| Adenovirus | Respiratory infections |
| Hepatitis B virus | Hepatitis B |
| Herpesviruses | Herpes simplex types 1 and 2 (oral and genital vesicles) |
| | Epstein-Barr virus (infectious mononucleosis) |
| | Varicella-zoster virus (chickenpox; herpes zoster) |
| | Cytomegalovirus (mononucleosis-like illness; hepatitis) |
| | Herpesvirus 8 (Kaposi sarcoma) |
| Papillomavirus | Warts; Genital condylomas (some strains cause cancer) |

| RNA Viruses | Diseases |
|---|---|
| Arboviruses | Encephalitis, various types, spread by mosquito |
| Enterovirus | Poliomyelitis |
| Norwalk virus (Norovirus) | Acute gastroenteritis |
| Measles virus | Measles |
| Mumps virus | Mumps |
| Rubella virus | German measles |
| Influenza viruses | Influenza |
| Various respiratory viruses | Respiratory infections (Influenza viruses; Rhinovirus; Rotavirus; Respiratory syncytial virus) |

## Mode of Action

A distinction is sometimes made between a viral infection and a viral disease. A condition in which a virus infects a cell without causing any evidence of cell injury is considered a *latent viral infection*. Many viruses are capable of coexisting with normal cells in lymphoid tissue and the gastrointestinal tract, and probably in other sites, without causing cellular injury. Such viruses are able to live for long periods within the cells of the infected host while they continually discharge virus particles. Other viruses are more virulent and regularly produce cell injury, manifested by necrosis and degeneration of the infected cell. This is called a *cytopathogenic effect*. Some cytopathogenic effects are shown in  Figure 5-5  and  Figure 5-6 . Some viruses induce cell hyperplasia and proliferation rather than cell necrosis. These effects are shown in  Figure 5-7  and  Figure 5-8 . Many viruses induce various combinations of cell damage and cell hyperplasia.

Under certain circumstances, a latent asymptomatic viral infection may become activated, leading to actual disease. The herpesvirus, which infects both the oral cavity and the genital tract, may persist in the tissues of the host for many years. The virus periodically becomes activated and causes crops of painful vesicles that may recur during an unrelated febrile illness, when the patient's immunologic defenses have been disrupted by a neoplasm or by various other diseases, or sometimes for no apparent reason ( Figure 5-9 ).

Another member of the herpes group of viruses is the *varicella-zoster virus*, named from its two different manifestations. The initial contact with the virus causes *chickenpox* (varicella), which is an extremely contagious disease characterized by an itchy skin rash that usually soon subsides without any serious complications. A person who has had chickenpox develops an immunity and cannot contact chickenpox again. However, the virus is not eradicated by the immune system and remains dormant within sensory nerve ganglia. Sometimes the virus becomes active again within a sensory ganglion many years later and travels down the sensory nerve to the skin where it causes a characteristic bandlike vesicular skin rash in the segment of skin supplied by the sensory nerve. The recurrent infection is *herpes zoster*, which is often called *shingles*. The term comes from a Latin word *cingulum* that means a belt or girdle, named from the beltlike band of skin vesicles along the course of a spinal nerve that partially girdles the trunk, as in  Figure 5-10 .

A live virus vaccine is available to immunize against chickenpox. A similar vaccine has been developed to help prevent herpes zoster in older adults who had chickenpox many years ago and harbor the virus in

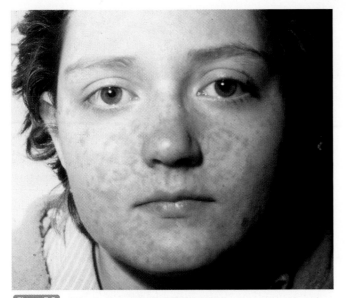

Figure 5-5    A young woman with German measles, illustrating skin rash.

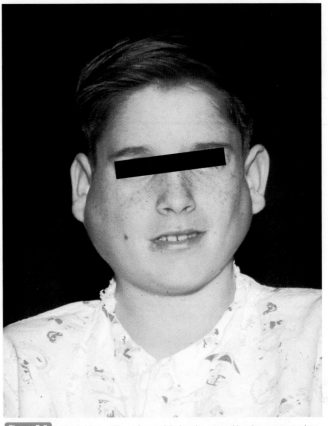

Figure 5-6    Marked swelling of parotid glands caused by the mumps virus.

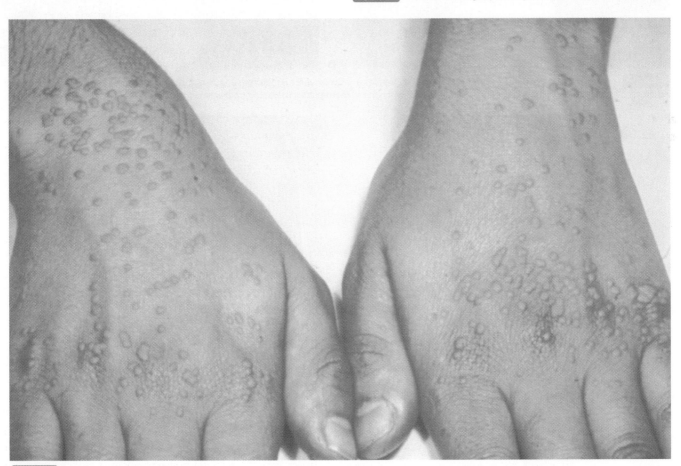

Figure 5-7    Multiple warts on skin of hands.

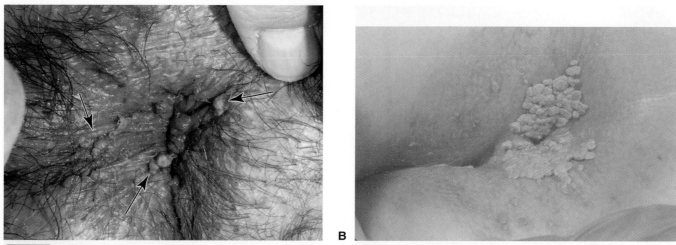

**Figure 5-8** Skin condylomas caused by papillomavirus. **A,** Condylomas around skin of anus (*arrows*). **B,** Large group of condylomas involving skin of buttocks around gluteal cleft.

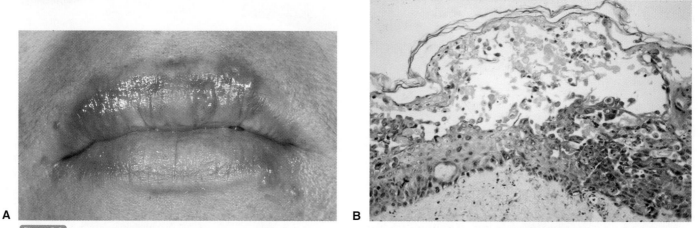

**Figure 5-9** Herpesvirus infection. **A,** Recurrent oral herpes caused by herpesvirus type 1. **B,** Section of small herpes blister (vesicle). The superficial skin layer is almost completely destroyed, and a superficial ulcer will form when the surface epithelium sloughs (original magnification × 100).

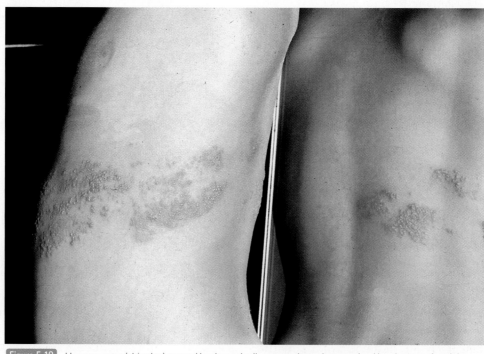

**Figure 5-10** Herpes zoster (shingles) caused by the varicella-zoster virus, characterized by clusters of vesicles that occur in a segment of skin (dermatome) supplied by a sensory nerve. The subject was photographed beside a mirror in order to illustrate the bandlike distribution of the rash in the segment of skin supplied by a spinal nerve.

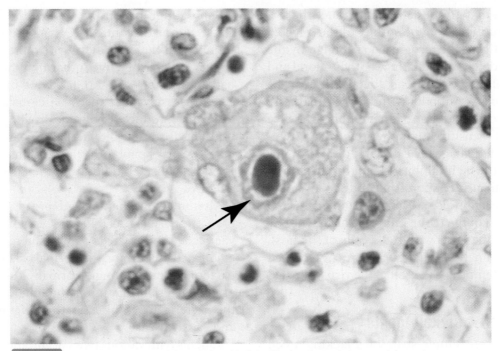

Large intranuclear inclusion within epithelial cell in the center of photograph (*arrow*).

sensory nerve ganglia. The vaccine stimulates the body's immune response against the dormant virus, like a booster injection of a vaccine, thereby reducing the likelihood that the virus will be able to reactivate and cause herpes zoster.

**Inclusion Bodies in Viral Disease**  Tissues that are infected with virus frequently contain spherical, densely staining structures called **inclusion bodies** ( Figure 5-11 ). These are present within the nucleus or the cytoplasm or both locations. Inclusion bodies consist of masses of virus or products of virus multiplication. The presence of inclusion bodies may be of considerable diagnostic aid in recognizing viral infection and determining the type of viral disease present.

## Defenses Against Viral Infections

The body responds to a viral infection by forming a protein substance called **interferon** and by activating humoral and cell-mediated defense mechanisms.

**Formation of Interferon**  Interferon is a general term for a group of carbohydrate-containing proteins produced by cells in response to viral infection and was named from its ability to "interfere" with viral multiplication. Interferon functions as a nonspecific, "broad-spectrum" antiviral agent. It inhibits not only the virus that induced its formation, but other viruses as well. This is in contrast with the behavior of a specific antiviral antibody, which reacts only to the virus that induced its formation. Interferons provide a rapid

"first-line" defense against a viral infection. By slowing viral growth during the early phase of the infection, the infected person is allowed time to mobilize humoral and cell-mediated responses directed against the invading virus.

In addition to their antiviral activity, interferons have other actions concerned with regulation of the immune system and cell growth. These functions are considered in Chapter 8.

**inclusion bodies**
Spherical structures in the nucleus or cytoplasm of virus-infected cells.

**interferon**  (in-tur-fēr′on) A broad-spectrum antiviral agent manufactured by various cells in the body.

**Humoral and Cell-Mediated Immunity in Viral Infections**  The body also forms specific antiviral antibodies that are capable of inactivating viruses and may actually destroy virus particles in the presence of complement. Antiviral antibodies cannot combine with the virus, however, unless the virus particles are discharged into the extracellular fluid where they are exposed to the action of the antibody. Consequently, antiviral antibodies are relatively inefficient in combating viruses that spread directly from cell to cell because the virus particles remain within the infected cells and are protected from the antibody. For example, persons who have recurrent fever blisters caused by the herpesvirus possess antibodies to the virus, but the antibody is often unable to eradicate the intracellular virus particles.

In addition to producing specific antiviral antibodies, the cell-mediated immune defenses of the host are directed against the virus-infected cells. This occurs because viruses that invade cells often induce the formation of new antigens on the surface of the infected cells. These antigens are recognized as foreign by the host's immune defenses and induce both humoral and cell-mediated immune reactions directed against the virus-infected cells. Antibodies are formed that affix to the infected cells and destroy them in the presence of complement. Sensitized lymphocytes release lymphokines, which damage the cells, and they also produce interferon, which inhibits the multiplication of viruses. Chemical mediators that induce an acute inflammatory reaction also are liberated. In many viral infections, much of the tissue injury is caused, not by proliferation of the virus within the cells of the host, but by the inflammation and tissue destruction caused by the body's attempts to rid itself of the virus-infected cells.

## Treatment with Antiviral Agents

Because viruses are simple structures lacking a cell wall, a cell membrane, and the complex "metabolic machinery" of bacteria, they are not susceptible to the disruptive actions of antibiotics. However, some chemotherapeutic agents that are active against viruses have been developed. In many cases, their mechanisms of action are similar to those of compounds used to treat cancer (Chapter 8). Unfortunately, many compounds that block viral multiplication also have adverse effects on the host cells and may be as toxic to the host as to the virus. For this reason, antiviral agents have had limited application in clinical medicine.

Some newer antiviral agents are less toxic and promise to be more useful. One such drug is effective against some infections caused by the herpes group of viruses. The drug is activated within the virus-infected cells by a viral enzyme to yield the active antiviral compound that selectively inhibits synthesis of viral DNA within the cells in which the virus is replicating. It does not interfere with the synthesis of host DNA, and this accounts for its low toxicity.

# Fungi

Fungi are plantlike organisms without chlorophyll and are subdivided into two large groups: yeasts and molds. Yeasts are small ovoid or spherical cells that reproduce by budding. Molds, when grown on suitable media at room temperature, form large colonies composed of multiple branching filamentous structures called hyphae (singular, hypha). The matted mass of hyphae, which is called a mycelium, is responsible for the characteristic appearance of the colony ( Figure 5-12 ).

Some fungi live on the skin and only occasionally cause minor discomfort. Others are found in small numbers in the oral cavity, gastrointestinal tract, and vagina, where they live in harmony with the normal bacterial flora. Most fungi have a limited ability to cause disease. Under special circumstances, however, fungi may produce serious localized or systemic infections in susceptible individuals. Two major factors predispose to systemic fungal infections: disturbance in the normal bacterial flora and impaired immunologic defenses.

After intensive therapy with broad-spectrum antibiotics, the normal bacterial flora of the oral cavity, colon, vagina, and other areas may be altered or completely eradicated, disturbing the normal balance between the bacterial flora and fungi. Normally, the predominance of the bacterial flora holds the fungi in check. When the bacteria are eliminated, the fungi may proliferate and cause disease.

Patients with various types of chronic debilitating diseases may be susceptible to fungal infections. Infections of this type are also encountered in patients whose immunologic defense mechanisms have been depressed by various drugs and chemicals or by radiation therapy. Patients with certain types of cancer, particularly those treated with cytotoxic drugs, may also develop systemic fungal infections.

## Superficial Fungal Infections

The common superficial fungal infections of the skin are caused by a group of fungi called **dermatophytes**, which grow on the skin. They cause itchy, scaling skin lesions on the scalp and on other parts of the body. Some have been given such picturesque, popular names as "athlete's foot" and "jock itch." A common superficial

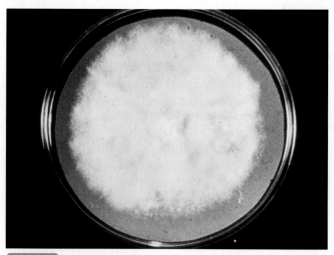

Figure 5-12   Appearance of fungus colony growing on a laboratory culture medium.

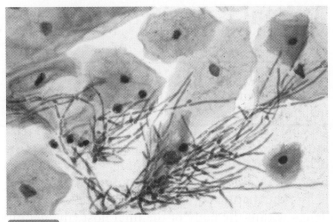

**Figure 5-13** A cluster of hyphae in a vaginal smear from a patient with a vaginal infection caused by *Candida albicans* (original magnification × 400).

fungal infection of the mucous membranes is caused by a yeastlike fungus called *Candida albicans*. This organism is a common cause of vaginal infections, producing symptoms of itching and vaginal discharge ( **Figure 5-13** ). Pregnant women and women taking oral contraceptive pills seem more susceptible to *Candida* infection, as are persons treated with broad-spectrum antibiotics such as tetracycline. A number of antifungal drugs are available that can be applied locally to treat infections caused by dermatophytes and *Candida*.

## Highly Pathogenic Fungi

Although most fungi are at best only potential pathogens of low virulence, two are highly infectious and frequently produce disease in humans. They can be identified by biopsy or by culture of infected tissues. The fungus *Histoplasma capsulatum*, which is found in many parts of the United States, causes the disease histoplasmosis. This organism is found in the soil. People become infected by inhaling dust containing spores of the fungus. In most cases, the fungus produces an acute, self-limited respiratory infection. Less commonly, the organism causes a more chronic pulmonary infection similar to tuberculosis. In some cases, a progressive, disseminated, sometimes fatal disease develops. Another fungus, *Coccidioides immitis*, which is found in parts of California and elsewhere in the southwestern part of the United States, causes the disease *coccidioidomycosis*. As in the case of histoplasmosis, humans become infected by inhaling dust that contains fungus spores. The symptoms are similar to those of histoplasmosis. Coccidioidomycosis is usually manifested as an acute pulmonary infection, but sometimes the fungus causes chronic or severe progressive systemic disease.

## Other Fungi of Medical Importance

Two other pathogenic fungi of medical importance are *Blastomyces dermatitidis*, which causes the disease *blastomycosis*, and *Cryptococcus neoformans*, which causes *cryptococcosis*. Infections caused by these organisms are less common than either histoplasmosis or coccidioidomycosis. Both organisms are found in the soil, and infection is caused by inhalation of dust containing the organisms.

Clinically, blastomycosis is similar to histoplasmosis and coccidioidomycosis. Most infections are acute and self-limited. Occasionally, the fungus causes a more chronic pulmonary infection ( **Figure 5-14** ), as illustrated in Case 5-1, or a widespread systemic disease.

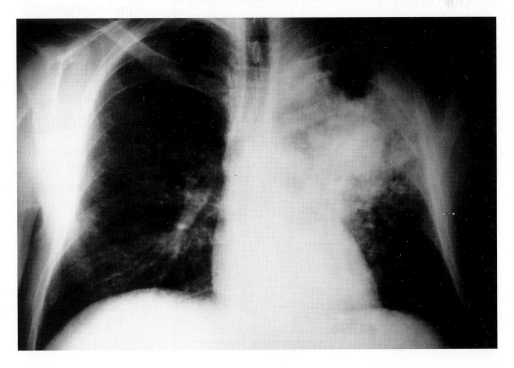

**Figure 5-14** Chest x-ray illustrating a blastomycosis of the left lung (*right side* of photograph), which appears as a dense (white) area occupying the upper part of the lung. The right lung (*left side* of photograph) appears normal (Case 5-2).

*Cryptococcus neoformans* is a yeastlike organism that has a large mucoid capsule. The organism initially causes a pulmonary infection but then may be transported in the bloodstream to the brain, where it causes a chronic meningitis. The organisms can be identified in smears and cultures of spinal fluid.

## Treatment of Systemic Fungal Infections

Acute pulmonary infections caused by fungi frequently subside spontaneously and many do not require treatment with antifungal antibiotics, but chronic or progressive systemic fungal infections require antibiotic treatment, as illustrated by the following cases.

### Case Study 5-1

A 39-year-old diabetic man was admitted to the hospital with cough and fever, and a chest x-ray revealed a large area of consolidation in the left lung (Figure 5-14). Bronchial biopsy revealed nonspecific chronic inflammation, but cultures revealed growth of *Blastomyces dermatitidis*. The patient responded to treatment with antifungal antibiotics.

### Case Study 5-2

A young man who had resided for a short time in the southwestern United States consulted his physician and was found to have a dense infiltrate in the upper lobe of the lung with the formation of a cavity, suggesting tuberculosis. However, cultures of sputum for tubercle bacilli were negative. A specimen from the affected area was obtained by means of a flexible bronchoscope, and material for culture was also obtained. *Coccidioides immitis* was cultured from the involved area. Biopsy revealed only nonspecific chronic inflammation. No organisms were identified in the biopsy specimen. The patient was treated with an antifungal antibiotic and made an uneventful recovery.

# Animal Parasites and Their Host

Animal parasites are organisms that have become adapted to living within or on the body of another animal, called the host. These organisms are no longer capable of a free-living existence. Many animal parasites have a complex life cycle. An immature form of a parasite may spend a part of its cycle within the body of an animal or fish (the intermediate host) before the mature parasite eventually takes up residence within the body of the final host (the definitive host). In general, many animal parasites live within the intestinal tract and discharge eggs in the feces. Transmission is favored by conditions of poor sanitation and by relatively high temperature and humidity, which enhance survival of the parasite in its infective stage. Therefore, many parasitic infections are common in tropical climates but are much less frequent in cold or temperate climates. Specific drugs are available to treat almost all parasitic infections effectively. Animal parasites may be classified into three large groups:

1. *Protozoa*, which are simple, one-celled organisms
2. *Metazoa*, which are more complex, multicellular structures
3. *Arthropods*, which are small insects

# Protozoal Infections

Some of the more important protozoal infections in humans include:

1. Malaria, caused by various species of *Plasmodium*
2. Babesiosis, usually caused by *Babesia microti*, a malarialike parasite
3. Amebic dysentery, caused by a pathogenic ameba, *Entamoeba histolytica*
4. Genital tract trichomonad infections, caused by the parasite *Trichomonas vaginalis*
5. *Giardiasis*, caused by *Giardia lamblia*, which infects the small intestine
6. Toxoplasmosis, caused by *Toxoplasma gondii*, which may infect the fetus and cause congenital malformations
7. Cryptosporidiosis, caused by a parasite called *Cryptosporidium parvum*, which parasitizes the intestinal tract and can cause severe diarrhea
8. Pneumocystis pneumonia, caused by an organism now called *Pneumocystis jiroveci* (previously called *Pneumocystis carinii*), a parasite that does not cause disease in immunocompetent persons but causes

a severe, sometimes fatal pulmonary infection in persons with acquired immune deficiency syndrome (AIDS). The pulmonary disease is considered in Chapter 12.

## Malaria

Malaria is caused by several species of the protozoan parasite *Plasmodium*, which has a complicated life cycle. The parasite is transmitted to humans by the bite of the Anopheles mosquito, which breeds in swampy lowland areas. The name malaria dates to the time when the disease was thought to be caused by breathing night air near lowland marshes and swampy areas (*malo* = bad + *aria* = air). After the parasite and its mosquito vector were recognized, it became apparent that the marshy areas were mosquito breeding grounds, and the evening hours were the times when the mosquitoes were most active.

The parasites first begin their development within the liver and then invade the red blood cells of the host. There they multiply, feeding on the hemoglobin, which becomes degraded to a product called malarial pigment. Soon, the rapidly multiplying parasites destroy the red cells that they have invaded, releasing masses of new parasites along with red-cell debris and malarial pigment into the circulation. This event is associated with an elevated temperature and a shaking chill ("chills and fever"). The newly liberated parasites in turn attack other red cells, and the cycles of invasion–multiplication–red-cell destruction continue. The time taken for each species of parasite to complete its cycle is quite constant. Consequently, the episodes of chills and fever tend to occur at regular intervals every 48 or 72 hours, depending on the species. Besides suffering repeated, periodic chills and fever, infected individuals frequently become anemic because of the excessive red-cell destruction. Often their spleens also enlarge because phagocytic cells in the spleen proliferate and become filled with debris and malarial pigment. In one type of malaria, clumps of parasitized red cells may plug small blood vessels in the brain, heart, or other vital organs. This serious complication impedes blood flow to the affected organs and may be fatal. Diagnosis of malaria is established by demonstrating the parasite in properly prepared and stained slides made from the blood of the infected patient.

Malaria is a major health problem in many parts of the world. It is widespread in many third world countries, including parts of Africa, Asia, Central America, and South America. Most cases of malaria in the United States are contracted by persons who have traveled to areas where malaria occurs frequently and become ill after returning home. Various antimalarial drugs are available to prevent infection when traveling in an endemic area and to treat an established infection. Unfortunately, parasites are becoming resistant to some antimalarial drugs, which makes treatment more difficult.

### Case Study 5-3

An American family had been vacationing in a resort outside the United States. After returning to their own country, several members became ill with chills and fever. Examination of the blood smears revealed malarial parasites. The affected family members received a course of antimalarial therapy and made an uneventful recovery.

## Babesiosis

Babesiae are tick-borne protozoal parasites that infect a wide variety of wild and domestic animals and birds, and they sometimes also infect people. The first documented infections in the United States occurred in Nantucket Island in Massachusetts, but now babesia infections are more widely distributed throughout the United States. In North America, the organism that infects people is *Babesia microti*, which is usually transmitted from small rodents to people by the same ticks that transmit Lyme disease. The organism parasitizes red cells where the babesiae multiply and eventually rupture the parasitized red cells, releasing the parasites to invade and proliferate in other red cells. The *Babesia microti* infection causes a malarialike illness characterized by chills, fever, and anemia resulting from destruction of red cells by the parasites. The diagnosis of the infection is established by identifying the parasites within the infected red cells, which must be distinguished from malaria parasites, which they resemble. The severity of the babesial infection varies in different individuals, and the blood filtration function of the spleen plays an important role in controlling the infection by eliminating many of the parasites as blood flows through the spleen. Most infected individuals have a mild illness and recover without complications. However, if the infected person has had a splenectomy, the proliferation of the parasites is unchecked by the spleen, and these unfortunate persons develop a severe and sometimes fatal infection. Several drugs are available to treat the infection.

## Amebiasis

Amebiasis is an infection of the intestinal tract by a pathogenic ameba, *Entamoeba histolytica*. The life cycle of the parasite includes an active, motile, vegetative phase (called a trophozoite) and a relatively resistant cystic phase. Humans become infected by ingesting cysts of the parasite in contaminated food and water. The motile phase of the parasite develops from the cyst and invades the mucosa of the colon, producing mucosal ulcers and causing symptoms of inflammation of the colon. Occasionally, the amebas are carried to the liver in the portal circulation and may cause amebic hepatitis or amebic liver abscess.

## Genital Tract Infections Caused by Trichomonads

The trichomonads are small motile parasites. One species, *Trichomonas vaginalis*, sometimes causes an acute inflammation of the vagina characterized by itching, burning, and a profuse, frothy vaginal discharge. The infection can be transmitted to the male by sexual intercourse and causes an inflammation of the urethra.

## Giardiasis

*Giardia lamblia* is a small, pear-shaped parasite that inhabits the duodenum and upper jejunum. The parasite attaches to the mucosa, causing an intestinal inflammation manifested by crampy abdominal pain, distention, and watery diarrhea. Parasites are present in the stools of infected individuals, and the disease is usually transmitted by means of contaminated food and water. Several epidemics of *Giardia* infection caused by contaminated water supplies have occurred in the United States.

### Case Study 5-4

A young woman complained of vaginal itching and profuse vaginal discharge. Examination revealed redness of the vaginal mucosa and abundant yellow vaginal secretions. Microscopic examination revealed large numbers of trichomonads and leukocytes in the secretions ( Figure 5-15 ). The patient was treated with an antiparasitic drug (metronidazole). Because the disease is transmitted by sexual intercourse, the patient's sexual partner also was treated.

## Toxoplasmosis

*Toxoplasma gondii* is a small intracellular parasite that infects a large number of birds and animals, as well as humans. Many cats are infected with the parasite and excrete an infectious form of the organism in their stools. The parasite is frequently present in the flesh of cattle and many other animals. People acquire *Toxoplasma* infections by ingesting raw or partially cooked meat that is infected with the parasite or by contact with infected cats that excrete in their feces an infectious form of the parasite called an oocyst. Usually the infection does not cause symptoms in healthy adults. About 50 percent of the adult population has

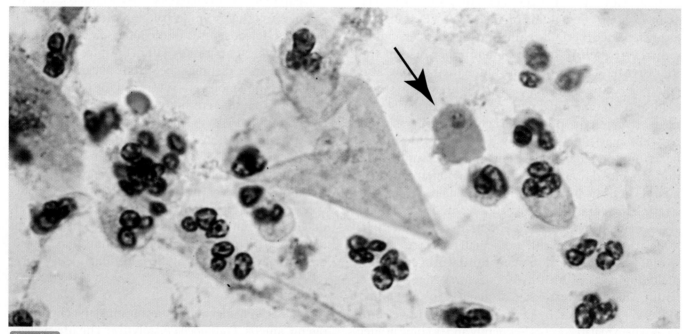

Figure 5-15   Vaginal secretions from a woman with a trichomonad infection, illustrating a parasite (*arrow*) and many neutrophils (original magnification × 400).

had a previous inapparent infection and is immune. The importance of toxoplasmosis is related to its effect on the fetus. If a susceptible (nonimmune) woman acquires a *Toxoplasma* infection during pregnancy, the parasite may be transmitted to the fetus. Infection of the fetus causes severe injury to fetal tissues and often leads to congenital malformations that are described in Chapter 7.

Toxoplasmosis is also a risk to immunocompromised persons, as are other parasitic infections. The disease may result either from a first exposure to the parasite or from reactivation of an infection acquired many years previously, as illustrated by the following case.

### Case Study 5-5

A 55-year-old HIV-antibody-positive man consulted his physician because of recent onset of confusion, dizziness, and seizures. Neurologic examination was normal, but CT scans of the head revealed multiple spherical nodules throughout both cerebral hemispheres. Examination of the spinal fluid was normal. Biopsy of one of the nodules revealed the characteristic appearance of toxoplasmosis, which was associated with some surrounding cerebral edema and reactive proliferation of astrocytes ( Figure 5-16 ). The toxoplasmosis was considered to be a reactivation of a prior infection, and appropriate treatment was started to control the infection.

## Cryptosporidiosis

*Cryptosporidium parvum*, an organism closely related to *Toxoplasma*, has been recognized recently as a very important cause of severe diarrhea in both immunocompetent and immunocompromised persons. The organism infects cattle, other farm animals, and people who excrete in their fecal material large numbers of the infectious forms of the parasites called oocysts. Fecal material from farm animals can contaminate surface water flowing into rivers and lakes, and oocysts have been identified in a large number of surface water samples tested throughout the United States. The infectious oocyst has a thick wall and is quite small, only about half the size of a red blood cell. It is highly resistant to chlorination of water supplies and can be removed from municipal water supplies only by filtration. People can become infected by ingesting oocysts in unfiltered municipal water supplies, from oocyst-contaminated water in swimming pools, or by person-to-person fecal-oral transmission in the same way that other intestinal infections are transmitted. The infection is easily transmitted person to person in households and in child day-care facilities.

When oocysts are ingested, the cyst wall disintegrates in the intestinal tract, releasing the infectious parasite, which multiplies and infects the intestinal epithelial cells. The parasite is very infectious. Only a few oocysts are enough to cause an infection, and persons with diarrhea excrete large numbers of oocysts in their stool. Persons with normal immune defenses experience an acute self-limited diarrhea when infected with the parasite, but persons with AIDS and other immunocompromised persons develop a severe chronic life-threatening diarrhea. Unfortunately, there is no specific treatment for the infection.

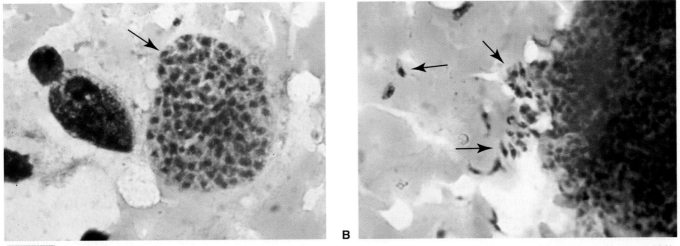

**A**  **B**

Figure 5-16  A cerebral toxoplasmosis demonstrated by brain biopsy. **A,** Cyst composed of a large cluster of organisms (*arrow*) (original magnification × 400). **B,** Higher magnification view illustrating disruption of the cyst wall with extruded sickle-shaped parasites (*arrow*) (original magnification × 1000).

## Table 5-4 Common Protozoal Infections

| Disease | Source of Infection | Manifestations | Diagnosis | Treatment |
|---|---|---|---|---|
| Malaria | Mosquito bite | Chills and fever Anemia | Identify parasite in red cells | Antimalarial drugs |
| Babesiosis | Deer tick bite | Chills and fever Anemia | Identify parasite in red cells | Various drugs available |
| Amebiasis | Ingestion of parasite in contaminated food or water | Cramps and diarrhea. Sometimes hepatitis. | Identify parasite or cysts in stool | Various drugs available |
| Giardiasis | Ingestion of parasite in contaminated food or water | Cramps and diarrhea | Identify parasite in stool. Other tests also available | Antiparasite drug (metronidazole) |
| Cryptosporidiosis | Food or water contaminated with parasite cysts. Recreational water (swimming pools) | Cramps and diarrhea | Identify parasite cysts in stool | No antiparasite drugs available. Treat symptoms |
| Trichomoniasis | Vaginal secretions containing parasite | Profuse vaginal discharge | Identify parasite in vaginal secretions | Antiparasite drug (metronidazole) |
| Toxoplasmosis | Eating meat containing parasites. Contact with feces of infected cats | Causes disease in AIDS patients. Pregnant woman may transmit infection to fetus. | Identify parasite (usually biopsy required) | Drugs available to prevent disease in AIDS patients. Otherwise no treatment required |
| Pneumocystis infection | Organisms normally present in respiratory tract Asymptomatic in persons with normal immune system | Causes pneumonia in persons with impaired immune system, often in persons with AIDS | Identify parasite in lung biopsy or bronchial secretions | Several different effective antibiotics available for treatment |

Several large epidemics of cryptosporidiosis have been traced to municipal water supplies where filtration of water to eliminate oocysts either was not performed or was inadequate. Small, swimming-pool–related epidemics have been reported. In these cases, the oocyst contamination of the pool water was caused by persons with cryptosporidial diarrhea using the pool; oocysts contaminating the perianal skin of these people were released into the pool water and infected other swimmers.

## Pulmonary Pneumocystis Infection

This condition occurs in immunocompromised persons, especially in persons with AIDS. The pulmonary disease is considered in Chapter 12.

Table 5-4 summarizes the manifestations, diagnosis, and treatment of the common protozoal infections considered in this section.

# Metazoal Infections

The three large groups of metazoal parasites are

1. Roundworms
2. Tapeworms
3. Flukes

## Roundworms

The three most important roundworms that parasitize human beings are the *Ascaris*, the pinworm, and the *Trichinella* worm.

***Ascaris*** The *Ascaris lumbricoides* is the most commonly encountered parasitic worm, infecting an estimated one billion people worldwide. It is a large roundworm, about the size of a large earthworm, that lives in the intestinal tract and discharges eggs in the feces. Direct person-to-person transmission of *Ascaris* eggs does not occur because the eggs expelled in feces are immature, and a 2- to 3-week maturation period is required before the eggs become infectious. Maturation of the immature eggs usually occurs in the soil, as when fecal material is defecated on the ground if toilet facilities are not available or if a child is not toilet trained, or when fecal material is used to fertilize the soil for growing vegetables or other farm products, as is done in some countries. The mature eggs can survive in the soil for many years, and later contact with egg-contaminated soil may transfer eggs to hands, then to food or beverages, and finally into the intestinal tract.

When mature *Ascaris* eggs are ingested, the larval worms are released from the eggs within the intestinal tract, and the small larval worms burrow through the intestine, enter the circulatory system, and are carried in the circulation throughout the body. They are then filtered out in various organs and tissues. The larvae that lodge in the lung burrow through the alveolar walls and migrate into the bronchi, are coughed up, and eventually are swallowed, finding their way again into the small intestine where they grow to maturity. The stage characterized by the passage of *Ascaris* larvae through the lungs and other tissues is called *the phase of larval migration* and may be associated with fever, cough, and inflammation of the lungs. Adult worms living in the small intestine may at times wander from their usual location. They may migrate upward and be coughed up or vomited, or they may pass out through the nose. At times, they may enter and block the bile ducts or plug the appendix. Rarely, a large mass of worms may completely block the lumen of the small intestine. An *Ascaris* infection is identified by detecting worm eggs in the fecal material of an infected person or by identifying an adult worm as illustrated in Cases 5-6 and 5-7, which illustrate the migratory behavior of the *Ascaris* worm.

## Case Study 5-6

A young woman complained of a "funny feeling" in the back of her throat and coughed up a large *Ascaris* worm. The organism, which normally inhabits the small intestine, had migrated through the stomach and esophagus into the pharynx and was subsequently expelled ( Figure 5-17 ).

## Case Study 5-7

A child was admitted to the hospital with symptoms suggesting acute appendicitis, and an appendectomy was performed. When the base of the appendix was cut away from the colon during the removal, an *Ascaris* was found stuck in the appendix and was transected during the removal of the appendix ( Figure 5-18 ). The symptoms of appendicitis apparently had been caused by the worm lodged in the lumen of the appendix.

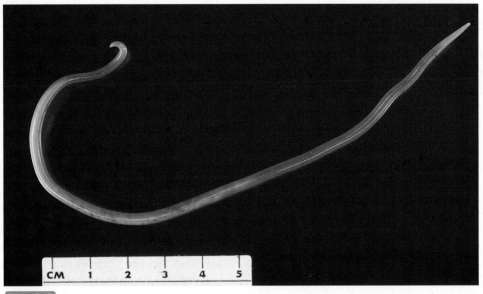

Figure 5-17   Large *Ascaris* that migrated into back of patient's throat and was coughed up.

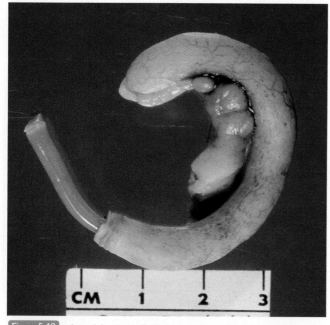

Figure 5-18 *Ascaris* in appendix that caused symptoms suggesting appendicitis. The head of a worm had entered the appendix, and the worm was transected when the appendix was removed.

Dogs and cats may be infected with a similar type of roundworm; the animal worm occasionally causes disease in humans. Infection by the animal worm is most common in children who are in close contact with an infected animal. The children transfer the eggs to their mouths by means of contaminated hands, toys, or other objects. The eggs hatch within the intestinal tract, and the larvae invade the tissues of the host, undergoing a phase of larval migration, which may be associated with systemic symptoms. However, the larvae that have been ingested by a foreign host are eventually destroyed within the tissues of the host and never reach maturity within the intestinal tract.

**Pinworms** The small roundworm *Enterobius vermicularis* is usually called simply the *pinworm* because of its small size, which generally measures less than 1 centimeter in length. Pinworm infections are very common, second only to *Ascaris* infections in frequency, and often infect children, who may harbor a large number of worms in their intestinal tract. Often the infection spreads from the child to the rest of the family members. The infection is acquired from ingesting worm eggs that are transferred to the hands from contaminated bedclothes or other objects. The worms hatch in the duodenum and then travel to the colon, where they take up residence. Female egg-laden worms migrate out of the colon through the anus, often at night while the child is asleep, and deposit their eggs on the perianal skin. Sometimes recently deposited eggs may hatch near the anus, and worms on the

perianal skin may travel back through the anus into the colon. Occasionally a worm may migrate into the vagina instead of the anus, and may travel through the genital tract until it is eventually destroyed by the body's defenses, but this is uncommon.

The main symptoms of pinworm infection are intense anal and perianal itching caused by irritation resulting from the migration of the worm. Pinworm eggs are usually not found in fecal material. The diagnosis of a pinworm infection is made by identifying the eggs deposited by migrating worms on the perianal skin. Usually a piece of Scotch Tape is applied to the skin, and any pinworm eggs present stick to the tape. Then the sticky side of the tape is attached to a glass slide, and the slide is examined microscopically for pinworm eggs. Sometimes a worm that has left the colon to deposit eggs can be identified by examining the perianal skin, as illustrated in Case 5-8. The disease is more a nuisance than a threat to life, as illustrated by the following case.

### Case Study 5-8

An 8-year-old girl, who had recently attended a slumber party at a neighbor's house, began to experience perianal and vulvar itching, which at times awakened her at night. On one such occasion, her mother examined the perineum after she had been awakened by the itching and found a small 1-centimeter-long worm moving around the perianal area. The mother collected the worm on a piece of Scotch Tape and brought it to her physician for evaluation.

It was a pinworm, and the eggs within the worm had the typical appearance of pinworm eggs. She was treated with an appropriate medication to eradicate the worms, and the other family members were also treated.

**Trichinella** Another small roundworm, *Trichinella spiralis*, causes a severe parasitic infection called *trichinosis*. The organism parasitizes not only humans, but also a wide variety of animals. Larval forms of the *Trichinella* are encapsulated as small cystic structures within the muscles of the infected human or animal host. People usually become infected by eating improperly cooked pork or meat from another *Trichinella*-infected animal. After the infected meat has been ingested, the larvae are released from their cysts and develop into mature parasitic worms in the small intestine. The worms then burrow into the intestinal mucosa and produce larvae, which gain access to the circulation and are carried throughout the body. They are filtered out in various tissues, where they incite an intense inflammatory reaction. The parasites that lodge in the muscles of the infected individual become encapsulated, forming small cysts within the muscle ( Figure 5-19 ). These cysts are the infectious form of the parasite. The phase of larval migration is associated with severe systemic symptoms, and there may also be symptoms referable to disturbed function of organs that have been heavily infiltrated by the parasites. Extremely heavy parasitic infestations may be fatal.

## Tapeworms

Tapeworms are long, ribbonlike worms that sometimes grow to a length of several feet. They inhabit the intestinal tract. In general, most tapeworms cause no great inconvenience to the individual carrying them except for depriving the host of the food that nourishes the worm. Three species of tapeworms are recognized: the pork tapeworm, the beef tapeworm, and the fish tapeworm. Humans become infected by eating the flesh of an infected animal that contains the larval form of the parasite.

## Flukes

Flukes are thick, fleshy, short worms that are provided with suckers for the attachment to the host. They have a complex life cycle involving one or more intermediate hosts. Flukes are classified according to the area of the body in which the development of the adult flukes is completed and the eggs are deposited. Some species of flukes live within the intestinal tract; others live within the liver; and one species lives within the lung. Some flukes, called *schistosomes* or blood flukes, live within the portal venous system and its tributaries or within the veins draining the bladder, where they cause serious damage to the surrounding tissues. Fluke infections are an important cause of illness and disability in some Asiatic countries, but human blood-fluke infections are not seen in the United States or Canada.

Although serious blood-fluke infections do not occur in North America, some animal schistosomes can infect humans, but they are more a nuisance than a cause of serious illness. Birds and mammals, infected with their own specific species of schistosomes, excrete them in their droppings into lakes and other bodies of water, where they develop into the infectious form of the parasite. People who swim in bird or animal schistosome-contaminated lakes may be "attacked" by the parasites, which can penetrate the skin of the swimmers. The parasites cause discrete areas of acute itchy inflammation at the site where they entered the skin. They cannot cause a systemic infection, however, because humans are not the normal host for the parasite, and the parasites are destroyed in the skin by the body's immune defenses. The condition is called *schistosome dermatitis* but is more commonly referred to as "swimmers' itch." Many lakes in North America and some saltwater beaches are infested by bird or animal schistosomes, and the problems they cause are illustrated in Case 5-9.

Table 5-5 summarizes the features of these common metazoal parasites.

**Arthropods** There are two common parasitic skin infestations: scabies and lice. Both are transmitted by close physical contact and are often spread by sexual contact. Both infestations respond promptly to treatment with antiparasitic medications applied to the skin.

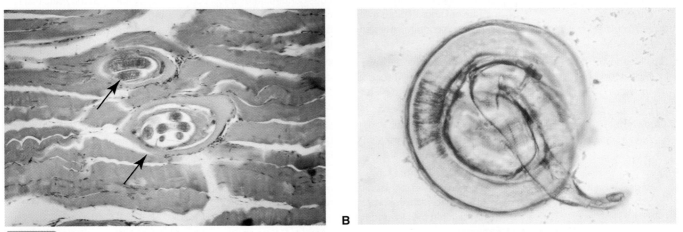

A B

Figure 5-19 Trichinosis. **A,** Biopsy of skeletal muscle showing encysted larvae surrounded by fibrous capsules. Each cyst measures about 1 millimeter in diameter (original magnification × 100). **B,** Higher magnification view of unstained coiled larva with the capsule removed (original magnification × 400).

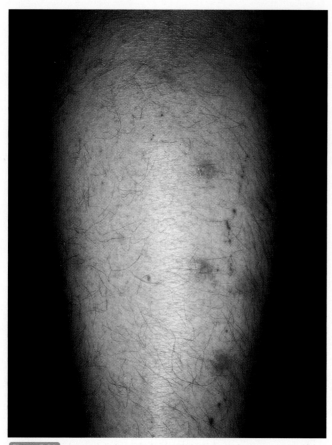

Figure 5-20 "Swimmers' itch." Multiple discrete areas of inflammation caused by animal schistosomes penetrating skin of calf.

### Case Study 5-9

A middle-aged man, who had a summer cabin in Wisconsin, spent the morning swimming and working on his dock. Soon afterward he developed multiple very itchy nodules on the skin of his legs ( Figure 5-20 ). He consulted a physician who diagnosed "swimmers' itch" and prescribed some medication to relieve the itching.

**Scabies**  Scabies is caused by a small parasite called *Sarcoptes scabiei*, which burrows in the superficial layers of the skin, where it lays eggs that hatch in a few days. The infestation causes intense itching. The tracks made by the parasites as they burrow in the skin appear as fine, wavy, dark lines in the skin measuring from 1 millimeter to 1 centimeter in length. Common sites of involvement are the base of the fingers, the wrists, the armpits, the skin around the nipples, and the skin around the belt line.

**Lice**  Of the various types of lice that may infest the body, the most common and best known is the crab louse (*Phthirus pubis*), which lives in the anal and

## Table 5-5    Characteristics of Common Metazoal Parasites

| Parasite | Source of Infection | Parasite Characteristics | Result of Infection |
|---|---|---|---|
| Large roundworm<br>*Ascaris lumbricoides* | Eggs expelled in stool require 2–3 weeks before eggs are infectious. Infection acquired from eggs in soil by hands directly to mouth or by egg contaminated food or beverages. | Larvae hatch in bowel, enter bloodstream, lodge in tissues, travel from lung to trachea and into throat, are swallowed, and mature in bowel. | Mature worms move around in bowel, may block appendix or bile duct, or several worms may form a ball that blocks the intestine. |
| Pinworm<br>*Enterobius vermicularis* | Worms live in colon and migrate out anus at night to lay eggs, which contaminate perianal tissues. | Eggs contaminate hands, bed clothes, and other surfaces. Eggs on hands spread infection through families and to others. | Heavy infection may cause itching and disturb sleep. Occasionally, worm may migrate into vagina instead of anus. |
| Small roundworm<br>*Trichinella spiralis* | Cyst of parasite in flesh of animals. Eating improperly cooked meat releases larvae to mature in small intestine. | Worms produce larvae that enter bloodstream and lodge in tissues. Larvae in muscle form cysts. | Larval migration causes severe inflammation in affected organs. Heavy infection may be very hazardous. |
| *Tapeworm*<br>*Taenia species* | Long ribbonlike worms acquired from eating meat of infected beef, pork, or fish. | Larvae mature in intestine, can become several feet long, and live for a long time. | Worms consume our food but usually don't cause any major problems. |
| Fluke<br>Bird or animal<br>*Schistosomes* | Complex life cycle that forms the infectious form of the parasite. Hazardous schistosomes do not occur in the United States. | Schistosome can invade skin of person swimming in contaminated water. | Schistosome lesions called "swimmers' itch" but systemic infection does not occur. |

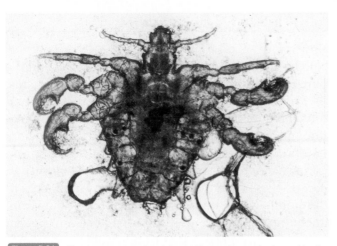

The appearance of crab louse, illustrating turtle-shaped body with three pairs of claws. The size is about 1 millimeter.

genital hairs ( Figure 5-21 ). The organism also causes intense itching. The louse lays eggs that become attached to the hair shafts. Diagnosis is established by identifying either the parasite or the eggs.

## Case Study 5-10

A young man complained of intense itching in the pubic area. Examination revealed small crab lice in the pubic hair (Figure 5-21) and numerous eggs attached to the hair shafts. Both the patient and his sexual partner were treated with an antiparasitic drug (Kwell).

# CHAPTER REVIEW

## Summary

We are surrounded by large numbers of microorganisms of various types, but only a few are harmful. Bacteria are widely distributed in our environments. They come in all sizes and shapes, and they are classified on their structure, staining reaction, biochemical characteristics, and antigenic structure. Although most are not pathogenic, some can be quite hazardous, including species of staphylococci, streptococci, *Neisseria*, various aerobic and anaerobic spore-forming bacteria, the acid-fast organisms that cause tuberculosis, and the spiral organisms that cause syphilis and Lyme disease. Many bacterial infections respond to antibiotics, and antibiotic sensitivity tests help us to select the most appropriate antibiotic to treat a serious infection. Unfortunately, many pathogens have become quite resistant to multiple antibiotics by developing adaptations to thwart the action of the antibiotic on the bacterial cell, and resistant organisms can pass their resistance genes to other bacteria, which further complicates treatment of infections.

Other groups of microorganisms that respond to antibiotics include chlamydiae that can only live inside a cell and form inclusion bodies in the infected cells. Rickettsiae and ehrlichiae are transmitted by insect bites and multiply in endothelial cells or white blood cells, and mycoplasmas are fragile bacteria lacking a cell wall but nevertheless can cause a type of pneumonia.

Viruses are simple structures that contain very few enzymes; they must "take over" the cells of the host in order to survive and multiply. Once established, many viruses persist indefinitely in the host tissues and may become active periodically to cause problems. Viruses are classified based on their structure as either DNA or RNA viruses, as well as on their size and their effects on the infected host. Relatively few antiviral agents are available against viruses, and some are moderately toxic.

Fungi are another large group of organisms. A few cause superficial skin and mucous membrane infections that are easy to treat with antifungal agents. A few cause acute pulmonary infections resulting from inhaling fungus spores present in the environment, such as histoplasmosis and coccidiodomycosis. Systemic fungus infections may be very hazardous to elderly adults or persons whose immune systems have been compromised.

Many parasitic infections are relatively common in the United States and Canada. Two different organisms parasitize and destroy red cells. Malaria is transmitted by mosquitoes, and babesiosis is transmitted from rodents to people by ticks. Both cause a febrile illness, and both can be very serious. One species of malaria is potentially fatal, and babesiosis in a splenectomized person is also very hazardous. Diagnosis is established by demonstrating the parasite in infected red cells. Amebiasis is less common and the parasite causes small colon ulcers and inflammation in the colon, often with diarrhea. The disease may be complicated by spread of the parasite from the colon to the liver via the portal venous drainage, leading to amebic hepatitis or liver abscess.

Trichomonad infection of the vagina causes vaginal discomfort and a profuse vaginal discharge in which the parasites can be identified, and can be treated with a drug effective against the parasite; the woman's sexual partner should also be treated to prevent a recurrent infection transmitted from her partner back to her.

Giardiasis is a common parasitic infection in many animals, and can be transmitted from animals to people by contact with water contaminated by feces from infected animals. Fecal-oral transmission via contaminated food or water may also transmit the infection. Campers and backpackers drinking untreated supposedly pure mountain stream water (contaminated by infected animal feces) are often infected. Toxoplasmosis is usually contacted from eating incompletely cooked meat from infected animals, or from contact with cats that excrete an infectious form of the parasite (oocyst) in their feces. A recently infected pregnant woman may transmit the parasite to her unborn child, which can cause severe fetal damage (described in Chapter 7). Cryptosporidiosis is caused by a small hardy parasite that is not destroyed by chlorination of water supplies, and requires filtration of water to eliminate the parasite. Several large outbreaks have occurred from unfiltered municipal water supplies. The illness causes an acute diarrhea that usually subsides in a short time, but persons whose immune system is impaired may not be able to eradicate the parasite.

The large roundworm *Ascaris lumbricoides* and the pinworm are the two most common worm infections. *Ascaris* infection is not transmitted by the fecal-oral route because the eggs excreted in the feces are immature and must mature for several weeks in the soil before they become infectious. Consequently the usual spread is from hands having contact with soil containing mature *Ascaris* eggs. Then the hands carry the *Ascaris* eggs to the mouth, which leads to the infection. The pinworm, in contrast, is easy to transmit from person to person via contact with bedclothes or other objects contaminated with pinworm eggs, and spread among family members occurs frequently. Trichinosis is a serious condition resulting from eating improperly cooked meat from an infected animal. The encysted larvae in the meat are released when the food is eaten, setting off a chain of events leading to migration of larvae in the circulation that damages the tissues in which they lodge. A heavy infection is always serious and potentially lethal.

Tapeworm infections are less common and usually not serious. The worms live for a long time, eat our food, but most species usually don't cause major problems. Serious fluke infections don't occur in the United States or Canada, but a bird or animal schistosome causes "swimmers' itch" (schistosome dermatitis) from swimming in lakes contaminated by bird or animal schistosomes that invade the skin, where they cause inflammation and itching, but are destroyed by the body's immune defenses. Scabies and crab lice are a nuisance but not a health hazard.

## Questions for Review

1. How are bacteria classified?
2. What is the Gram-stain test procedure? What important diseases are caused by the following bacteria: staphylococci, beta streptococci, pneumococci, gonococci, and acid-fast bacteria?
3. What is meant by the following terms: *granulomatous inflammation*, *gram-positive organism*, and *Legionella*?
4. How do antibiotics inhibit the growth of bacteria? How does penicillin kill bacteria?
5. How do bacteria become resistant to an antibiotic?
6. What are some of the potential harmful effects of antibiotics?
7. What is meant by the following terms: *competitive inhibition*, *sensitivity test*, *resistant organism*, and *cell membrane*?
8. What is a latent (asymptomatic) viral infection?
9. What factors render a patient susceptible to an infection by a fungus of low pathogenicity?
10. What are the names of the two highly pathogenic fungi? What type of disease do they cause?
11. A young woman receives a course of antibiotics and soon afterward develops a vaginal infection caused by a fungus. Why?
12. What are some of the more important protozoal infections?
13. How is malaria transmitted?
14. What is trichinosis? How is it transmitted?
15. Name three important worm infections. What are their manifestations?
16. What are "crabs"? What symptoms do they cause? How are they acquired?
17. How do people become infected with pinworms? How do they acquire an *Ascaris* infection?

## Supplementary Reading

Centers for Disease Control and Prevention. 1994. Cryptosporidium infections associated with swimming pools—Dane County, Wisconsin, 1993. *Morbidity and Mortality Weekly Report* 43:561–63.

Members of a swim team became infected from a swimming pool. Measures to prevent such infections are discussed.

Centers for Disease Control and Prevention. 2000. Coccidioidomycosis in travelers returning from Mexico—Pennsylvania. *Morbidity and Mortality Weekly Report* 49:1004–6.

Thirty-five church members from two cities in Pennsylvania spent a week in Mexico to construct a church, and 27 developed acute coccidioidomycosis (CM) within 2 weeks after returning home.

Travel to endemic areas is becoming more frequent and presents a special risk to elderly and persons with impaired immunity, who may develop severe pulmonary disease or widely disseminated disease.

Centers for Disease Control and Prevention. 2001. Coccidioidomycosis in workers at an archeological site—Dinosaur National Monument, Utah, June–July 2001. *Morbidity and Mortality Weekly Report* 50:1005–8.

Under the direction of National Park Service (NPS) archaeologists, six student volunteers and two leaders worked at an archaeological site. All eight team members and two NPS archaeologists developed acute coccidioidomycosis with pulmonary symptoms and abnormal chest x-rays, and eight were hospitalized.

Centers for Disease Control and Prevention. 2001. Update: Outbreak of acute febrile respiratory illness among college students—Acapulco, Mexico, March 2001. *Morbidity and Mortality Weekly Report* 50:359–60.

Two hundred twenty-nine students from 44 colleges in 22 states who went to Acapulco in Mexico during spring break developed acute histoplasmosis characterized by cough, shortness of breath, chest pain, or headache. They stayed at several different hotels during spring break but one hotel was associated with the largest number of cases.

Chen, X., Keithly, J. S., Paya, C. V., and LaRusso, N. F. 2002. Cryptosporidiosis. *New England Journal of Medicine* 346:1723–80.

An update on the organism's life cycle, clinical features, diagnosis, and management.

Hayes, E. B., Matte, T. D., O'Brien, T. R., et al. 1989. Large community outbreak of cryptosporidiosis as a result of contamination of filtered water supply. *New England Journal of Medicine* 320:1372–76.

Parasites in municipal supply caused a large outbreak affecting 13,000 residents of a community in Georgia due to a defective filtration system.

Kimberlin, D. W., and Whitley, R. J. 2007. Varicella-zoster vaccine for prevention of herpes zoster. *New England Journal of Medicine* 356;1338–43.

An active live virus vaccine has been developed to immunize against chickenpox. A somewhat similar vaccine is available to help prevent herpes zoster in older adults who had chickenpox many years ago.

Klevins, R. M., Morrison, M., Nadle, M. A., et al. 2007. Invasive methicillin-resistant *Staphylococcus aureus* infections in the United States. *Journal of the American Medical Association* 298:1763–71.

Invasive methicillin-resistant staphylococcal infections (MRSA) were classified as either health-care associated (in hospitals or related health-care facilities) or in the community (affecting patients without health-care risk factors for MRSA). Invasive MRSA is a major public-health problem related to health care but has spread into the community and is no longer confined to health-care institutions.

MacKenzie, W. R., et al. 1994. A massive outbreak in Milwaukee of cryptosporidium infection transmitted through the public water supply. *New England Journal of Medicine* 331:161–67.

Documents a huge outbreak with some deaths related to this parasite in unfiltered water.

Phares, C., Lynfield, R., Farley, M., et al. 2008. Epidemiology of invasive group B streptococcal disease in the United States, 1999–2005. *Journal of the American Medical Association* 299:2056–64.

Disease-prevention guidelines have reduced the frequency of B streptococcal disease in infants, but have been associated with a greater number of invasive streptococcal disease cases in older children and adults, as well as in pregnant women.

# Interactive Activities

## Matching 1

Match the parasite in the right column with the clinical manifestations in the left column.

| Manifestations | Organism |
|---|---|
| 1. "Swimmers' itch" | A. Pinworms |
| 2. Profuse vaginal discharge | B. *Plasmodium* species |
| 3. Maternal infection may injure the fetus of pregnant women | C. Crab louse |
| 4. Severe diarrhea after eating a meal of rice and ground beef | D. *Ascaris* worm |
| 5. Person coughs up a large roundworm | E. *Trichomonas* |
| 6. Diarrhea after swimming in chlorinated swimming pool | F. *Cryptosporidium* |
| 7. Chills and fever after returning from trip to region where malaria is endemic | G. Pathogenic ameba |
| 8. Perianal itching awakens child at night | H. *Toxoplasma* |
| 9. Marked itching of pubic skin | I. *Schistosomes* |
| 10. Malarialike illness in person who has had the spleen removed | J. Babesiosis |

## Matching 2

Match the disease in the right column with the responsible organism in the left column.

| Organism | Disease |
|---|---|
| 1. Group A beta streptococcus | A. Severe throat infection |
| 2. Group B beta streptococcus | B. Warts |
| 3. Hemolytic staphylococcus | C. Infection of newborn infant |
| 4. Human papillomavirus | D. "Fever blisters" |
| 5. *Histoplasma capsulatum* | E. Pulmonary infection |
| 6. Herpesvirus | F. Germ warfare agent |
| 7. Varicella-zoster virus | G. Wound infection |
| 8. Mumps virus | H. Skin rash |
| 9. *Bacillus anthracis* | I. Parotid gland infection |
| 10. Meningococcus (*Neisseria meningitidis*) | J. Meningitis |

## Matching 3

Match the organism in the left column with the disease or condition in the right column.

| Organism | Disease |
|---|---|
| 1. *Brucella* | A. Paralysis from eating toxin-containing food |
| 2. *Borrelia* | B. A febrile illness transmitted to people from unpasteurized milk or tissues of infected animal |
| 3. *Ehrlichiae* | C. Causes a febrile illness with skin lesion |
| 4. *Clostridium botulinum* | D. Causes bubonic plague |
| 5. *Yersinia* | E. A tick-transmitted rickettsialike agent that infects white blood cells |

## True or False

Indicate whether the following statements are true or false by indicating T or F at the end of the statement.

1. Most fungi are highly pathogenic and frequently cause disease in humans.＿＿＿

2. Some viruses persist indefinitely in the tissues of the host and become activated periodically, causing disease.＿＿＿

3. Histoplasmosis results from the bite of an infected rodent.＿＿＿

4. A newborn infant may become infected with a group B beta hemolytic streptococcus from the mother's birth canal during delivery.＿＿＿

5. Chlamydia may be transmitted by sexual intercourse, and may infect the cervix and fallopian tubes.＿＿＿

6. *Ascaris* infection may result from eating food prepared by a person with an *Ascaris* infection.＿＿＿

7. Cryptosporidiosis is characterized by an infection of the lungs.＿＿＿

8. Malaria is transmitted by mosquitoes.＿＿＿

9. Babesiosis is characterized by a malarialike febrile illness.＿＿＿

10. Toxoplasmosis is characterized by a profuse vaginal discharge.＿＿＿

## Critical Thinking

1. Nancy Lee has developed oral herpes and has some vesicles and blisters around her mouth. She is concerned that the herpes infection will make her susceptible to developing herpes zoster as well. What would you tell her?

2. Eric Johansen spent spring break at a hotel in Mexico, and heard from news reports that a number of students at the hotel became ill with a respiratory infection that was diagnosed as acute histoplasmosis. He wants to know how the infection was acquired and whether he also is at risk of developing the infection. What should he do?

3. Susan Castro's son Michael experienced abdominal pain interpreted as appendicitis and his appendix was removed. A large roundworm was found plugging the lumen of the appendix, which was the cause of Michael's symptoms. Susan asks you what she should do now. What would you tell her?

4. John Jones experienced recent onset of pubic itching and he suspects that he may have crab lice. How can he determine whether the itching is caused by crab lice? If the itching is caused by lice, what should he do? Can the condition be transmitted to another person?

# 6 Communicable Diseases

## Methods of Transmission and Control

An infectious disease that is readily transmitted from person to person is considered a **communicable disease**. Such a disease is said to be **endemic** (*en* = within + *demos* = population) if small numbers of cases are continually present in the population. It reaches **epidemic** proportions (*epi* = upon + *demos* = population) when relatively large numbers of people are affected. Sometimes an endemic disease may flare up and assume epidemic proportions.

## Methods of Transmission

A communicable disease may be transmitted from person to person by either direct or indirect methods. Direct transmission is either by direct physical contact or by means of droplet spread, such as by coughing or sneezing. Indirect transmission of an infectious agent

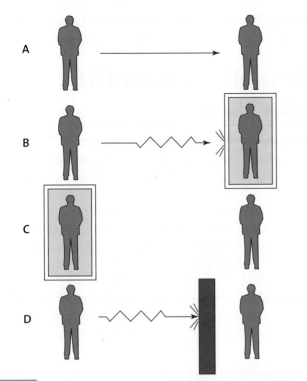

**Figure 6-1** Methods of eradicating or controlling a communicable disease. **A,** Unimpeded direct or indirect transmission of a communicable disease from person to person. **B,** Immunization protects a susceptible person by conferring resistance to infection. **C,** Isolation and prompt treatment of the infected person prevent the spread of disease to susceptible persons. **D,** Control of means of indirect transmission blocks spread of infectious agent.

is accomplished by some intermediary mechanism, such as transmission in contaminated water or by means of insects. A few communicable diseases are primarily diseases of animals and are transmitted to humans only incidentally.

For a communicable disease to perpetuate itself, there must be a continuous transmission of the infectious agent from person to person by either direct or indirect methods. Therefore, in order to eradicate or control the disease, the chain of transmission must be broken at some point ( Figure 6-1 ).

# Methods of Control

This section deals with some of the methods that can be applied to control communicable diseases. In practice, multiple methods of control are applied whenever possible.

## Immunization

If a large proportion of the population can be immunized against a communicable disease, the disease will eventually die out because there will be very few susceptible persons in the population. Smallpox is an example of a disease that has been eliminated worldwide because of widespread immunization. Poliomyelitis is another disease that has been virtually eradicated in the United

States as a result of widespread immunization of persons at risk.

Immunization can also be used to protect susceptible persons entering a foreign country where a communicable disease is endemic. The immunized person will no longer be susceptible to the disease, even though the disease is widespread in the native population.

**communicable disease**
A disease transmitted from person to person.

**endemic disease**
(en-dem´ik)
A communicable disease in which small numbers of cases are continually present in a population.

**epidemic disease**
(ep-i-dem´ik)
A communicable disease affecting concurrently large numbers of persons in a population.

## Identification, Isolation, and Treatment of Infected Persons

Sick persons are identified and treated promptly in order to shorten the time during which they can infect others. Isolation of infected persons prevents contact with susceptible persons and stops the spread of the disease. Identification, isolation, and treatment are the primary methods used to control diseases when effective methods of immunization are not available. In some cases, these measures are difficult to accomplish because some diseases produce relatively few symptoms in the infected individual. For example, the person infected with tuberculosis or a sexually transmitted disease may spread the disease to others, but his or her own disease may not be recognized and treated because the person does not feel ill and does not seek medical treatment.

## Control of Means of Indirect Transmission

Various control measures can be instituted, depending on the manner by which the infectious agent is transmitted. Where the transmission is by means of contaminated food or water, methods of control include chlorination of water supplies and establishment of effective sewage treatment facilities, control of food handlers, and standards for monitoring the manufacture and distribution of commercially prepared foods. When a disease is transmitted by insects, either between people or between infected animals and people, it is necessary to eradicate or control the insects that transmit the disease. When a disease is spread from animals to people, control of the animal source of infection also is required.

## Requirements for Effective Control

Application of effective control measures requires knowing the cause of the disease and its method of transmission. If this information is not available, control measures are often ineffective. For example, bubonic plague, the "black death" of the Middle Ages, decimated entire populations because the people understood neither the cause of the disease nor how it was transmitted and therefore were unable to protect themselves from its ravages. We now know that plague is primarily a disease of rats and other rodents, that it is caused by a bacterium, and that it is transmitted to people by insects. In some cases, the plague bacillus causes a pulmonary infection in people. When this occurs, direct transmission from person to person can be through droplet spread, causing an extremely contagious and highly fatal pulmonary infection called *pneumonic plague*. In some parts of the United States, plague infection still persists in some rodent populations, but plague is no longer a serious problem because the disease can be largely prevented in people by controlling the infected animal population and by instituting measures that prevent close contact between potentially infected rodents and people. Trans-

mission from person to person is prevented by prompt isolation and treatment of infected persons.

# Sexually Transmitted Diseases

Sexually transmitted diseases are communicable diseases that spread primarily by sexual contact and have reached epidemic proportions. They can be transmitted by sexual relations between heterosexual partners and by sexual acts between individuals of the same sex. The four major sexually transmitted diseases are syphilis, gonorrhea, genital herpes infection, and genital chlamydial infections (Table 6-1). In a class by itself because of its devastating consequences and high mortality is the **acquired immune deficiency syndrome (AIDS)**, which is transmitted by both homosexual and heterosexual contacts and by blood and secretions from infected persons.

## Table 6-1   Comparison of Four Major Sexually Transmitted Diseases

|  | Syphilis | Gonorrhea | Herpes | Chlamydia |
|---|---|---|---|---|
| Organism | *Treponema pallidum* | Gonococcus (*Neisseria gonorrhoeae*) | Herpesvirus | *Chlamydia trachomatis* |
| Major clinical manifestations | Primary: chancre<br>Secondary: systemic infection with skin rash and enlarged lymph nodes<br>Tertiary: late destructive lesions in internal organs | Urethritis<br>Cervicitis<br>Pharyngitis<br>Infection of rectal mucosa (proctitis) | Superficial vesicles and ulcers on external genitalia and in genital tract<br>Regional lymph nodes often enlarged and tender | Cervicitis<br>Urethritis |
| Tests used to establish diagnosis | Demonstration of treponemas in chancre<br>Serologic tests | Culture of organisms from sites of infection<br>Nonculture tests also available | Demonstration of intranuclear inclusions in infected cells<br>Virus cultures<br>Serologic tests in some cases | Detection of chlamydial antigens in cervical/urethral secretions<br>Fluorescence microscopy<br>Cultures<br>Nonculture tests also available |
| Major complications | Damage to cardiovascular system and nervous system in tertiary syphilis may be fatal | Disseminated bloodstream infection<br>Tubal infection with impaired fertility<br>Spread of infection to prostate and epididymides | Spread from infected mother to infant | Tubal infection with impaired fertility<br>Epididymitis |
| Treatment | Antibiotics | Antibiotics | Antiviral drug shortens infection but not curative | Antibiotics |

Other common but less serious sexually transmitted diseases, considered in Chapter 5, are anal and genital warts (condylomas) caused by the papillomavirus, trichomonal vaginitis caused by the protozoan parasite *Trichomonas vaginalis*, as well as scabies and crab lice caused by arthropod parasites.

## Syphilis

Syphilis, caused by the spirochete *Treponema pallidum*, is a very serious sexually transmitted disease because it may cause severe damage in almost any organ of the body. If the disease is not treated, it progresses through three stages called primary, secondary, and tertiary syphilis. Each stage has its own characteristic clinical manifestations.

**Primary Syphilis**   Contact with an infected partner enables the treponemas to penetrate the mucous membranes of the genital tract, oral cavity, or rectal mucosa, or to be introduced through a break in the skin. The organisms multiply rapidly and spread throughout the body. After an incubation period of several weeks, a small ulcer called a *chancre* develops at the site of inoculation. It is easily seen if it is on the penis or vulva, but it may be undetected if it is within the vagina, oral cavity, or rectum.

The chancre, which is swarming with treponemas and is highly infectious, persists for about 4 to 6 weeks and eventually heals even if the disease is untreated. Even though the chancre has healed, however, the treponemas are widely disseminated through the body and continue to multiply.

**Secondary Syphilis**   The secondary stage of syphilis begins several months after the chancre has healed. The infected individual develops manifestations of a systemic infection characterized by elevated temperature, enlargement of lymph nodes, a skin rash, and shallow ulcers on the mucous membranes of the oral cavity and genital tract. This stage of the disease also is extremely infectious because the skin and mucous-membrane lesions contain large numbers of treponemas. The secondary stage persists for several weeks and, like the chancre, eventually subsides even if no treatment is administered. Some subjects experience one or more recurrences of secondary syphilis, but each recurrence subsides spontaneously.

**Tertiary Syphilis**   After the second stage subsides, the infected individual appears well for a variable period of time, but the organisms are still active and may cause irreparable damage to the cardiovascular and nervous systems and to other organs as well. Often the wall of the ascending aorta is damaged by the treponemas, which causes the weakened aortic wall to dilate. Consequently the aortic valve leaflets attached to the dilated aortic wall can't function normally, which leads to aortic insufficiency. The weakened aortic wall may balloon out, forming an aortic aneurysm that may rupture. Degeneration of fiber tracts in the spinal cord caused by syphilis impairs sensation and disturbs walking. Damage to the brain by the treponemas causes mental deterioration and eventual paralysis. The late manifestations of the disease, which can appear as long as 20 years after the initial infection, are called *tertiary syphilis*. This stage is not generally communicable because the organisms are relatively few and are confined to the internal organs.

**Diagnosis and Treatment**   Two different types of laboratory tests are used to diagnose syphilis:

1. Demonstration of treponemas, by means of microscopic examination, in fluid squeezed from the ulcerated surface of the chancre. Specialized techniques and equipment are required.
2. Blood tests, called serologic tests for syphilis, detect the various antibodies produced in response to a treponemal infection. The serologic tests become positive soon after the chancre appears and remain positive for many years.

Both types of tests are widely used; each has specific applications and limitations. Microscopic examination of material from a suspected chancre establishes the diagnosis of syphilis several weeks before a blood test will show positive results. On the other hand, if the chancre is in an inaccessible location and escapes detection, a positive blood test may be the only indication of syphilis in an individual who does not exhibit symptoms of active infection.

Syphilis can be treated successfully by penicillin and some other antibiotics. Treatment stops the progression of the disease and prevents serious late complications.

**Congenital Syphilis**   A syphilitic mother may transmit the disease to her unborn infant. The intrauterine infection may cause death of the fetus, or the infant may be born with congenital syphilis. The treponemas seem to be less able to pass through the placenta to infect the fetus during the first few months of pregnancy. Early in pregnancy the placental villi are covered by a double layer of epithelium and contain more connective tissue compared with their appearance later in pregnancy, which may account for their reduced permeability. An infected mother should be treated as soon as the maternal infection is identified without regard to the stage of her pregnancy, but it is unlikely that the fetus will be infected if treatment is started during the early months of the pregnancy.

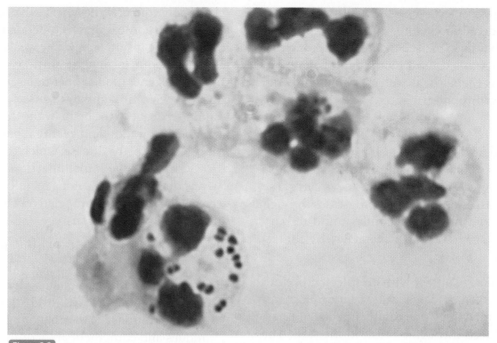

**Figure 6-2** Gram stain of pus from the urethra, illustrating many gram-negative intracellular diplococci characteristic of gonorrhea (original magnification × 1000).

## Gonorrhea

Gonorrhea, caused by the gonococcus *Neisseria gonorrhoeae*, is one of the most common communicable diseases (Figure 6-2). The organism primarily infects mucosal surfaces: the linings of the urethra, genital tract, pharynx, and rectum. Symptoms of infection appear about a week after exposure, and the clinical manifestations differ in the two sexes.

**Gonorrhea in the Female**  In the female, the gonococci infect chiefly the mucosa of the uterine cervix and the urethral mucosa. The gonococcal infection may also spread into Bartholin's glands, which are located adjacent to the vaginal orifice. The cervical infection usually causes profuse vaginal discharge; the urethral involvement is manifested by pain and burning on urination. Some women, however, have few or no symptoms of infection but are nevertheless capable of transmitting the disease to their sexual partners. The gonococcal infection may also spread upward from the cervix through the uterus into the fallopian tubes, where it causes an acute salpingitis (*salpinx* = tube). Sometimes the tubal infection is followed by the formation of an abscess within the fallopian tube or an abscess involving both the tube and the adjacent ovary.

Gonococcal salpingitis is manifested by abdominal pain and tenderness together with elevated temperature and leukocytosis. Scarring following the tubal infection may delay transport of the fertilized ovum through the fallopian tube, causing the pregnancy to develop in the tube instead of the uterus, a condition called an ectopic pregnancy (described in Chapter 14). Complete obstruction of both tubes by scar tissue completely blocks the transport of a fertilized ovum through the tubes and leads to sterility.

**Gonorrhea in the Male**  In the male, gonococci cause an acute inflammation of the mucosa of the anterior part of the urethra. The infection is usually manifested by a purulent urethral discharge and considerable pain on urination, but occasionally the infected male may have relatively few symptoms, although he is still capable of infecting others. However, gonorrhea is less likely to be asymptomatic in men than in women.

From the anterior urethra, the infection often spreads by direct extension into the posterior urethra, prostate, seminal vesicles, vasa deferentia, and epididymides. An infection in both epididymides and vasa deferentia may lead to sterility because the scarring after the infection may obstruct the duct system and thus block transport of sperm into the seminal fluid.

**Extragenital Gonorrhea**  Recently, the incidence of gonococcal infection in extragenital sites has increased. Gonoccocal infection of the rectal mucosa causes anorectal pain and tenderness associated with purulent bloody mucoid discharge from the rectum. Rectal infection results from contamination of the rectal mucosa either by infected vaginal secretions or from anal intercourse. Gonococcal infection of the pharynx

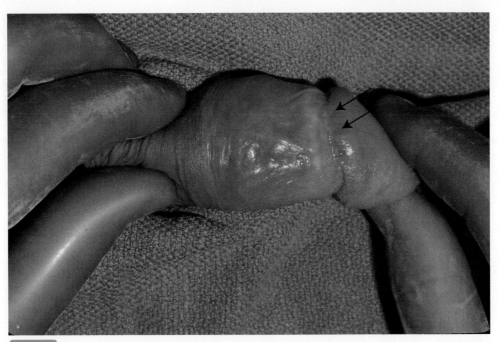

**Figure 6-3** Several small superficial herpetic ulcers on shaft of penis behind glans (*arrows*).

and tonsils results from oral–genital sex acts. The infection may be asymptomatic but often causes a sore throat.

**Disseminated Gonococcal Infection** In a small proportion of infected patients, the organism gains access to the bloodstream and spreads throughout the body. This serious complication is characterized by elevated temperature, joint pain, multiple small abscesses in the skin, and sometimes infections of the joints, tendons, heart valves, and covering of the brain (meninges).

**Diagnosis and Treatment** Diagnosis of gonorrhea is established by culturing gonococci from suspected sites of infection: urethra, cervix, rectum, and pharynx. Gonococci may also be cultured from the bloodstream in disseminated gonococcal infection. A non–culture-based test to identify gonococci (called a nucleic acid amplification test) is also available. The test is based on the identification of groups of nucleic acids in the organism. Formerly, most infections responded to penicillin. Now many strains produce an enzyme (penicillinase) that inactivates penicillin so that the antibiotic is ineffective, and some strains have also become resistant to other antibiotics as well. Consequently, selection of an appropriate antibiotic to treat a gonococcal infection is more difficult than in the past.

## Herpes

The herpes simplex virus is one of several herpesviruses that infect people. There are two forms of the herpes simplex virus, designated type 1 and 2. Type 1 herpes usually infects the oral mucous membrane, where it causes the familiar fever blisters. Most individuals are infected in childhood, and most adults have antibodies to the virus, indicating a previous infection. Type 2 herpesvirus usually infects the genital tract, and infections usually occur after puberty. However, the two types are not restricted in their distribution. Type 1 virus may cause genital infections, and type 2 virus may infect the oropharyngeal mucous membrane.

The lesions caused by the viral infection usually appear within a week after sexual exposure. They consist of clusters of very small, painful blisters (vesicles) that soon rupture, forming painful shallow ulcers that often coalesce. The lesions contain large quantities of virus and are infectious to sexual contacts. Usually the lymph nodes draining the infected areas are swollen and tender. In men, the vesicles usually appear on the glans or shaft of the penis ( Figure 6-3 ). In women, the lesions may be quite extensive ( Figure 6-4 ). They may be on the vulva, in the vagina, or on the cervix. Vulvar lesions are quite painful, but those deep in the vagina or on the cervix may cause little discomfort because these regions are relatively insensitive. The ulcers heal slowly in a few weeks. However, the virus persists in the tissues of the infected person and may flare up periodically, causing recurrent infections. Some patients have repeated flare-ups for several years after the initial infection.

Active herpetic ulcers shed large amounts of virus, and sexual partners of patients with active lesions are readily infected. Unfortunately, patients without active

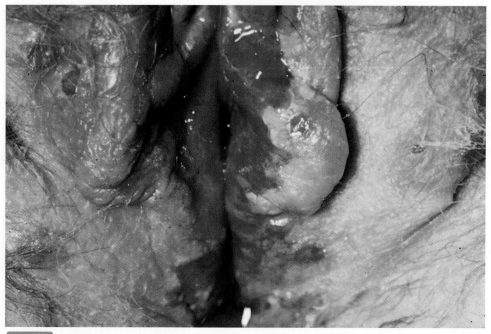

Figure 6-4   Multiple confluent ulcers of vulva as a result of herpes.

lesions also may excrete small amounts of virus periodically and infect their sexual partners even though they have no lesions or symptoms of infection.

**Diagnosis and Treatment**   Herpes can usually be suspected from the clinical appearance of the lesions and can be confirmed by smears obtained from the lesions, which reveal the characteristic intranuclear inclusions in infected cells (Figure 6-5). The most reliable diagnostic test is a culture of the virus from the ulcers and vesicles, and facilities for virus culture are now widely available.

Antiviral drugs are available that shorten the course and reduce the severity of an acute infection, but do not eradicate the virus.

## Genital Chlamydial Infections

Genital tract infections caused by *Chlamydia trachomatis* (Chapter 5) are now the most common sexually transmitted disease, and it has been estimated that there are between 3 and 4 million new cases each year. Part of this increase reflects the availability of new diagnostic tests that enable the physician to recognize

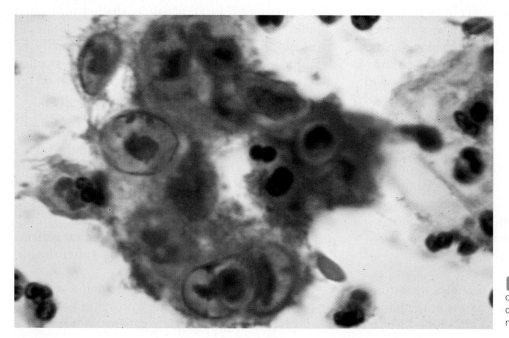

Figure 6-5   Vaginal smear illustrating clusters of herpes-infected epithelial cells containing intranuclear inclusions (original magnification × 1000).

chlamydial infections in patients who have few symptoms and whose cases probably would previously have gone undetected.

Chlamydia causes much the same type of inflammation and clinical symptoms as gonorrhea. In women, the initial infection is usually in the uterine cervix and is associated with moderate vaginal discharge. Men often develop acute inflammation of the urethra associated with frequency and burning on urination, which is called nongonococcal urethritis. Like gonorrhea, the chlamydial infection may spread to the fallopian tubes in women, followed by scarring and impaired fertility, and may cause acute epididymitis in men. As in gonorrhea, many infected persons may have no symptoms of infection but are still able to infect their sexual partners and may develop complications related to the spread of the infection to other parts of the genital tract.

**Diagnosis and Treatment** Highly sensitive specific tests can detect chlamydial antigens in cervical secretions and secretions from the male urethra, and tests can also be performed on urine. Nucleic acid amplification tests, similar to the tests used to identify gonococci, can also be used to diagnose a chlamydial infection by identifying characteristic groups of chlamydial nucleic acids. The infection responds to tetracycline antibiotics. Both the client and his or her partner should be treated.

# Human Immunodeficiency Virus Infections and AIDS

AIDS is a devastating disease that cripples the body's immune system by attacking and destroying helper T lymphocytes, making the affected persons susceptible to a number of unusual infections and malignant tumors. Although HIV infection is often regarded as a sexually transmitted disease, many HIV infections are transmitted in other ways.

The first cases of the disease that we now call AIDS were identified in 1981 in a small group of homosexual men with an unusual lung infection. HIV was identified in 1983, and a blood test to detect HIV infection became available in 1985. Today we know a lot about the virus and how it damages the immune system, and we know how to avoid becoming infected. We can slow the multiplication of the virus and we can arrest the progression of the disease that it causes but we cannot completely eliminate the virus from the body of an infected person.

## HIV and Its Target

HIV is an RNA virus that belongs to a class of viruses called *retroviruses*. The viral RNA and an important enzyme called *reverse transcriptase* are enclosed within a protein coat (capsid), forming the core of the virus. The core is surrounded by an envelope, composed of a double layer of lipid molecules, that was acquired from the cell membrane of the infected cell when the virus budded from the cell. When the virus binds to the cell, the virus envelope fuses with the cell membrane, and the virus enters the cell. Once inside the cell, the virus makes a DNA copy of its own RNA genetic material by means of its reverse transcriptase enzyme, and the DNA copy is inserted into the genetic material of the infected cell, a process assisted by another viral enzyme called *HIV integrase*, and the viral genes direct the synthesis and assembly of more virus. The final stages of virus production requires a viral enzyme called *HIV protease*, which cuts and assembles the virus protein into small segments that surround the viral RNA, forming the infectious virus particles that bud from the infected cells. As the virus particles bud from the cells, they become coated by part of the cell membranes of the infected cells. The newly formed virus particles attack other susceptible cells within the lymphoid tissue throughout the body, where the virus replicates (proliferates) and releases more virus particles to infect still more susceptible cells.

## Manifestations of HIV Infection

During the early stages of the infection, large amounts of virus can be detected in the blood and body fluids of the infected person, and large numbers of virus-infected lymphocytes are present in lymph nodes and other lymphoid tissue throughout the body. During this phase, many infected persons develop a mild febrile illness. The body responds to the infection by forming anti-HIV antibodies and by generating cytotoxic T lymphocytes. The amount of virus in the blood and body fluids declines as the acute phase of the infection subsides, but unfortunately, the body's defenses are not able to eliminate the virus, and the infection enters a more chronic phase. However, there is no latent or dormant phase where the virus remains inactive. Very large numbers of virus particles are produced continuously that infect and destroy helper T (CD4+) cells. Large numbers of virus particles also circulate in the bloodstream, and the amount of virus in the blood correlates with the magnitude of the infection in the body's lymphoid tissue.

The body responds to the destruction of helper T cells by stepping up production of more helper T cells to replace those killed by the virus. Cytotoxic (CD8+) T cells directed against the virus proliferate in an attempt

| Table 6-2 | Sequence of Events in HIV Infections and Their Significance |
| --- | --- |
| **Event** | **Significance** |
| HIV invades CD4+ cells and becomes part of cell DNA | Individual is infected for life |
| Virus proliferates in infected cells and sheds virus particles | Virus present in blood and body fluids |
| Body forms anti-HIV antibody | Antibody is a marker of infection but is not protective |
| Progressive destruction of helper T cells | Compromised cell-mediated immunity |
| Immune defenses collapse | Opportunistic infections Neoplasms |

**opportunistic infection** (op-por-too-nis´tik) An infection in an immunocompromised person caused by an organism that is normally nonpathogenic or of limited pathogenicity.

to restrain the viral multiplication and the helper T-cell destruction. Without treatment the rate at which CD4+ cells are replaced cannot keep up with the rate of destruction, and the functions of the immune system begin to decline.

Generally, anti-HIV antibodies appear from 1 to as long as 6 months after the initial infection. Unfortunately, the antibodies cannot eradicate the virus or reduce its infectivity. Nevertheless, a confirmed positive test for virus antibodies is a useful test to indicate that a person has been infected with HIV, is infectious to others, and is at risk of damage to the immune system from the infection. Table 6-2 summarizes the sequence of events in HIV infection and their significance.

## Measurement of Viral RNA and CD4+ Lymphocytes as an Index of Disease Progression

Although HIV replicates in lymph nodes and not in the blood, the amount of viral RNA in the blood reflects the extent of viral replication in the lymphoid tissue throughout the body and can vary from over a million virus particles per milliliter of blood plasma in a patient with an acute infection to extremely low levels in a patient being treated successfully with agents effective against the virus.

A determination of the number of helper T lymphocytes in the blood allows one to estimate the extent of damage to the immune system. Normally, there are from about 800 to 1200 helper T (CD4+) lymphocytes per microliter of blood, but this number declines progressively as the disease advances. When this number falls to about 500 cells per microliter of blood, the

patient becomes at risk of opportunistic infections, and by the time the helper T-lymphocyte count falls below 200 per microliter, the infected person is at very high risk of major complications from the disease.

## Complications of AIDS

The impaired cell-mediated immunity leads to two very serious problems: a greatly increased susceptibility to infection and a predisposition to various malignant tumors.

**Infections** Many of the viruses, fungi, parasites, and other pathogens that attack AIDS patients do not usually cause disease in healthy persons. (Infections of this type are often called **opportunistic infections** because the pathogens normally do not have an *opportunity* to cause serious disease in persons whose immune systems are intact.) One of the most common AIDS-related opportunistic infections is pneumonia caused by the protozoan parasite *Pneumocystis jiroveci* (Chapter 12). Another relatively common and serious systemic infection is caused by a normally nonpathogenic acid-fast bacterium called *Mycobacterium avium* complex. Other serious infections are the parasitic infections *toxoplasmosis* and *cryptosporidiosis*, described in Chapter 5.

AIDS patients are also at risk for acquiring widespread, rapidly progressive tuberculosis or histoplasmosis, infections that normally are held in check by persons with normal immune systems. Many of the symptoms exhibited by patients with AIDS such as fever, cough, shortness of breath, weight loss, and enlarged lymph nodes are the result of the severe pulmonary infections. Table 6-3 lists some of the more common, severe, and often life-threatening infections in AIDS patients.

**Malignant Tumors** The malignant tumors common in AIDS patients also are related to failure of the immune system, which helps to protect persons from tumors as well as infections (Chapter 8). The most common malignant tumor in AIDS patients, that is rare in other persons, is Kaposi's sarcoma, that is caused by a herpes-

| Table 6-3 | Common Infections in AIDS Patients |
| --- | --- |
| Viruses | Herpes, cytomegalovirus, Epstein-Barr virus (infectious mononucleosis) |
| Fungi | Histoplasmosis, coccidioidomycosis, aspergillosis, *Candida* infections |
| Protozoa | *Pneumocystis* pneumonia, amebiasis, cryptosporidiosis, toxoplasmosis |
| Mycobacteria | Tuberculosis, *Mycobacterium avium* complex infections |

virus designated *human herpesvirus 8*. This tumor, which is composed of immature connective-tissue cells (fibroblasts) and blood capillaries intermixed with inflammatory and phagocytic cells, forms hemorrhagic nodules in the skin, mouth, lymph nodes, and internal organs (Figure 6-6). Malignant tumors of B lymphocytes also are common, as are cancers of the mouth, rectum, and uterine cervix.

## Prevalence of HIV Infection and AIDS in High-Risk Groups

The distribution of AIDS cases among the various high-risk groups is indicated in Table 6-4. Most AIDS cases are found in homosexual or bisexual males and intravenous drug abusers, and these two groups make up about 77 percent of all AIDS cases. Heterosexual contacts of HIV-infected persons make up another 11 percent of the total, and heterosexually transmitted HIV is increasing, as is the percentage of AIDS cases occurring in women, related to intravenous drug use or heterosexual activity with an infected partner. In young people ages 13 to 19, almost half the infections occur in females. Persons with hemophilia who received antihemophilic globulin, persons who received a blood transfusion, and persons with other sources of infection make up the balance. The percentages of asymptomatic HIV-positive infected persons in these groups are similar to the percentages of AIDS patients in these groups, as would be expected.

| Table 6-4 | Distribution of AIDS Cases by Risk Group | |
|---|---|
| **Risk Group** | **Percentage of Total AIDS Cases** |
| Homosexual and bisexual men | 46 |
| Homosexual and bisexual men who are also intravenous drug users | 6 |
| Heterosexual drug abusers | 25 |
| Heterosexual contacts of HIV-infected persons | 11 |
| Hemophiliacs | 1 |
| Blood transfusion recipients | 1 |
| Other sources of infection | 10 |

*Source:* Centers for Disease Control and Prevention. *HIV/AIDS Surveillance Report.* Volume 13, No. 2.

There are also some striking ethnic differences in the prevalence of HIV infections and AIDS. There is a disproportionately large number of AIDS cases in minority groups.

**HIV Transmission by Blood and Body Fluids** Transmission of the virus requires contact with body fluids containing virus-infected cells or free virus particles. The amount of virus in body fluids varies with the stage of the disease and the source of the body fluids. Blood, seminal fluid, cervical and vaginal secretions,

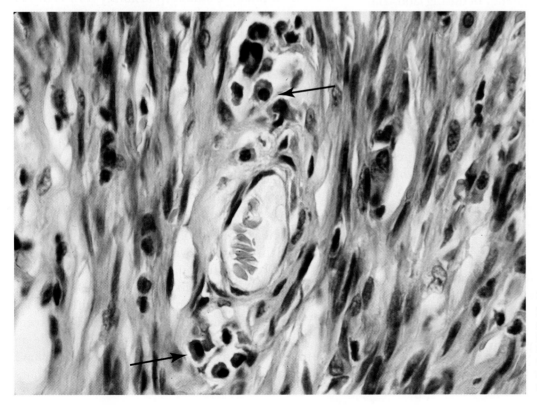

Figure 6-6 Kaposi's sarcoma, illustrating proliferating spindle-shaped connective-tissue cells (fibroblasts) surrounding a small blood vessel in the center of the field. Plasma cells (*arrows*) are intermixed with connective-tissue cells (original magnification × 400).

and breast milk generally contain large amounts of virus and are considered quite infectious, whereas urine, stool, saliva, tears, and perspiration usually contain little virus and are much less infectious. Transmission of the virus is usually either by sexual contact or by means of infected blood or blood products, but the virus may also be passed from an infected mother to her newborn infant.

**Sexual Transmission**  Among male homosexuals and bisexuals, transmission of the virus is chiefly by anal intercourse, which injures anal tissues and permits intermixing of infected blood and seminal fluid. Heterosexual partners of infected persons become infected by sexual intercourse because semen of infected males and vaginal secretions of infected women contain the virus. Many prostitutes of both sexes are infected, either from drug abuse or sexual contacts; sexual contacts with prostitutes are very risky. In some countries, the infection is transmitted chiefly by heterosexual intercourse, and both sexes are equally affected.

**Transmission by Blood and Blood Products**  Intravenous drug abusers become infected by sharing needles and syringes contaminated with blood from an infected person. Most transfusion recipients were infected from contaminated blood received before laboratory tests were available to screen donors for evidence of infection.

**Mother-to-Infant Transmission**  The infection of the fetus may occur during pregnancy or during labor and delivery, or the newborn infant may be infected through breastfeeding. The risk of HIV infection can be greatly reduced by treating the mother with antiviral drugs during pregnancy beginning at 14-weeks gestation, and continuing treatment through labor and delivery, with delivery preferably by cesarean section. The infant also receives oral antiviral therapy for 6 weeks after delivery, and no breastfeeding is permitted because breast milk may contain virus. This regimen can reduce the infant HIV infection rate to about 5 percent, which is a marked improvement when compared with an estimated 30 percent infant infection rate if no maternal and infant antiviral treatment are given. We do not know the possible late effects of the antiviral drugs on the infant. Children exposed to antiviral drugs to prevent HIV infection require long-term follow-up in order to detect any possible late harmful effects caused by the drugs.

## Prevention and Control of HIV Infection

Individuals infected with the virus are at risk of late complications, which eventually occur in a significant

| Table 6-5 | Groups at High Risk of Immunodeficiency Virus Infection |
|---|---|

1. Homosexual or bisexual men
2. Present or past intravenous drug abusers
3. Persons with clinical or laboratory evidence of HIV infection
4. Persons born in countries where heterosexual transmission plays the major role in spreading the infection
5. Male or female prostitutes and their sexual partners
6. Sexual partners of infected persons
7. Persons with hemophilia who have received blood products
8. Newborn infants of infected or high-risk mothers

number of persons. Infections and tumors in AIDS patients can be treated, but treatment of the underlying viral infection has been hampered by lack of a drug that can eliminate the virus. Several drugs are available that can impede viral replication and slow the progression of the disease. Much effort is being directed toward finding ways to control or eradicate the virus and toward developing a vaccine to immunize against the virus, but at present, there are no major breakthroughs on the horizon. The only really effective way to control the disease is to prevent further spread of the infection. This means that each individual must assume responsibility for his or her own behavior if the relentless spread of the disease is to be contained.

1. Uninfected persons should avoid sexual contacts with persons in high-risk groups or known to be infected with the virus (Table 6-5).

2. Members of high-risk groups should limit their number of sexual partners, practice "safe sex," which requires the use of condoms to reduce the risk of transmitting the infection, and avoid sexual practices such as unprotected anal intercourse and oral–genital contact, which can spread the virus.

3. Persons at high risk of infection should not donate blood, in order to prevent transmission of the virus by blood transfusion. Blood banks now screen donor blood for antibodies to the AIDS virus (as well as the hepatitis virus) and reject the blood for transfusion if antibodies are detected. The screening tests, however, will not reliably exclude all infected donors because some persons who have been infected recently may not have yet formed antibodies.

4. Infected women planning to become pregnant should consider the risks of pregnancy based on the stage of the HIV disease, the risks of mother-to-infant transmission of HIV, which can be greatly reduced but not completely eliminated by antiviral drugs, and the unknown long-term effects of the antiviral drugs on the infant.

## Treatment of HIV Infection

**When to Treat** When to start treatment requires one to balance the advantages of suppressing viral multiplication against the cost, side effects, and inconvenience of treatment. Intensive treatment of HIV infection is called *highly active antiretroviral therapy* (HAART), which involves multiple drugs that must be taken on a precise schedule for life in order to arrest the progression of the disease. Side effects related to the drugs are relatively frequent and may be severe, and drug resistance may occur, especially if the multiple drugs are not taken as prescribed. However, effective antiviral therapy inhibits viral multiplication, reduces the amount of virus in the circulation, and helps the immune system to recover.

The current goal of treatment is to suppress virus replication completely for as long as possible by using a potent combination of antiviral drugs, with periodic determination of the number of virus particles in the blood to measure response to therapy.

In general, most physicians believe that persons with high concentrations of virus in their blood should be treated even though the number of CD4+ cells in the blood is still normal and they have no symptoms of infection. Persons with a large amount of virus in their blood have a large amount of replicating virus in their lymphoid tissue that is destroying their CD4+ cells. Suppressing virus multiplication helps preserve the function of the immune system and hopefully will prevent or delay many of the late complications of the disease.

**Drugs to Treat HIV Infections** Many drugs are now available to treat HIV infections, and more are being developed. Treatment schedules are being revised continually as new drugs are developed and as physicians gain experience with the advantages and side effects of various drug combinations. These drugs fall into three main groups.

Each class of drug attacks a different phase in the HIV life cycle. Generally, a combination of three drugs is given. Such combinations usually are very effective for inhibiting viral replication and maintaining the function of the immune system, and can help restore an immune system that has already been damaged by the virus. Although combination drug therapy can reduce the level of virus in the circulation to extremely low or undetectable levels, such therapy cannot eradicate the virus in the lymphoid tissues of the body.

# Case Studies

The following three cases illustrate some of the clinical features and medical problems encountered in AIDS patients.

### Case Study 6-1

A 62-year-old woman, whose husband has hemophilia and had been treated with antihemophilic globulin, was hospitalized because of low-grade fever, cough, sweating, and a 35-pound weight loss over the previous 6 weeks. A chest x-ray revealed a bilateral pneumonia. A blood test for antibodies to the AIDS virus was positive, and lung biopsy obtained by bronchoscopy revealed *Pneumocystis jiroveci* pneumonia. The patient was treated with appropriate antibiotics.

This patient had been infected with HIV through sexual intercourse with her husband, who had become infected previously from blood products used to treat his hemophilia.

### Case Study 6-2

A 39-year-old homosexual male with multiple sexual partners and a positive test for antibodies to the AIDS virus had been treated on several occasions for *Candida* infections of the mouth and intermittent chronic diarrhea. Recently, he developed a red vascular nodule in his oral cavity that was biopsied and interpreted as Kaposi's sarcoma. The implications of this diagnosis were explained to the patient, and he was advised of the precautions necessary to prevent the spread of the HIV infection to others. He was referred to another physician for further treatment.

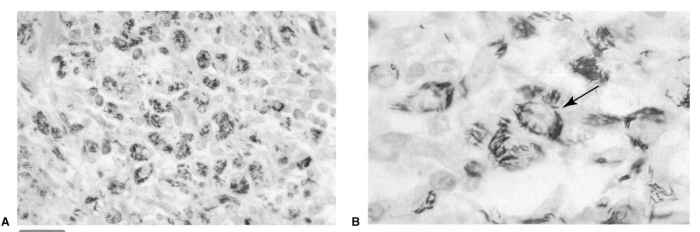

**Figure 6-7** Disseminated *Mycobacterium avium* complex infection (Case 6-3). **A,** Acid-fast organisms that fill the cytoplasm of large mononuclear phagocytes (macrophages) throughout the node, as demonstrated by special stains. **B,** High-magnification view of the mycobacteria. The nucleus of a mononuclear phagocyte (*arrow*) surrounded by masses of organisms in the cytoplasm appears in the center of the field. Large clumps of organisms fill the cytoplasm of other phagocytes in the field, obscuring the nuclei of the phagocytes (original magnification × 1000).

## Case Study 6-3

A 30-year-old HIV-positive homosexual male had been treated previously for various AIDS-related complications. Recently, he had experienced fever, fatigue, and weight loss. Physical examination revealed many large lymph nodes in the neck, armpits, and groin. A chest x-ray revealed no evidence of pneumonia. A lymph node biopsy revealed large numbers of mononuclear phagocytic cells filling the lymph node, and special stains revealed that the phagocytes were packed with acid-fast organisms (Figure 6-7). A biopsy of the bone marrow revealed similar focal clusters of mononuclear cells within the marrow, and marrow culture yielded *Mycobacterium avium complex*. Treatment with appropriate antibiotics was begun.

# CHAPTER REVIEW

## Summary

Communicable diseases can be transmitted by direct contact with an infected person, or indirectly by contaminated food, water, or by insects or animals. Control measures involve immunization to block susceptibility to the infection, identification and treatment of infected persons to prevent spread of the infection, and control of indirect transmission sources by a safe water and food supply and control of insects or animals that are potential sources of infection.

The major sexually transmitted diseases (STDs) are syphilis, gonorrhea, chlamydial infections, and herpes infections. Syphilis is well known, and an untreated infection has three distinct stages. Primary syphilis is manifested by a chancre, which is highly infectious and can be recognized if visible on the external genitalia but may escape detection if located in the mouth, vagina, or rectum. The organisms can be identified by special techniques in the fluid expressed from the chancre. If untreated the chancre will eventually heal, but the organisms have already spread through the body and a serologic test for syphilis is positive. The second stage is represented by fever, enlarged lymph nodes, and often a skin rash, which will also relent even without treatment. The third stage occurs years later and is characterized by severe destructive lesions affecting the central nervous system and the cardiovascular system. The disease responds to penicillin therapy but cannot repair the organ damage in the late stage of the disease.

Gonorrhea and chlamydial infections involve the mucous membranes: oral, genital, and urethral. The gonococcus can also travel in the bloodstream to infect bone (osteomyelitis), and heart valves (gonococcal endocarditis), and may also cause small pimplelike skin lesions. The infections respond to antibiotic therapy, although the gonococcus is becoming more resistant and is more difficult to treat than it was in previous years. In women both the gonococcus and chlamydia may extend into the fallopian tubes to cause an infection (salpingitis) followed by damage to the tubes that may impair fertility.

Herpes affects the oral (type 1) and genital (type 2) mucosa, but they are not restricted in their distribution. Once established, the infections may recur periodically in the same location that had been infected previously. Even a person without any demonstrable herpes lesions may shed virus periodically and infect a sexual partner. Some drugs can shorten the course of an infection but do not destroy the virus.

HIV infection and AIDS are in a separate category because of the way HIV behaves and the problems it causes. Transmission is by blood and body fluids, and the infection rate is high in homosexuals and intravenous drug users who share needles. Heterosexual transmission is becoming more frequent, and in some communities and age groups, both sexes are equally represented. Minority groups have a significantly higher infection rate than do other population groups. Modern therapy has changed AIDS from a fatal disease to a more chronic disease that can be controlled for many years but can't be cured. Many HIV-infected women are choosing to become pregnant, and the fetus also may become infected. Intensive treatment of the mother during pregnancy, labor, and delivery preferably by cesarean section, no nursing of the infant, and treatment of the infant after delivery have reduced the likelihood of infection of the infant. However, the long-term effects of the antiretroviral therapy on the infant are unknown.

## Questions for Review

1. How are bacteria classified, as described in Chapter 5?
2. What is meant by the following terms: *epidemic disease*, *endemic disease*, *immunization*, and *sexually transmitted disease*?
3. How is syphilis transmitted? What are its clinical manifestations?
4. How is gonorrhea transmitted? What are its clinical manifestations?
5. What are the manifestations of herpes infection of the genital tract?
6. What are the manifestations of chlamydial infection of the genital tract? How are chlamydial infections diagnosed and treated?
7. What is AIDS? What is its cause? What are its clinical manifestations? What groups are at high risk of infection, and how do they become infected? How can the spread of the infection be prevented or minimized?
8. What is the significance of a positive test for HIV antibody?

## Supplementary Reading

Bhaskaran, K., Hamouda, O., Sannes, M., et al. 2008. Changes in the risk of death after HIV seroconversion compared with mortality in the general population. *Journal of the American Medical Association* 300:51–59.

Mortality rates for HIV-infected persons have become much closer to mortality rates in the general population for the first 5 years after becoming infected, apparently related to the introduction of highly active antiretroviral therapy. This is not sustained after 5 years, probably due to problems related to drug toxicity, HIV drug resistance, and less adherence to therapy.

Centers for Disease Control and Prevention. 2002. U.S. Public Health Service Task Force recommendations for use of antiretroviral drugs in pregnant HIV-1 infected women for maternal health and interventions to reduce perinatal HIV-1 transmission in the United States. *Morbidity and Mortality Weekly Report* 51 (No. RR-18):1–38.

Current recommendations for treatment of pregnant women to prevent mother-to-infant transmission of HIV, as discussed in this chapter.

Goulder, P. J. R., and Walker, B. D. 2002. HIV-1 superinfection: A word of caution. *New England Journal of Medicine* 347:756–58.

An HIV-1 infection with one strain of virus does not protect against a new infection with a different strain of virus, and the infection with a new virus strain may precipitate a rapid progression of HIV disease. To prevent a second infection with a different virus strain, an HIV-positive person should use the same "safe-sex" precautions that an uninfected person should use.

Hirschel, B., and Calmy, A. 2008. Initial treatment of HIV infection—An embarrassment of riches. *New England Journal of Medicine* 358:2170–72.

> Describes current guidelines for HIV treatment. Elimination of the virus is not possible and therefore lifelong continuous treatment is necessary to maintain inhibition of viral multiplication. Intermittent treatment is always followed by rebound of virus proliferation. New drugs are being developed, new drug combinations are being evaluated, and new ways to impede virus proliferation are being evaluated.

Kovacs, J. A., and Masur, H. 2000. Prophylaxis against opportunistic infections in patients with human immunodeficiency infections. *New England Journal of Medicine* 342:1416–29.

> Persons with counts above 200 CD4 cells are at low risk of opportunistic infections. No prophylactic therapy is 100 percent effective; prophylaxis is available

against many infections, and maintenance therapy is usually required. However, additional maintenance antituberculosis treatment is not required if a patient has been treated successfully for tuberculosis. Relapses are rare among treated patients with drug-sensitive tuberculosis, but such patients may acquire a new infection with a drug-resistant tubercle bacillus.

Stephenson, J. 2003. Growing, evolving HIV/AIDS pandemic is producing social and economic fallout. *Journal of the American Medical Association* 289:31–33.

> An estimated 42 million people are now infected worldwide, and about half the people living with HIV are women. The increase of infected women reflects the epidemic in sub-Saharan Africa where heterosexual transmission predominates. Heterosexually transmitted HIV has also increased in the United States. More than half the HIV infections among people 13 to 19 years old were among females, with a disproportionate percentage African American.

## Interactive Activities

### True or False

Indicate whether the following statements are true or false by writing T or F at the end of the statement.

1. Herpes may infect both the oral cavity and the genital tract._____
2. The initial attack of herpes confers permanent immunity._____
3. Syphilis responds to penicillin therapy._____
4. A syphilitic chancre is highly infectious and can be identified on the genitalia, but may not be visible in other locations._____
5. The gonococcus may infect heart valves and bone as well as the genital tract._____
6. A chlamydial infection spreading to the fallopian tubes may cause a tubal infection that may damage the tubes and impair future fertility._____
7. Highly active antiretroviral therapy (HAART) suppresses viral multiplication and may improve the function of the immune system, but can't eradicate the virus._____
8. In order to control a disease, one needs to know what causes the disease and how the disease spreads._____
9. An HIV-infected mother may nurse her newborn infant because the virus is not present in breast milk._____
10. An endemic disease is one in which the rate of infection in the population is stable, neither increasing nor decreasing periodically._____

### Critical Thinking

1. A woman had a chlamydia test of her cervical secretions performed, and the test was positive. She is concerned about the consequences of the infection. What would you tell her about the consequences of the infection, the risk of infecting her partner, and the steps she should take to eradicate the infection.
2. A young woman is HIV positive and does not feel ill. She would like to marry and raise a family. Should she tell a future partner that she is HIV positive? What can she do to minimize the risk of infecting a future partner? If she becomes pregnant what is the risk of infecting her baby, and can she minimize her risk? Will her baby have to be treated? Can she nurse her baby?
3. A 35-year-old woman had unprotected sexual intercourse with a man she met at a party. About a week later she didn't feel well and had moderate pain in her left hip. She consulted a physician who aspirated fluid from the hip joint which was then cultured and reported as a gonococcal infection. She doesn't understand how a hip infection could have resulted from sexual contact. What would you tell her?

# Congenital and Hereditary Diseases

1. List the common causes of congenital malformations and their approximate incidence.

2. List four abnormalities of sex chromosomes, and describe their clinical manifestations.

3. Describe some of the common genetic abnormalities, and explain their methods of transmission.

4. Compare the methods of transmission and clinical manifestations of phenylketonuria and hemophilia.

5. Describe some of the more important malformations resulting from intrauterine injury.

6. Explain the process of amniocentesis.

7. Explain multifactorial inheritance. Give an example of a multifactorial defect, and describe the relevant factors.

8. List the causes of Down syndrome, and describe its clinical manifestations. Give reasons why it is important to identify a carrier of a 14/21 chromosome translocation.

9. Understand the various methods available to make a diagnosis of a congenital abnormality in the fetus.

# Causes of Congenital Malformations

There are many congenital and hereditary diseases. Their clinical manifestations range from minor, inconsequential defects to severe malformations that are incompatible with extrauterine life. A *hereditary* or *genetic* disease may be defined as one resulting from a chromosome abnormality or a defective gene. The term **congenital** disease or malformation refers to any abnormality that is present at birth (*congenitus* = with birth), even though it may not be detected until some time after birth; this broad category encompasses all abnormalities caused by disturbed prenatal development, regardless of their nature. Congenital defects are recognized in about 2 to 3 percent of all newborn infants. In an additional 2 to 3 percent, developmental defects are not recognized at birth but become apparent as the infants grow older. Major malformations are also found in from 25 to 50 percent of spontaneously aborted embryos and fetuses and in stillborn infants.

Four major factors are known to induce congenital malformations:

1. Chromosomal abnormalities
2. Abnormalities of individual genes
3. Intrauterine injury to the embryo or fetus by drugs, radiation, maternal infection, or other harmful environmental factors
4. Environmental factors acting on a genetically predisposed embryo

# Chromosomal Abnormalities

Chromosomal abnormalities leading to congenital malformations may result from failure of homologous chromosomes in the germ cells to separate normally, or abnormal breaks and rearrangements of chromosomes in the germ cells as they are maturing (gametogenesis), and occasionally from failure of chromosomes to separate normally in the fertilized ovum (zygote) as the cells divide by mitosis during early prenatal development.

## Chromosome Nondisjunction During Gametogenesis

Occasionally, homologous chromosomes in germ cells fail to separate from one another in either the first or the second meiotic division. This is called *nondisjunction*. It causes abnormalities in the distribution of chromosomes between germ cells ( Figure 7-1 ). One of the two germ cells derived from the abnormal chromosome division has an extra chromosome, and the other cell lacks a chromosome. Nondisjunction may involve either the sex chromosomes or the autosomes. If it occurs during gametogenesis, one daughter cell will have 24 chromosomes, and the other will have 22. If a gamete having an abnormal number of chromosomes fuses with a normal gamete during fertilization, the resulting zygote will either have an extra chromosome or be lacking one of the homologous pairs of chromosomes. The presence of an extra chromosome in a cell is called a **trisomy** (*tri* = three + *soma* = body) of the chromosome present in triplicate. Absence of a chromosome is called a **monosomy** (*mono* = one) of the missing chromosome.

## Chromosome Deletions and Translocations During Gametogenesis

Sometimes a chromosome breaks in the course of meiosis, and the broken piece is lost from the cell. This is called a *chromosome deletion*. In other cases, the broken piece is not lost but becomes attached to another nonhomologous chromosome with which it is carried along during meiosis. A misplaced chromosome or part of a chromosome attached to another chromosome is called a *translocation* (*trans* = across + *locus* = place).

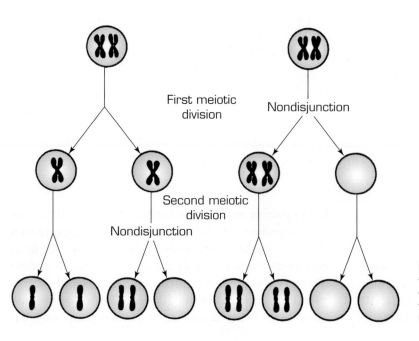

First meiotic division

Nondisjunction

Second meiotic division

Nondisjunction

Figure 7-1 Effects of nondisjunction in meiosis, leading to formation of gametes with an extra or missing chromosome. Only the chromosome pair involved in nondisjunction is illustrated. **Left,** Nondisjunction at second meiotic division. **Right,** Nondisjunction at first meiotic division.

## Case Study 7-1

A mother gave birth to an infant with multiple congenital abnormalities and had two subsequent pregnancies. Both terminated in spontaneous abortions about 8 weeks after conception. Chromosome studies were performed on the parents, the live-born infant, and the two aborted fetuses. The mother's karyotype was normal. The father's karyotype revealed that one chromosome 7 had broken and the detached piece had become attached (translocated) to chromosome 21. In this case, the father was the carrier of a chromosomal abnormality that did not disturb the function of his own cells because all of the genetic material was present in his cells. However, the translocation did result in the formation of chromosomally abnormal gametes that led to multiple congenital abnormalities in one live-born infant and two subsequent spontaneous abortions.

Figure 7-2 illustrates how the chromosomes from these parents can be distributed during fertilization, and the possible effects on the pregnancy. A normal fetus could have resulted if the fertilizing sperm had contained normal chromosome 7 and normal chromosome 21 (A), and also would have resulted from fertilization by a sperm containing the deficient chromosome 7 along with the chromosome 21 containing the translocated piece of chromosome 7 (the 7-21 translocation chromosome) because the amount of genetic material was normal even though the chromosomes were not normal (D). However, the fetus would be a carrier of the translocation chromosome, as was the father. Fertilization by a sperm containing a normal chromosome 7 and the chromosome 21 containing the translocated piece of chromosome 7 (the 7-21 tranlocation chromosome) would lead to an excess of genetic material in the zygote (B) resulting in congenital abnormalities. If the fertilizing sperm contained the deficient chromosome 7 (lacking its full component of genetic material) along with a normal chromosome 21, the total amount of genetic material in the zygote would be deficient, resulting in a spontaneous abortion (C).

In a *reciprocal translocation*, pieces of chromosomes (containing different sets of genes) are reciprocally exchanged between two nonhomologous chromosomes. Such an accident does not disturb the function of the cell because there is no loss or gain of genetic material. However, if the translocation occurs in a germ cell, an egg or sperm containing either a deficiency or an excess of chromosomal material may form during meiosis. If such a chromosomally abnormal gamete unites with a normal gamete during fertilization, the fertilized ovum (*zygote*) contains an abnormal amount of chromosomal material. Many abnormal zygotes are spontaneously aborted, but some survive and give rise to defective fetuses, as illustrated by the following case from the medical literature.

The literature contains many descriptions of clinical abnormalities that are associated with extra chromosomes, chromosome translocation, or loss of entire chromosomes or portions of chromosomes. Identification of chromosomal abnormalities is possible when the chromosomes are abnormal in size or configuration or when an abnormality is identified in the band pattern on the arms of the chromosomes.

## Chromosome Nondisjunction in the Zygote

Failures of chromosome separation are not restricted to germ cells. Sometimes the chromosomes fail to separate *during mitosis* in one of the cells of the zygote during prenatal development. When this occurs during mitosis, the cell lacking the chromosome is unable to survive but the cell with the extra chromosome continues to divide along with the other chromosomally normal cells. As a result, the embryo eventually becomes composed of a population of normal cells and another population of cells having a chromosome trisomy (Figure 7-3). The relative proportions of the two cell types depend on how early in prenatal development the chromosome nondisjunction occurred. A person composed of two or more types of cells is called a *chromosomal mosaic* or, simply, a *mosaic*, and the condition is called *chromosomal mosaicism*. (A mosaic is a picture composed of tiles or stones of different colors and shapes. By analogy, the term is also applied to persons who are "constructed" of different kinds of cells.)

## Sex Chromosome Abnormalities

When expressing the number of chromosomes in a cell, it is customary to indicate first the total number of chromosomes in the cell and then indicate the sex chromosomes. For example, a normal male is designated 46,XY and a normal female is 46,XX. Variations from the normal number of sex chromosomes are often

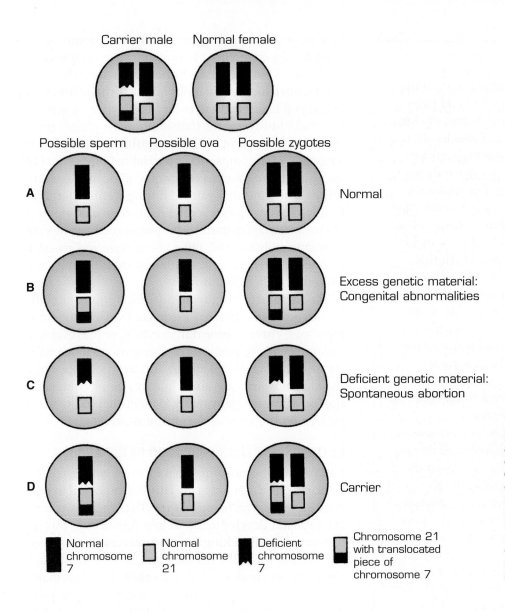

Carrier male    Normal female

Possible sperm    Possible ova    Possible zygotes

A    Normal

B    Excess genetic material:
Congenital abnormalities

C    Deficient genetic material:
Spontaneous abortion

D    Carrier

Normal chromosome 7    Normal chromosome 21    Deficient chromosome 7    Chromosome 21 with translocated piece of chromosome 7

Figure 7-2    Possible results when sperm of a 7-21 translocation carrier fertilizes a normal ovum. A, Normal chromosomes 7 and 21 (normal fetus). B, Normal chromosome 7 and chromosome 21 containing translocated piece of chromosome 7 (excess genetic material). C, Deficient chromosome 7 with normal chromosome 21 (deficient genetic material). D, Deficient chromosome 7 and chromosome 21 containing the translocated piece of chromosome 7 (abnormal chromosomes but normal genetic material).

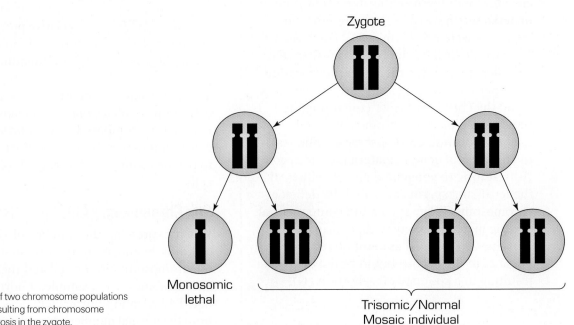

Zygote

Monosomic lethal

Trisomic/Normal Mosaic individual

Figure 7-3    Formation of two chromosome populations (chromosome mosaic) resulting from chromosome nondisjunction during mitosis in the zygote.

associated with some reduction of intelligence. The Y chromosome directs masculine sexual differentiation, and its presence is almost invariably associated with a male body configuration regardless of the number of X chromosomes present. An extra Y chromosome does not cause any significant changes in the appearance of the affected individual, because the Y chromosome carries little genetic material other than genes concerned with male sexual differentiation. If the Y chromosome is absent, the body configuration is female.

The effect of extra X chromosomes depends on the sex of the individual. The presence of one or more extra X chromosomes adversely affects masculine development but has very little effect on the female, because the additional X chromosomes are inactivated and appear as extra sex chromatin bodies attached to the nuclear membrane of the cell.

Several syndromes result from abnormalities in the number or structure of the sex chromosomes. The two most common that occur in the female are (1) *Turner syndrome*, which usually results from an absence of one X chromosome (genotype 45,X), and (2) *triple X syndrome*, which results from an extra X chromosome (genotype 47,XXX).

The two most common syndromes in the male are (1) *Klinefelter syndrome*, which results from an extra X chromosome (genotype 47,XXY), and (2) the *XYY syndrome*, which results from an extra Y chromosome (genotype 47,XYY).

The principal characteristics of these syndromes are summarized in Table 7-1 .

**Turner Syndrome** Turner syndrome, which results from an X chromosome abnormality, occurs less often than other sex chromosome abnormalities because most embryos lacking an X chromosome are aborted spontaneously. The reported frequency of about 1 in 2500 female births represents only the very small proportion of the embryos surviving to be born alive. Most persons

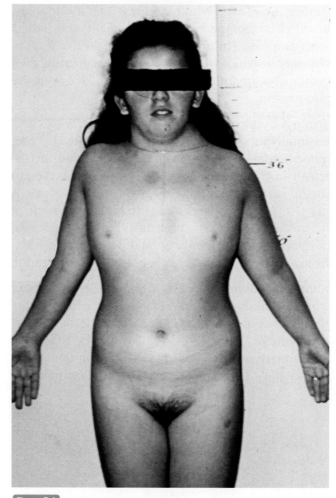

Figure 7-4   Child with Turner syndrome, illustrating a broad neck resulting from prominent lateral skin folds, a broad chest with widely spaced nipples, and a short stature.

with Turner syndrome have only 45 chromosomes because they lack one X chromosome (designated 45,X), and their cells lack a sex chromatin (Barr) body.

Figure 7-4 illustrates the appearance of a girl with Turner syndrome. The body configuration is female but abnormal. Characteristic features include short

| Table 7-1 | Syndromes Resulting from an Abnormal Complement of Sex Chromosomes |

| | Usual Genotype | Approximate Incidence | Unusual Number of Barr Bodies | Unusual Number of Y Fluorescent Bodies | Fertility |
|---|---|---|---|---|---|
| Turner syndrome | 45,X | 1:2500 females | 0 | 0 | Sterile |
| Triple X syndrome | 47,XXX | 1:850 females | 2 | 0 | Usually not impaired |
| Klinefelter syndrome | 47,XXY | 1:750 males | 1 | 1 | Usually sterile |
| XYY syndrome | 47,XYY | 1:850 males | 0 | 2 | Usually not impaired |

stature, broad neck with prominent lateral skin folds, broad chest lacking breast development, and widely spaced nipples. The uterus is small, and the ovaries consist only of bands of fibrous tissue. Frequently, congenital abnormalities of the cardiovascular system are also present.

**Triple X Syndrome** The presence of an extra X chromosome in the cells of the female is a relatively common abnormality. It has an incidence of about 1 in 850 female births. Usually there are no specific abnormalities of body form because the extra X chromosome is inactivated and appears on the nuclear membrane of the cell as an extra sex chromatin (Barr) body. Sexual development is generally normal. Fertility and intelligence may be either normal or somewhat decreased.

**Klinefelter Syndrome** Having an incidence of about 1 in 750 male births, Klinefelter syndrome results from the presence of extra X chromosomes in the male (usual genotype 47,XXY). **Figure 7-5** illustrates the characteristic appearance of a subject with this chromosomal abnormality. The external genital organs are male, but the testicles are atrophic. Usually, no spermatozoa are produced, and the individual is sterile. The body configuration is somewhat feminine, and there may be slight breast hypertrophy. Intelligence tends to be subnormal; however, many men with Klinefelter syndrome function reasonably well in society, and some are able to hold responsible positions. Because of the extra X chromosome, the cells contain a sex chromatin body (Barr body) as well as a Y fluorescent body.

**XYY Syndrome** The sex chromosomal abnormality known as XYY syndrome has an incidence of about 1 in 850 male births. It may be associated with some reduction of fertility and intelligence. The individuals are usually taller than normal, but there are no specific abnormalities of body configuration.

**The Fragile X Syndrome (X-Linked Mental Deficiency)** This condition, although not related to an excess or deficiency of a sex chromosome, is associated with a characteristic abnormality of the X chromosome and is second only to Down syndrome as a major cause of mental deficiency. The X chromosome abnormality is a constricted area on the long arm of the chromosome near its tip, causing the tip of the long arm to look like a small round knob connected to the rest of the chromosome by a narrow stalklike constriction. The constricted area is quite fragile compared with the rest of the chromosome and is often broken in the course of preparing a chromosome karyotype, which is how the designation "fragile X chromosome" originated.

The gene responsible for the fragile X syndrome has been identified and named *FMR1* (for Fragile X Mental Retardation-1) or simply *fragile X gene*, and the gene product is called *fragile X mental retardation protein* (FMRP). In normal persons, the first part of the fragile X gene contains groups (sequences) of the three nucleotides cytosine–guanine–guanine arranged in that order from six to as many as 50 times (CGG repeating sequences, often just called *repeats*). *A greater number of repeats is abnormal* and the larger the number, the more severe the mental deficiency.

Because the fragile X syndrome follows an X-linked pattern of inheritance, women carrying the fragile X gene can pass it to both daughters and sons, but men carrying it can pass it only to their daughters. The effect of the fragile X on the offspring depends on which parent transmitted it. When a woman transmits the gene, the number of CGG repeats in the transmitted X chromosome becomes greatly increased (amplified), and the degree of mental deficiency in the offspring who received the chromosome may be more marked than that of the mother who transmitted the fragile X gene. In contrast, when a man carrying the fragile X

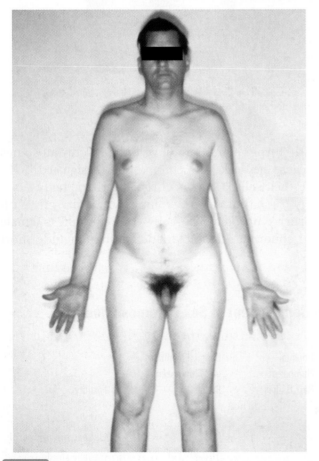

**Figure 7-5** Klinefelter syndrome. The patient's body configuration is male, although there is slight breast hypertrophy (photograph courtesy of Dr. Robert Gorlin).

passes it to his daughter, the number of CGG repeating sequences in the fragile X gene that the daughter receives does not increase significantly, and the severity of the mental deficiency in the daughter may be no greater than that of the father.

A diagnosis of fragile X syndrome should be considered in any mentally retarded person. The preferred diagnostic test is DNA analysis, which can identify a greatly increased number of CGG repeats in the gene characteristic of the fragile X syndrome.

## Autosomal Abnormalities

Absence of an autosome results in the loss of so many genes that development is generally not possible and the embryo is aborted. Deletion of a small part of an autosome may be compatible with development, but it usually results in multiple severe congenital abnormalities in the infant. The most common autosomal trisomy seen in newborn infants is that of the small chromosome 21, which causes *Down syndrome*. Trisomy of a larger chromosome, such as chromosome 13 or chromosome 18, is less frequent and is associated with multiple severe congenital malformations. Trisomy of other large autosomes is almost invariably lethal.

**Down Syndrome**  Down syndrome is the most common chromosomal abnormality, having an incidence of about 1 in 600 births. It is characterized by mental deficiency and a characteristic facial expression caused by the upward-slanting eyes and the prominent skin folds extending from the base of the nose to the inner aspects of the eyebrows ( Figure 7-6 ). Other abnormalities of body form are also seen. Congenital cardiac malformations occur frequently, as do major congenital defects in other organ systems. The reported incidence of 1 in 600 births represents only the proportion of abnormal fetuses surviving to term. About 70 percent of trisomy 21 fetuses do not survive to be live born.

Down syndrome may arise as a result of three possible conditions:

1. Nondisjunction during gametogenesis, leading to the formation of an abnormal gamete containing an extra chromosome 21
2. An extra chromosome 21 acquired as part of a translocation chromosome (*translocation Down syndrome*)
3. Nondisjunction occurring in the zygote (*mosaic Down syndrome*)

**Nondisjunction During Gametogenesis**  In about 95 percent of cases, Down syndrome results from nondisjunction of chromosome 21 during oogenesis, which causes the formation of an ovum containing an extra chromosome 21. Fertilization by a normal sperm

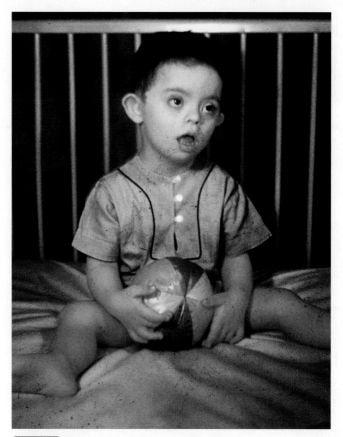

Figure 7-6  Child with Down syndrome.

produces a zygote containing 47 chromosomes, with chromosome 21 being present in triplicate. Down syndrome resulting from nondisjunction during oogenesis increases in frequency with advancing maternal age. The incidence is as high as 1 in 50 in the offspring of women over 40 years of age.

**Translocation Down Syndrome**  In a small number of persons with Down syndrome, the extra chromosome 21 is attached to another chromosome, usually chromosome 14. Although the total number of chromosomes is not increased in these individuals, one of the chromosomes is actually a composite chromosome resulting from the fusion of chromosome 21 with another chromosome; consequently, the affected person has genetic material that is equivalent to 47 chromosomes. Chromosome studies performed on the parents of children with translocation Down syndrome often reveal normal chromosomes in the cells of both parents. In these instances, the translocation apparently occurred as an accident in a germ cell of one parent during gametogenesis and is not present in other germ cells or in somatic cells. In other instances, the translocation chromosome can be identified in the karyotype of one of the parents, who is a carrier of the abnormal chromosome. The carrier parent has only 45 chromosomes

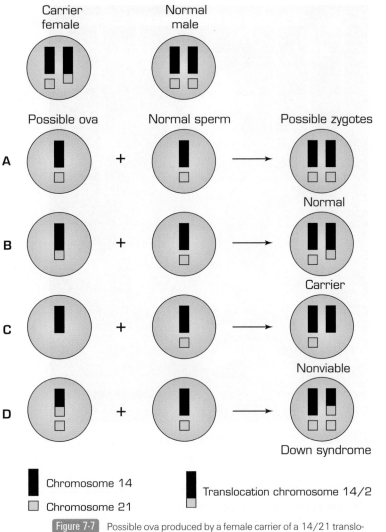

Carrier female    Normal male

Possible ova    Normal sperm    Possible zygotes

A    +    →

Normal

B    +    →

Carrier

C    +    →

Nonviable

D    +    →

Down syndrome

■ Chromosome 14
☐ Chromosome 21

▮ Translocation chromosome 14/2

**Figure 7-7** Possible ova produced by a female carrier of a 14/21 translocation chromosome and possible zygotes that could result from fertilization by normal sperm.

because one chromosome is represented by a fusion of chromosome 21 with another chromosome.

The recognition of a translocation carrier is important because the carrier is capable of transmitting the abnormal chromosome to his or her children, resulting in translocation Down syndrome. **Figure 7-7** illustrates the possible outcome of a pregnancy involving a female carrier of a 14/21 translocation chromosome. As indicated, the ova of the carrier parent can possess any one of four chromosome types, depending on how chromosomes 14 and 21 are distributed in the oocyte. Because there is only one chromosome 14 that can be distributed to the ovum independent of chromosome 21, an ovum can receive either the normal chromosome 14 (ova A and C) or the translocation chromosome (ova B and D). Because only one chromosome 21 can be distributed to the ovum (the other being carried with chromosome 14 as the translocation chromosome), some ova will receive the single chromosome 21 (ova

A and D), but others will fail to receive this chromosome (ova B and C). The consequences of fertilization of these various possible ova by normal spermatozoa are indicated. In the first example (A), union of a normal ovum with a normal sperm produces a normal zygote containing 46 chromosomes.

In the second example (B), a zygote containing 45 chromosomes results from fertilization, one chromosome being represented by the translocation chromosome. The individual derived from this zygote will be normal but will be a carrier of the translocation chromosome. In example C, the zygote lacks one chromosome 21 and is unable to survive. Fertilization of the ovum containing the translocation chromosome (example D) produces a zygote containing an excess of chromosome 21 material, resulting in a translocation Down syndrome.

**Nondisjunction in the Zygote: Mosaic Down Syndrome** In a few individuals with Down syndrome, only some of the cells exhibit the characteristic trisomy 21. Other cells have a normal component of chromosomes. This type of Down syndrome, which is called mosaic Down syndrome, results from nondisjunction of chromosome 21 in a cell during the early divisions of the zygote. The cell in which nondisjunction occurs gives rise to one daughter cell lacking chromosome 21 and another cell having an extra chromosome 21. The cell having only one chromosome 21 fails to survive, but the trisomy 21 cell continues to divide, forming more trisomy 21 cells that multiply along with the normal cells of the zygote. (Refer to Figure 7-3 illustrating chromosome mosaicism.) Individuals with mosaic Down syndrome suffer less disability than those in whom all of the cells contain an extra chromosome 21.

**Trisomy of Other Autosomes** Trisomy of chromosome 13 is associated with multiple severe developmental abnormalities, the most conspicuous being cleft lip and palate, abnormal development of the skull and brain, abnormal eye development, congenital heart defects, and polydactyly (extra fingers and toes). Trisomy of chromosome 18 also is associated with multiple severe congenital malformations. Both chromosomal trisomies are usually fatal in the neonatal period or in early infancy.

# Genetically Transmitted Diseases

Genetically determined diseases are the result of abnormalities of individual genes on the chromosome. The chromosomes themselves appear normal, and the

## Table 7-2  Mode of Inheritance, Pathogenesis, and Major Manifestations of Some Common Genetic Diseases

| Abnormality | Mode of Inheritance | Defect | Manifestations |
|---|---|---|---|
| Phenylketonuria | Recessive | Phenylalanine hydroxylase deficiency | Mental retardation |
| Tay-Sachs disease | Recessive | Hexosaminidase A deficiency | Mental retardation, motor weakness, blindness |
| Cystic fibrosis of pancreas | Recessive | Dysfunction of mucous and sweat glands, thick mucus obstructs bronchioles, pancreatic ducts, and bile ducts | Chronic bronchopulmonary infections as a result of bronchial obstruction by mucus; pancreatic and liver dysfunction as a result of thick mucous obstruction of excretory ducts |
| Achondroplasia | Dominant | Disordered bone growth at ends of long bones (epiphyses) | Dwarfism with disproportionately short limbs |
| Congenital polycystic kidney disease (one type) | Dominant | Maldevelopment of nephrons and collecting tubules causes formation of multiple cysts in kidneys | Renal failure |
| Multiple neurofibromatosis | Dominant | Multiple tumors arise from peripheral nerves | Disfigurement and deformities caused by tumors; predisposition to malignant change in tumors |
| Sickle cell trait | Codominant | Red cells contain mixture of normal (A) and sickle (S) hemoglobin | None |
| Sickle cell anemia | Codominant | Red cells contain no normal hemoglobin | Severe anemia and obstruction of blood flow to organs by masses of sickled red cells |
| Hemophilia | X-linked recessive | Deficiency of protein required for normal coagulation of blood | Uncontrolled bleeding into joints and internal organs after minor injuries |

chromosome karyotype is normal. Transmission of the abnormal gene is from parent to offspring, following the well-established patterns of inheritance described in Chapter 2.

Genes direct many functions within the cell. Some genes direct the synthesis of proteins. These may be proteins that form the structure of the cell (*structural proteins*) or enzymes that are necessary for cell function. Other genes function by regulating the activity of the genes that direct protein synthesis. Normally, genes are stable and are passed without change from parent to offspring. Occasionally, a gene undergoes a change called a *gene mutation*, which may occur spontaneously or as a result of exposure to chemicals or radiation. After a mutation has occurred in a germ cell, it can be transmitted from parent to offspring.

Sometimes a gene mutation that induces only a minor change in the structure of a protein may cause a serious change in its properties. For example, sickle hemoglobin (hemoglobin S) differs from normal hemoglobin (hemoglobin A) only in a single amino acid but undergoes crystallization within the red blood cells when the oxygen content of the blood is reduced.

If a mutation involves genes that control the synthesis of an enzyme, the enzyme may be defective and may lack functional activity. Metabolic processes regulated by the enzyme are disturbed, and the cell is unable to function normally. Most hereditary diseases are transmitted on autosomes. A few are carried on sex chromosomes ( Table 7-2 ).

## Autosomal Dominant Inheritance

A dominant gene expresses itself in the heterozygous state. If either parent carries an abnormal dominant gene, either the abnormal gene or the corresponding normal allele may be passed to the offspring. Consequently, there is one chance in two that the offspring will receive the abnormal gene and will be affected with the hereditary disease. A common example of a genetic disease transmitted in this manner is *achondroplasia*, a type of dwarfism in which the limbs are disproportionately short (Chapter 22). A second example is one type of *congenital polycystic kidney disease*, which is characterized by the formation of multiple cysts throughout both kidneys that progressively enlarge and eventually destroy renal function (Chapter 15).

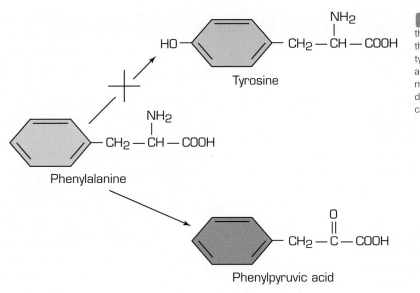

Tyrosine

NH₂

Phenylalanine

Phenylpyruvic acid

**Figure 7-8** Metabolic defects in phenylketonuria. Infants with this disorder lack the enzyme phenylalanine hydroxylase, and their bodies are unable to hydroxylate phenylalanine to form tyrosine. Some phenylalanine is converted into phenylpyruvic acid (substitution of a keto group for the amino group in the molecule) by other metabolic pathways. Permanent mental deficiency results from disturbed phenylalanine metabolism and can be prevented by restricting dietary intake of phenylalanine.

A third genetic disease of this type is *multiple neurofibromatosis*, a condition characterized by the formation of multiple tumors that arise from peripheral nerves (Chapter 21).

## Autosomal Recessive Inheritance

A trait transmitted as an autosomal recessive is expressed only in the homozygous individual. Many diseases characterized by an enzyme deficiency within the cell are transmitted in this manner. The hereditary disease results only if both alleles are abnormal and no enzyme is produced. Therefore, in order for the offspring to be affected, both parents must carry the abnormal gene, and both must transmit the gene to the offspring. Consequently, when both parents carry an abnormal recessive gene, there is one chance in four that the mother will give birth to an abnormal infant who is homozygous for the defective gene. If only one parent transmits the recessive gene, the infant will be a carrier of the abnormal gene but will be normal because the normal allele will direct the synthesis of enough enzymes to keep the cell functioning normally. Two of the more important genetic diseases in this category are *phenylketonuria* and *Tay-Sachs disease*.

**Phenylketonuria** Phenylalanine is an essential amino acid present in dietary protein. Much of it is converted in the body to tyrosine, which the body uses to make thyroid hormone, melanin, and other important compounds. A deficiency of the enzyme *phenylalanine hydroxylase*, which is required for normal metabolism of the amino acid phenylalanine, causes a disease called phenylketonuria. The enzyme deficiency causes no difficulty while the infant is still within the uterus being nourished by the mother. Soon after birth,

however, the infant begins to drink milk. Because milk protein contains abundant phenylalanine, which the infant is unable to metabolize, this amino acid accumulates in the infant's blood and is excreted in the urine. The affected infant is able to convert some phenylalanine into phenylpyruvic acid (and other metabolites) by means of other metabolic pathways that do not require phenylalanine hydroxylase ( Figure 7-8 ). Phenylpyruvic acid accumulates in the blood and is excreted in the urine along with phenylalanine. Permanent mental deficiency results from the disturbed phenylalanine metabolism, but it can be prevented by restricting the dietary intake of phenylalanine. Phenylketonuria can be detected in the newborn infant by means of a screening laboratory test capable of detecting the elevated level of phenylalanine in the blood. This disease is a cause of preventable mental deficiency; thus, a routine screening test to detect phenylketonuria is an important requirement for all newborn infants.

**Tay-Sachs Disease** Tay-Sachs disease occurs primarily in the offspring of Jewish parents who carry the defective gene. The clinical manifestations result from absence of a lysosomal enzyme called *hexosaminidase A*. The enzyme deficiency causes a lipid called a *ganglioside* to accumulate within the lysosomes of nerve cells in the brain, spinal cord, autonomic nervous system, and retina of the eye, causing cell dysfunction and eventually degeneration of the affected nerve cells. Clinically, the disease is characterized by progressive mental deterioration, neurologic dysfunction, and blindness. Onset of symptoms begins by about 6 months of age, and the disease is invariably fatal by the time the child is 3 or 4 years old.

Carriers of the abnormal gene can be detected by means of the low levels of hexosaminidase A in their serum and in their leukocytes. Tests for this enzyme can be used for screening. Surveys have indicated that the carrier rate is relatively high in some Jewish populations (those of Eastern European origin). In these groups, about 1 in 30 individuals carries the abnormal gene.

Tay-Sachs disease can be diagnosed prenatally by examining fetal cells obtained by amniocentesis. The applications and limitations of this diagnostic procedure are described later in this chapter.

**Other Genetic Diseases** Two other relatively common and important diseases that are transmitted by autosomal recessive inheritance are *cystic fibrosis of the pancreas* and *hemochromatosis*. Cystic fibrosis, manifested by dysfunction of mucous and sweat glands, is considered in Chapter 16 in conjunction with diseases of the pancreas. Hemochromatosis is characterized by excessive absorption of iron, which accumulates within the body and disrupts organ functions and is considered in Chapter 11.

## Codominant Inheritance

If both alleles of a pair are fully expressed in the heterozygous state, the genes are said to be *codominant*. This type of transmission is illustrated by the genes responsible for the synthesis of *sickle (S) hemoglobin* and other abnormal hemoglobins. These genes are alleles of the gene that directs the synthesis of normal (A) hemoglobin. An individual heterozygous for the sickle hemoglobin gene will have approximately equal quantities of sickle hemoglobin and normal hemoglobin in the red cells. This condition is called *sickle cell trait* and usually causes no serious difficulties. Significant clinical manifestations are apparent, however, if the individual is homozygous for the sickle cell gene, and no normal hemoglobin is formed. This leads to a serious hereditary anemia called *sickle cell anemia*. This subject is considered in Chapter 11.

## X-Linked Inheritance

A few hereditary diseases are transmitted on the X chromosome. The best-known example is the disease *hemophilia*, which is caused by a deficiency of protein called *antihemophilic globulin*, which is required for normal blood coagulation. This disease is described in Chapter 9. The female parent carries the defective gene on one of her X chromosomes and can transmit either the normal X chromosome or the one containing the defective gene to her offspring. The child will be normal if the normal X chromosome is received. If the mother transmits the abnormal X chromosome, its effect depends on the sex of the offspring. A female child will appear normal because the defective gene on the X chromosome is paired with a normal allele on the other X chromosome. However, she will be a carrier of the abnormal gene and can transmit it to her own children. In contrast, a male child will have hemophilia. Because a male has only one X chromosome, he lacks the normal allele possessed by a female carrier. Consequently, the abnormal X-linked gene functions like a dominant gene when paired with the Y chromosome.

Although female carriers of the mutant gene appear normal and generally produce adequate antihemophilic globulin, they produce less than normal amounts of this protein. The subnormal production is related to the random inactivation of one of the X chromosomes, as described in Chapter 2. Consequently, a carrier female has two populations of cells concerned with synthesis of antihemophilic globulin. Synthesis is normal in the cells in which the X chromosome containing the mutant gene is inactivated but deficient in the cells in which the X chromosome containing the normal gene is inactivated. The amount of antihemophilic globulin produced by a carrier female depends on the relative proportions of the two cell types: functioning cells that produce antihemophilic globulin, and nonfunctional cells in which the functional gene is carried on the X chromosome that has been inactivated.

# Intrauterine Injury

The embryo or fetus may be injured by drugs, radiation, or an infection that disrupts prenatal development and leads to congenital malformations. The effects of the injury inflicted on the developing embryo vary, depending on the nature of the harmful agent and the stage of gestation. The embryonic period from the third to the eighth week after conception, when the organ systems are forming, is the time when the embryo is most vulnerable to the injurious effects of environmental agents.

## Harmful Drugs and Chemicals

Many drugs are known to harm the developing embryo. The classic example is thalidomide, which was widely used in Europe in the 1960s to treat nausea and vomiting associated with pregnancy (morning sickness) but was never marketed in the United States. The drug produced a highly characteristic malformation in which the bones of the extremities were much reduced or absent, the hands or feet arising from the trunk ( Figure 7-9 ). Either upper or lower limbs or all four extremities were affected, depending on the time when

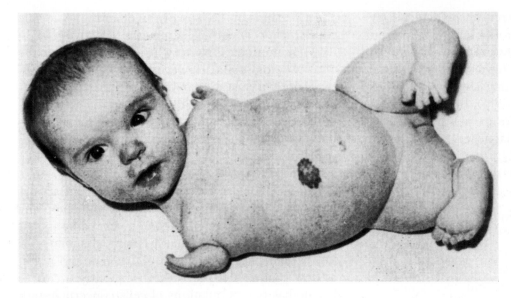

**Figure 7-9** Characteristic limb deformities caused by thalidomide. (From Tausig, H. B. 1962. Study of German outbreak of phocomelia: Thalidomide syndrome. *Journal of the American Medical Association* 180:1106–14. Copyright 1962, American Medical Association. Used with permission.)

the drug was taken during pregnancy. In addition to causing limb defects, the drug also caused malformations of the heart, gastrointestinal tract, eyes, and ears. The correlation between thalidomide and congenital malformations was eventually determined because of the unusual type of limb malformations produced by the drug but, unfortunately, not until thousands of infants had been damaged by this drug. The thalidomide tragedy clearly demonstrated to the medical profession the disastrous effects of a supposedly innocuous drug taken by a mother during a critical phase of embryonic development.

Many other drugs, although less hazardous than thalidomide, may also cause congenital malformations. Currently, all drugs used in the United States are rated in five categories by the United States Food and Drug Administration (FDA) according to the degree of possible risk to the fetus balanced against the drug's potential benefit to the patient (Table 7-3).

Ratings range from "A" for drugs that are generally considered safe for use in pregnancy through "D" for drugs that may injure the fetus but are of enough benefit to the patient that the benefit of the drug to the patient outweighs the risk to the fetus. "X"-rated drugs are contraindicated in pregnancy because the severe risk to the fetus outweighs any possible benefit to the patient.

Even cigarettes and alcoholic beverages are not without risk. Cigarette smoking leads to retarded intrauterine growth with birth of smaller than normal infants and premature births. Heavy alcohol consumption during pregnancy can result in a characteristic pattern of developmental abnormalities called *fetal alcohol syndrome*. Affected infants are both physically and mentally retarded, exhibit abnormal cranial and facial development, and may have other congenital malformations affecting the genital tract and cardiovascular system. Consequently, women with severe drinking

| Table 7-3 | Five Categories of All Drugs Used in the United States Rated by the FDA According to Degree of Possible Risk to the Fetus |
|---|---|
| **Category** | **Interpretation** |
| A | No risk to fetus demonstrated in well-controlled studies in humans. |
| B | No evidence of risk to fetus. Either animal studies show risk but human studies do not or there are no adequate human studies but animal studies do not indicate risk. |
| C | Risk to fetus cannot be ruled out. No human studies available to assess risk. Animal studies either are not available or indicate possible risk. |
| D | Positive evidence of risk to fetus; however, drug is needed to treat patients, and no safer alternative drug is available. Potential benefit to patients outweighs risk to fetus. |
| X | Absolutely contraindicated in pregnancy. Severe risk to fetus greatly outweighs any possible benefit to patients. |

problems should be cautioned to not become pregnant until their alcoholism is controlled. Even small amounts of alcohol may put the fetus at risk, and it is generally considered unsafe for a pregnant woman to consume any alcohol during pregnancy.

Drugs such as heroin, methadone, and cocaine used by a pregnant woman impair fetal growth and development and may lead to congenital malformation, as well as to addiction in both the fetus and the mother. The infant born to an addicted mother may experience narcotic withdrawal symptoms within a few days after delivery. Maternal cocaine use may also disturb blood flow through the placenta, leading to intrauterine fetal death, as described in Chapter 14.

Because of the established relation between drugs and congenital defects, most physicians recommend that pregnant women refrain from indiscriminate use of drugs or other medications, especially during the early part of pregnancy when the embryo is especially vulnerable. Many new drugs and antibiotics are not recommended for use in pregnancy because the possible effects of the drugs on the developing embryo are not known.

## Radiation

Exposure of a pregnant woman to radiation may harm the fetus. Consequently, x-ray examinations or diagnostic tests using radioactive materials are avoided during pregnancy.

## Maternal Infections

Some infections acquired by a pregnant woman may injure the developing fetus. Three infectious agents are known to be important causes of congenital malformations and may also cause a chronic systemic infection of the fetus:

1. The virus of German measles (*rubella*)
2. The virus of cytomegalic inclusion disease (*cytomegalovirus*)
3. The protozoan parasite *Toxoplasma gondii*

**Rubella**  Rubella is a mild illness; 90 percent of women of childbearing age have already had the disease in childhood, or have been immunized and are immune. If a susceptible woman acquires rubella during pregnancy, the virus may infect the embryo, leading to either spontaneous abortion of severely affected embryos or congenital malformations in many of the embryos that survive. Common malformations resulting from prenatal rubella infection include congenital cataracts, cardiac malformations, deafness, and neurologic disturbances. The earlier the infection occurs in the pregnancy, the greater is the hazard to the developing embryo. The

virus may also cause a chronic progressive infection in the fetus. When this occurs, the affected infant is born with evidence of an active systemic disease characterized by enlargement of the liver and spleen, anemia, and reduced numbers of platelets in the blood. The low platelet levels usually lead to multiple small hemorrhages in the skin. Rubella virus can be isolated from the tissues and secretions of the infected infants. It may persist in the infant's tissues for 6 months or longer after delivery.

**Cytomegalic Inclusion Disease**  The name of the cytomegalovirus (*cyto* = cell + *megalos* = large) derives from its characteristic property of producing marked enlargement of the cells it infects. The infected cells also contain characteristic large, basophilic, intranuclear inclusions, causing the virus-infected cell to have a distinctly characteristic histologic appearance ( Figure 7-10 ). Cytomegalovirus infection is very common and is usually asymptomatic. More than 50 percent of women of childbearing age have had a previous cytomegalovirus infection and have formed antibodies

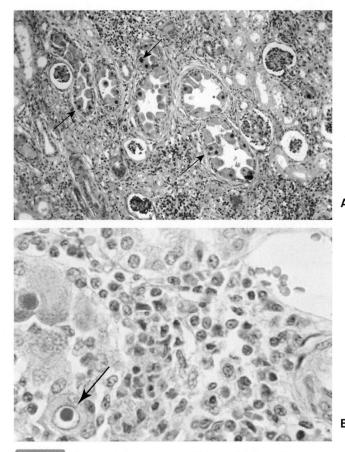

**A**

**B**

Figure 7-10  Characteristic appearance of kidney cells infected by cytomegalovirus. **A,** Many large virus inclusions within enlarged kidney tubule cells (arrows) (original magnification × 100). **B,** High-magnification view illustrating virus-infected cells (arrow) in kidney tubules with many chronic inflammatory cells in adjacent tissue (original magnification × 400).

against the virus, but latent cytomegalovirus persists within the tissues of the infected woman and may become reactivated during pregnancy, leading to intermittent excretion of virus in cervical and vaginal secretions throughout the pregnancy. The fetus may become infected either from a new maternal infection acquired during pregnancy or from reactivation of a prior maternal infection. A newly acquired maternal infection poses the greatest risk to the fetus. The virus may cause severe fetal damage characterized by injury to the brain and eyes, leading to failure of the brain to develop normally (*microcephaly*), mental retardation, and blindness. The cytomegalovirus may also cause a chronic systemic infection of the fetus similar to that caused by the rubella virus, and the virus can be identified in the tissues of the infected infant.

A reactivation of a previous maternal infection is less hazardous to the fetus and may produce only relatively mild symptoms.

**Other Virus Diseases in Pregnancy** The herpes simplex virus, the same virus that causes fever blisters, may at times cause congenital infections similar to those produced by cytomegalovirus, leading to malformations of the nervous system. Some other viruses may occasionally be transmitted to the fetus and cause disease in the fetus, but they are not usually associated with congenital malformations.

**Toxoplasmosis** *Toxoplasma gondii* is a small, ovoid, intracellular parasite described in Chapter 5. Adults acquired the infection by eating raw or partially cooked meat that is infected with the parasite or by contact with infected cats, which excrete an infectious form of the organism (oocysts) in their feces. As with cytomegalovirus infection, more than 50 percent of women of childbearing age have had a previous inapparent infection and have formed antibodies to the parasite. These women are immune, and the prior infection does not put the fetus at risk.

A hazard to the fetus exists if a susceptible mother acquires the infection during pregnancy. In the fetus, the parasite causes severe injury to the brain and eyes, leading to abnormal development of the brain (*microcephaly*); obstruction of the ventricles of the brain, causing *hydrocephalus* (Chapter 21); and visual disturbances or blindness. The infected fetus may be born with evidence of a systemic *Toxoplasma* infection that is clinically quite similar to that caused by rubella and the cytomegalovirus.

It is possible to determine by laboratory tests whether a pregnant woman is susceptible to *Toxoplasma*. A susceptible pregnant woman should avoid eating incompletely cooked meat and should exercise caution in contact with cats. Pregnant women with cats are generally advised to adopt the following precautions.

1. Wash hands after handling cats, especially before eating.
2. Have the cat-litter box emptied daily by someone else (to avoid contact with oocysts).
3. Do not permit indoor cats to go outside because cats allowed to roam outdoors have a higher risk of acquiring a *Toxoplasma* infection.
4. Do not allow outdoor cats or stray cats to enter the house because they are very likely to be infected with *Toxoplasma*.
5. Do not feed cats raw meat products because they may become infected in this way.

The following case illustrates the clinical features of a systemic infection of the fetus that resulted from an inapparent infection of the mother during pregnancy (Figure 7-11).

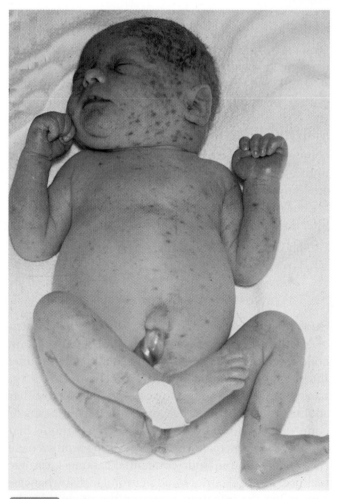

**Figure 7-11** Severe systemic disease in newborn infant caused by an inapparent infection of the mother during pregnancy, as described in Case 7-2.

Rubella virus, cytomegalovirus, *Toxoplasma*, and occasionally the herpesvirus all produce a similar type of infection in the fetus, and it may not be possible to determine clinically which agent caused the disease unless the infectious agent can be identified by histologic examination, culture, or serologic methods.

**Case Study 7-2**

An infant girl was born prematurely at 36 weeks' gestation. Her skin was covered with numerous small hemorrhages, and the abdomen was markedly distended because of extreme enlargement of her liver and spleen. She was moderately anemic and the platelet count was greatly reduced. The infant was considered to be seriously ill with a prenatal infection acquired from the mother. Diagnostic possibilities considered were congenital rubella, cytomegalic inclusion disease, systemic herpesvirus infection, or toxoplasmosis. The infant died of the widespread infection before further diagnostic studies could be performed. The autopsy revealed that the infection was caused by the cytomegalovirus.

# Multifactorial Inheritance

Many congenital defects do not result from single gene abnormalities and are not entirely caused by environmental factors. Rather, they result from the combined effects of multiple genes interacting with environmental agents. This type of inheritance is called multifactorial inheritance.

Some of the common defects in which inheritance is multifactorial include cleft lip and palate, some congenital cardiac malformations, clubfoot, congenital dislocation of the hip, and certain congenital abnormalities of the nervous system called *anencephaly* and *spina bifida*. These multifactorial malformations have an incidence among newborn infants of from 1 in 500 to 1 in 2000, depending on the malformation. The incidence is much higher, approximately 1 in 25, if one parent has the same type of congenital malformation or if other children born to the same parents have the malformation. This is because the genes that the parents are transmitting render their offspring more susceptible to disturbances in embryologic development, leading to specific types of congenital abnormalities.

# Prenatal Diagnosis of Congential Abnormalities

A wide variety of approaches are available to identify congenital abnormalities in the fetus. They fall into several groups:

1. Tests on maternal blood to screen for possible fetal abnormalities. The first group of tests measured the concentration of three substances that are normally present in the blood of pregnant women. Abnormal results may indicate a fetal abnormality. One of the first maternal blood screening tests measured a protein called *alpha fetoprotein* (AFP). The protein, produced by the fetus, diffuses into the amnionic fluid and then into the mother's blood. AFP is elevated when the fetus has a major central nervous system abnormality called an open neural tube defect, as described in Chapter 21. Later it was observed that maternal blood AFP is often lower than normal when the mother is carrying a fetus with Down syndrome or a trisomy of some other autosome, although we do not know why this occurs. Additional screening laboratory tests were also added, often supplemented by an ultrasound examination of the fetus in an attempt to identify features suggestive of Down syndrome. Currently, screening tests are offered to all pregnant women, not just older women who are at higher risk of chromosomal abnormalities. Screening tests, however, may not detect all abnormal fetuses, and may also at times yield false-positive results. Consequently, positive screening test results always should be confirmed by chromosome studies on fetal cells obtained by amniocentesis or by a procedure called chorionic villus sampling.

2. Examination of amnionic fluid. Products secreted into the fluid by the fetus, such as AFP, may indicate a congenital fetal abnormality. An abnormal volume of amnionic fluid may also indicate a fetal abnormality.

3. Examination of fetal cells. Fetal cells can be obtained by amniocentesis or by chorionic villus sampling. Cytogenetic studies of fetal cells can detect chromosomal abnormalities. Genetic abnormalities can also be identified by biochemical tests performed on fetal cells or by analysis of DNA obtained from fetal cells.

4. Ultrasound examination of the fetus. By about 16-weeks' gestation, ultrasound examination, described in Chapter 1, can visualize the limbs and all of the major organs, including the brain and spinal cord, kidneys, bladder, and heart. The

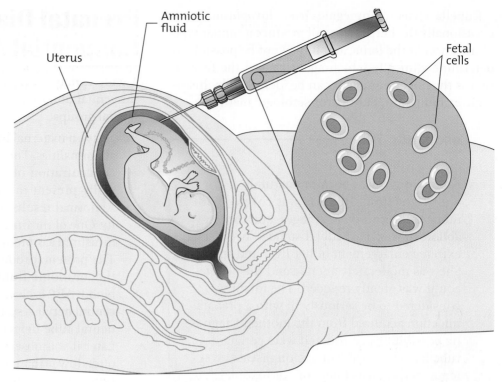

**Figure 7-12** Amniocentesis. Amnionic fluid containing some free cells derived from the fetus is withdrawn. The fetal cells can be grown in tissue culture so that their karyotype and many of their metabolic functions can be determined. Studies of fetal DNA can also be performed in selected cases (from Alters, S. 2000. *Biology, understanding life,* 3rd ed. Boston: Jones and Bartlett Publishers).

examination can detect major structural abnormalities of the nervous system called neural tube defects (anencephaly and spina bifida) and congenital hydrocephalus (Chapter 21). Other structural abnormalities can also be identified, including such defects as congenital obstruction of the urinary tract, failure of the kidneys to develop, or failure of the limbs to form normally.

An ultrasound examination usually is also performed before amniocentesis or chorionic villus sampling in order to check for any fetal abnormalities, to locate the position of the placenta, and to guide placement of the needle for aspirating amnionic fluid during amniocentesis.

## Amniocentesis

Fetal cells can be easily obtained from amnionic fluid because the cells in the fluid are of fetal origin. The cells can be grown in the laboratory by tissue culture techniques, and the karyotype of the cells can be determined. In this way, abnormalities in the number or structure of the fetal chromosomes can be determined and analysis of fetal DNA makes it possible to identify a large number of genetic diseases, including those listed in Table 7-2. The list of genetic diseases that can be identified prenatally continues to grow along with the rapid advances in the field of molecular genetics. One can also determine the concentration in amnionic fluid of

AFP, which is high when the fetus has a neural tube defect. This subject is considered in Chapter 21.

Amniocentesis is usually performed between the 14th and 18th week of pregnancy, although amniocentesis as early as the 12th to 13th week of pregnancy is available in some medical centers ( Figure 7-12 ). A needle is inserted through the mother's abdominal wall directly into the amnionic sac, and a small amount of amnionic fluid is withdrawn. Table 7-4 summarizes the main indications for the procedure. At present, the main use of amniocentesis is to confirm a chromosomal abnormality suggested by abnormal prenatal screening tests, or to determine the karyotype of the fetus carried by an older woman over the age of 35 who has declined prenatal screening tests. Some older women decline screening tests because even the most comprehensive screening tests can't detect all effected fetuses. These women want to be absolutely certain that their fetus will not have Down syndrome or some other chromosome abnormality, which can only be guaranteed by examination of fetal chromosomes obtained by amniocentesis or chorionic villus sampling

If an abnormal fetus is identified by means of a prenatal amnionic fluid study, the parents are advised of the nature of the abnormality and its possible effects on the offspring. They must then reach a decision as to whether to terminate the pregnancy or allow it to continue to term.

| Table 7-4 | **Main Indications for Amniocentesis or Chorionic Villus Sampling** |

1. Maternal age over 35 years
2. Previous infant born with Down syndrome or other chromosomal abnormality
3. Known translocation chromosome carrier, or other chromosome abnormality in either parent
4. Risk of fetal genetic disease that can be detected by fetal cell biochemical or DNA analysis
5. Maternal blood tests (triple screen) indicating increased risk of fetal chromosome abnormality

## Chorionic Villus Sampling

Chorionic villus sampling also can be used to obtain fetal cells for evaluation and in general provides the same type of information as does amniocentesis, although no amnionic fluid is obtained for chemical examination. (Chorionic villi are frondlike structures that form part of the placenta and attach to the lining of the uterus, described in Chapter 14.) The usual procedure involves passing a small catheter through the cervix to the site where the villi are attached to the uterus and suctioning out a small quantity of villi with a syringe.

Chorionic villus sampling has some advantages over aminocentesis because it can be performed at 8- to 10-weeks' gestation, which is earlier than amniocentesis can be performed, and results can be obtained earlier. If a congenital abnormality is detected and the patient wants to terminate the pregnancy, the abortion can be performed earlier in pregnancy, which carries less risk than one performed midway through the pregnancy. However, chorionic villus sampling is technically more difficult than amniocentesis, and complications from the procedure leading to spontaneous abortion are more frequent than with amniocentesis. Moreover, in some instances, chorionic villus sampling may injure the embryo. There appears to be a slight increase of limb deformities in fetuses that have undergone chorionic villus sampling early in pregnancy.

# CHAPTER REVIEW

## Summary

There are four major causes of congenital abnormalities. The first are chromosome abnormalities characterized by trisomies, deletions, and translocations, such as Turner syndrome, Klinefelter syndrome, and the fragile X syndrome. Autosomal chromosome abnormalities include Down syndrome resulting from nondisjunction of chromosome 21. A second group is characterized by abnormalities involving individual genes that result in abnormal structural proteins or enzymes. Transmission may be dominant, recessive, codominant, or transmitted on the X chromosome leading to effects determined by the gender of the fetus who receives the abnormal X chromosome. A third group of congenital abnormalities is caused by intrauterine injury from such conditions as drugs taken by the mother, maternal infections such as German measles and other infections described in this section, or radiation. The fourth group results from the interaction of multiple genes transmitted as a set from each parent in association with some environmental factors. Abnormalities such as cleft lip and palate and congenital dislocation of the hip fall into this category.

Prenatal diagnosis of congenital abnormalities includes screening blood tests that may suggest the probability of a congenital abnormality, but which must be confirmed by a more definitive test. The definitive test involves examining the chromosomes by either amniocentesis, which can be performed as early as 12 weeks' gestation, or chorionic villus sampling, which can be performed even earlier at 8 to 10 weeks' gestation, but has some disadvantages. Culture of amnionic cells can yield dividing fetal cells that can be used to construct a karyotype. Analysis of fetal DNA can provide a large amount of diagnostic information. The list of genetic diseases that can be identified prenatally continues to grow along with the rapid advances in the field of molecular genetics.

## Questions for Review

1. What are the consequences of chromosome nondisjunction? What is Down syndrome?
2. What is the karyotype of an individual with Down syndrome? Klinefelter syndrome? Turner syndrome? What is the fragile X syndrome?
3. What is the approximate incidence of congenital abnormalities? What are the major causes of congenital abnormalities? What types of maternal infections may cause congenital abnormalities in the infant?
4. What is amniocentesis? How is it used in prenatal diagnosis of congenital malformations? What type of congenital malformations may be detected by this method? In which group of patients is amniocentesis most widely used?

## Supplementary Reading

Bass, H. N., et al. 1973. Two different chromosome abnormalities resulting from a translocation carrier father. *Journal of Pediatrics* 83:1034–40.

> Describes the transmission of abnormal sets of genes to offspring from a father who is a carrier of a balanced translocation. (See Case 7-1 described in this chapter.)

Berkowitz, R. L., Roberts, J., and Minkoff, H. 2006. Challenging the strategy of maternal age-based prenatal genetic counseling. *Journal of the American Medical Association* 295:1446–48.

> Although older women have a greater risk of conceiving an infant with Down syndrome, most Down syndrome infants are born to younger women because they conceive a larger proportion of infants. Restricting prenatal detection to older women will fail to detect many Down syndrome infants. Many effective prenatal screening tests can be offered to younger women, with a confirmatory amniocentesis if the screening tests suggest a chromosomal abnormality.

Centers for Disease Control and Prevention. 1995. Chorionic villus sampling and amniocentesis: Recommendations for prenatal counseling. *Morbidity and Mortality Weekly Report* 44 (No. RR-9):1–11.

> Chorionic villus sampling carries a small risk of limb deformities probably caused by disruption of the blood supply to the limbs related to the procedure. Risk is from 0.03 to 0.10 percent, with greater risk if the procedure is performed prior to 10-weeks' gestation. The procedure also carries a greater risk of spontaneous abortion than does amniocentesis.

Centers for Disease Control and Prevention. 2002. Barriers to dietary control among pregnant women with phenylketonuria—United States, 1998–2002. *Morbidity and Mortality Weekly Report* 51:117–20.

> Untreated phenylketonuria (PKU) leads to severe mental retardation in an infant, which can be prevented by phenylalanine-restricted diets. Many affected women often discontinue their dietary restrictions as they get older. When a woman with PKU on a regular diet becomes pregnant the infant has a very high risk of mental retardation, which can be prevented by adhering to a restricted diet. A woman contemplating pregnancy should resume a PKU-restricted diet to protect her unborn infant. A phenylalanine-restricted diet is relatively expensive, which can be a financial burden on the woman, and methods to help defray some of the cost of a phenylalanine-restricted diet are essential to ensure compliance.

Cooper, R. S., Kaufman, J. S., and Ward, R. 2003. Race and genomics. *New England Journal of Medicine* 348:1166–70.

> There are large biologic differences in populations, and genomics may help define what the differences are and how the differences affect responses to environmental agents.

Hagerman, R. J., and Hagerman, P. J. 2008. Testing for fragile X gene mutations throughout the life span. *Journal of the American Medical Association* 300:2419–21.

> Describes the fragile X mental retardation gene and the CGG triplet repeat enlargement. Persons with a full mutation have both intellectual and developmental disability and may be associated with neurologic dysfunction in older adults. Autistic behavior is seen in most affected boys.

Migeon, B. R. 2006. The role of X chromosome inactivation and cellular mosaicism in women's health and in sex-specific diseases. *Journal of the American Medical Association* 295:1428–33.

Females are mosaics, having a mixture of genes expressing either their mother's or father's X-linked genes. Often the mosaicism is advantageous because it ameliorates the deleterious effects of X-linked gene mutation. Most X-linked mutations produce male-only diseases, but occasionally the gene interactions may lead to female-specific disease manifestations.

Simpson, J. L. 2005. Choosing the best prenatal screening protocol. *New England Journal of Medicine* 353:2068–70.

Most pregnant women prefer the option of prenatal screening for Down syndrome and avoiding the possible risk of amniocentesis. However, if the woman's goal of screening is 100 percent detection of trisomies, even the most comprehensive screening cannot guarantee this result, and amniocentesis or chorionic villus sampling may be preferable.

Sybert, V. P., and McCauley, E. 2004. Turner's syndrome. *New England Journal of Medicine* 351:1227–38.

The syndrome is caused by missing all or part of an X chromosome. Diagnostic characteristics and clinical features are described. Most affected persons have normal intelligence but about 70 percent have learning disabilities. Many have congenital cardiovascular abnormalities, most commonly aortic coarctation and bicuspid aortic valve. Prenatal diagnosis of Turner syndrome is possible by ulttrasound demonstration of fetal edema.

# Interactive Activities

## Multiple Choice

1. Which of the following statements about the fragile X syndrome is INCORRECT?
   A. Causes mental deficiency.
   B. Affects gene on X chromosome.
   C. Characterized by an excessive number of cytosine–guanine–guanine triplet repeating sequences that disrupt gene function.
   D. There is no relationship between the number of triplet repeats and the severity of the mental deficiency.
   E. Diagnosis made by DNA analysis of cells from the affected person.

2. Which of the following conditions is NOT an indication for amniocentesis?
   A. A 25-year-old pregnant woman with no family history of a genetic disease or chromosome abnormality wants an amniocentesis to be sure that she has no unsuspected genetic or chromosomal abnormality that could affect her fetus.
   B. History of a previous infant born with Down syndrome or other chromosomal abnormality.
   C. The woman is known to be a carrier of a translocation chromosome carrier, or one of her parents has a chromosome abnormality.
   D. The woman has a risk of genetic disease that can be detected by fetal cell biochemical or DNA analysis.
   E. Maternal screening blood tests indicate an increased risk of a fetal abnormality.

3. All of the following statements about chromosomal mosaicism are correct EXCEPT:
   A. The affected person has more than one population of chromosomally distinct cells.
   B. Mosaicism results from chromosome nondisjunction occurring in the ovum prior to fertilization.
   C. Mosaicism results from chromosome nondisjunction during a mitotic division of the fertilized ovum (zygote).
   D. Persons with mosaic Down syndrome often have less disability than those in whom all the cells contain an extra chromosome 21.
   E. Mosaicism may occur in association with other chromosomal abnormalities as well as Down syndrome.

## True or False

1. Most persons with Turner syndrome have only a single X chromosome (45,X). _____
2. Most cases of Down syndrome result from chromosome nondisjunction during mitosis. _____
3. An increased concentration of alpha fetoprotein in maternal blood or amnionic fluid suggests that the fetus has Down syndrome. _____
4. Most infants with Down syndrome are born to mothers who are carriers of a chromosome 21 that is attached to another chromosome (translocation carrier). _____

5. A neural tube defect (anencephaly or spina bifida) usually can be identified in an affected fetus by means of an ultrasound examination performed at about 16 weeks gestation. ___

## Matching
Match the congenital abnormality with its method of inheritance.

| Congenital Abnormality | Method of Inheritance |
| --- | --- |
| 1. Achondroplasia | A. Sex-linked transmission |
| 2. Hemophilia | B. Autosomal dominant transmission |
| 3. Sickle cell trait | C. Autosomal recessive transmission |
| 4. Phenylketonuria | D. Codominant inheritance transmission |

## Critical Thinking

1. Mary Jones has a brother with hemophilia. She wants to know how the disease is transmitted and whether she will also be affected. What would you tell her?
2. Susan Smith is a 38-year-old woman who is in the second month of her pregnancy. She is concerned that her baby might have Down syndrome. What should she do? What would you tell her?
3. Nancy Brown is pregnant and has developed a urinary tract infection. She wonders whether it is safe to take an antibiotic because she does not want to risk harming her developing fetus. What would you tell her? What should she do?

# Tumors

**8**

1. Compare the general characteristics of benign and malignant tumors. Explain how tumors are named. List the common exceptions to standard terminology.

2. Summarize the features of the principal types of lymphoma.

3. Differentiate between infiltrating and in situ carcinoma. Explain the role of the Pap smear in early diagnosis of neoplasm.

4. Explain how leukemia is classified. Describe the clinical manifestations of each type and its response to treatment.

5. Differentiate myeloma from leukemia. Describe its clinical manifestations, and explain how it is diagnosed.

6. Explain the mechanisms of the body's immunologic defenses against tumor.

7. Summarize the principal ways used to treat tumors, including advantages, disadvantages, and common side effects of each method.

8. Describe the applications and limitations of tumor-associated antigens in the diagnosis and treatment of patients with tumors.

9. Compare the incidence and survival rates for various types of malignant tumors. Explain the mechanisms of late recurrence. Define the role of adjuvant therapy in preventing late recurrence.

10. Understand the role of activated oncogenes and disturbance in suppressor gene function in the pathogenesis of tumors.

# Tumors: Disturbed Cell Growth

Normal life processes are characterized by continuous growth and maturation of cells, and all cells are subject to control mechanisms that regulate their growth rate. This ongoing growth process serves the purpose of replacing cells that have been injured or have undergone degenerative changes. In contrast, a neoplasm (*neo* = new + *plasm* = growth) is an overgrowth of cells that serves no useful purpose. Neoplasms appear not to be subject to the control mechanisms that normally regulate cell growth and differentiation.

# Tumors

## Classification and Nomenclature

The terms *neoplasm* and *tumor* have essentially the same meaning and may be used interchangeably. There are two large classes of neoplasms:

1. Benign tumors
2. Malignant tumors

Table 8-1 compares the major characteristics of the two classes.

## Comparison of Benign and Malignant Tumors

Generally, a benign tumor grows slowly and remains localized. Although it pushes surrounding normal tissue aside, it does not infiltrate surrounding tissues or spread by blood and lymphatic channels to distant sites. Usually, a benign tumor can be completely removed surgically without difficulty (Figure 8-1 and Figure 8-2). Histologically, the cells in a benign tumor

**metastasis**
The spread of cancer cells from the primary site of origin to a distant site within the body.

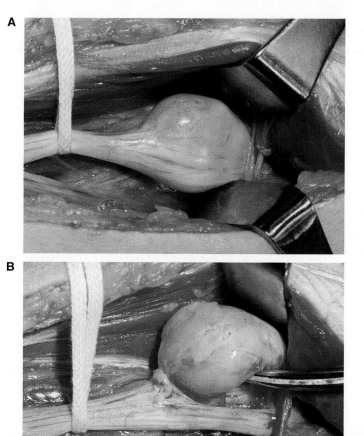

A

B

Figure 8-1    A, Benign tumor (neuroma) arising from the sciatic nerve. B, Tumor dissected from surrounding nerve. The cleavage plane is easily established, indicating that the tumor is sharply circumscribed and does not infiltrate the adjacent nerve.

appear mature and closely resemble the normal cells from which the tumor was derived.

In contrast to a benign tumor, a malignant neoplasm is composed of fewer well-differentiated cells (Figure 8-3), grows more rapidly, and infiltrates the surrounding tissues rather than growing by expansion (Figure 8-4). Frequently, the infiltrating strands of tumor find their way into the vascular and lymphatic channels. Bits of tumor may be carried in the lymphatics to reach the lymph nodes, where they establish secondary sites of tumor growth not connected with the original tumor (Figure 8-5). Eventually, the tumor may spread widely throughout the lymphatic channels. Tumor cells may also gain access to the bloodstream and be carried to distant sites, leading to secondary tumor deposits throughout the body. The process by which a tumor spreads some distance from the primary site is called **metastasis** (*meta* = beyond + *stasis* = standing), and the secondary deposits are called *metastatic tumors*

| Table 8-1 | Comparison of Benign and Malignant Tumors | |
|---|---|---|
| | Benign Tumor | Malignant Tumor |
| Growth rate | Slow | Rapid |
| Character of growth | Expansion | Infiltration |
| Tumor spread | Remains localized | Metastasis by bloodstream and lymphatics |
| Cell differentiation | Well differentiated | Poorly differentiated |

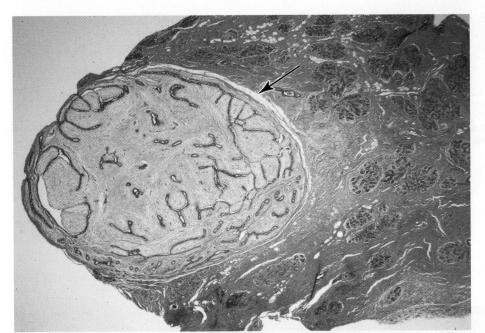

Low-magnification photomicrograph of benign breast tumor (fibroadenoma). Note the sharp demarcation between the tumor and surrounding breast tissue (*arrow*).

**A**

**B**

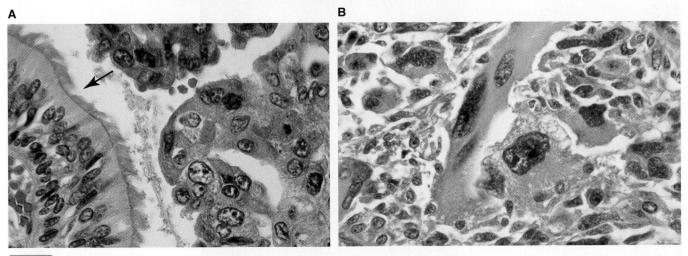

Figure 8-3 Cellular abnormalities in malignant tumors. **A,** Biopsy of a bronchus from a patient with lung carcinoma, comparing normal respiratory epithelium (*arrow*) with clusters of neoplastic cells from a lung carcinoma. Cancer cells grow in a haphazard pattern and exhibit great variation in size and structure. **B,** Malignant tumor of smooth muscle (leiomyosarcoma) illustrating large, bizarre, elongated tumor cells showing little resemblance to normal smooth muscle cells from which the tumor arose.

**A**

**B**

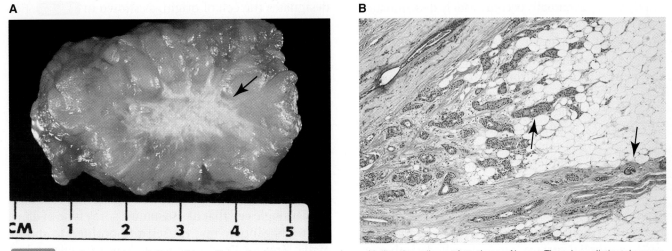

Figure 8-4 Breast carcinoma. **A,** Breast biopsy illustrating breast carcinoma (*arrow*) infiltrating adjacent fatty tissue of breast. There is no distinct demarcation between tumor and normal tissue. **B,** Low-magnification photograph illustrating the margin of infiltrating breast carcinoma. Small clusters of tumor cells (*arrows*) infiltrate adipose tissues of breast (original magnification × 20).

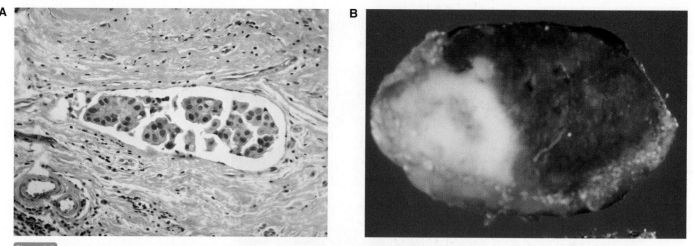

**Figure 8-5** Lymphatic spread of carcinoma. **A,** Cluster of tumor cells in lymphatic vessel (original magnification × 400). **B,** Deposit of metastatic carcinoma (white mass within node) that has spread via lymphatic channels into a small regional lymph node.

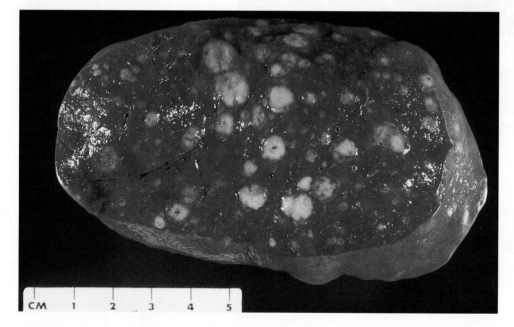

**Figure 8-6** Multiple nodules of metastatic carcinoma in spleen.

(Figure 8-6). If a malignant tumor is not eradicated promptly, it may eventually become widely disseminated throughout the body and may kill the patient. Benign tumors do not metastasize.

Tumors are named and classified according to the cells and tissues from which they originate. Therefore, understanding the primary tissue classifications explained in Chapter 2 is helpful in understanding the names of tumors. Tumor nomenclature is not completely uniform, but certain generalizations are possible.

## Benign Tumors

A benign tumor that projects from an epithelial surface is usually called a **polyp** or **papilloma** (Figure 8-7). Most other benign tumors

are named by adding the suffix *oma* to the prefix that designates the cell of origin, as shown in Table 8-2. For example, a benign tumor arising from glandular epithelium is called an **adenoma**. A benign tumor of blood vessels is an *angioma*, and one arising from cartilage is designated a *chondroma*.

## Malignant Tumors

There are many types of malignant tumors, but all can be classified into three groups: (1) carcinomas, (2) sarcomas, or (3) leukemias. The term *cancer* is a word used to indicate any type of malignant tumor.

It is generally agreed that a malignant tumor starts from a single cell that has sustained some type of damage to its genome that causes it to proliferate abnormally, first forming a clone of identical cells and, if unchecked, eventually developing into a distinct tumor.

**polyp**
A descriptive term for a benign tumor projecting from an epithelial surface.

**papilloma** (pap-pil-ō′muh) A descriptive term for a benign tumor projecting from an epithelial surface.

**adenoma** (ad-en-ō′muh) A benign tumor arising from glands.

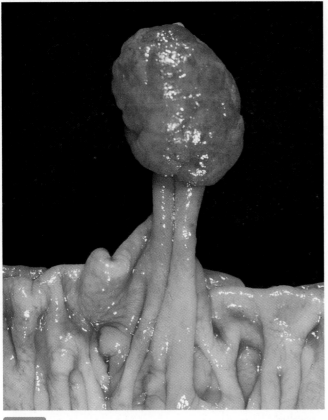

Benign polyp of colon.

### Table 8-2 — Common Prefixes Used to Name Tumors

| Prefix | Meaning |
| --- | --- |
| Adeno- | Gland |
| Angio- | Vessels (type not specified) |
| Chondro- | Cartilage |
| Fibro- | Fibrous tissue |
| Hemangio- | Blood vessels |
| Lymphangio- | Lymph vessels |
| Lipo- | Fat |
| Myo- | Muscle |
| Neuro- | Nerve |
| Osteo- | Bone |

Cells of malignant tumors exhibit behavior that is quite different from that of normal cells. They do not respond to normal growth regulatory signals from other cells, and they continue to proliferate when there is no need to do so. As they grow, they acquire properties that allow them to flourish at the expense of the surrounding normal cells. They secrete enzymes that break down normal cell and tissue barriers, which allows them to infiltrate into adjacent tissues, invade lymphatic channels and blood vessels, and eventually spread throughout the body. Moreover, the proliferating tumor cells do not "wear out" and die after a specific number of cell divisions, as normal cells do. They become "immortal" and can proliferate indefinitely.

A **carcinoma** is any malignant tumor arising from surface, glandular, or parenchymal (organ) epithelium. (The term is not applied, however, to malignant tumors of endothelium or mesothelium, which behave more like malignant connective-tissue tumors.) A carcinoma is classified further by designating the type of epithelium from which it arose. For example, a malignant tumor arising from the transitional epithelium of the urinary bladder is called a transitional cell carcinoma of the bladder. A carcinoma arising from the glandular epithelium of the pancreas is termed an adenocarcinoma of the pancreas (*aden* = gland), and a tumor arising from the squamous epithelium of the esophagus is called a squamous cell carcinoma of the esophagus.

**Sarcoma** is a general term referring to a malignant tumor arising from primary tissues other than surface, glandular, or parenchymal (organ) epithelium. The exact type of sarcoma is specified by prefixing the term designating the cell of origin. For example, a malignant tumor of cartilage is designated as a chondrosarcoma. Fibrosarcoma, liposarcoma, myosarcoma, osteosarcoma, and angiosarcoma indicate, respectively, malignant tumors of fibroblasts, fat cells, muscle cells, bone-forming cells, and blood vessels.

The term **leukemia** is applied to any neoplasm of blood-forming tissues. Neoplasms arising from the precursors of white blood cells usually do not form solid tumors. Instead, the abnormal cells proliferate diffusely within the bone marrow, where they overgrow and crowd out the normal blood-forming cells. The neoplastic cells also "spill over" into the bloodstream, and large numbers of abnormal cells circulate in the peripheral blood.

Table 8-3 summarizes the general principles used to name both benign and malignant tumors.

## Variations in Terminology

There are some inconsistencies and exceptions to the general principles of nomenclature. Exceptions are encountered in the naming of lymphoid tumors, skin tumors arising from pigment-producing cells within the epidermis, certain tumors of mixed cellular

**carcinoma** (kär-sin-ō′-mah) A malignant tumor derived from epithelial cells.

**sarcoma** (sar-kō′muh) A malignant tumor arising from connective and supporting tissues.

**leukemia** (lōō-kē′me′-yuh) A neoplastic proliferation of leukocytes.

| Table 8-3 | General Principles of Naming Tumors |
| --- | --- |
| **General Term** | **Meaning** |
| Polyp, papilloma | Any benign tumor projecting from surface epithelium. |
| _____ + oma (suffix) | A benign tumor. The prefix designates primary tissue of origin. |
| Carcinoma | Malignant tumor arising from surface, glandular, or parenchymal epithelium (but not endothelium or mesothelium). |
| Sarcoma | Malignant tumor of any primary tissue other than surface, glandular, and parenchymal epithelium. |
| Leukemia | Neoplasm of blood cells. |

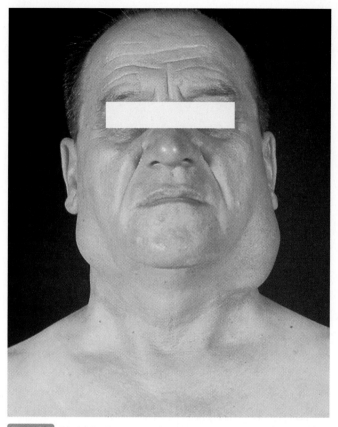

**Figure 8-8** Marked enlargement of cervical lymph nodes as a result of malignant lymphoma.

components, and certain types of tumors composed of primitive cells seen in children. In other cases, names of tumors seem to follow no rules or general principles. The student should not be unduly concerned about the exceptions or unusual situations but should attempt to grasp the general principles of naming tumors.

**Lymphoid Tumors** All neoplasms of lymphoid tissue are called **lymphomas**. With extremely rare exceptions, these tumors are malignant (Figure 8-8). Therefore, the term lymphoma without qualification refers to a malignant, not a benign, tumor. Often, to avoid confusion, the term malignant lymphoma, rather than simply lymphoma, is used.

Lymphomas are subdivided into two major groups: Hodgkin's lymphoma, more often called **Hodgkin's disease**, and non-Hodgkin's lymphoma. Hodgkin's lymphoma has several features that are quite different from other lymphomas. The disease frequently occurs in young adults, in contrast to non-Hodgkin's lymphoma, which usually affects much older persons. The disease usually starts in a single lymph node or small group of nodes and then spreads to adjacent nodes before eventually spreading to other parts of the body. The tumor has a variable histologic appearance consisting of large atypical cells intermixed with lymphocytes, plasma cells, eosinophils, and fibrous tissue. A person with Hodgkin's lymphoma usually first becomes aware of a painless enlargement of a single lymph node or group of nodes. In more advanced cases, several groups of nodes may be involved. Patients with early localized disease are usually treated by radiation therapy,

**lymphoma**
(limf-ō′muh) A neoplasm of lymphoid cells.

**Hodgkin's disease** One type of lymphoma.

which cures most patients. Patients with more advanced disease are treated by anticancer chemotherapy sometimes supplemented by radiation therapy, and many patients respond well to treatment.

All other lymphomas are grouped together under the general term of non-Hodgkin's lymphomas. Most are B cell lymphomas that are quite variable in their appearance, behavior, and prognosis. Most patients have widespread disease by the time the lymphoma is diagnosed, and it is difficult to cure the lymphoma because the tumor cells have already spread throughout the body. Some tumors are very aggressive and grow rapidly, whereas other tumors that appear somewhat similar grow more slowly. Some lymphomas respond reasonably well to specific anticancer drugs, whereas others do not. Moreover, some lymphomas, which initially were composed of mature, slowly growing cells, may transform abruptly into aggressive rapidly growing tumors composed of very immature cells.

The variable appearance and sometimes poor correlation between histologic appearance and biologic behavior have created difficulties when attempting to classify lymphomas. Various classifications have been proposed to provide a better guide to prognosis and treatment.

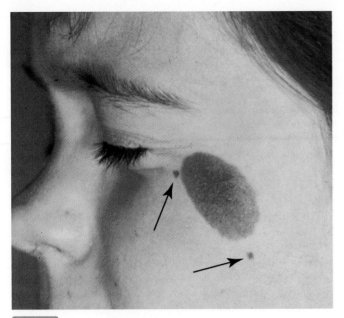

**Figure 8-9** Benign nevi of skin. A large nevus is near the eye, and two smaller adjacent nevi are shown (*arrows*).

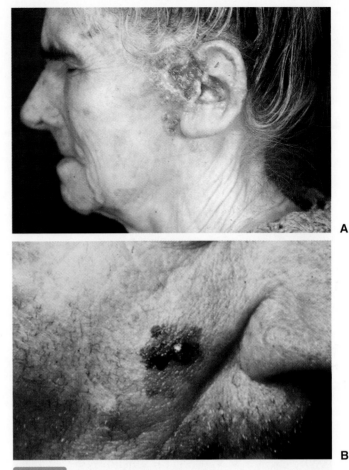

**Figure 8-10A** Common skin cancers caused by excessive sun exposure. **A,** Cancer arising from keratinocytes (basal cell carcinoma). **B,** Cancer arising from melanocytes (malignant melanoma).

**Skin Tumors** Most skin tumors arise either from the keratin-forming cells or from the pigment-producing cells of the epidermis. The keratin-forming cells are called **keratinocytes.** The deepest layer of keratinocytes adjacent to the dermis consists of cuboidal cells called basal cells that proliferate and give rise to the upper layers of cells, which are called squamous cells. Interspersed among the keratinocytes are the skin cells that normally produce pigment and are responsible for normal skin color. These are called **melanocytes,** and the black pigment that they produce is called **melanin.** The common benign pigmented skin lesion that is derived from melanin-producing cells is called a *nevus,* a Latin word that means "birthmark" (Figure 8-9). The malignant counterpart is called a melanoma (or malignant melanoma); the name being derived from the pigment elaborated by the cells.

Keratinocytes can give rise to benign proliferations, called keratoses, and two types of skin carcinomas. One type, called a basal cell carcinoma, is composed of clusters of infiltrating cells that resemble the normal basal cells of the epidermis. It is a rather indolent, slowly growing tumor that can be locally destructive but rarely metastasizes (Figure 8-10A). The other type, composed of abnormal infiltrating squamous cells, is called a squamous cell carcinoma and is a more aggressive tumor that sometimes metastasizes. Both types generally can be cured by complete surgical excision and carry a very good prognosis. Excessive sunlight exposure predisposes to the development of all types of skin cancer, including the potentially lethal melanoma

(Figure 8-10B), and also predisposes to the development of some types of keratoses, as well as causing skin damage and premature aging of the skin.

**Tumors of Mixed Components (Teratomas)** A **teratoma** is a tumor derived from cells that have the potential of differentiating into many different types of tissue (bone, muscle, glands, epithelium, brain tissue, and hair). Frequently, such tumors consist of poorly organized mixtures of many tissues. Teratomas often arise in the reproductive tract but may also develop in some other locations. Because a teratoma may be either benign or malignant, one must specify the type, calling the tumor either a benign teratoma or a malignant teratoma. A common type of cystic benign teratoma arising in the ovary is usually called a dermoid cyst (Figure 8-11).

**Childhood Primitive Cell Tumors** Certain unusual and relatively rare tumors encountered in children

**keratinocyte** (ker-u-tin′ō-cyte) A keratin-forming cell in the epidermis.

**melanocyte** (me-lan′o-cyte) Melanin-producing cell in the epidermis.

**melanin** Dark pigment found in the skin, in the middle coat of the eye, and in some other regions.

**teratoma** (tār-uh-tō′muh) A tumor of mixed cell components.

Tumors **137**

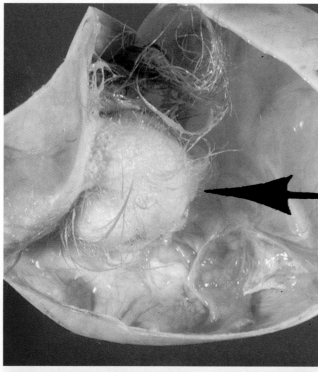

A

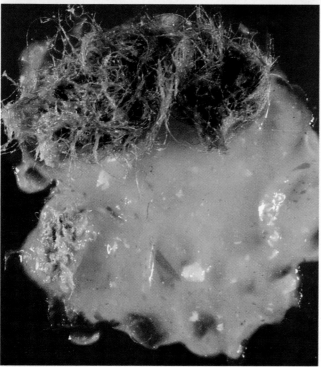

B

**Figure 8-11** **A,** Cystic teratoma (dermoid cyst) of ovary. The cyst is lined by skin containing sweat and sebaceous (oil secreting) glands, and the skin surface is covered by hair. The *arrow* indicates a nodule in the cyst wall containing fat, muscle, and bone. **B,** Contents of cyst, consisting of matted hair and oil derived from skin lining the cyst.

may arise in the brain, retina of the eye, adrenal gland, kidney, liver, or genital tract. Primitive cell tumors of this type are named from the site of origin, with the suffix *blastoma* added (*blast* = a primitive cell + *oma* = tumor). Thus, a primitive cell tumor arising from the

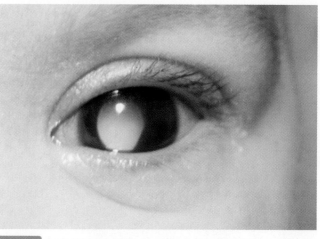

**Figure 8-12** Retinoblastoma of an eye that appears as a pale mass of tissue seen through the dilated pupil.

retina of the eye is a retinoblastoma (Figure 8-12) and one of hepatic origin is called a hepatoblastoma. A primitive cell tumor of the kidney is a nephroblastoma.

## Necrosis in Tumors

Tumors derive their blood supply from the tissues they invade. Malignant tumors frequently induce new blood vessels to proliferate in the adjacent normal tissues to supply the demands of the growing tumor. However, a malignant tumor may outgrow its blood supply. When this occurs, the parts of the tumor with the poorest blood supply undergo necrosis (Figure 8-13). If the tumor is growing within an organ such as the lung or kidney and is surrounded by normal tissue, the blood supply is best at the junction of tumor and adjacent normal tissue and poorest in the center of the tumor, which often degenerates (Figure 8-14A). In contrast,

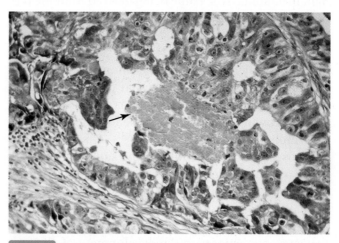

**Figure 8-13** Central necrosis (*arrow*) within cells of a breast carcinoma arising from duct epithelium.

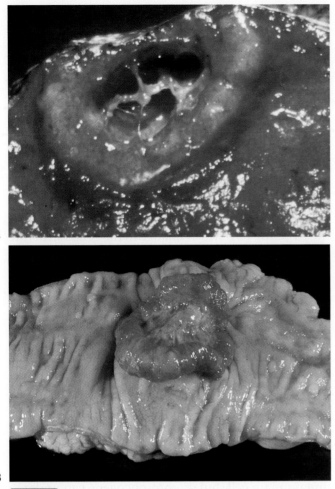

A

B

Figure 8-14  **A,** Carcinoma of lung with central necrosis. **B,** Carcinoma of colon exhibiting superficial ulceration.

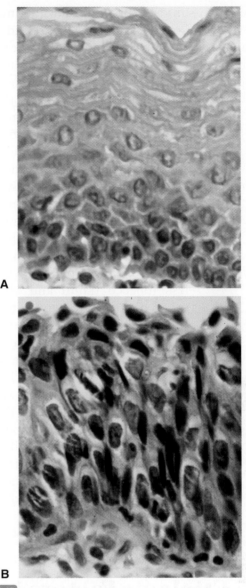

A

B

Figure 8-15  Normal cervical stratified squamous epithelium **A,** compared with in situ carcinoma of cervix. **B,** Note the nuclear abnormalities characteristic of carcinoma. The tumor has not yet infiltrated the underlying tissues (original magnification × 400).

if the malignant tumor is growing outward from an epithelial surface, such as the colon, the best blood supply is at the base of the tumor. The poorest blood supply is at the surface, which frequently becomes necrotic and sloughs, leaving a shallow crater covered with degenerated tissue and inflammatory exudate (Figure 8-14B). Often, small blood vessels are exposed in the ulcerated base of the tumor. Blood may ooze continuously from these vessels, eventually leading to anemia from chronic blood loss. Sometimes the ulcerated tumor may be the source of a severe hemorrhage.

## Noninfiltrating (in Situ) Carcinoma

Infiltration and metastasis are two characteristic features of malignant tumors. However, we now know that many carcinomas arising from surface epithelium remain localized within the epithelium for many years before evidence of infiltration into the deeper tissues or spread to distant sites becomes apparent. This has been well documented for squamous cell carcinoma of the cervix (Figure 8-15). Noninfiltrating tumors have also

been recognized in many other locations, including the breast, urinary tract, colon, and skin. The term *carcinoma in situ* (in-site carcinoma) is used for this type of neoplasm. In situ carcinoma can be completely cured by surgical excision or other treatment that eradicates the abnormal epithelium, and this is the stage most favorable to successful treatment.

## Precancerous Conditions

Sometimes the term *precancerous* is used when referring to conditions that have a high likelihood of eventually developing into cancer. Prolonged exposure to sunlight, for example, not only causes premature aging of the skin, but also causes small, crusted, scaly patches to develop on sun-exposed skin, called **actinic keratoses** ("actinic" refers to sun rays). Untreated, many keratoses eventually develop into skin cancers. Another precancerous condition resulting from prolonged sun exposure is a frecklelike proliferation of melanin-producing cells in the skin called **lentigo maligna** (a Latin term meaning "malignant freckle"). They are so named because many eventually become transformed into melanomas. Precancerous, thick white patches descriptively called **leukoplakia** (*leuko* = white + *plakia* = patch) may develop in the mucous membranes of the mouth as a result of exposure to tobacco tars from pipe or cigar smoking or from use of smokeless tobacco (snuff and chewing tobacco) and may give rise to squamous cell cancers of the oral cavity. Somewhat similar precancerous changes may take place in the epithelium of the vulva (Chapter 13) and may eventuate into vulvar cancer. Some types of colon polyps that are prone to malignant change are also considered precancerous. There are many precancerous conditions, of which these are only a few examples. Precancerous conditions should always be treated appropriately in order to prevent malignant change, which occurs in many, but not all, cases.

# Etiologic Factors in Neoplastic Disease

## Viruses

Many types of tumors in animals are caused by viruses and can be readily transmitted by appropriate methods to animals of the same or a different species. In some instances, a single type of virus is capable of producing many different types of tumors in various species of animals. At least some of the cancers in humans also appear to be caused by viruses. Kaposi's sarcoma in AIDS patients is caused by a herpesvirus, designated human herpesvirus 8 (HHV-8). Some strains of the papillomavirus that cause genital condylomas (Chapter 13) predispose to cervical carcinoma and are also responsible for some squamous cell carcinomas of the mouth, throat, and larynx. Chronic viral hepatitis (Chapter 16) predisposes to primary carcinoma of the liver. Some types of nasopha-

ryngeal carcinoma and some types of lymphoma appear to be related to Epstein-Barr virus infections, the virus that causes infectious mononucleosis.

## Gene and Chromosomal Abnormalities

The basic process common to all neoplasms is an alteration of the genes on the chromosomes of a cell so that the cell no longer responds to normal control mechanisms and proceeds to proliferate without regard for the needs of the body. In the body, many billions of cells are dividing all the time. They are also continually subjected to radiation, various chemical carcinogens (cancer-producing substances), or other agents that can alter the structure of genes. A change in the gene's structure is called a **mutation** (*muto* = change), and the mutated gene may function differently from a normal gene.

Three large groups of genes play important roles in regulating cell functions, and derangements of these genes are associated with formation of tumors. The first group comprises **proto-oncogenes**. The second group consists of **tumor suppressor genes**, and the third group is the **DNA repair genes** ( Table 8-4 ).

**Proto-Oncogenes** Human chromosomes contain a number of normal "growth genes" that promote some aspect of cell growth, differentiation, or mitotic activity. They are called *proto-oncogenes*. A proto-oncogene is a normal gene that regulates some normal growth function in a cell, but a proto-oncogene can undergo a mutation or become translocated to another chromosome where its functions are deranged. Either event can convert a normally functioning proto-oncogene into an oncogene (*onkos* = tumor), an abnormally functioning gene that stimulates cell growth excessively and leads to unrestrained cell proliferation. An oncogene is a "gene that causes cancer."

| Table 8-4 | Gene Mutations That Disrupt Cell Function | |
|---|---|---|
| Gene | Normal Function | Malfunction |
| Proto-oncogene | Promotes normal cell growth | Point mutation, amplification, or translocation forms an oncogene, resulting in unrestrained cell growth |
| Paired tumor suppressor genes | Inhibit cell proliferation | Both genes inactivated in same cell promotes cell proliferation |
| Paired DNA repair genes | Correct errors in DNA duplication | Gene inactivation increases mutation rate |

Conversion of a proto-oncogene into an oncogene (activation of an oncogene) may consist of a change in only a single nucleotide in the DNA of the gene, which is called a point mutation, or the mutation may generate multiple copies of the same gene, called gene amplification, which greatly increases the activity of the gene. Translocation to another chromosome activates an oncogene because of the way in which genes are related on individual chromosomes. A specific gene, such as one that regulates some aspect of cell growth or mitotic activity, is influenced by other nearby genes that either suppress or stimulate its activities. Cell growth and differentiation are normal when the proto-oncogene ("growth gene") and its neighbors function together in an orderly manner, but may be deranged if this relation is disturbed. For example, the translocation may bring the proto-oncogene to a new location on another chromosome where it is freed from the inhibitory genes that formerly controlled its activities. Alternatively, the translocation may bring the proto-oncogene to a new location on another chromosome adjacent to another gene that stimulates its functions.

**Tumor Suppressor Genes** These are groups of different genes that function to suppress cell proliferation. Loss of suppressor gene function by mutation or another event disrupts cell functions and can lead to unrestrained cell growth. Suppressor genes exist in pairs at corresponding gene loci on homologous chromosomes, and both suppressor genes must cease to function before the cell malfunctions.

**DNA Repair Genes** DNA repair genes are part of the cell's "quality control" and repair system. These genes regulate the processes that monitor and repair any errors in DNA duplication that may occur when the cell's chromosomes are duplicated in the course of cell division; they are also concerned with the repair of DNA that has been damaged by radiation, chemicals, or other environmental agents. Any change in the normal arrangement of DNA nucleotides on the DNA chain constitutes a DNA mutation. Consequently, failure of DNA repair gene function increases the likelihood of DNA mutations within the affected cell. A high mutation rate within cells predisposes to tumors because some mutations may affect cell functions that promote unrestrained cell growth.

Like tumor suppressor genes, DNA repair genes also exist in pairs in homologous chromosomes, and both must become nonfunctional before the repair functions regulated by the genes are compromised. Persons with an inherited mutation of a DNA repair gene are at increased risk of some tumors because if a spontaneous mutation of the other gene occurs, the affected cell is no longer able to regulate cell growth properly. Uncontrolled cell proliferation results and gives rise to a tumor.

***Multistep Progression of Genetic Changes Leading to Cancer*** In most cases, cancers do not result from mutation of a single gene, but rather are the result of multiple genetic "insults" to the genome characterized by activation of oncogenes along with loss of function of one or more tumor suppressor genes. The transition, for example, from a benign polyp of the colon to an invasive colon cancer requires activation of an oncogene (called *ras*) and inactivation of three distinct tumor suppressor genes (designated *APC*, *DCC*, and *p53*).

After a cell has been deregulated and has formed a tumor, additional random genetic changes may take place in the tumor cells, which is indicative of the instability of the tumor cell genome. Often, individual genes may undergo additional mutations or they may reduplicate themselves by gene amplification, forming multiple copies of a single gene. Chromosomes may fragment; pieces of chromosomes may be lost from the cells or be translocated to other chromosomes. Some of these mutations in the unstable tumor cell genome may produce new mutant cells that exhibit more aggressive growth than the original tumor cells, and the new mutant may eventually outgrow the other cells in the tumor. Clinically, this event may be manifested by more rapid growth and aggressive behavior of the tumor, and often the tumor may become less responsive to the anticancer drugs that formerly could control it.

***Chromosomal Abnormalities*** Not all gene alterations that activate oncogenes or inactivate tumor suppressor genes can be identified from examination of the tumor cell chromosomes. Point mutations do not change chromosome structure, but translocations relocate large pieces of chromosomes and change their structure, as do deletions of chromosome material and amplification of individual genes. The best-known neoplasm-associated chromosomal abnormality, which is called *Philadelphia chromosome* (named after the city where it was discovered), can be demonstrated in the white cells of patients with one type of leukemia called chronic granulocytic leukema (described in the section on leukemia). The abnormality is a reciprocal translocation of broken end pieces between chromosomes 9 and 22. In this translocation, a proto-oncogene (designated *abl*) on chromosome 9 is moved to a position on chromosome 22. There it becomes fused with another gene (called *bcr*) to form a composite gene (*bcr/abl*) that directs the synthesis of an uncontrolled extremely active enzyme that promotes active cell growth and cell division. It is the excessive unregulated

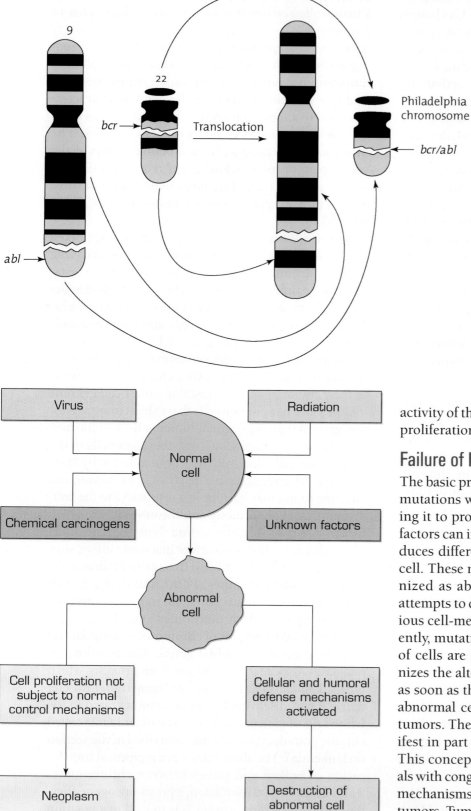

Figure 8-16 Reciprocal translocation between broken pieces of chromosomes 9 and 22, forming the Philadelphia chromosome containing the composite gene that disrupts normal cell functions.

Figure 8-17 Factors leading to neoplastic transformation of cells counterbalanced by immunologic defense against neoplasm. Conversion of a normal cell into an abnormal one requires activation of oncogenes and inactivation of tumor suppressor genes, which renders the cell unresponsive to normal control mechanisms that regulate cell growth. Generally, multiple step-by-step mutations are required to transform a normal cell into a cancer cell.

activity of this enzyme that stimulates the unrestrained proliferation of the leukemic cells (Figure 8-16).

## Failure of Immunologic Defenses

The basic processes common to all neoplasms are gene mutations within a cell that deregulate the cell, causing it to proliferate abnormally. Many environmental factors can induce mutations. A mutant cell often produces different cell proteins not present in a normal cell. These mutant-gene–encoded proteins are recognized as abnormal by the immune system, which attempts to destroy the abnormal cell by means of various cell-mediated and humoral mechanisms. Apparently, mutations leading to neoplastic transformation of cells are relatively common, but the body recognizes the altered cells as abnormal and destroys them as soon as they are formed. Only a tiny percentage of abnormal cells ever develop into clinically apparent tumors. Therefore, one may consider a tumor to manifest in part a failure of the body's immune defenses. This concept is supported by evidence that individuals with congenital deficiencies of immunologic defense mechanisms have a higher than expected incidence of tumors. Tumors also occur frequently in persons whose immune responses have been deliberately suppressed by drugs or other substances.

Figure 8-17 illustrates the interrelation of the factors concerned with the defense against tumors. On one hand, abnormal cells arise and tend to proliferate, leading to tumors. On the other hand, the immune-defense mechanisms destroy these abnormal cells before they can prove hazardous to the body. Tumors result when the defense mechanisms fail. Fortunately, in most instances, the immune surveillance system eliminates the "bad" cells as soon as they appear. Although the immune-defense mechanisms are quite efficient in eliminating abnormal cells before they develop into a tumor, they are much less effective in eliminating an established tumor.

## Heredity and Tumors

Although there is no strong hereditary predisposition to most common malignant tumors, hereditary factors do play a small role in some common tumors. A person whose parent or sibling has been afflicted with a breast, colon, or lung carcinoma has about a three times greater risk of developing a similar tumor than do other people. The predisposition is apparently the result of a multifactorial inheritance pattern in which the individual at risk has inherited sets of genes that influence some hormonal or enzyme-regulated biochemical process within the body that slightly increases the susceptibility to a specific cancer. The increased risk may be caused by genetic differences in various biochemical or physiologic activities that influence cell functions, such as

1. Differences in circulating hormone levels that could influence cell growth rates
2. Variations in the rate at which the cell can metabolize and inactivate cancer-causing chemicals to which the cells are exposed
3. Variations in the ability to repair DNA that has been damaged by injurious agents
4. Variations in the efficiency of the immune system in eliminating abnormal cells as they arise

Heredity does play an important role in some tumors. The classic example is retinoblastoma, an uncommon childhood tumor illustrated in Figure 8-12. This tumor is also a typical example of how tumor suppressor genes control cell function and how loss of control can cause a tumor. Retinoblastoma is a malignant tumor of primitive retinal cells occurring in infants and children that is caused by loss of function of tumor suppressor genes called *RB* genes. Normal *RB* genes exist in pairs, one on each of the homologous pair of chromosome 13, and both *RB* genes must be nonfunctional in a retinal cell before a tumor arises. About half the retinoblastomas are hereditary; the rest occur sporadically, without any hereditary predisposition. The hereditary form of retinoblastoma is prone to occur if a

child inherits a defective nonfunctional *RB* gene from a parent. The affected child has only a single-functioning *RB* gene in all body cells, including those in the retina, but the single-functioning *RB* gene is sufficient to maintain control of cell functions. However, if a chance mutation occurs in the remaining single-functional *RB* gene within a retinal cell, all *RB* gene function in the affected cell is lost. The affected cell then proliferates to form a clone of unregulated cells and eventually a malignant retinal tumor. Hereditary retinoblastomas may occur in both eyes because retinal cells in both eyes are equally vulnerable to similar random *RB* gene mutations in other single-functioning *RB* genes. In the sporadic form of retinoblastoma, both *RB* genes in the same retinal cell must undergo mutation in order to deregulate cell function and give rise to a retinoblastoma. Figure 8-18 summarizes the pathogenesis of this tumor. The hereditary form of neuroblastoma is considered to be transmitted as a Mendelian dominant trait because the transmission of a single

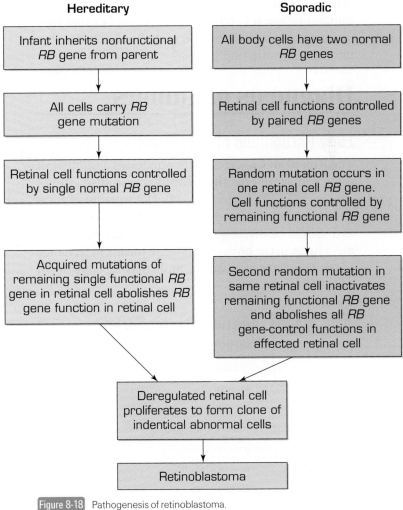

**Figure 8-18** Pathogenesis of retinoblastoma.

defective *RB* gene from parent to child places the child at very high risk of developing this tumor, even though the second *RB* gene must become nonfunctional in a retinal cell before the neoplasm actually arises.

Hereditary gene mutations are also responsible for a small percentage of breast carcinomas, and the affected persons are at increased risk of ovarian carcinoma as well. Two different genes are involved. Some hereditary breast and ovarian carcinomas can be traced to an inherited mutation of a tumor suppressor gene designated *BRCA1* (breast carcinoma 1), which has been localized to chromosome 17. Other cases are related to a mutation of a second tumor suppressor gene designated *BRCA2* (breast carcinoma 2), which is located on chromosome 13. The pathogenesis of hereditary breast and ovarian carcinoma related to either a *BRCA1* or *BRCA2* mutation is comparable to that of hereditary retinoblastoma caused by an inherited mutant *RB* gene as illustrated in Figure 8-18. *BRCA* mutations are considered to be inherited as dominant traits because the inheritance of a single *BRCA* mutant gene from either parent is responsible for the increased susceptibility to both breast and ovarian carcinomas. There are many other examples of tumors related to hereditary gene mutations, but it is important to remember that they make up only a small fraction of the benign and malignant tumors afflicting humans.

# Diagnosis of Tumors

## Early Recognition of Neoplasms

The American Cancer Society publicizes a number of signs and symptoms that should arouse suspicion of cancer ( Table 8-5 ). In general, any abnormality of form or function may be an early manifestation of a neoplasm and should be investigated by a physician. For example, a lump in the breast, an ulcer on the lip, or a change in the character of a wart or mole may be considered an abnormality of form. Menstrual bleeding in a postmenopausal woman or a change in bowel habits manifested by constipation or diarrhea is an abnormality of function.

A complete medical history and physical examination by the physician are the next steps in evaluating suspected abnormalities. The physical examination may include special studies such as an examination of the rectum and colon by means of a special instrument, a vaginal examination and Pap smear in women, examination of the esophagus and stomach with special devices, and various types of x-ray studies.

If a tumor is discovered, exact diagnosis requires biopsy or complete excision of the suspected tumor. Histologic examination of the tissue by the pathologist will provide an exact diagnosis and serve as a guide to further treatment. If the tumor is benign, simple excision is curative. If the tumor is malignant, a more extensive operation or another kind of treatment may be required.

## Cytologic Diagnosis of Neoplasms

Tumors shed abnormal cells from their surfaces, and these cells can be recognized in the body fluids and secretions that come into contact with the tumor ( Figure 8-19 ). Often the abnormal cells can be recognized

| Table 8-5 | American Cancer Society Warning Signals |
|---|---|
| 1. | Change in bowel or bladder habits |
| 2. | A sore that does not heal |
| 3. | Unusual bleeding or discharge |
| 4. | A thickening or lump in the breast or elsewhere |
| 5. | Indigestion or difficulty in swallowing |
| 6. | An obvious change in wart or mole |
| 7. | A nagging cough or hoarseness |

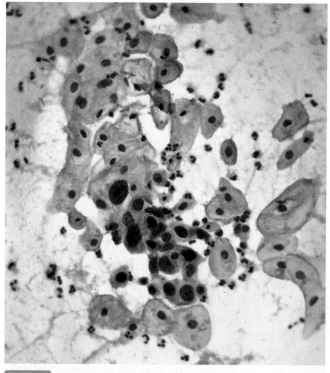

**Figure 8-19** Photomicrograph of Pap smear, illustrating cluster of abnormal cells from in situ carcinoma of cervix. Cells appear much different from adjacent normal squamous epithelial cells (original magnification × 160).

when the neoplasm is only microscopic in size and is still confined to the surface epithelium. These observations have been applied to the cytologic diagnosis of tumors. The method is named after the physician who played a large part in developing and applying cytologic methods, Dr. George Papanicolaou. The microscopic slides of the material prepared for cytologic examination are called Papanicolaou smears or, simply, Pap smears.

Widespread application of cytologic methods has led to much earlier detection of cervical carcinoma than had previously been possible and has played a significant role in reducing mortality from carcinoma of the uterine cervix. It should be emphasized, however, that an abnormal cervical Pap smear indicates only that the cervical epithelium is shedding atypical or abnormal cells. It does not necessarily indicate a diagnosis of cancer because some benign diseases are occasionally associated with desquamation of atypical cells. A Pap smear should be considered as a screening procedure, and an atypical or abnormal smear should be followed by further studies, which may include a biopsy and histologic examination of the tissue to establish an exact diagnosis. This subject is considered further in Chapter 13.

Cytologic methods can also be applied to the diagnosis of neoplasms in other locations by examining sputum, urine, breast secretions, and fluids obtained from the pleural or peritoneal cavities. However, cytology has been most valuable in the early diagnosis of cervical cancer.

**Cytologic Diagnosis by Fine-Needle Aspiration** Cells for cytologic study can also be obtained by aspirating material from organs or tissues by means of a thin needle with a narrow lumen attached to a syringe, and preparing slides from the aspirated material. Suspected tumors in the lung, liver, pancreas, kidney, and other internal organs also can be examined by fine-needle aspiration. When attempting aspiration from internal organs, one must precisely determine the location of the suspected tumor by means of a CT scan or other x-ray examination or by ultrasound and insert the needle into the suspected tumor under x-ray guidance.

## Frozen-Section Diagnosis of Neoplasms

Many times, it is important that a surgeon learn immediately whether a tumor discovered in the course of an operation is benign or malignant because the extent of resection performed may depend on the nature of the neoplasm. Often, the surgeon must also find out during the operation whether a tumor has been excised completely or whether it has spread to lymph nodes or distant sites. A pathologist can provide the surgeon with a rapid histologic diagnosis and other information by means of a special technique called a frozen section. In this method, a portion of the tumor or other tissue to be examined histologically is frozen solid at a subzero temperature. A thin section of the frozen tissue is cut by means of a special instrument called a microtome, and slides are prepared and stained. The slides can then be examined by the pathologist, and a rapid histologic diagnosis can be made. The entire procedure takes only a few minutes.

## Tumor-Associated Antigen Tests

Some cancers secrete substances called tumor-associated antigens. These are either absent from normal mature tissues or present only in trace amounts. Most tumor-associated antigens are carbohydrate–protein complexes (*glycoproteins*) that are secreted as a coating on the surface of the cancer cells. Some of the glycoprotein gains access to the circulation, where it can be detected by means of specialized laboratory tests performed on the blood of patients with cancer.

A well-known tumor-associated antigen is a substance called carcinoembryonic antigen (CEA), so named because it resembles a glycoprotein antigen secreted by the cells lining the fetal intestinal tract. It has been postulated that cancer cells elaborate CEA because they are immature and have acquired some properties of fetal cells that adult cells do not have (Figure 8-20).

Not all malignant tumors secrete CEA. Moreover, elevation of CEA levels is not specific for any one type of cancer. CEA is produced by most malignant tumors of the gastrointestinal tract and pancreas, but it is also secreted by many cancers of the breast and lung and by other cancers as well. The amount of CEA secreted is related to the size of the tumor. CEA is usually not

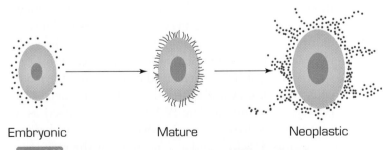

Embryonic      Mature      Neoplastic

**Figure 8-20** Relation of carcinoembryonic antigen (CEA) to embryonic cells. Embryonic cell (*left*) produces a specific type of carbohydrate–protein coating in its surface. Coating is replaced by a different type in a mature cell (*center*). Neoplastic cell (*right*) reverts to a more primitive state and resumes production of embryonic coating material, which enters circulation and often can be detected in blood of patient with invasive carcinoma.

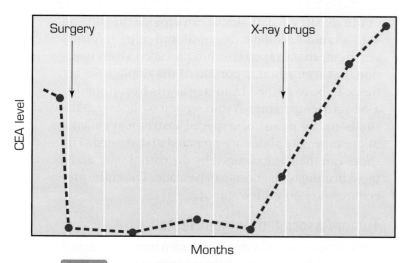

**Figure 8-21** The use of CEA to monitor response therapy. An elevated CEA level falls after resection of colon cancer and then rises when tumor recurs, indicating the need for additional treatment.

elevated in the blood of persons with small, early cancers, but the levels are often quite high in persons with large tumors or tumors that have metastasized. When CEA is elevated in a patient with cancer, the level falls after the tumor has been removed and often rises again if the tumor recurs or metastasizes (Figure 8-21). One can perform serial determinations of CEA to monitor the course of patients with CEA-secreting tumors. If CEA falls after removal of the tumor and later becomes elevated, this usually means that the tumor has recurred and indicates that additional treatment is needed. Slight elevations of CEA are sometimes detected in patients with diseases other than cancer. This does not detract from the usefulness of the CEA test, however, because the CEA levels are usually much lower than in patients with malignant tumors.

Other products secreted by tumor cells that can be used to monitor tumor growth are discussed in Chapter 15. They include *alpha fetoprotein*, a protein produced by fetal tissues but not normally produced by adult cells, and *human chorionic gonadotropin*, the hormone normally produced by the placenta in pregnancy, which are often elevated in patients with testicular carcinoma. Alpha fetoprotein is also frequently elevated in patients with primary carcinoma of the liver. *Prostate-specific antigen* (PSA), produced by prostatic epithelial cells, often is elevated in the bloodstream of men with prostatic carcinoma. The PSA test often is used as a screening test to detect early prostate carcinoma before symptoms develop, and also to monitor the response to treatment. Many other tumor-associated substances have been described (sometimes called tumor markers) that are used to monitor patients with various types of lung, breast, and ovarian carcinoma.

# Treatment of Tumors

Benign tumors are completely cured by surgical excision. Malignant tumors are much more difficult to treat. Four major forms of treatment are directed against malignant tumors:

1. Surgery
2. Radiotherapy
3. Hormones
4. Anticancer drugs (chemotherapy)

The method of treatment depends on the type of tumor and its extent, and sometimes several methods are combined. In many cases, treatment eradicates the cancer, and the patient is cured. In less favorable cases, cure is no longer possible, but the growth of the cancer is arrested and life is prolonged.

## Surgery

Many malignant tumors are treated by wide surgical excision of the tumor and the surrounding tissues, usually with removal of the regional lymph nodes that drain the tumor site. This treatment is successful if the tumor has not already spread to distant sites. Unfortunately, many cancers have already metastasized when first detected and may no longer be curable by surgery alone. Other methods of treatment must be used, frequently in combination with surgery.

## Radiotherapy

Malignant lymphomas and some epithelial tumors are quite radiosensitive and can be destroyed by radiotherapy rather than by surgical excision. In other cases, radiation and surgery are combined. For example, radiation may be administered preoperatively to reduce the size of a tumor, thereby facilitating its surgical resection; in other instances, radiotherapy is given after a malignant tumor has been resected (cut out) in order to destroy any cancer cells that may have been left behind. Radiotherapy is also used to control the growth of widespread tumors and to treat deposits of metastatic tumor that cause pain and disability. The treatment relieves symptoms and makes the patient more comfortable, even though the cancer is not curable.

## Hormone Therapy

Some malignant tumors require hormones for their growth and are called hormone responsive. They regress temporarily if deprived of the required hormone. For example, many prostate tumors require testosterone and are inhibited by removal of the testes, which eliminates the source of testosterone, or by administration of drugs that block the ability of the testes to produce testosterone. Many breast carcinomas in postmenopausal women are estrogen responsive and can be controlled by drugs that block estrogen so that the tumor cells are no longer stimulated by estrogen.

Adrenal cortical hormones (corticosteroids) also inhibit the growth of many malignant tumors. Corticosteroids inhibit protein synthesis, thereby suppressing the growth and division of the tumor cells. Tumors of the lymphatic tissues are especially susceptible to the effects of corticosteroids.

## Anticancer Drugs

Cancer cells, like normal cells, synthesize deoxyribonucleic acid (DNA) from various precursors. The DNA directs the production of the various forms of ribonucleic acid (messenger RNA, transfer RNA, and ribosomal RNA), and the RNA in turn takes part in the synthesis of enzymes and other proteins that are necessary for cell function. Anticancer drugs impede the growth and division of cells by disrupting some phase of this complex process.

Most anticancer drugs are quite toxic. They injure normal cells as well as cancer cells and must be administered very carefully in order to ensure maximum damage to tumor cells without irreparable injury to normal cells. Lymphoid tissue is quite susceptible to the destructive effects of these potent drugs, and consequently, one unavoidable side effect of anticancer drugs is impairment of cell-mediated and humoral immunity.

Recently, several less toxic and more cell-specific anticancer drugs have been developed that function by blocking the action of specific cell components that stimulate the tumor cells. Some of these drugs suppress tumor growth by blocking growth factor receptors on the surface of the tumor cells so that growth factors produced by normal cells cannot attach to the receptors and stimulate the tumor cells. Other drugs inhibit the functions of important intracellular proteins, such as the enzyme tyrosine kinase, that in various ways stimulate cell proliferation.

## Adjuvant Chemotherapy

Sometimes surgical resection of a cancer appears to be successful, but metastases appear several years later and eventually prove fatal. The operation fails to eradicate the tumor because small, unrecognized metastases have already spread throughout the body. Even though the main tumor has been removed, the minute metastases continue to grow until eventually they form many large, bulky deposits of metastatic tumor that kill the patient.

In order to forestall the development of late metastases, a current trend is to administer a course of anticancer drugs after surgical resection of some tumors. This is called adjuvant chemotherapy (*adjuvare* = to assist). The drugs destroy any small, undetected foci of metastatic tumor before they become large enough to produce clinical manifestations. In some cases, adjuvant chemotherapy combined with surgery appears to achieve better results than surgery alone. Many anticancer drugs are quite toxic, however, and the potential benefits of adjuvant chemotherapy must be weighed against the harmful effects of the drugs on normal tissues.

## Immunotherapy

The immune system has evolved in a number of ways to deal with abnormal cells that can proliferate and form tumors and to deal with established tumors.

1. Cytotoxic T cells recognize antigens on tumor cells that are displayed along with the cells' own MHC Class I proteins and can damage the tumor cells by secreting destructive cytokines.
2. Natural-killer lymphocytes can attack and destroy tumor cells without prior antigenic stimulation.
3. Activated macrophages can destroy tumor cells by phagocytosis and by secreting cytokines that damage the tumor cells, and also stimulate lymphocytes to attack the tumor cells.
4. Antibodies formed against tumor cell antigens can affix to tumor cells and activate complement; products of complement activation attract lymphocytes and macrophages that damage the cell membranes of the tumor cells.

Despite the array of immunologic defenses, many tumors circumvent or overwhelm the body's defenses, which become less effective and are no longer able to retard the growth of the tumor. In addition, the chemotherapy and irradiation used to treat tumors also suppress the body's immune responses. Various attempts have been made to stimulate the body's immune system so that it can deal more effectively with the tumor, which is called **immunotherapy**. Some types of immunotherapy have produced gratifying results in persons with specific types of widespread tumors when no other methods of treatment were able to control the tumor. Unfortunately, most patients treated with immunotherapy have advanced disease, and often the body's immune defenses are incapable of dealing with such large amounts of tumor even when stimulated by immunotherapy.

**immunotherapy**
(im′mu′-nō-ther′uh-pē)
Treatment given to retard growth of a disseminated malignant tumor by stimulating the body's own immune defenses.

# Leukemia

The term *leukemia* refers to a neoplasm of hematopoietic tissue. In contrast to solid tumors, which form nodular deposits, leukemic cells diffusely infiltrate the bone marrow and lymphoid tissues, spill over into the bloodstream, and infiltrate throughout the various organs of the body. The leukemic cells may be mostly mature, or they may be extremely primitive. The overproduction of white cells in leukemia may be revealed in the peripheral blood by a very high white blood count. In some cases of leukemia, however, the proliferation of the white cells is largely confined to the bone marrow, and there is no significant increase in the number of white cells in the bloodstream.

## Classification of Leukemia

Leukemia is classified on the basis of both the cell type and the maturity of the proliferating cells. Any type of hematopoietic cells can give rise to leukemia, but the most common types are granulocytic, monocytic, and lymphocytic. Leukemia developing from stem cells that would normally give rise to the leukocytes containing specific granules (neutrophils, eosinophils, and basophils) is called *granulocytic leukemia*. *Monocytic leukemia* develops from precursor cells that give rise to monocytes. *Lymphocytic leukemia* is derived from lymphoid precursor cells. Various subclassifications have been established within these major groups on the basis of the characteristics of the cell membranes and the enzymes present within the leukemic cells, as determined by highly specialized techniques.

If the leukemia cells are mostly primitive forms, the leukemia is classified as *acute leukemia* (Figure 8-22), and if the cells are mostly mature, the leukemia is classified as *chronic leukemia*. In chronic granulolcytic leukemia, most of the circulating cells are maturing granulocytes and neutrophils, and there are few primitive cells (Figure 8-23). In *chronic lymphocytic leukemia*, the circulating cells are mostly mature lymphocytes (Figure 8-24).

In most instances, the total number of white blood cells in the peripheral blood is significantly above normal. Occasionally, however, the marrow may be crowded with abnormal cells, but the number of white blood cells in the blood is normal or decreased.

Generally, the classifications by cell type and maturity are used together. Thus, one may speak of chronic granulocytic leukemia, acute lymphocytic leukemia, or acute monocytic leukemia.

## Clinical Features and Principles of Treatment

The clinical features of leukemia are of two kinds: those caused by impairment of bone marrow function

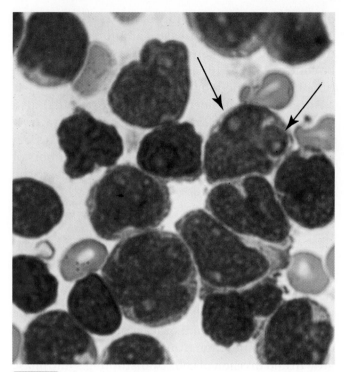

**Figure 8-22** A photomicrograph of a blood smear from a patient with acute leukemia. The nuclei of the white cells have fine chromatin structure and prominent nucleoli indicating immaturity (*arrows*). Nuclei are irregular in size and configuration (original magnification × 1000).

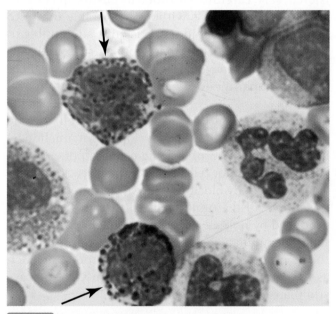

**Figure 8-23** Chronic granulocytic leukemia. Most of the cells in the photomicrograph are mature. Note the basophils (*arrows*), the eosinophil (*left of arrows*), and the two neutrophils (*right of arrows*) (original magnification × 1000).

and those caused by infiltration of the viscera by leukemic cells. The overgrowth of leukemic cells in the bone marrow often crowds out normal bone marrow cells. This leads to anemia as a result of inadequate red cell production, bleeding caused by thrombocytopenia, and infection resulting from inadequate

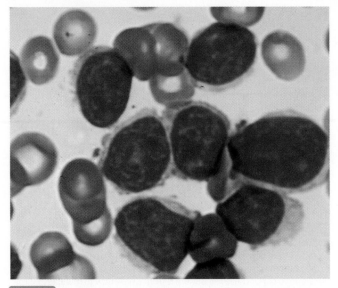

Figure 8-24 Chronic lymphocyctic leukemia. The dense nuclear chromatin structure indicates that the lymphocytes are mature (compare with Figure 10-26). The total white count is elevated (original magnification × 1000).

numbers of normal white blood cells, which are an important part of the body's defenses against pathogenic organisms.

The leukemic cells not only infiltrate the bone marrow, but also spread into the spleen, liver, lymph nodes, and other tissues. In chronic leukemia, the evolution of the disease proceeds at a relatively slow pace and often can be well controlled by treatment for long periods of time. Therefore, the patient with chronic leukemia may survive for many years in relatively good health. In contrast, acute leukemia is often a rapidly progressive disease. Symptoms of bone marrow infiltration and visceral infiltration make their appearance early and are quite conspicuous. In some patients with acute leukemia, the abnormal proliferation of the leukemic cells can be stopped for a variable period of time by various anticancer drugs, and the patient appears to have completely recovered. An arrest of the disease induced by therapy is called a remission. In many cases, however, the patient undergoes a relapse, and the disease ultimately proves fatal. Acute leukemia in children responds better to anticancer chemotherapy than acute leukemia in adults, and some children have been completely cured by intensive therapy.

Some patients with acute leukemia and chronic granulocytic leukemia can be treated successfully by bone marrow transplantation from a compatible donor. Marrow transplantation has also been used successfully to treat patients with multiple myeloma, widespread lymphoma affecting the bone marrow, and Hodgkin's disease when the bone marrow is infiltrated by the neoplasm. The marrow transplant is a foreign tissue, however, and the patient's own immunologic defenses must be suppressed in order for the transplanted marrow to survive.

Although marrow transplantation is an important advance, it is not always successful. Patients may develop life-threatening infections related to the immune system suppression required to maintain the transplant, and in some patients, the leukemia recurs despite the marrow transplant.

Not all leukemic patients are suitable candidates for bone marrow transplantations, and many patients require some type of chemotherapy. The types of chemotherapy drugs used and the treatment schedules are being evaluated and adjusted continually. As new drugs become available, their effectiveness and side effects are compared with drugs currently used, and treatment schedules may be readjusted as required in order to provide the maximum benefit to the patient.

## Precursors of Leukemia: The Myelodysplastic Syndromes

For many years it has been recognized that acute leukemia in older patients may not have an abrupt onset but is preceded by a period lasting from several months to several years in which the affected patients have only a moderate anemia, sometimes associated with reduced white cells (leukopenia) and low blood platelets (thrombocytopenia). Examination of the bone marrow of these patients reveals variable degrees of disturbed growth and maturation of red cells, white cell precursors, and megakaryocytes but not leukemia. Recently these conditions have been grouped together under the general term **myelodysplastic syndromes** (*myelo* = marrow + *dysplasia* = disturbed growth). Several different types have been described that differ somewhat in their clinical and hematologic manifestations. In general, the more severe the maturation disturbance in the bone marrow, the greater the likelihood that leukemia would eventually occur.

**myelodysplastic syndrome** (my'elo-dis-plas'tik) A disturbance of bone marrow function that is characterized by anemia, leukopenia, and thrombocytopenia and that may be a precursor to leukemia in some patients.

# Multiple Myeloma

Multiple myeloma is a neoplasm arising from plasma cells within the bone marrow (Figure 8-25). In many ways, it resembles leukemia, but the neoplastic plasma cell proliferation is generally confined to the bone marrow. Infiltration of the viscera by the abnormal plasma cells is unusual; outpouring of large numbers of plasma cells into the peripheral blood also is uncommon. The abnormal plasma cells either may infiltrate the bone

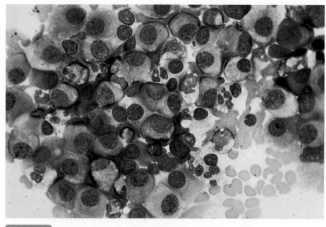

Figure 8-25 Photomicrograph illustrating aspirated bone marrow from a patient with multiple myeloma. Almost all cells are immature plasma cells containing large eccentric nuclei and abundant cytoplasm (original magnification × 400).

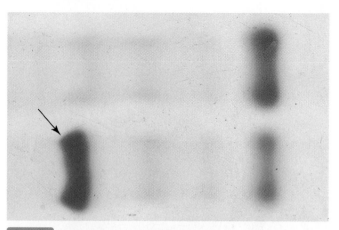

Figure 8-27 An examination of serum proteins by a special technique (electrophoresis) that separates serum proteins into various fractions. The *upper* pattern is from normal serum, with the dense albumin band at the *far right* in the photograph and the less intensely stained globulin bands *to the left* of the albumin band. The lower pattern is from a patient with multiple myeloma. The *arrow* indicates a densely stained homogeneous globulin band representing large amounts of a single type of globulin protein produced by the abnormal plasma cells.

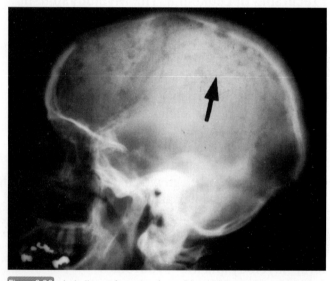

Figure 8-26 A skull x-ray from a patient with multiple myeloma. Multiple punched-out areas in skull bones (*arrow*) result from bone destruction caused by nodular masses of neoplastic plasma cells growing in bone marrow.

marrow diffusely or may form discrete tumors that weaken the bone, leading to spontaneous fractures, pain, and disability (Figure 8-26). Normal plasma cells produce antibody proteins (immunoglobulins), as described in Chapter 4. In myeloma, the neoplastic cells also often produce large amounts of protein. This greatly increases blood proteins and, correspondingly, blood viscosity. The protein produced by the myeloma cells is generally a single type of immunoglobulin, usually IgG. The myeloma protein can be identified in the blood (Figure 8-27). Masses of coagulated myeloma protein

may accumulate within the patient's own tissues, and thus the function of the affected tissues is severely impaired. Some patients with myeloma die of kidney failure because masses of protein produced by the plasma cells infiltrate the kidneys and block the renal tubules.

A number of different drugs and treatment schedules are used to treat myeloma. Thalidomide and similar drugs derived from thalidomide have been quite effective. Radiotherapy may also be useful for treating localized areas of bone destruction caused by myeloma.

# Survival Rates in Neoplastic Disease

Malignant neoplasms are a leading cause of disability and death. Cancer is second only to heart disease as a cause of death in the United States, accounting for 23 percent of all deaths in this country. Of the cancers affecting major organs, lung and prostate carcinoma are the most common malignant tumors in men, and breast carcinoma is the most frequent in women. Carcinoma of the intestine is quite common in both sexes. The survival rate for patients with malignant tumors depends on whether the disease has been diagnosed and treated early, before it has spread. The chances for survival are significantly reduced if the tumor has metastasized to regional lymph nodes or to distant sites.

## Table 8-6 — Malignant Neoplasms: 5-Year Survival Rates

| Type of Neoplasm | 5-Year Survival (%) White | 5-Year Survival (%) Black |
|---|---|---|
| Thyroid | 97 | 94 |
| Melanoma | 93 | 75 |
| Uterus, cervix | 73 | 63 |
| Uterus, body | 85 | 60 |
| Breast | 90 | 77 |
| Bladder | 82 | 65 |
| Larynx | 66 | 54 |
| Prostate | 100 | 98 |
| Hodgkin's disease | 87 | 81 |
| Colon-rectum | 65 | 55 |
| Kidney | 65 | 66 |
| Non-Hodgkin's lymphoma | 64 | 54 |
| Ovary | 45 | 39 |
| Multiple myeloma | 33 | 32 |
| Leukemia | 49 | 47 |
| Stomach | 22 | 23 |
| Lung | 15 | 12 |
| Esophagus | 16 | 11 |
| Pancreas | 5 | 5 |

Cases diagnosed 1996 to 2002. Survival for all ages with survival for whites and blacks listed separately. Average survival for both sexes used when neoplasm occurs in both sexes.

Source: Jemal, A., Siegel, R., Ward, E., et al. Cancer statistics, 2007 *CA: A Cancer Journal for Clinicians*. 57: 43–66. Extensive cancer data from the American Cancer Society, including most recent 5-year survival rates of cancers diagnosed 1996–2002.

The curability of the various types of cancer can be assessed in terms of 5-year survival rates, which range from 100 percent for prostate cancer and more than 95 percent for patients with thyroid cancer to a discouraging 5 percent for those with pancreatic carcinoma (Table 8-6). Attempts are being made continually to improve survival rates by means of earlier diagnosis and more effective therapy. Unfortunately, 5-year survival does not necessarily indicate that the patient is cured because some types of malignant tumors may recur and prove fatal many years after initial treatment. Breast carcinoma and malignant melanomas are two such tumors that are prone to late recurrence. For breast carcinoma, for example, the overall 5-year survival rate in one large group of patients followed for many years was approximately 65 percent (although more recent 5-year survival data indicated in Table 8-6 reveal higher survival rates). The 10-year rate in this group is only 50 percent because of late recurrences and metastases. Even after 10 years, a small proportion of patients eventually die of their original tumor (Figure 8-28). In such cases, the tumor had already spread by the time it was first recognized and treated, but the metastatic deposits were held in check by the body's immune defense mechanisms. The recurrence was caused by an eventual failure of the body's defenses, which allowed the tumor to become reactivated. However, current breast cancer treatment methods (called adjuvant therapy) described in Chapter 13 have greatly reduced the likelihood of late recurrences and metastases.

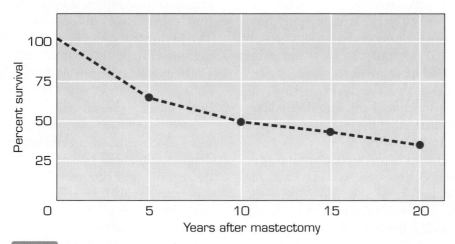

**Figure 8-28** Continuing mortality from breast carcinoma after mastectomy, as described in text. (Data from Berg, J. W., and Robbins, G. F. 1996. Factors influencing short- and long-term survival of breast cancer patients. *Surgery, Gynecology, and Obstetrics* 122:1311–16.

# CHAPTER REVIEW

## Summary

A tumor is an overgrowth of cells that serves no useful purpose, and is not subject to the normal control mechanisms that regulate cell proliferation. Benign tumors are composed of well-differentiated cells that grow slowly, are well circumscribed, and do not extend beyond the location where they are growing. They are named from the tissue from which the tumor arose with the suffix *oma* added, such as *aden* (gland) + *oma* (tumor) = *adenoma*. Alternatively, a tumor on a narrow base projecting from an epithelial surface can be called a polyp or papilloma. In contrast, a malignant tumor is characterized by immature cells that grow faster, infiltrate surrounding tissues, and may spread (metastasize) to other areas in the body. The general term *cancer* applies to any malignant tumor. The more precise terms are *carcinoma*, referring to a tumor arising from epithelium, glands, or organs with excretory or secretory functions; *sarcoma* refers to a tumor arising from other tissues such as muscle, nerve, bone, cartilage, and connective tissue. *Leukemia* designates a tumor of blood cells. Our immune system helps protect us from malignant tumors by recognizing and destroying abnormal cells before they begin to proliferate and form a tumor, but is less effective at destroying an established tumor.

Generally benign tumors are easy to treat and are not hazardous to the affected person. In contrast, malignant tumors are more difficult to treat when they have spread to involve other parts of the body. Many malignant tumors begin as a localized neoplastic proliferation that remains confined to the surface epithelium for many years before becoming invasive. This growth phase, which is called noninfiltrating carcinoma or carcinoma in situ, is the most favorable stage for cure. Once the tumor extends into the deeper tissues, the cells can extend into lymphatic channels and blood vessels, and can spread throughout the body, a stage much more difficult to treat successfully.

Many factors are known to predispose to tumors or cause tumors, such as viruses, gene and chromosome abnormalities, and failure of the body's immune defenses to destroy abnormal cells that arise during cell division. Heredity also plays a role. Although there is no strong hereditary predisposition to most tumors, some are caused by hereditary gene mutations, such as those that predispose to breast and ovarian carcinoma, and the gene mutation responsible for the childhood tumor retinoblastoma. Many gene mutations or chromosome abnormalities may deregulate cells, causing cells to proliferate excessively. Three different groups of genes regulate cell functions and tumors may arise if their regulatory functions are disrupted: (1) Proto-oncogenes are normal genes that regulate cell growth, but may convert to oncogenes that stimulate unrestrained cell proliferation; (2) tumor suppressor genes, which occur in pairs at corresponding sites on homologous chromosomes, inhibit excess cell proliferation, and both must fail to function before excessive cell growth occurs; (3) DNA repair genes, which also exist in pairs like tumor suppressor genes, monitor DNA strands produced during cell division, and also repair DNA that has been damaged by radiation, chemicals, or other environmental agents, thereby preventing potentially harmful mutations that may deregulate a cell and cause a tumor.

Chromosome abnormalities, such as deletions or translocations, may cause problems by changing the relationships of the genes on the affected chromosomes so that they no longer function properly. One of the best known is the Philadelphia chromosome that is a reciprocal translocation of chromosome segments between chromosomes 9 and 22, which causes one type of leukemia.

Leukemia is a neoplastic proliferation of white blood cells in the bone marrow, which disrupts production of normal red cells, white cells, and platelets. The neoplastic cells overflow into the bloodstream and infiltrate other tissues and organs throughout the body. The proliferation can be controlled but is usually difficult to cure. Multiple myeloma is a plasma cell neoplasm characterized by nodular tumor deposits in the bone marrow and excess proliferation of protein by the neoplastic plasma cells.

Early recognition of a malignant tumor permits early more effective treatment and improves prognosis. Early diagnosis is aided by appropriate screening tests to detect a possible tumor, such as Pap smears and mammograms, as well as seeking medical evaluation if abnormal signs or symptoms are detected that suggest a possible tumor.

Treatment of a malignant tumor begins with a biopsy that identifies the presence of a tumor and its characteristics, and also suggests the type of treatment that is most likely to be successful. Surgical resection of the tumor and the regional lymph nodes is often effective. Some tumors respond best to radiation therapy. Sometimes both methods of treatment are used to eradicate a tumor. Anticancer drugs can be used to destroy or control tumors, and are also used as adjuvant therapy after surgical treatment to prevent late recurrences of the tumor. Hormones are also used to retard growth of some tumors. Hormone-dependent tumors can often be controlled by depriving the tumor of the required hormone that stimulates its growth, such as estrogen when dealing with an estrogen-dependent tumor.

## Questions for Review

1. What are the major differences between a benign and a malignant tumor (see Table 8-1)?
2. How are tumors named? What are the common prefixes used in naming tumors? How would you name the following tumors: a benign tumor of fat; a malignant tumor of muscle; a malignant tumor of squamous epithelium; a benign tumor of glandular epithelium arising from the surface of the colon and projecting into the lumen; and a malignant tumor of cartilage?
3. How does the body defend itself against abnormal cells that arise spontaneously in the course of cell division? What is the consequence of failure of these defense mechanisms (see Figure 8-17)?
4. What is a lymphoma? What is the difference between a nevus and a melanoma? What is a teratoma?
5. What is a Pap smear? How is it used in the early diagnosis of tumors? What is the significance of a Pap smear containing atypical cells?
6. What is a frozen section? How is it used in the diagnosis of tumors? How are neoplasms treated?
7. What is leukemia? What are its major clinical manifestations? How is leukemia classified? What is the difference between multiple myeloma and leukemia?

## Supplementary Reading

Connors, J. M. 2005. Radioimmunotherapy: Hot new treatment for lymphoma. *New England Journal of Medicine* 352:496–97.

> Most patients with B cell lymphomas have widespread disease by the time the lymphoma is diagnosed, and it is difficult to cure the lymphoma because the tumor cells have already spread throughout the body. Recently, antibodies directed against B cells and labeled with a radioisotope have been used to seek out and destroy the B-lymphoma cells wherever they are located in the body. Studies on a selected group of patients have yielded encouraging results.

Croce, C. M. 2008. Oncogenes and cancer. *New England Journal of Medicine* 358:502–11.

> Cancer is caused by alteration of oncogenes, tumor suppressor genes, and DNA repair genes. Another group called micro-RNA genes are also involved. They are short, single RNA strands that regulate gene expression by attaching to messenger RNA, which blocks its function and also degrades the messenger RNA, thereby disrupting processes controlling cell growth.

Dantal, J., and Soulillou, J. P. 2005. Immunosuppressive drugs and risk of cancer after organ transplantation. *New England Journal of Medicine* 352:1371–72.

> Immunosuppressive therapy, which is essential for survival of organ transplants, has some important limitations: infections and cancer related to immunosuppression. Many of the cancers result from activation of oncogenic viruses: lymphomas related to EB virus, Kaposi's sarcoma caused by human herpesvirus 8, and skin cancer caused by human papillomavirus. Most immunosuppressive agents favor cancer development, but a few actually reduce cancer risk by suppressing cell proliferation. Hopefully, effective combinations of immunosuppressive drugs can prevent organ rejection and also reduce cancer risk.

Finn, O. J. 2008. Cancer immunology. *New England Journal of Medicine* 358:2704–15.

> A description of the various ways that immunotherapy can stimulate the immune system to inhibit or control tumor growth. Describes ways that self-antigens can convert to tumor antigens.

Hahn, W. C., and Weinberg, R. A. 2002. Rules for making tumor cells. *New England Journal of Medicine* 347:1593–1603.

> Development of cancer in humans involves a complex succession of events that evolves over many years, characterized by deregulation of cell function caused by mutant tumor suppressor genes and activated oncogenes. Many of these genes affect cell growth and differentiation, and mutation-generated malfunction eventually leads to tumors.

Hoagland, H. C. 1995. Myelodysplastic (preleukemia) syndromes: The bone marrow factory failure problem. *Mayo Clinic Proceedings* 70:673–77.

> A review of classification, manifestations, diagnosis, and treatment.

Jemal, A., Siegel, R., et al. 2008. Cancer statistics, 2007. *CA: A Cancer Journal for Clinicians* 57:43–66.

> Extensive cancer data from the American Cancer Society, including 5-year survival rates of cancer diagnosed 1996–2002. Data cited in Table 8-6.

# Interactive Activities

## True or False

Indicate whether the following statements are true or false by writing T or F at the end of the statement.

1. A liposarcoma is a malignant tumor of glandular epithelium. ____
2. Tumor suppressor genes inhibit excessive cell proliferation that may lead to a tumor. ____
3. An angiosarcoma is a malignant blood vessel tumor. ____
4. Hodgkin's disease is a precancerous condition caused by a virus. ____
5. Most anticancer drugs given to treat malignant tumors may also damage normal cells. ____
6. An in situ carcinoma is a malignant epithelial tumor confined to the surface epithelium that has not yet invaded the tissue beneath the epithelium (subepithelial tissue). ____
7. Multiple myeloma is a neoplasm composed of abnormal plasma cells. ____
8. Adjuvant chemotherapy consists of anticancer chemotherapy given after surgical resection of a malignant tumor in order to prevent late recurrence of a previously treated tumor. ____
9. The Philadelphia chromosome occurs only in persons who live in Philadelphia. ____
10. A myosarcoma is a malignant tumor arising from muscle cells. ____

## Matching

Match the tumor with its characteristic features.

1. Polyp
2. Retinoblastoma
3. Acute leukemia
4. Hodgkin's disease
5. In situ carcinoma of uterine cervix
6. Multiple myeloma

A. A noninvasive malignant epithelial tumor
B. A protein-producing malignant tumor of plasma cells
C. A malignant eye tumor
D. One type of malignant lymphoma
E. A benign epithelial tumor
F. A malignant tumor of white blood cells

## Critical Thinking

1. Mary Jones is having a cervical Pap smear and doesn't know the purpose of the test. What would you tell her?
2. Paul Smith has an anemia. His white blood cell count is greatly elevated and consists almost entirely of mature lymphocytes. The number of platelets in his blood is also much lower than normal. He is concerned that he might have leukemia and asks what you think about his blood studies. What would you tell him?
3. Peter Jones has heard that persons whose immune system does not function properly are more likely to develop tumors than persons whose immune system functions normally. He asks you whether this is true, and if it is true, how does the immune system help protect us? What would you tell him?

# Blood Coagulation Abnormalities and Circulatory Disturbances

## LEARNING OBJECTIVES

1. Describe the functions of blood vessels and platelets in controlling bleeding.

2. Explain the three phases of coagulation, and list the coagulation factors involved.

3. Describe the laboratory tests used to evaluate hemostasis.

4. List the most common clinically significant disturbances of hemostasis, and describe their clinical manifestations.

5. Describe the causes and effects of venous thrombosis.

6. Explain the pathogenesis of pulmonary embolism. Describe the clinical manifestations and compare the methods of diagnosis.

7. Describe the causes and effects of arterial thrombosis.

8. List the four factors regulating the circulation of fluid between capillaries and interstitial tissue. Explain the major clinical disturbances leading to edema.

9. Describe the pathogenesis of the hypercoagulable state sometimes seen in patients with carcinoma.

10. What is shock? What diseases or conditions can cause shock?

# Hemostasis

If a person cuts his or her finger with a knife, the cut bleeds, but the bleeding soon stops and healing ensues. The body has a complex mechanism for causing blood to clot when and where it is necessary, while keeping the blood fluid within the capillaries and larger blood vessels.

# Factors Concerned with Hemostasis

The proper functioning of the hemostatic mechanism depends on the proper integrated functioning of the five major factors that affect hemostasis:

1. Integrity of the small blood vessels
2. Adequate numbers of structurally and functionally normal platelets
3. Normal amounts of coagulation factors (proteins present in small quantities in the blood plasma)
4. Normal amounts of coagulation inhibitors
5. Adequate amounts of calcium ions in the blood

## Blood Vessels and Platelets

The small blood vessels and blood platelets function together to prevent bleeding. The small blood vessels are the body's first line of defense. If a blood vessel is injured, it automatically contracts (reflex vasoconstriction), narrowing its caliber and facilitating closure of the vessel by a blood clot. Injury to the vessel also leads to disruption of the endothelium, exposing the underlying connective tissue. Platelets accumulate and adhere to the site of injury, where they perform three important functions:

1. They plug the defect in the vessel wall.
2. They liberate chemical compounds (vasoconstrictors) that cause the vessel to contract and compounds that cause platelets to aggregate.
3. They release substances (*phospholipids*) that initiate the process of blood coagulation.

Platelets, which play an essential role in blood coagulation, are very small fragments of the cytoplasm from large precursor cells in the bone marrow called *megakaryocytes*. Platelets have an average survival in the circulation of about 10 days, and when they wear out, they are removed by macrophages in the spleen.

Platelets contain contractile proteins and various enzyme systems that produce products essential for normal platelet functions. When platelets come in contact with

**petechia**
(pe-tē'-kē-y-uh) A small pinpoint hemorrhage caused by decreased platelets, abnormal platelet function, or capillary defect.

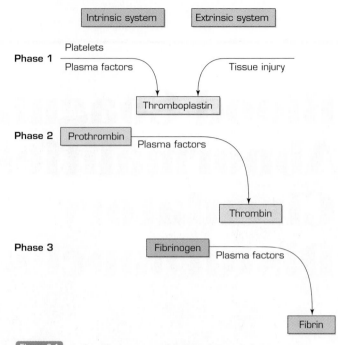

**Figure 9-1** A simplified concept of the blood coagulation process.

a roughened or damaged endothelial surface, they undergo a dramatic change. They swell and become sticky. Long processes (pseudopods) extend from their cytoplasm, and they release various products that cause further platelet swelling and platelet aggregation to form a platelet plug. Activated platelets also interact with blood coagulation proteins to start the coagulation process, as illustrated in **Figure 9-1**.

Platelets play a very important part in preventing bleeding from capillaries. Small breaks in the walls of capillaries occur frequently, but the defects are promptly sealed by platelets, and bleeding does not occur. However, if the quantity of platelets in the blood is seriously reduced, as occurs in some diseases, the "platelet sealing mechanism" is impaired. As a result, the affected individual develops multiple small pinpoint areas of bleeding (called **petechiae** or *petechial hemorrhages*) in the skin and deeper tissues resulting from leakage of blood through minute defects in the capillary endothelium.

## Plasma Coagulation Factors

The blood plasma contains several different proteins called *coagulation factors*, which are designated by both name and Roman numerals (**Table 9-1**). When these factors are activated, they interact to produce a blood clot. The process of blood coagulation is a chain reaction in which each component of the chain is formed from an inactive precursor in the blood, and each activated component in turn activates the next member of the chain. The process has been compared with what happens when the first in a long chain of dominoes is knocked

## Table 9-1  Coagulation Factors

| Factor Number | Name | Functions |
|---|---|---|
| I | Fibrinogen | Protein synthesized in liver; converted into fibrin in Phase 3 |
| II | Prothrombin | Protein synthesized in liver (requires vitamin K); converted into thrombin in Phase 2 |
| III | Tissue thromboplastin | Released from damaged tissue; required in extrinsic Phase 1 |
| IV | Calcium ions | Required throughout entire clotting sequence |
| V | Proaccelerin (labile factor) | Protein synthesized in liver; required to form prothrombin activator in both intrinsic and extrinsic Phase 1 |
| VII | Serum prothrombin conversion accelerator (stable factor, proconvertin) | Protein synthesized in liver (requires vitamin K); functions in extrinsic Phase 1 |
| VIII | Antihemophilic factor (antihemophilic globulin) | Protein synthesized in liver; required for intrinsic Phase 1 |
| IX | Plasma thromboplastin component | Protein synthesized in liver (requires vitamin K); required for intrinsic Phase 1 |
| X | Stuart factor (Stuart-Prower factor) | Protein synthesized in liver (requires vitamin K); required to form prothrombin activator in both intrinsic and extrinsic Phase 1 |
| XI | Plasma thromboplastin antecedent | Protein synthesized in liver; required for intrinsic Phase 1 |
| XII | Hageman factor | Protein required for intrinsic Phase 1 |
| XIII | Fibrin-stabilizing factor | Protein required to stabilize the fibrin strands in Phase 3 |

over. Tipping the first domino represents the initiation of the clotting mechanism, and the fall of the last domino represents the formation of a firm blood clot.

The process of blood coagulation is a highly complex and bewildering sequence of interactions involving plasma and tissue components, platelets, and calcium. Its details are not required to understand how the system functions. At the risk of oversimplifying its complexities, however, it is convenient to divide it into three phases for descriptive purposes (Figure 9-1).

Phase 1 leads to the formation of *thromboplastin*, which may be produced by either of two different mechanisms. One mechanism depends on the interaction of platelets and plasma coagulation factors. If the wall of a blood vessel is injured, platelets accumulate at the site and release a phospholipid that interacts with plasma components to form thromboplastin. This is called the *intrinsic system* because the thromboplastin is produced from substances present in the bloodstream. Tissues also have thromboplastic activity, and thromboplastin is also liberated from injured tissues. This is called the *extrinsic system* because the thromboplastin is not derived from the blood but primarily from tissue outside of the vascular compartment.

Actually, the intrinsic and extrinsic pathways are not completely independent. Usually both pathways are activated at the same time when tissues are injured, and both pathways interact to initiate the blood clotting process.

The conversion of *prothrombin* into *thrombin* takes place in phase 2. The thromboplastin formed in either the intrinsic or the extrinsic system interacts with additional plasma factors and platelet phospholipid to form a complex (thromboplastia) that converts the prothrombin into thrombin. Prothrombin is a protein manufactured in the liver. It is split into several fragments by thromboplastin. One of these is the active component **thrombin**, an enzyme capable of digesting protein. The formation of thrombin from prothrombin requires other plasma coagulation factors (called accessory factors) that function by speeding the rate of the conversion.

Phase 3 leads to the conversion of *fibrinogen* into *fibrin* by thrombin. Fibrinogen is a high molecular weight protein produced by the liver. Thrombin splits off a part of the fibrinogen molecule, forming a smaller molecule called **fibrin monomer**. The fibrin monomer molecules then become joined end to end (polymerized) to form long strands of fibrin, and the fibrin strands also become linked together side to side. Another plasma factor (*fibrin stabilizing factor*) acts by strengthening the bonds between the fibrin molecules and increasing the strength of the fibrin clot. The

**thrombin**  A coagulation factor formed by activation of prothrombin in the process of blood coagulation.

**fibrin monomer**  (mä′nō-mer) A derivative of fibrinogen that polymerizes to form the fibrin clot during blood coagulation.

blood clot is the end stage in the clotting process. It consists of an interlacing meshwork of fibrin threads containing entrapped plasma, red cells, white cells, and platelets.

## Coagulation Inhibitors and Fibrinolysins

Coagulation factors are counterbalanced by various coagulation inhibitors that restrict the clotting process to a limited area.

An equally important control system is one that dissolves fibrin after it has formed. A precursor compound in blood plasma called *plasminogen* (profibrinolysin) is activated to form *plasmin* (fibrinolysin), which dissolves fibrin in blood clots. The fibrinolytic system is activated at the same time that the coagulation process is initiated, and thrombin produced in the coagulation process also activates this system. Another important plasminogen activator is a substance called *tissue plasminogen activator*, which is released from endothelial cells in the region where the clot is forming. As described in Chapter 10, one of the ways to restore blood flow through a coronary artery obstructed by a thrombus is to administer intravenously tissue plasminogen activator or another plasminogen activator called streptokinase to dissolve the blood clot in the coronary artery of a patient who has had a recent heart attack. Prompt administration of one of these plasminogen activators within a few hours after onset of symptoms dissolves the clot and restores flow through the artery, which minimizes heart muscle damage resulting from the blockage.

## Calcium and Blood Coagulation

Adequate amounts of calcium ions ($Ca^{2+}$) are required in all phases of blood coagulation, and blood will not clot in the absence of calcium. However, there are no diseases in which a disturbance of blood coagulation results from an abnormally low level of blood calcium, because calcium levels sufficiently low to affect blood coagulation would be incompatible with life.

# Clinical Disturbances of Blood Coagulation

Disturbances of blood coagulation may be classified as one of four major categories:

1. Abnormalities of small blood vessels
2. Abnormalities of platelet numbers function
3. Deficiency of one or more of the plasma coagulation factors
4. Liberation of thromboplastic material into the circulation

## Abnormalities of Small Blood Vessels

Some rare diseases characterized by abnormal bleeding have been found to result from abnormal function of the small blood vessels. Normally, small blood vessels contract after injury, helping to seal the defect by a blood clot. Sometimes this function is defective, leading to excessive bleeding. In a few other rare diseases, the small blood vessels are abnormally formed and cannot function properly.

## Abnormalities of Platelet Numbers or Function

A decrease in platelets is called **thrombocytopenia** (*thrombus* = clot + *cyte* = cell + *penia* = deficiency). This decrease may be a result of injury or disease of the bone marrow, which damages the megakaryocytes in the marrow, the precursor cells of the platelets. In other cases, thrombocytopenia occurs because the bone marrow has been infiltrated by leukemic cells or by cancer cells that have spread to the skeletal system and the megakaryocytes have been crowded out by the abnormal cells. Thrombocytopenia may also occur if antiplatelet autoantibodies destroy the platelets in the peripheral blood, as seen in some autoimmune diseases. Sometimes platelets are normal in quantity but abnormal in function, and so they are ineffective in initiating the clotting process.

Bleeding associated with defective or inadequate platelets is generally manifested by small petechial hemorrhages rather than by large areas of hemorrhage ( Figure 9-2A ).

## Deficiency of Plasma Coagulation Factors

Deficiencies of plasma coagulation factors often lead to large areas of hemorrhage called hematomas (*heme* = blood + *oma* = swelling), as illustrated in Figure 9-2B . Deficiencies of factors concerned with the first phase of coagulation are usually hereditary and are relatively rare. Only three hereditary bleeding diseases occur with any frequency. Hemophilia, an X-linked hereditary disease affecting males, is the most common and best known. Clinically, the disease is characterized by episodes of hemorrhage in joints and internal organs after minor injury. There are two forms of hemophilia. Both have the same clinical manifestations and X-linked method of transmission. The most common type, which is called hemophilia A or classic hemophilia, is characterized by a decrease in coagulation factor VIII, which is also called antihemophilic factor. Its method of inheritance was considered in Chapter 7. The less common form of hemophilia is called hemophilia B or Christmas disease. It is caused by a deficiency of coagulation factor IX, which is also called Christmas factor (named after an affected patient, not the holiday). Both factors

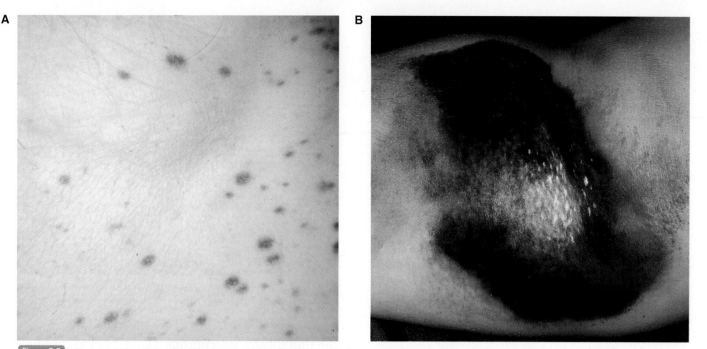

**Figure 9-2** Characteristics of bleeding in patients with disturbed hemostatic function. **A,** Petechial hemorrhages indicating thrombocytopenia or disturbed platelet function. **B,** A large hemorrhage (hematoma) associated with a deficiency of plasma coagulation factors.

VIII and IX, which are produced in the liver, are required in the first phase of coagulation.

A third hereditary bleeding disease is called von Willebrand disease and is usually transmitted as a Mendelian dominant trait. This disease also is characterized by excessive bleeding after a minor injury, but usually the bleeding is not in the joints, as is so characteristic of hemophilia. The manifestations of von Willebrand disease result from a deficiency of a large protein molecule that is produced primarily by the endothelial cells lining blood vessels. This factor is required in order for platelets to adhere to the vessel wall at the site of injury. The protein is also released into the bloodstream, where it forms a complex in the circulation with factor VIII, and it is needed in order to maintain a normal level of factor VIII in the blood.

Von Willebrand's factor functions by adhering to the vessel wall where the endothelium is disrupted, forming a latticelike framework that allows platelets and coagulation factors to adhere, interact, and form a blood clot.

The level of factor VIII is low in patients with von Willebrand disease, as it is in hemophilia A, but for a different reason. Patients with von Willebrand disease can synthesize factor VIII, but an adequate level of von Willebrand's factor is required to form a complex with factor VIII and maintain a normal amount of factor VIII in the circulation. The factor VIII deficiency in von Willebrand disease occurs because the affected persons lack adequate amounts of circulating von Willebrand's factor with which the factor VIII can combine.

Because von Willebrand's factor is also required in order for platelets to adhere at the site of vascular injury, some platelet functions also are disturbed in persons with this disease, which can be identified by special laboratory tests.

Patients with hemophilia A, hemophilia B, and von Willebrand disease who have bleeding episodes can be treated by administration of factor concentrates prepared by recombinant DNA technology.

Disturbances affecting the second phase of blood coagulation result from a deficiency of prothrombin or various accessory coagulation factors that are required for the conversion of prothrombin into thrombin. These factors are produced in the liver, and vitamin K is required for the synthesis of most of these factors (called vitamin K-dependent factors). Vitamin K is present in many foods (Chapter 18) and is also synthesized by intestinal bacteria. It is a fat-soluble vitamin, and bile is required for its absorption.

A disturbance of blood coagulation caused by a deficiency of prothrombin or related factors suggests four possibilities:

1. Administration of anticoagulant drugs
2. Inadequate synthesis of vitamin K
3. Inadequate absorption of vitamin K
4. Severe liver disease

Anticoagulant drugs such as Coumadin and similar compounds are sometimes used to treat patients who have shown an increased tendency to develop blood clots in their leg veins. These drugs are also sometimes given to patients with some types of heart disease. Anticoagulant drugs act by inhibiting the synthesis of biochemically active vitamin K-dependent factors. Inadequate synthesis of vitamin K also occurs if the intestinal bacteria have been eradicated by prolonged antibiotic therapy. This condition sometimes occurs in seriously ill hospitalized patients who are not eating food that provides a source of vitamin K, and no longer have colon bacteria to make vitamin K.

The most common cause of inadequate vitamin K is blockage of the common bile duct by a gallstone or tumor, preventing bile from entering the intestine. Bile acts as a biologic detergent to emulsify fat into small globules so that pancreatic lipase can digest the fat more efficiently and also promote absorption of the digested fat. If bile cannot flow into the duodenum, fat digestion and absorption are impaired, which also impairs absorption of vitamin K.

Patients with severe liver diseases have deficiencies of prothrombin and other vitamin K-dependent blood coagulation factors because the liver is so badly damaged that it can no longer synthesize adequate amounts of coagulation factors even though vitamin K is available.

Intramuscular administration of vitamin K corrects coagulation disturbances resulting from Coumadin anticoagulants, inadequate synthesis of vitamin K, or insufficient absorption of the vitamin. The coagulation disturbance associated with severe liver disease does not respond to vitamin K because the diseased liver is no longer capable of synthesizing sufficient coagulation factors to provide efficient hemostasis.

## Liberation of Thromboplastic Material into the Circulation

In a number of diseases associated with shock, overwhelming bacterial infection, or extensive necrosis of tissue, products of tissue necrosis and other substances with thromboplastic activity are liberated into the circulation, leading to widespread intravascular coagulation of the blood ( Figure 9-3 ). In the process of clotting, platelets and the various plasma coagulation factors are utilized, and the levels of these components in the blood drop precipitously.

In order to defend itself against widespread intravascular clotting, the body activates

**disseminated intravascular coagulation syndrome**
A disturbance of blood coagulation as a result of activation of the coagulation mechanism and simultaneous clot lysis.

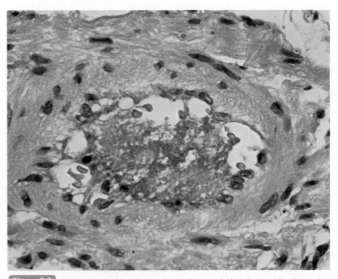

Figure 9-3    Fibrin thrombus in small blood vessel of patient with disseminated intravascular coagulation syndrome (original magnification × 400).

the fibrinolysin system; this dissolves clots and prevents potentially lethal obstruction of the circulatory system by massive intravascular coagulation. The breakdown products produced during degradation of the fibrin act as additional inhibitors of the clotting process. The net effect of these various events is a bleeding disturbance, sometimes in a patient already seriously ill because of an underlying disease that caused the blood-clotting mechanism to be activated. This abnormal bleeding state is called the **disseminated intravascular coagulation syndrome**, often abbreviated DIC. Figure 9-4 summarizes the pathogenesis of this bleeding syndrome.

## Laboratory Tests to Evaluate Hemostasis

Several laboratory tests can evaluate the overall efficiency of the coagulation process, detect the presence of inhibitors of coagulation, and estimate the number and function of the platelets ( Figure 9-5 ).

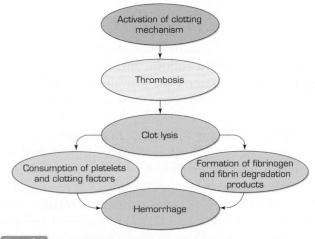

Figure 9-4    Pathogenesis of disseminated intravascular coagulation syndrome.

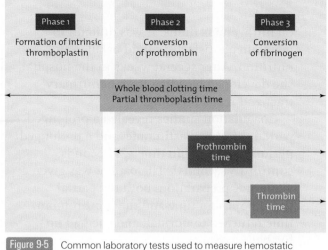

Phase 1
Formation of intrinsic thromboplastin

Phase 2
Conversion of prothrombin

Phase 3
Conversion of fibrinogen

Whole blood clotting time
Partial thromboplastin time

Prothrombin time

Thrombin time

**Figure 9-5** Common laboratory tests used to measure hemostatic function, indicating the phases of the clotting mechanism measured by the various tests.

The number of platelets in the blood can be estimated by examining the blood smear, and more precise data can be obtained by a numerical platelet count. Special tests also are available to evaluate platelet function. The function of the capillaries in the hemostatic process is evaluated by the bleeding time, which reflects the time it takes for a small, standardized skin incision to stop bleeding.

A few relatively simple tests can be used to evaluate the various proteins concerned with blood coagulation (coagulation factors). The time it takes for blood to clot in a test tube under standard conditions is a crude and relatively insensitive test that measures the overall efficiency of the clotting process. Three other tests are more often used to evaluate the coagulation system. The tests, which are performed on plasma obtained from blood collected in tubes containing an anticoagulant, are the partial thromboplastin time, the prothrombin time, and the thrombin time. Each test measures a different phase of the coagulation process. When the tests are used together, one can assess separately each of the three phases of blood coagulation and can identify the location of the coagulation factor deficiency if any of the tests yield an abnormal result.

The **partial thromboplastin time (PTT) test** measures the time it takes for blood plasma to clot after a lipid substance is added to the plasma along with calcium to start the clotting process. The lipid added is similar to the lipid material released from platelets to initiate the first phase of blood coagulation, which in turn is followed by activation of the second and third phases of the coagulation process. If a plasma factor in any of the three coagulation phases is deficient, the coagulation process is slowed, and the partial thromboplastin time is prolonged.

The **prothrombin time test** measures the time it takes for blood plasma to clot after adding a commercially available preparation of thromboplastin made from animal brain tissue along with calcium to start the coagulation. The thromboplastin added to start the reaction is essentially the same material as the thromboplastin produced by the interaction of platelets and plasma coagulation factors in the first phase of blood coagulation. A normal prothrombin time test indicates that the second and third phases of blood coagulation are normal. If the prothrombin time is prolonged, an abnormality in either the second or third stages of coagulation is indicated. The abnormality cannot be in the first phase of blood coagulation because the first phase is concerned with the formation of intrinsic thromboplastin, and thromboplastin has already been supplied as the test reagent. The first phase has been bypassed, and the test is only measuring the coagulation factors involved in the second and third phases.

The prothrombin time test is commonly used to monitor the effect of Coumadin anticoagulants administered to patients in order to reduce the coagulability of the blood.

The **thrombin time** test bypasses the first two phases of blood Coagulation. One determines the clotting time of plasma after the addition of thrombin, which is normally generated in the second phase of the clotting process. Therefore, the test primarily measures the level of fibrinogen, which may be deficient in some conditions. The level of fibrinogen can also be measured directly by other tests, and one can also test for fibrinogen and fibrin breakdown products, which are increased if fibrinolysis is excessive.

In the event that abnormalities are detected in any phase of coagulation, it is necessary to determine whether they have occurred because a coagulation factor is deficient or because an inhibitor is impairing the action of the factor. If necessary, one can also determine the concentrations of the various factors.

## Case Studies

The following cases illustrate the spectrum of coagulation abnormalities encountered in clinical medicine. The cases also illustrate how laboratory tests can help to determine the nature of the abnormality and suggest a proper course of treatment.

**partial thromboplastin time (PTT) test** (throm-bō-plas′tin) A test that measures the overall efficiency of the blood coagulation process.

**prothrombin time test** A test that measures that phase of the coagulation mechanism after the formation of thromboplastin.

**thrombin time** A laboratory test measurement that determines the concentration of fibrinogen in the blood by determining the clotting time of the blood plasma after addition of thrombin.

## Case Study 9-1

**Factor VIII Deficiency** A 10-month-old child was admitted to the hospital through the emergency room because he was bleeding profusely from a cut under the lip that he received when falling. The history revealed easy bruising since birth but no episodes of bleeding into the joints, and the child was considered by the parents to be in good health.

Physical examination revealed ecchymoses over the left chest and a small bruise on the abdomen. Small bruises were noted on both lower extremities. Laboratory studies revealed moderate anemia and normal platelets. Coagulation studies revealed a normal plasma prothrombin time, but the partial thromboplastin time was significantly prolonged.

The bleeding was controlled by applying pressure for about 10 minutes. The next day, the child had a tarry stool, apparently caused by swallowed blood. After this, the stools became normal in color, and no further bleeding was noted.

In this case, the abnormal partial thromboplastin time indicated an abnormality of blood coagulation, but the normal prothrombin time indicated that the abnormality was not in the second or third stages of coagulation. Therefore, the defect must have been in the first phase, which suggests either hemophilia or von Willebrand disease as diagnostic possibilities. Further tests showed a very low level of factor VIII (antihemophilic factor), and additional diagnostic tests established the diagnosis of von Willebrand disease.

## Case Study 9-2

**Vitamin K Deficiency** A 55-year-old woman was admitted to the hospital with a severe staphylococcal pneumonia that was complicated by an accumulation of pus in the left pleural cavity. She received intensive antibiotic therapy. She was unable to take food or fluid orally because of severe nausea and vomiting and was maintained almost entirely on intravenous fluids. It was difficult to maintain a satisfactory fluid balance and nutrition. After several weeks in the hospital, she developed bleeding from her urinary tract and rectal bleeding.

Coagulation studies revealed a prolonged partial thromboplastin time, and a prolonged plasma prothrombin time (27 seconds, control 13 seconds). The patient was given a vitamin K preparation. Both the partial thromboplastin time and the prothrombin time returned to normal, and she had no further bleeding.

In this case, the coagulation data indicate an acquired depression of vitamin K-dependent coagulation factors primarily caused by inadequate food intake to provide vitamin K coupled with deficient synthesis of vitamin K by intestinal bacteria, which were eliminated by the intensive antibiotic treatment. The excellent response to vitamin K confirmed the diagnosis.

## Case Study 9-3

**Chronic Liver Disease** A 57-year-old man was admitted to the hospital because of bleeding from his urinary tract. Blood coagulation studies revealed that both the partial thromboplastin time and prothrombin time tests were prolonged. Other studies revealed that his liver function was very abnormal. The prothrombin time did not return to normal after administration of a vitamin K preparation. A needle biopsy of the liver revealed a type of chronic liver disease called cirrhosis (Chapter 16).

Here the abnormality was localized to the second stage of blood coagulation. Failure to respond to vitamin K suggested chronic liver disease rather than vitamin K deficiency or a decrease in coagulation factors caused by anticoagulant therapy. The needle biopsy confirmed the presence of chronic liver disease.

**Case Study 9-4**

> **Disseminated Intravascular Coagulation Syndrome Caused by a Retained Dead Fetus**
> A 36-year-old pregnant woman was admitted to the hospital at 38 weeks' gestation. She had not felt fetal movement for the previous month, and no fetal heart tones were detected by her physician. Coagulation studies revealed prolonged partial thromboplastin time and prothrombin time. Fibrinogen was markedly reduced. The patient's blood contained high levels of fibrinogen and fibrin degradation products. Labor was induced, and delivery was accomplished with very little loss of blood. The next day, the fibrinogen returned to normal, and all coagulation studies were within normal limits.
>
> In this case, all of the coagulation factors were decreased because they had been used up in the coagulation process induced by release of thromboplastic material into the maternal circulation from the retained dead fetus. The high levels of fibrinogen and fibrin degradation products were the result of activation of the fibrinolytic system, the body's defense against a potentially lethal intravascular coagulation process.

# Circulatory Disturbances: Thrombosis and Embolism

Normally, blood does not clot within the vascular system. Under unusual circumstances, however, intravascular clotting may occur because of one or more of the following factors:

1. Slowing or stasis of the blood flow
2. Damage to the walls of the blood vessel
3. An increase in the coagulability of the blood

An intravascular clot is called a thrombus; the condition is termed **thrombosis**. Intravascular thrombi may form within veins or arteries and occasionally within the heart itself. A clot in the vascular system may become detached and may be carried in the circulation. Such a clot is termed an *embolus* (*embolos* = plug or stopper); the condition is termed **embolism**. Depending on where the blood clot was formed initially, the embolus may be carried into either the pulmonary circulation or the systemic arterial circulation. Eventually, it is arrested in an artery of smaller caliber than the diameter of the clot. When the embolus plugs the vessel, it blocks the blood flow to the tissue beyond (distal to) the obstruction, and the damaged tissue may undergo necrosis if the collateral blood supply is inadequate. The area of tissue breakdown is called an infarct or *infarction*.

> **thrombosis** A blood clot formed within the vascular system.
> **embolism** (em´bō-lizm) A condition in which a plug composed of a detached clot, mass of bacteria, or other foreign material (*embolus*) occludes a blood vessel.

# Venous Thrombosis and Pulmonary Embolism

Formation of blood clots within leg veins is primarily a result of slowing or stasis of the blood in the veins. This is likely to occur during periods of prolonged bed rest or after a cramped position has been maintained for a long period of time. Under these circumstances, the "milking action" of the leg musculature, which normally promotes venous return, is impaired, leading to stasis of the blood. Varicose veins or any condition preventing normal emptying of veins predisposes an individual to thrombosis by causing venous stasis.

Postoperative thrombosis in leg veins is a common problem because blood coagulation factors usually increase as a result of tissue injury or necrosis from any cause. The surgical patient is susceptible to venous thrombosis because of the combined effects of venous stasis resulting from inactivity and increased blood coagulability resulting from an increased concentration of coagulation factors. A venous thrombosis may partially block venous return in the leg, making the leg swell. However, the major complication of venous thrombosis is related to detachment of the clot from the wall of the vein. The thrombus often is not firmly attached to the vein wall. It may break loose, forming an embolus that is carried rapidly up the inferior vena cava into the right side of the heart. From there it is ejected into the pulmonary artery, where it may become lodged in either the main pulmonary artery or one of its branches. The clinical manifestations of a pulmonary embolism depend on the size of the embolus and where it lodges in the pulmonary artery.

## Large Pulmonary Emboli

A large embolus that completely blocks the main pulmonary artery or its two major branches obstructs the flow of blood through the lungs ( Figure 9-6 ). The right

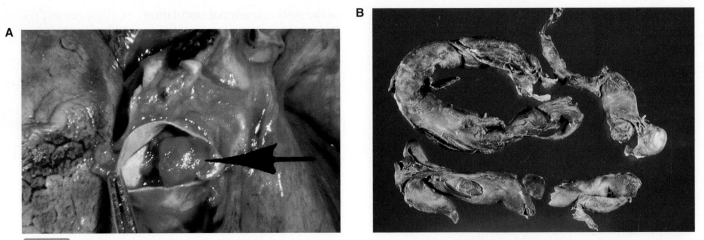

**Figure 9-6** Massive pulmonary embolism. **A,** Main pulmonary artery occluded by an embolus (*arrow*). **B,** Several emboli filled both pulmonary arteries and obstructed blood flow to lungs.

side of the heart becomes overdistended with blood because blood cannot be expelled into the lungs. The pulmonary artery leading to (proximal to) the obstructing embolus also becomes overdistended with blood, and the pressure in the pulmonary artery rises. Because less blood flows through the lungs into the left side of the heart, the left ventricle is unable to pump an adequate volume of blood to the brain and other vital organs. The systemic blood pressure falls, and the patient may go into shock. Blood still flows into the lungs from the bronchial arteries, which arise from the descending aorta and interconnect with the pulmonary arteries by means of collateral channels. This flow normally prevents infarction of the lung ( Figure 9-7 ).

Clinically, the patient becomes very short of breath, and the skin and mucous membranes assume a bluish coloration (cyanosis) because of inadequate oxygena-tion of the blood. If the massive embolism is not immediately fatal, some blood may be able to flow around the embolus and circulate through the lungs, because the caliber of the pulmonary artery is increased by overdistention, and the high arterial pressure forces blood around the site of obstruction. In favorable circumstances, the embolus is eventually dissolved by the body's normal clot-dissolving mechanisms, and blood flow through the pulmonary artery is restored. In unfavorable cases, however, thrombus material builds up on the surface of the obstructing embolus and enlarges it. The sluggishly flowing blood in the branches of the pulmonary artery distal to the obstructing embolus may also become thrombosed. These events further impair pulmonary blood flow and may ultimately cause death several days after the initial embolization.

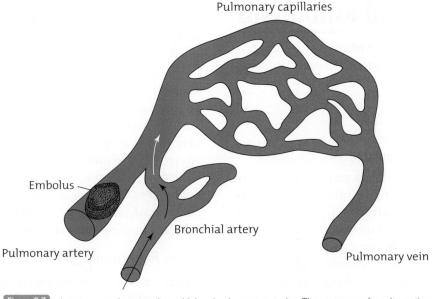

Pulmonary capillaries

Embolus

Bronchial artery

Pulmonary artery

Pulmonary vein

**Figure 9-7** Anastomoses between bronchial and pulmonary arteries. The presence of an alternative pathway for blood flow often prevents infarction of the lung when the pulmonary artery is blocked by an embolus.

## Small Pulmonary Emboli

If emboli are small, they may pass through the main pulmonary arteries and become impacted in the peripheral branches, usually in the arteries supplying the lower lobes of the lungs. Smaller emboli impede the flow of blood through the lungs and raise pulmonary artery pressure, but they have a less devastating effect than large emboli. Frequently, the segment of lung supplied by the obstructed pulmonary artery undergoes necrosis, resulting in a pulmonary infarct. The alveolar septa break down, and blood flows from the ruptured capillaries into the pulmonary alveoli, which become distended with blood. The typical infarct is a wedge-shaped hemorrhagic area that extends to the pleural surface (Figure 9-8). Infarction does not always follow a pulmonary embolism because anastomoses between the bronchial artery and pulmonary artery distal to the obstruction provide an alternative pathway for blood flow. If the pulmonary venous pressure is elevated, however, as occurs in heart failure or when the lungs are poorly expanded, an adequate collateral circulation often does not develop, which leads to a pulmonary infarct.

The clinical manifestations of smaller pulmonary emboli are quite variable and are frequently minimal if the lung does not become infarcted. Common symptoms of pulmonary infarction are difficulty in breathing (dyspnea), pleuritic chest pain, cough, and expectoration of bloody sputum. The chest pain occurs because the pleura overlying the infarct become inflamed and rubs against the overlying parietal pleura as the lung expands and contracts during respiration. The cough is caused by irritation of the bronchi in the injured area. The bloody sputum appears because blood escapes from the infarcted segment of lung into the bronchi and is subsequently coughed up.

## Diagnosis of Pulmonary Embolism

A diagnosis of pulmonary embolism requires a high index of suspicion. Unexplained dyspnea, cough, or pleuritic chest pain in a predisposed patient may be the only manifestations of a pulmonary embolism. These symptoms should alert the physician to undertake further diagnostic studies. Some of the more useful studies are chest x-ray, radioisotope lung scans, and pulmonary angiography using either a standard

**A**
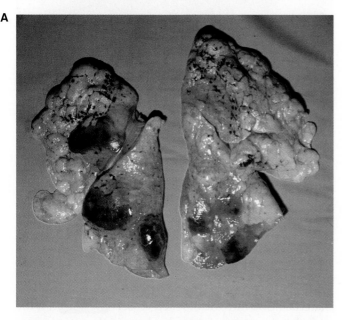

**B**
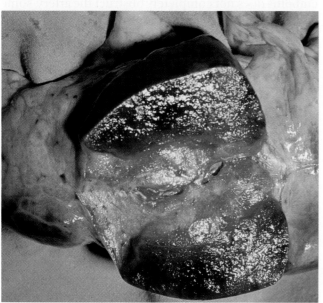

**C**
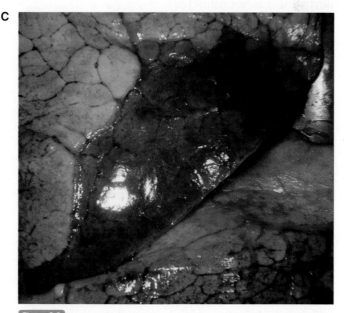

Figure 9-8  A, Multiple hemorrhagic pulmonary infarcts in both lungs. B, Closer view of infarct illustrating typical wedge-shaped hemorrhagic area that extends to pleural surface. C, Cut surface of pulmonary infarct, illustrating the hemorrhage in the infarcted lung segment, and the sharp demarcation between infarct and adjacent normal lung tissue.

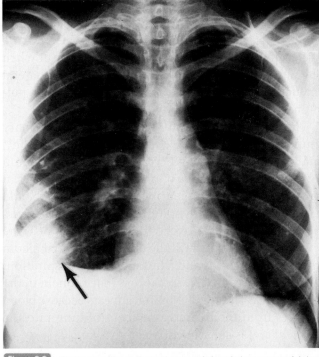

Figure 9-9 Chest x-ray illustrating pulmonary infarct in lower part of right lung (*left side* of photograph), which appears as an area of increased density (*arrow*). The opposite lung appears normal.

radiologic method or a computed tomography (CT) procedure.

**Chest X-Ray** If the embolus has caused a pulmonary infarction, a routine chest x-ray will often demonstrate the infarct, which appears as a wedge-shaped area of increased density in the lung ( Figure 9-9 ). Because emboli cannot be visualized on x-ray films, the lung will appear normal if it is not infarcted.

**Radioisotope Lung Scan** To perform a radioisotope lung scan, one first injects a peripheral vein with a solution labeled with a radioisotope. The injected material flows through the lung, is filtered out in the pulmonary capillaries, and the radioactivity in the lungs is recorded. When blood flow to a part of the lung is blocked by an embolism, the isotope does not flow into the part of the lung supplied by the blocked artery.

**Pulmonary Angiography** The definitive diagnostic method to identify a pulmonary embolism is a pulmonary angiogram, which directly visualizes the pulmonary artery and its branches. A catheter is inserted into a vein in the arm and advanced up the vein and through the superior vena cava into the right side of the heart, and out the pulmonary artery. A radiopaque material is then injected into the artery through the catheter, and the flow of the material through the pulmonary arteries is visualized by means of serial x-ray films. If the pulmonary artery or one of its branches is completely obstructed by an embolus, no contrast

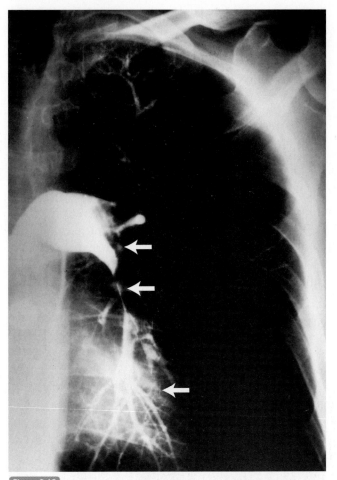

Figure 9-10 An angiogram used to identify pulmonary embolism illustrated by view of the left lung and pulmonary artery. A catheter has been inserted into the pulmonary artery and radiopaque contrast material injected. Flow of contrast material is almost completely blocked (*upper arrow*) by a large pulmonary embolus obstructing the left main pulmonary artery. Only a thin trickle of contrast material flows around the embolus (*middle arrow*) to fill the pulmonary artery branches supplying part of the lower lobe (*lower arrow*).

material flows into the blocked vessel ( Figure 9-10 ). If the embolus does not completely obstruct the artery, some contrast medium flows around the embolus, which appears as a filling defect in the column of contrast material within the partially occluded vessel. New advanced CT equipment can provide similar information and does not require insertion of a catheter into the pulmonary artery, although an intravenous injection of radiopaque contrast material is required. The equipment can monitor the flow of contrast material through the pulmonary artery and its branches and can detect an obstruction of blood flow within the pulmonary circulation, indicating a pulmonary embolus.

## Treatment of Pulmonary Embolism

Treatment of patients with pulmonary embolism includes general supportive care and administration of anticoagulants. Heparin, which has an immediate effect, is generally used initially, followed by administration

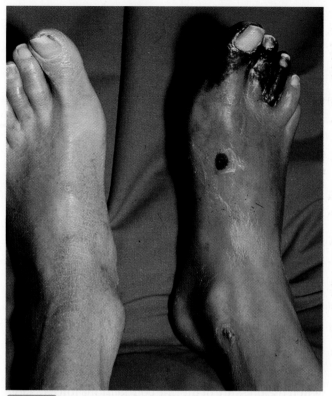

**Figure 9-11** Gangrene of right foot as a result of arterial obstruction.

of Coumadin-type anticoagulants, which act by depressing hepatic synthesis of coagulation factors. The purpose of anticoagulant therapy is twofold: (1) to prevent recurrent pulmonary emboli by preventing the formation of more thrombi in leg and pelvic veins, and (2) to prevent thrombus formation in branches of the pulmonary artery distal to the embolism. If adequate therapy is given, further thromboembolism is prevented, and the embolus will slowly dissolve. Rarely, if the patient has sustained a massive embolus and is in critical condition because blood flow through a main pulmonary artery is blocked, it is necessary to remove the embolus surgically or dissolve the embolus rapidly by administering clot-dissolving (thrombolytic) drugs. These are the same drugs that are given to a heart attack patient in order to dissolve a thrombus blocking a coronary artery (Chapter 10).

## Arterial Thrombosis

Blood flow in arteries is rapid, and intravascular pressure is high; so stasis of blood is not a factor in arterial thrombosis. The main cause of arterial thrombosis is injury to the wall of the vessel, usually secondary to arteriosclerosis. The arteriosclerotic deposits cause ulceration and roughening of the lining of the artery, and thrombi form on the roughened area. The effects of arterial thrombus formation depend on the location and size of the artery that has become obstructed. Blockage of a coronary artery frequently causes infarction of the heart muscle and consequent *heart attack.* Occlusion of an artery to the brain leads to infarction of a portion of the brain, commonly called a *stroke.* If a major artery supplying the leg is occluded, the extremity undergoes necrosis, usually called **gangrene** ( Figure 9-11 ). This term may be confusing because the same word is used to describe *gas gangrene,* which is an infection caused by anaerobic spore-forming bacilli called **Clostridia**.

> **gangrene** (gang-grēn′) Term has two different meanings. Refers to (1) infection caused by gas-forming anaerobic bacteria (*gas gangrene*) or (2) necrosis of an extremity caused by interruption of its blood supply (*ischemic gangrene*).
>
> **Clostridia** (klä-strid′ē-yum) Anaerobic gram-positive spore-forming rod-shaped bacteria.

## Intracardiac Thrombosis

Occasionally, blood clots may form within the heart itself. Thrombi may form within the atrial appendages when heart function is abnormal, as in heart failure, or when the atria are not contracting normally. Thrombi may also form on the surfaces of heart valves that have been damaged as a result of disease. Occasionally, thrombi may form on the internal lining of the ventricle adjacent to an area where the heart muscle has been damaged by thrombosis of a coronary artery (a "heart attack"). Intracardiac thrombi may become dislodged and may be carried into the systemic circulation, resulting in infarction of the spleen, kidneys, brain, or other organs. The symptoms produced depend on the size and location of the infarction.

## Thrombosis Caused by Increased Blood Coagulability

In some conditions, the concentration of various blood coagulation factors is elevated, increasing the coagulability of the blood and predisposing the individual to intravascular clotting. After injury or operation, products of tissue necrosis that have thromboplastic activity, stimulate the synthesis of many clotting factors. This increases the likelihood of postoperative thrombosis in leg veins.

The estrogen in contraceptive pills has also been found to stimulate synthesis of coagulation factors, raising their concentration and predisposing the women who use the pills to both venous and arterial thrombosis. This observation has led to concern about the safety of "the Pill" when used for a long period of time, but the risk of thrombosis related to oral contraceptives is less of a problem when using the currently available pills that contain a much lower concentration of estrogen and progestin.

## Thrombosis in Patients with Cancer

Many patients with advanced cancer have elevated platelets and increased concentrations of coagulation factors in their blood, which predisposes them to both venous and arterial thromboses. This tendency results from the release of thromboplastic materials into the circulation from areas of degeneration and necrosis within the tumor. This is the same basic mechanism that induces hemorrhage in patients with a disseminated intravascular coagulation syndrome. The variations in clinical manifestations result from differences in the rate at which the thromboplastic material enters the circulation. In the acute process, a large quantity of thromboplastic material is rapidly released into the circulation. Platelets and coagulation factors are consumed faster than they can be replenished, and bleeding results. In patients with widespread cancer, the thromboplastic material is liberated slowly but continuously from the tumor. The blood coagulation mechanism is activated, leading to intravascular thrombosis followed by clot lysis. Production of coagulation factors and platelets increases in response to an increased demand, but the body overcompensates. Production exceeds destruction, which leads to a hypercoagulable state. Figure 9-12 compares these two processes.

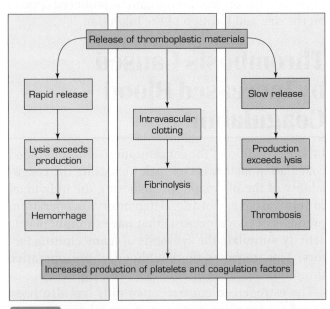

Figure 9-12  Pathogenesis of hypercoagulable state that occurs in patients with cancer, contrasted with the pathogenesis of disseminated intravascular coagulation syndrome. Different clinical manifestations reflect differing rates of fibrinolysis and compensatory regeneration of hemostatic components.

# Embolism as a Result of Foreign Material

Most emboli are caused by blood clots, but other materials occasionally gain access to the circulation. Fat, air, and foreign particles within the vascular system may sometimes cause serious difficulties.

## Fat Embolism

After a severe bone fracture, fatty bone marrow and surrounding adipose tissue may be disrupted. The emulsified fat globules may be sucked into the veins and carried into the lungs, leading to widespread obstruction of the pulmonary capillaries. Some of the fat may be carried through the pulmonary capillaries and may reach the systemic circulation, eventually blocking small blood vessels in the brain and other organs.

## Amnionic Fluid Embolism

This condition is an uncommon but devastating complication of pregnancy that usually occurs during labor when the pressure of uterine contractions forces a large volume of amnionic fluid through a tear in fetal membranes into a torn uterine vein at the site of a cervical or uterine laceration. The amnionic fluid, which contains desquamated fetal epithelial cells and hair, fatty material (vernix), debris from the fetal respiratory and gastrointestinal tract, and thromboplastic material, is carried in the maternal venous circulation to the lungs, where it plugs the pulmonary capillaries. Manifestations are severe dyspnea, shock, and often an acute disseminated intravascular coagulation syndrome induced by the thromboplastic material in the amnionic fluid (Figure 9-12).

## Air Embolism

Sometimes a large amount of air is sucked into the venous circulation after a chest wound with injury to the lung. The air is carried to the heart and accumulates in the right heart chambers, preventing filling of the heart by returning venous blood. As a result, the heart is unable to pump blood, and the individual dies rapidly of circulatory failure.

# Edema

The term *edema* refers to accumulation of fluid in the interstitial tissues. Edema is most conspicuous in the skin and subcutaneous tissues of the dependent parts of the body and is usually noted first in the legs and ankles. When the edematous tissue is compressed by indenting the tissue with the fingertips, the fluid is pushed aside, leaving a pit or indentation that gradually refills with fluid. This characteristic is responsible for the common term *pitting edema*. Fluid may also accumulate in the pleural cavity (hydrothorax) or in the peritoneal cavity (ascites).

Edema may result from any condition in which the circulation of extracellular fluid between the capillaries and the interstitial tissues becomes disturbed.

## Factors Regulating Fluid Flow Between Capillaries and Interstitial Tissue

The flow of fluid through the interstitial space depends on four factors:

1. The *capillary hydrostatic pressure*, which tends to filter fluid from the blood through the capillary endothelium.
2. The *permeability of the capillaries*, which determines the ease with which the fluid can pass through the capillary endothelium.
3. The *osmotic pressure* exerted by the proteins in the blood plasma (called *colloid osmotic pressure*), which tends to attract fluid from the interstitial space back into the vascular compartment. Osmotic pressure is the property causing fluid to migrate in the direction of a higher concentration of molecules. The osmotic pressure of the plasma depends primarily on the concentration of the plasma proteins. Because the capillaries are impermeable to protein, the protein tends to draw water from the interstitial fluid into the capillaries and to hold it there.
4. The presence of open *lymphatic channels*, which collect some of the fluid forced out of the capillaries by the hydrostatic pressure of the blood and return the fluid to the circulation.

Figure 9-13 illustrates the mechanism by which fluid flow is regulated through interstitial tissues.

**Flow of Fluid into and out of Capillaries** Movement of fluid in and out of capillaries is determined by the hydrostatic pressure of the blood that "pushes" fluid out of the capillaries, which is opposed by the osmotic pressure caused by the blood proteins, primarily albumin, within the capillary blood that "pulls" fluid back into the capillaries. The capillary endothelium acts as a semipermeable membrane that limits the rate at which fluid is filtered from the blood. At the arterial end of the capillary, the hydrostatic pressure is higher than the osmotic pressure, which causes fluid to be filtered through the endothelium of the capillaries into the interstitial space. At the venous end of the capillary, the hydrostatic pressure is lower than the colloid osmotic pressure, and fluid tends to move back into

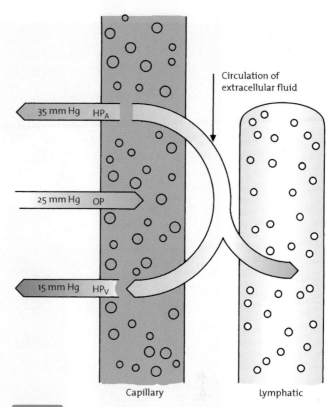

Figure 9-13 Factors regulating the flow of fluid through the interstitial tissues, as described in the text. $HP_A$, hydrostatic pressure at the arterial end of the capillary. $HP_V$, hydrostatic pressure at the venous end of the capillary. OP, osmotic pressure. Pressures are indicated in millimeters of mercury (mm Hg). Fluid is forced from the arterial end of the capillary because the hydrostatic pressure exceeds the osmotic pressure. At the venous end of the capillary, the hydrostatic pressure is lower than the osmotic pressure and fluid returns. Lymphatic channels also collect some of the fluid forced from the capillaries by the hydrostatic pressure.

the capillaries. In this way, the fluid containing dissolved nutrients is carried from the blood into the interstitial tissues to nourish the cells, and waste products are returned to the circulation for excretion. Some of the fluid is also returned to the bloodstream by lymphatic vessels.

## Pathogenesis and Classification of Edema

**Increased Capillary Permeability** Normally, the endothelium of the capillaries limits the amount of fluid filtered from the blood. If the capillaries are excessively permeable, filtration of fluid into the interstitial space is greater than normal. Increased capillary permeability is responsible for the swelling of the tissues associated with an acute inflammation as illustrated in Chapter 3 (Figures 3-3 and 3-12).

**Low Plasma Proteins** If the concentration of plasma proteins is decreased, the colloid osmotic pressure is reduced correspondingly. Consequently, less fluid is attracted back into the capillaries, and the fluid accumulates in the tissues. A low concentration of plasma

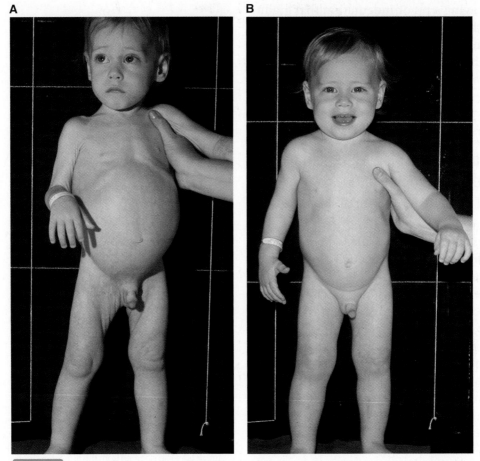

**Figure 9-14** Edema resulting from low plasma proteins as a result of malnutrition. **A,** Child prior to treatment, illustrating emaciation, abdominal distention caused by accumulation of fluid in the peritoneal cavity, and edema of legs. **B,** Same child after treatment by a nutritious high-protein diet.

proteins may result from excessive loss of plasma proteins in the urine, as occurs in patients with some types of kidney disease or from inadequate synthesis of plasma proteins as a result of malnutrition or starvation ( Figure 9-14 ). Hypoproteinemia caused by inadequate protein intake may be encountered in patients with chronic debilitating diseases who are unable to eat an adequate amount of food and in patients with intestinal diseases in whom assimilation of food is impaired.

**Increased Hydrostatic Pressure** Increased pressure in the veins draining the capillaries is transmitted back to the capillaries, and is reflected as a higher than normal pressure at the venous end of the capillaries. As a result, more fluid is filtered from the capillaries, causing it to accumulate in the tissues. Often the increased venous pressure is a manifestation of heart failure, and the pressure is elevated in all the systemic veins ( Figure 9-15A ). However, a localized increase in venous pressure may be encountered if a vein draining a part of the body becomes obstructed by a blood clot that fills the lumen ( Figure 9-15B ), or if the draining vein is

compressed in the thigh or pelvis so that venous return is impeded.

**Lymphatic Obstruction** Sometimes lymphatic channels draining a part of the body become obstructed because of disease. The obstruction blocks a pathway by which fluid is returned from the interstitial space into the circulation and leads to edema in the region that is normally drained by the obstructed lymphatic vessels ( Figure 9-16 ).

# Shock

Shock is a general term to describe any condition in which the blood pressure is too low to provide adequate blood flow to the body cells and organs, and is a serious potentially life-threatening condition. Shock may result from:

1. A *low blood volume* leading to a corresponding drop in blood pressure (hypovolemic shock)
2. An inadequate or *impaired cardiac pumping function* that reduces cardiac output (cardiogenic shock)

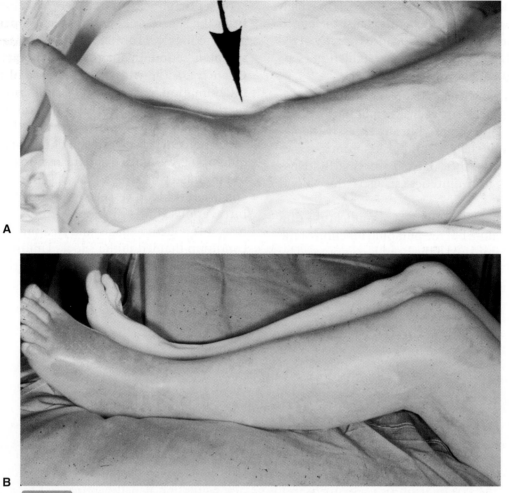

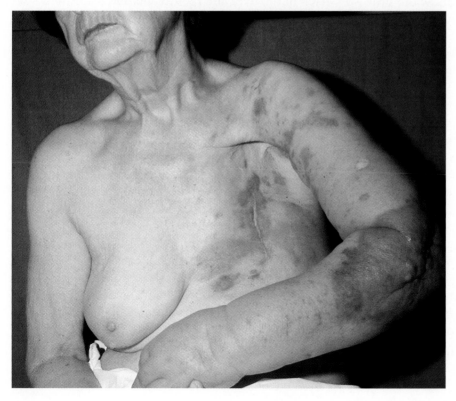

**Figure 9-15** **A,** Marked pitting edema of leg (*arrow*) as a result of chronic heart failure. **B,** Localized edema of left leg caused by venous obstruction. Right leg appears normal.

**Figure 9-16** Severe edema of arm resulting from long-standing lymphatic obstruction. The patient had a radical operation for breast carcinoma many years previously. Scarring in the axilla blocked lymphatic drainage from the arm, leading to chronic edema. The dark discolored areas in the skin of the chest wall and upper limb are caused by a malignant tumor of lymphatic vessels (lymphangiosarcoma), which sometimes complicates chronic lymphedema.

**3.** *Excessive dilation of the body's blood vessels* in which the volume of circulating blood is insufficient to fill adequately the greatly *expanded capacity of the blood vessels* resulting from the vasodilation (septic shock and anaphylactic shock)

Most cases of hypovolemic (low blood volume) shock result from a large hemorrhage that significantly reduces the circulating blood volume, but any excessive depletion of body fluids such as fluid losses from a severe burn, from severe diarrhea, or from excessive fluid loss in urine resulting from diuretics can also reduce blood volume.

Cardiogenic shock usually is a complication of a myocardial infarction, but the pumping function of the heart can also be impaired if the heart is compressed by accumulation of blood or fluid within the pericardial sac, which prevents adequate filling of the heart in diastole.

In septic shock the marked vasodilation results from the severe infection in which microbial toxins and mediators of inflammation are released at the site of infection. In anaphylactic shock (described in Chapter 5), the widespread release of mediators of inflammation from mast cells and basophils leads to marked vasodilation that is often followed by circulatory collapse.

The outcome of shock depends on its cause, and how quickly it is recognized and treated. Treatment consists of administering drugs that raise blood pressure by constricting blood vessels, restoring blood volume by intravenous fluids or blood if the shock is caused by a severe hemorrhage, and treating the underlying condition that led to the shock. Unfortunately, septic shock or cardiogenic shock in an elderly patient with other medical problems has a very poor prognosis.

# CHAPTER REVIEW

## Summary

Many factors contribute to hemostasis. It is convenient to divide the coagulation process into three phases: (1) the formation of thromboplastin, (2) the conversion of prothrombin to thrombin, and (3) the conversion of fibrinogen to fibrin. Laboratory tests can help pinpoint the coagulation phase that is disturbed; localization of the coagulation abnormality helps determine the likely cause of the coagulation disturbance, and also helps guide therapy. A few relatively rare diseases are characterized by defective blood vessel structure or function, but most blood coagulation problems are caused by deficiencies of plasma coagulation factors or platelets. Insufficient platelets (thrombocytopenia) may result from disease of the bone marrow where platelets are produced, or from autoantibodies and drugs that damage the platelets. Usually thrombocytopenia is characterized by small petechial hemorrhages rather than a large hemorrhage (hematoma).

A deficiency of a coagulation factor localized to the first phase of coagulation is usually hereditary and the three common deficiencies are classic hemophilia (hemophilia A) and Christmas disease (hemophilia B), which are transmitted on the X chromosome, and von Willebrand disease, which follows an autosomal dominant transmission. These diseases can't be cured but can be treated successfully.

Coagulation problems related to the second phase of coagulation usually are caused by a deficiency of prothrombin and related coagulation factors that are made in the liver and require vitamin K for their synthesis. Deficiencies result from (1) administration of a Coumadin anticoagulant drug that inhibits hepatic synthesis of the coagulation factors and is given to decrease the coagulability of the blood in patients with conditions in whom this is desirable, (2) a deficiency of vitamin K caused by inadequate food intake coupled with loss of intestinal bacteria that produce the vitamin, or inadequate absorption of the fat-soluble vitamin, which is not well absorbed when fat absorption is impaired by disease, and (3) severe liver disease because the damaged liver is unable to produce adequate amounts of these coagulation factors even though vitamin K is adequate.

Another coagulation problem arises when large amounts of thromboplastic material are released into the bloodstream of patients as a result of shock, sepsis, or tissue necrosis. The thromboplastic material activates the coagulation system, which leads to widespread thrombosis within small blood vessels. The thrombi are promptly lysed by the body's fibrinolytic system, but the widespread intravascular thrombosis depletes platelets and plasma coagulation factors that are used up as the clots are formed and rapidly dissolved by fibrinolysin. The condition is called disseminated intravascular coagulation (or simply DIC).

Blood clots may also form in large veins related to slow blood flow or stasis of blood in veins sometimes associated with an increased concentration of coagulation factors. Clots in leg veins may break loose and travel as emboli to block pulmonary arteries or their branches, leading to impaired blood flow to the lungs or pulmonary infarcts. Chest x-ray and angiography help make the proper diagnosis.

Thrombi in arteries are usually caused by formation of a thrombus at the site of an atheromatous plaque, obstructing blood flow to the brain (stroke), heart (myocardial infarct), large arteries in the lower limb (necrosis of a limb that may require amputation), or other organs. Treatment consists of removing the blockage by various means.

Several factors regulate movement of fluid between capillaries and the fluid in the interstitial tissues: (1) the capillary hydrostatic pressure, (2) the capillary permeability, (3) the osmotic pressure of the blood plasma, which is related to the concentration of albumin in the blood, and (4) the amount of fluid removed from the interstitial fluids by lymphatic vessels. Derangement of this system leads to accumulation of excess fluid in the tissues, which is called edema. Treatment involves correcting the derangement.

Shock results from a precipitous fall in blood pressure that leads to inadequate circulation of blood to the tissues and is classified by its pathogenesis. Hypovolemic shock results from low blood volume; cardiogenic shock occurs when the failing heart can't pump effectively; septic shock and anaphylactic shock result from excessive dilation of the blood vessels to such an extent that the volume of blood in the circulation is unable to adequately fill the greatly expanded capacity of the vascular system. As a result the blood pressure falls. Treatment is directed to restoring blood pressure by whatever methods are most appropriate.

## Questions for Review

1. How does blood clot?
2. What are some of the common disturbances of blood coagulation?
3. What is thrombocytopenia? What type of bleeding is produced when platelets are reduced? What types of diseases are associated with thrombocytopenia?
4. What types of diseases produce abnormalities in the first phase of blood coagulation?
5. What is the consequence of liberation of thromboplastic material into the circulation?
6. What laboratory tests are used to evaluate the coagulation of blood?
7. A patient with a bleeding tendency has a prolonged partial thromboplastin time with a normal prothrombin time. In what phase of the clotting process is the disturbance located? Name one possible disease that could produce these findings.
8. What are the effects of Coumadin anticoagulants on the clotting mechanism? How do they work? What laboratory test can be used to monitor the effect of the anticoagulant?
9. What is the difference between a thrombus and an embolus? What is an infarct?
10. What factors predispose to venous thrombosis? What is the major complication of a thrombus in a leg vein?
11. What factors predispose to arterial thrombosis?
12. What are the causes and effects of intracardiac thrombi?
13. What conditions predispose to thrombosis by increasing the coagulability of the blood?
14. What factors regulate the flow of fluid between capillaries and interstitial tissue? What are the major causes of edema?
15. What coagulation disturbances may be encountered in patients with tumors?
16. What is the difference between a pulmonary embolus and a pulmonary infarct? What are the clinical manifestations of a pulmonary infarct?
17. What is shock, and what are its causes?

# Supplementary Reading

Alperin, J. B. 1987. Coagulopathy caused by vitamin K deficiency in critically ill hospitalized patients. *Journal of the American Medical Association* 258:1916–19.

Vitamin K deficiency in hospitalized patients is common and can be misdiagnosed as disseminated intravascular coagulation syndrome. It can be prevented by prophylactic vitamin K in seriously ill patients receiving antibiotics.

Aster, R. H., and Bougie, D.W. 2007. Drug-induced immune thrombocytopenia. *New England Journal of Medicine* 357:380–87.

There are many causes of thrombocytopenia that may disrupt the blood coagulation process, including autoantibodies directed against platelets as well as many drugs and medications. The diagnosis of drug-induced thrombocytopenia is often overlooked or considered to be autoimmune thrombocytopenia. Stopping the causative drug or medication restores platelet numbers and platelet function.

Blom, J. W., Doggen, C. J. M., Osanto, S., and Rosendaal, F. R. 2005. Malignancies, prothrombotic mutations, and the risk of venous thrombosis. *Journal of the American Medical Association* 293:715–22.

Patients with cancer have a sevenfold greater risk of venous thrombosis than a comparable control group of patients, especially in the first few months after diagnosis and in the presence of distant metastases. Two hereditary gene mutations increase the risk even more by greatly increasing the coagulability of the blood. One is a relatively common mutation of a gene coding for the synthesis of coagulation factor V called factor V Leiden. Normal factor V is inactivated by a coagulation inhibitor called protein C during coagulation of the blood, but factor V Leiden is less efficiently inhibited. Mutation of another gene that regulates prothrombin synthesis leads to a higher than normal concentration of prothrombin in the blood.

Francis, C. W. 2007. Prophylaxis for thromboembolism in hospitalized medical patients. *New England Journal of Medicine* 356:1438–44.

Anticoagulant prophylaxis reduces the risk of asymptomatic deep vein thrombosis in hospitalized patients, which suggests that the risk of pulmonary emboli is reduced. Several different drugs are suitable.

Goldhaber, S. Z. 2005. Multislice computed tomography for pulmonary embolism: A technological marvel. *New England Journal of Medicine* 352:1812–14.

CT scanning of the chest has revolutionized the diagnostic approach to pulmonary embolism and has largely replaced radioisotope lung scans to evaluate suspected pulmonary emboli.

Laposata, M., Van Cott, E. M., and Lev, M. H. 2007. A 40-year-old woman with epistaxis, hematemesis, and altered mental status. *New England Journal of Medicine* 356:174–82.

A complex and well-studied case of a blood coagulation disturbance caused by accidental or deliberate ingestion of a Coumadin-type anticoagulant with a very high potency and long duration of action (brodifacoum, a highly toxic pesticide used as a rat poison), which responded to intensive vitamin K therapy and a prothrombin complex concentrate. Treatment was complicated by a disseminated intravascular coagulation syndrome. A good discussion of the effect of Coumadin anticoagulants on vitamin K-dependent coagulation factors, and management of a disseminated intravascular coagulation syndrome. The patient recovered.

# Interactive Activities

## True or False

Indicate whether the following statements are true or false by writing T or F at the end of the statement.

1. A marked platelet deficiency usually causes a large area of hemorrhage._____
2. The usual source of pulmonary emboli is thrombi in leg veins._____
3. Hemophilia and von Willebrand disease are both associated with a reduced antihemophilic globulin in the bloodstream._____
4. A prothrombin time test measures the concentration of prothrombin and some other blood coagulation factors made in the liver._____
5. Coumadin anticoagulant drugs inhibit synthesis of plasma coagulation factors made in the liver._____
6. A patient who sustains a pulmonary embolus always has a pulmonary infarction._____
7. Contraceptive pills increase the concentration of plasma coagulation factors in the bloodstream._____
8. Persons with chronic liver disease usually have an increased concentration of blood coagulation factors, which predisposes them to formation of intravascular thrombi._____
9. Shock may result from excessive dilation of blood vessels in the circulatory system so that the volume of blood in the circulation is unable to adequately fill the dilated vessels._____
10. Obstruction of lymphatic vessels in the axilla (armpit) doesn't cause edema of the upper limb because blood vessels return to the bloodstream all the fluid expelled from capillaries._____

## Matching

Match the edema-causing condition in the left column with the disease that caused the condition in the right column.

| Condition | Cause |
|---|---|
| 1. Reduced capillary osmotic pressure | A. Swollen face resulting from a bee sting |
| 2. Increased capillary permeability | B. Chronic heart failure |
| 3. Increased capillary hydrostatic pressure | C. Malnutrition with low blood proteins |
| 4. Obstruction of lymphatic vessels | D. Scarring in the axilla caused by surgical removal of axillary lymph nodes |

## Select the Proper Answer

Several factors predispose to formation of blood clots within blood vessels. They are

A. sluggish flow of blood within a blood vessel
B. damage to the wall of the blood vessel
C. increased coagulability of the blood

Which of these factors is of greatest importance in the following situations?

1. A thrombus formed in a coronary artery in which the lining (intima) is damaged by accumulation of cholesterol and other lipids in the arterial wall._____
2. A thrombus that formed in the artery of a healthy young woman taking birth control pills._____
3. A thrombus in the leg vein of a healthy middle aged man who recently completed a 10-hour airplane flight._____

## Critical Thinking

1. Mary Anderson is a 32-year-old woman who would like to defer a pregnancy until she completes her course work to obtain a PhD degree. She smokes about one pack of cigarettes per day but is planning to cut down or stop. Her blood pressure is 130/86 and she considers herself healthy. She is considering using contraceptive pills and asks your advice. What would you tell her?
2. John Anderson is a 54-year-old executive who heard that an associate working in another department developed a blood clot in his leg after a long airplane trip. He asks you why this developed, what problems could result from the leg vein clot, and how he could prevent a blood clot if he takes a long airplane trip. What would you tell him?

# 10 The Cardiovascular System

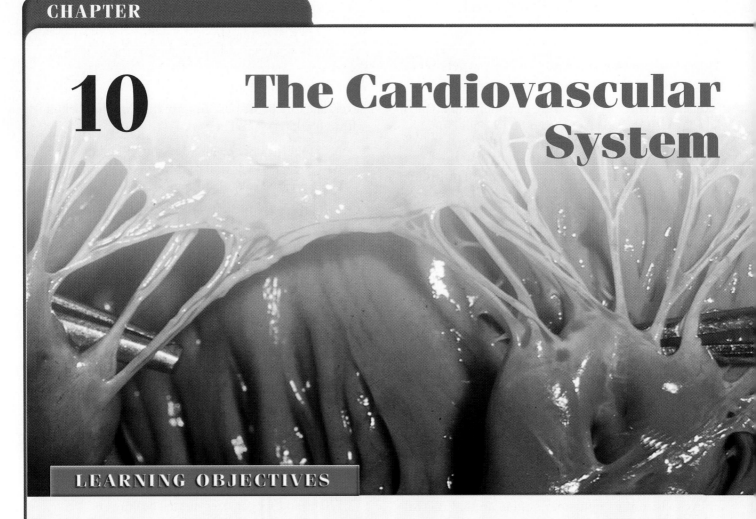

## LEARNING OBJECTIVES

1. Explain the basic anatomy and physiology of the heart as they relate to the common types of heart disease.
2. Describe the common causes of congenital heart disease and valvular heart disease. Explain the effects. Outline the methods of treating congenital and acquired valvular heart disease.
3. Describe the pathogenesis of coronary heart disease. List the four important risk factors. Describe the clinical manifestations of coronary heart disease. Explain the methods of treatment and their rationales.
4. List the major complications of myocardial infarction and describe their clinical manifestations.
5. Explain the general principles applied to the diagnosis and treatment of coronary heart disease and myocardial infarction.
6. Explain the current concepts regarding the effect of diet on coronary heart disease. Describe how cholesterol is transported by lipoproteins. Distinguish between "good" and "bad" cholesterol.
7. Describe the adverse effects of hypertension on the cardiovascular system and the kidneys.
8. Differentiate between pathogenesis of acute and chronic heart failure. Describe the pathogenesis of each, and list the principles of treatment.
9. Differentiate between the pathogenesis and clinical manifestations of arteriosclerotic and dissecting aneurysms of the aorta. Explain the principles of treatment.
10. List the common diseases affecting veins, their clinical manifestations, and methods of treatment.

# Cardiac Structure and Function

The heart is a muscular pump that propels blood through the lungs and to the peripheral tissues. Heart disease is caused by a disturbance in the function of the cardiac pump. A working knowledge of the normal structure and function of the heart is essential to an understanding of the various types of heart disease.

# Normal Cardiac Function

## Cardiac Chambers

The heart is divided by partitions into four chambers, the right and left atria, and the right and left ventricles. No direct communication exists between the right and left halves of the heart, and it is convenient clinically to consider each half of the heart as an independent structure. The "right heart" circulates blood into the pulmonary artery and through the lungs (the pulmonary circulation); the "left heart" pumps blood into the aorta for distribution to the various organs and tissues of the body (the systemic circulation).

## Cardiac Valves

The flow of blood into and out of the cardiac chambers is controlled by a system of valves that normally permits flow in only one direction. The **atrioventricular (AV) valves** are flaplike valves surrounding the orifices between the atria and the ventricles. The free margins of the valves are connected to the papillary muscles of the ventricular walls by narrow, stringlike bands of fibrous tissue called the **chordae tendineae** ( Figure 10-1 ). These bands prevent the valves from prolapsing into the atria during ventricular systole. The semilunar valves surrounding the orifices of the aorta and pulmonary artery are positioned so that the free margins of the valves face upward. This structural arrangement defines cuplike pockets between the free margins of the valves and the roots of the blood vessels to which the valves are attached ( Figure 10-2 ).

When the heart relaxes in diastole, the chordae produce tension on the valves and pull the atrioventricular valves apart. When the ventricles contract, the chordae are no longer under tension, and the force of the blood flow pushes the valves together so that no blood flows from the ventricles into the atria. During ventricular contraction, the semilunar valves are forced apart by the jets of blood leaving the ventricles. When ventricular contraction ceases, the weight of the column of ejected blood forces the valves back into position, preventing reflux of blood into the ventricles during diastole. The atrioventricular and semilunar valves function reciprocally. Ventricular contraction relaxes tension on the chordae, causing the atrioventricular valves to close at the same time that the jets of blood open the semilunar valves. Closure of the semilunar valves in diastole is also associated with opening of the atrioventricular valves. The two sounds heard in sequence followed by a pause when listening to heart sounds with a stethoscope result from closure of the atrioventricular valves followed by closure of the semilunar valves, and the pause represents diastole.

> **atrioventricular (AV) valve** (a′trē-o-ven-trik′ū-lar) The flaplike heart valve located between the atrium and ventricle.
>
> **chordae tendineae** (kor′dāten-din′ē-ā) Fibrous cords that extend from the free margins of the atrioventricular valves to attach to the papillary muscles.

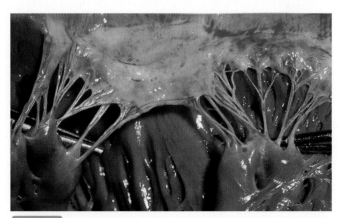

**Figure 10-1** Normal mitral valve, illustrating thin chordae extending from valve leaflets to papillary muscles.

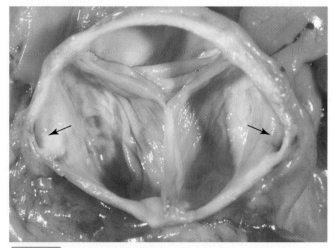

**Figure 10-2** Aortic valve viewed from above, illustrating a cup-shaped configuration of valve leaflets. Note the openings of coronary arteries (*arrows*) arising from base of aorta adjacent to aortic valve leaflets.

Figure 10-3 illustrates the reciprocal action of the two sets of valves, which is responsible for the unidirectional flow required for normal cardiac function.

## Blood Supply to the Heart

**The Left and Right Coronary Arteries**  The heart is supplied by two large coronary arteries that arise from the aortic sinuses at the root of the aorta ( Figure 10-4 ). The left main coronary artery is a short vessel that soon divides into two major branches. The left anterior descending artery descends to supply the front of the heart and the anterior part of the interventricular septum. The left circumflex artery swings to the left (*circum* = around + *flex* = bend) to supply the left side of the heart. The right coronary artery swings to the right, supplying the right side of the heart, and then descends to supply the back of the heart and the posterior part of the interventricular septum. Each coronary artery gives off many branches that supply the heart muscle. The terminal branches of the coronary arteries frequently communicate with each other by means of connections called **anastomoses**. Because of these connections, obstruction of one of the arteries does not necessarily completely interrupt the blood flow to the tissues supplied by the blocked vessel. There may be enough blood flow through anastomoses with other arteries to supply the heart muscle. This is called a **collateral circulation**.

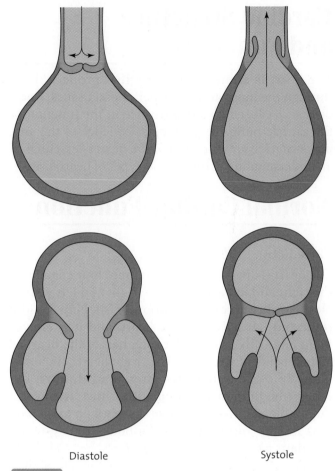

Diastole        Systole

**Figure 10-3**  Reciprocal action of atrioventricular and semilunar valves, resulting in unidirectional blood flow.

## A Closer Look

*The discovery of the stethoscope was directly related to problems a physician experienced when attempting to examine an obese patient.*

The story begins in 1819 when a French physician named René Laennec was examining a very overweight woman with heart disease. At that time a physician listened to heart sounds and heart murmurs by placing his ear directly against the patient's chest. The sounds were more difficult to hear in an overweight or obese patient, and sometimes the ear-to-chest examination procedure embarrassed both the woman patient and the physician.

During his examination, Laennec was unable to hear heart sounds clearly because of the woman's obesity. Recalling some principles regarding sound transmission, he picked up a thick pile of papers, which he rolled into a hollow tube. He pressed one end of the tube to the patient's chest and the other end to his ear, and was delighted at how much better he could hear the sounds. Soon afterward he constructed a hollow wooden tube similar to the roll of paper he had used previously, which he called a stethoscope (from *stethos* = chest + *skopos* = viewing or examining). Soon he also used his stethoscope to examine the lungs as well as the heart, and was able to correlate the sounds he heard with the type of pulmonary or cardiac disease demonstrated at autopsy in patients who did not survive. Eventually the instrument was modified by adding two separate ear pieces which evolved into the modern stethoscope in use today.

Laennec made many additional contributions to medicine, including descriptions of chronic liver disease (which he called cirrhosis), peritonitis, tuberculosis, and malignant melanoma. However, he is known best for the stethoscope. Unfortunately Laennec developed pulmonary tuberculosis, and the diagnosis was made by his physician-nephew, using the stethoscope that René Laennec had developed. He died of tuberculosis in 1826 at the age of 45.

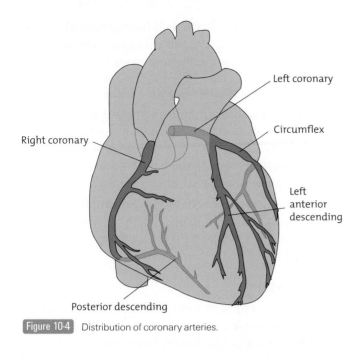

Figure 10-4   Distribution of coronary arteries.

## Conduction System of the Heart

The impulses that cause the heart to beat are initiated and propagated by groups of specialized muscle cells that depolarize spontaneously, which is called the conduction system of the heart ( Figure 10-5 ). Impulses normally are generated in the **sinoatrial (SA) node**, also called simply the sinus node, which is located in the right atrium near the opening of the superior vena cava. Small bundles of fibers called internodal tracts connect the SA node to the atrioventricular (AV) node that is located in the lower posterior part of the atrial septum. The

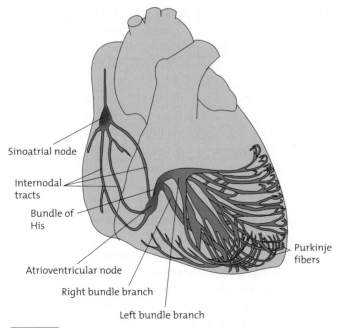

Figure 10-5   Diagram of the cardiac conduction system. The cardiac impulse originates in the SA node and is conducted to the ventricles via the internodal tracts, the AV node, the Bundle of His, and the right and left bundle branches, which terminate in the network of Purkinje fibers.

atrioventricular bundle (Bundle of His) is the continuation of the AV node that transmits the impulse to the ventricles by passing through a small opening in the fibrous connective tissue separating the atrial from the ventricular muscle (the fibrous framework of the heart). After entering the ventricles, the AV bundle divides into right and left bundle branches in the upper part of the interventricular septum and the branches descend in the septum to terminate as Purkinje fibers that activate the heart muscle. The autonomic nervous system also influences the depolarization rate set by the conduction system. Sympathetic nervous system impulses increase the rate and parasympathetic impulses slow it. The normal rhythm established by the cardiac conduction system is often called a normal sinus rhythm to indicate that it is controlled by the SA node.

Although any part of the conduction system can depolarize spontaneously and generate an impulse, the SA node normally functions as the cardiac pacemaker because it depolarizes about 60 to 70 times per minute, which in turn depolarizes the other parts of the conduction system. However, if impulse transmission from the SA node is interrupted by damage to the conduction system, the AV node that discharges at about 50 times per minute can take over; if the AV node fails, then the bundle or bundle branches can initiate impulses but at a still slower rate of about 30 to 40 times per minute.

## The Cardiac Cycle

The sequence of events that occurs during a single contraction and relaxation of the cardiac chambers is called a **cardiac cycle**. Contraction of a chamber is called systole (a Greek word meaning *contraction* or *shortening*), which is followed by diastole (which means *between contractions*). Atrial systole and diastole are followed by ventricular systole and diastole. During diastole, both the atria and ventricles are relaxed. In a normal person at rest, each ventricle in diastole contains about 120 ml of blood, and most of the blood filling the ventricles in diastole flows passively into the ventricles through the open atrioventricular valves. Atrial systole delivers an additional 30 ml of blood into the ventricles. If the heart rate is normal, the additional blood

**anastomosis**
(ä-nas-ta-mō′sis) A communication between two blood vessels or other tubular structures. Also refers to a surgical connection of two hollow tubular structures, such as the divided ends of the intestine or a blood vessel (*surgical anastomosis*).

**collateral circulation**
An accessory circulation capable of delivering blood to a tissue when the main circulation is blocked, as by a thrombus or embolus.

**sinoatrial (SA) node**   (sign-o-atrial′)
The part of the cardiac conduction system that depolarizes at the fastest rate, thereby functioning as the cardiac pacemaker to regulate the heart rate; also called *sinus node*.

**cardiac cycle**   The sequence of events during a single contraction and relaxation of the atria and ventricles.

pumped into the ventricles by atrial contractions is not essential for reasonably normal cardiac function because most of the blood filling the ventricles has already entered the ventricles before the atria contract. Atrial systole delivers a relatively small additional amount. However, as the heart rate increases, the duration of diastole shortens. Less time is available for passive filling of the ventricles, and atrial systole makes a much greater contribution to ventricular filling by actively pumping blood into the ventricles when the heart beats rapidly. Atrial systole is followed by ventricular systole, which ejects blood into the aorta at high pressure and into the pulmonary artery at much lower pressure.

When considering cardiac function it is helpful to remember a few useful concepts:

1. Each ventricle at rest fills during diastole with about 120 ml of blood (the end-diastolic volume). Normally only about 70 ml is ejected during systole, which is called the **stroke volume**, leaving about 50 ml within the ventricle (end-systolic volume). The percentage of the ventricular volume ejected during systole is called the **ejection fraction**, which is normally about 60 percent of the ventricular volume. This measurement is often used to evaluate the efficiency of the cardiac pump when evaluating patients with heart failure.

2. **Cardiac output** is the output of blood from a single ventricle in 1 minute, and is the product of the stroke volume (about 70 ml) multiplied by the heart rate (about 72 beats per minute), which equals about 5000 ml per minute. This is approximately the total blood volume of the average adult.

3. During vigorous activity, the normal heart of a healthy young person can double its stroke volume and greatly increase its heart rate, which can increase cardiac output from four to seven times over resting cardiac output.

## Blood Vessels

The heart pumps blood into a system of conduction, distribution, and collection tubes that differ in both their structure and function. It is convenient to consider them as four separate groups:

1. Large elastic arteries conduct the blood to various locations throughout the body. They distend as blood is ejected from the heart during systole and recoil during diastole to maintain flow between contractions.

2. Arterioles are smaller vessels having muscular walls that function like a nozzle on a garden hose to regulate flow from the large arteries into the capillaries. They lower the pressure and dampen the amplitude of the pulsations.

3. Capillaries are thin endothelium-lined channels that deliver nutrients to cells and remove waste products.

4. Veins return blood to the heart under low pressure and usually travel with the arteries.

A separate system of channels carrying fluid called lymph is part of the lymphatic system. Its functions and relation to the circulatory system are considered in Chapter 11.

## Blood Pressure

The force of ventricular contraction delivers deoxygenated venous blood into the pulmonary artery at low pressure to be oxygenated in the lungs, and into the aorta at much higher pressure to deliver oxygenated blood throughout the body. The pressure within the arteries varies rhythmically with the beating of the heart, and the high pressures generated by the left ventricle are the pressures measured using a blood pressure cuff applied to the brachial artery. The highest pressure is reached during ventricular contraction as blood is ejected into the aorta and its branches (systolic pressure). The pressure is lowest when the ventricles are relaxed (diastolic pressure), and the recoil of the stretched arteries provides the force to propel the blood between contractions. The peripheral arterioles regulate the rate of blood flow into the capillaries by varying the degree of arteriolar constriction. In many respects, the effect is analogous to the resistance to outflow of water from a garden hose, which can be varied by tightening or loosening the nozzle on the hose. Because of the resistance offered by the arterioles, the blood pressure during cardiac diastole does not fall to zero but declines slowly as blood leaves the large arteries through the arterioles into the capillaries.

The elasticity of the large arteries also influences the systolic pressure. Some of the pressure rise caused by the blood ejected from the ventricle is absorbed by the stretch of the arteries so that the systolic pressure does not rise as high as would occur if the arteries were more rigid and unable to stretch normally.

In summary, the systolic blood pressure is a measure of the force of ventricular contraction as blood is ejected into the large arteries. The diastolic pressure is a measure of the rate of "run off" of blood into the capillaries, which is governed by the peripheral resistance caused by the small arterioles throughout the body. The mean (average) pressure of blood in the large arteries is approximately midway between systolic and diastolic pressure.

## The Electrocardiogram

The **electrocardiogram** (ECG) records the electrical activity of the heart as measured on the surface of the body by means of electrodes attached to the legs, arms, and chest. Voltage differences are recorded as a series of upward (positive) and downward (negative) deflections that form a characteristic pattern of deflections named in order: P, Q, R, S, and T ( Figure 10-6 ). The P wave reflects the initial wave of depolarization associated with atrial systole. The Q, R, and S waves, called collectively the QRS complex, reflect the depolarization of the ventricles, which is followed by ventricular systole. The T wave represents repolarization of the ventricles during diastole. The time interval from the beginning of the P wave to the beginning of the QRS complex, which is called the PR interval, reflects the time required for the depolarization wave to pass through the AV bundle from the atria to the ventricles.

Usually the positive and negative deflections are recorded on calibrated graph paper, each horizontal line representing a standard voltage difference and each vertical line representing a standard time interval. However, the ECG tracing also can be displayed on a fluorescent screen, as when continuously monitoring a patient in a coronary care unit.

The ECG is a valuable diagnostic aid that can identify characteristic disturbances in the heart rate or rhythm and abnormalities in the conduction of impulses through the heart. The ECG can also identify heart muscle injury, as occurs following a heart attack, and can also determine the extent of the damage to the heart muscle.

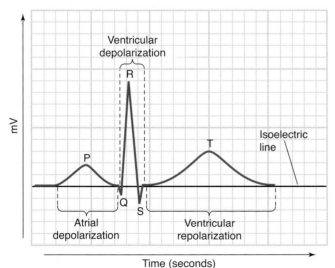

mV

Ventricular
depolarization

R

P

Q

S

T

Isoelectric
line

Atrial
depolarization

Ventricular
repolarization

Time (seconds)

Figure 10-6  Characteristic features of a normal electrocardiogram.

# Cardiac Arrhythmias

The orderly depolarization and repolarization of the conduction system that directs the contraction and relaxation of the atria and ventricles does not always function perfectly, which leads to disturbances in the heart rate or rhythm that are called cardiac arrhythmias.

## Atrial Fibrillation

One of the more common abnormal cardiac rhythms is a condition called atrial fibrillation (AF) in which the atria fail to contract normally. The condition often occurs in older persons, especially those with cardiovascular disease or chronic pulmonary disease, but may also occur in persons whose thyroid glands produce an excess of thyroid hormone (hyperthyroidism) and in a few other conditions. Occasionally AF occurs in apparently normal healthy persons for no apparent reason.

AF is characterized by multiple uncoordinated areas of atrial depolarization that causes the atria to quiver ineffectively instead of contracting normally. The abnormal atrial impulses are also relayed to the AV node, which is unable to respond to such a large number of stimuli, but the impulses reaching the ventricles often cause the heart to beat irregularly at about 140 to 160 times per minute. At such a fast ventricular contraction rate the duration of diastole is very short, which compromises ventricular filling. The cardiac output falls, which may not be well tolerated by a person with preexisting cardiovascular disease. Some of the ventricular contractions occur before the ventricles are adequately filled with blood, and the volume of blood ejected may not always be enough to be detected as a pulse in the radial artery at the wrist. Consequently, the radial pulse detects fewer beats per minute than the number of ventricular contractions per minute heard with a stethoscope placed on the chest. This discrepancy is called a pulse deficit. The diagnosis of atrial fibrillation is made by examination of the ECG, which reveals a lack of P waves indicating that the atria are not contracting normally and is associated with some variability in the QRS complexes related to the variable ventricular stroke volumes, as manifested by the pulse deficit ( Figure 10-7A ).

**electrocardiogram**
(ē lek-trō-kär′dē-ō-gram)
A technique for measuring the serial changes in the electrical activity of the heart during the various phases of the cardiac cycle. (Often called ECG or EKG.)

## Treatment of Atrial Fibrillation

The first treatment step is to give a drug to slow the heart rate, which provides more time for passive ventricular filling during diastole. When the heart rate

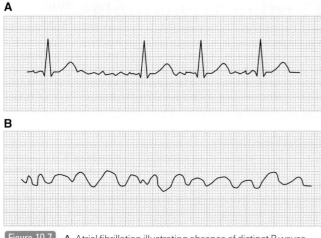

**Figure 10-7** **A,** Atrial fibrillation illustrating absence of distinct P waves together with irregular ventricular rate, usually 140 to 160 beats per minute. **B,** Ventricular fibrillation illustrating extremely abnormal chaotic cardiac rhythm without any evidence of synchronized electrical impulses. (From Garcia, T. B., and N. E. Holtz, 2003. *Introduction to 12-Lead ECG.* Boston: Jones and Bartlett.)

has been slowed, the next step is to restore a normal heart rhythm by terminating the fibrillation. This can be accomplished either by the application of an electrical shock by paddles applied to the patient's chest to terminate the arrhythmia, or by means of drugs that disrupt the formation and transmission of the abnormal impulses. After a normal rhythm has been established, the patient may need to continue taking some medication to maintain the normal rhythm.

## Ventricular Fibrillation

In contrast to atrial fibrillation, ventricular fibrillation is incompatible with life because the ventricles are unable to contract normally and the circulation ceases ( Figure 10-7B ). Ventricular fibrillation sometimes occurs following a heart attack. If recognized promptly, it is often possible to stop the fibrillation by delivering an electric shock to the heart by means of electrodes applied to the chest. The procedure usually causes the ventricles to resume normal contractions.

## Heart Block

Heart block is a delay or complete interruption of impulse transmission from the atria to the ventricles that often results from damage to the conduction system resulting from heart disease. This may be manifested as a delayed conduction of impulses to partial or complete block of impulse transmission. In the most severe form (complete heart block) conduction of impulses through the AV bundle is completely interrupted, which is treated by inserting a cardiac pacemaker to stimulate regular ventricular contractions. Many different types of pacemakers are available, each type having specific applications.

# Heart Disease as a Disturbance of Pump Function

For a pump to function properly, several conditions are required:

1. The pump must be properly constructed so that it is free of mechanical defects.
2. The pump must have a system of valves that are properly synchronized to allow unidirectional flow. If valves do not function properly, the force of the pump stroke is dissipated, and effective pumping is impaired.
3. The pump must have an adequate fuel supply. It will not run properly if the fuel line is dirty or plugged.
4. The pump must be used within its rated capacity. One must not use a pump rated at 3 horsepower to perform a job requiring a 10-horsepower pump. Either the pump will not function at all, or it will wear out very rapidly.
5. The pump motor must function smoothly and efficiently. If the motor functions erratically, the efficiency of the pump is reduced greatly.

The heart is a muscular pump that is subject to the same requirements as any mechanical pump. Each type of heart disease can be roughly compared with one of the derangements that would impair the function of a mechanical pump ( Table 10-1 ).

Congenital heart disease corresponds to faulty pump construction. The term *valvular heart disease* indicates that heart valves have been damaged by disease and fail to open and close properly. It is comparable to a malfunction in the unidirectional valve system of a mechanical pump. Coronary heart disease is a result of deposits of fatty material in the arterial walls that narrow their lumens and eventually may completely block the flow of blood through the arteries. This type of heart disease corresponds to failure of a mechanical pump

| **Table 10-1** | **Heart Disease Compared with Mechanical Pump Dysfunctions** |
|---|---|
| **Mechanical Abnormality** | **Comparable Heart Disease** |
| Faulty pump construction | Congenital heart disease |
| Faulty unidirectional valves | Valvular heart disease |
| Dirty or plugged fuel line | Coronary heart disease |
| Overloaded pump | Hypertensive heart disease |
| Malfunctioning pump | Primary myocardial disease |

caused by a dirty or plugged fuel line. Hypertensive heart disease results when the heart is forced to pump blood at high pressure against an excessively high resistance in the peripheral arterioles and corresponds to overloading a mechanical pump. Primary myocardial disease corresponds to malfunction of the pump motor.

# Congenital Heart Disease

## Cardiac Development and Prenatal Blood Flow

The heart undergoes a complex developmental sequence. It is formed from a tube that undergoes segmental dilatations and constrictions along with considerable growth and change in configuration. Eventually the individual chambers, valves, and large arteries develop, culminating in the final structural characteristics of a normal fully developed heart.

As the heart is developing, the blood flow through the fetal heart differs from its final postdelivery flow pattern. Much of the blood flow in the pulmonary artery is diverted away from the lungs, which are nonfunctional in the fetus, and used instead to supply other fetal tissues. The two pathways that bypass the lungs are the ductus arteriosus and the foramen ovale.

The ductus arteriosus is a large communication connecting the pulmonary artery with the aorta that shunts much of the blood pumped into the pulmonary artery directly into the aorta. When the infant is born and begins to breathe air, the ductus constricts, which blocks blood flow through the ductus arteriosus. Consequently, pulmonary artery blood can flow only into the newly expanded lungs, and the nonfunctional ductus arteriosus eventually becomes converted into a fibrous cord called the *ligamentum arteriosum*.

The foramen ovale is an opening in the atrial septum connecting the two atria that is covered by a flap of atrial tissue on the left atrial side of the septum. In this position, the flap functions as a one-way valve that allows blood to flow from right atrium into left atrium, which bypasses blood flow from the right atrium into the right ventricle and nonfunctional lungs, but does not allow flow in the opposite direction ( Figure 10-8 ). The right-to-left flow is determined by pressure differences between the two chambers. In the fetus the blood pressure is higher in the right atrium than in the left atrium because only a relatively small volume of blood flows through the lungs and is returned to the left atrium. Most is directed into the aorta through the ductus arteriosus. After birth the left atrial pressure rises when the lungs expand and a large volume of blood flows through the lungs and into the left atrium. The higher left atrial pressure presses the flap

valve against the left atrial surface of the septum, closing the communication between the atria. Usually, the tissue flap fuses with the atrial septum to form a solid partition between the two atria. Often the fusion is incomplete but no flow of blood from right to left atria is possible as long as the left atrial pressure exceeds the pressure in the right atrium, which holds the flap against the atrial septum.

## Pathogenesis and Manifestations of Congenital Heart Disease

Sometimes the heart fails to develop normally. Partitions between cardiac chambers may be defective. The cardiac valves may be malformed, or the large vessels entering and leaving the heart may not communicate normally with the appropriate atrium or ventricle. Some viral infections, such as German measles or other maternal illnesses during the early phases of fetal development, may cause improper development of the heart as well as other organs. Some chromosomal abnormalities, such as Down syndrome, also are frequently associated with abnormal cardiac development. Genetic factors may also account for some cardiac abnormalities, but often the reason for a congenital abnormality cannot be determined.

The effect of a structural abnormality depends on the nature of the defect and its effect on the circulation of blood. Most persons with congenital heart abnormalities have a heart murmur that is caused by turbulent flow of blood within the heart related to the cardiac malformation. Many congenital heart abnormalities result from abnormal communications between the systemic and pulmonary circulations that permit blood to be shunted between the adjacent chambers. The amount of blood shunted and the direction of the shunt depend on the size of the opening between the chambers, and the blood pressure difference between the chambers determines the direction of flow.

Most shunts are left-to-right shunts from left cardiac chambers (systemic circulation) into right cardiac chambers (pulmonary circulation). A left-to-right shunt mixes oxygenated blood from the left cardiac chambers with deoxygenated blood in the right chambers, but the admixture does not affect the oxygen content of the blood delivered to the tissues by the left ventricle. The amount of blood shunted depends on the size of the septal defect. A small defect shunts very little blood and has no significant effect on cardiovascular function. However, a large septal defect can shunt a large volume of blood, putting an additional burden on the right ventricle that is overfilled by the shunted blood. The larger volume of blood pumped into the lungs raises the pulmonary blood pressure, which eventually damages the lungs by causing thickening and narrowing of the pulmonary blood vessels. As the pulmonary vascular damage progresses and the pulmonary artery pressure continues to rises, the right ventricle has to work even harder to overcome the increasing resistance to blood flow through the lungs.

In contrast, right-to-left shunts mix poorly oxygenated blood from the right cardiac chambers with normally oxygenated blood contained in the left cardiac chambers, which reduces the oxygen content of the blood pumped by the left ventricle to supply the body. The affected person's activities usually are severely restricted by the poorly oxygenated arterial blood. The skin and mucous membranes acquire a blue color called **cyanosis**, which is caused by the admixture of deoxygenated blood that appears blue, in contrast to the bright red appearance of normally oxygenated arterial blood. Congenital cardiovascular abnormalities associated with cyanosis are grouped together under the general term *cyanotic congenital heart disease.*

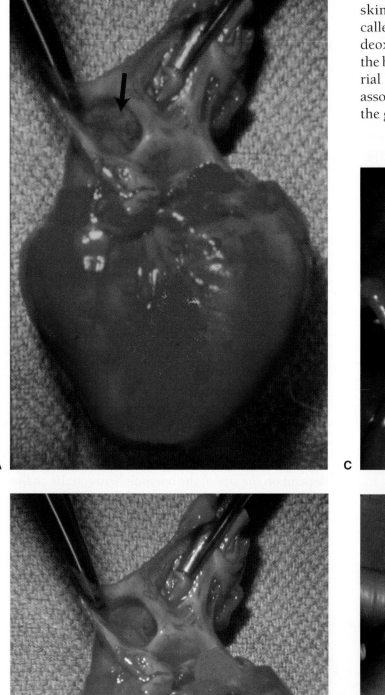

A

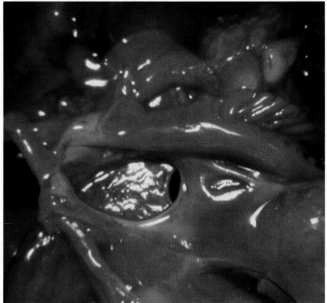

C

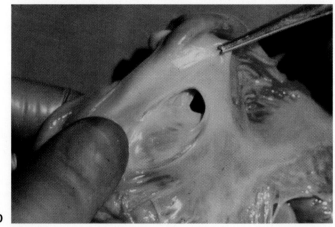

B

D

Figure 10-8 Structure and function of the foramen ovale. **A,** Overview of fetal heart with the right atrium opened to show the atrial septum. The foramen ovale appears as a depression in the right atrial surface of the septum (*arrow*). **B,** Closer view of foramen ovale illustrating flap of atrial septum tissue forming the base of the foramen that would be displaced toward the left atrium by the higher pressure of blood in the right atrium, allowing blood to flow into the left atrium. **C,** View of septal surface of the fetal right atrium stretched to reveal the free margin of the flap of septal tissue that would be displaced by the higher right atrial pressure in the fetus, allowing blood to flow into the left atrium. **D,** Similar view of stretched right atrium from adult heart with patent foramen ovale to illustrate how a high right atrial pressure allows blood to flow from right to left atrium but normally would prevent left-to-right blood flow when the flap is in its normal position.

# Common Cardiovascular Abnormalities

The more common and important cardiovascular abnormalities fall into four major groups.

1. Failure of the normal fetal bypass channels to close
2. Atrial and ventricular septal defects
3. Abnormalities that obstruct blood flow through the heart, pulmonary artery, or aorta
4. Abnormal formation of the aorta and pulmonary artery, or abnormal connection of the arteries to the appropriate ventricles

## Patent Ductus Arteriosus

Normally the ductus closes spontaneously soon after birth in full-term infants. A large patent ductus shunts blood from the aorta into the pulmonary artery and causes the same clinical manifestations and complications as an intracardiac left-to-right shunt, and is treated by surgical closure of the ductus.

## Patent Foramen Ovale

The foramen ovale normally becomes nonfunctional after birth, caused by the rapid postdelivery changes in atrial pressures, as described previously. In newborn infants the foramen ovale may remain patent and functional if the infant has a congenital cardiac abnormality that is associated with a high right atrial pressure, which forces right-to-left blood flow through the foramen ovale.

In many adults the flap valve does not fuse completely with the atrial septum, but the foramen ovale remains nonfunctional as long as the left atrial pressure remains higher than the right atrial pressure.

## Atrial and Ventricular Septal Defects

Usually an atrial septal defect results from defective development of the partitions that divide the atria, and the defect is located in the middle of the septum at the site usually occupied by the foramen ovale. Small defects in children often close spontaneously. Larger defects should be closed, which usually can be accomplished using a device inserted into the heart through a peripheral vein. Sometimes an open surgical procedure is required to place a patch over the defect.

Ventricular septal defects are also very common ( Figure 10-9 ). Many are less than 3 millimeters in diameter and often close spontaneously. Larger defects need to be closed surgically because of the harmful effects of a large left-to-right shunt on the heart and pulmonary blood vessels, as described previously.

## Pulmonary or Aortic Valve Stenosis

Abnormal development of the semilunar valve leaflets narrows the valve opening, which can vary from 2 to 10 millimeters in diameter, and the degree of obstruction depends on the diameter of the orifice ( Figure 10-10 ). Pulmonary stenosis obstructs outflow from the right ventricle, and aortic stenosis impedes outflow from the left ventricle. Treatment consists of dilating the valve opening by inserting a balloonlike device into the narrow valve opening.

**cyanosis**
A blue tinge of the skin and mucous membranes that results from an excessively large amount of reduced hemoglobin in the blood when blood oxygenation is insufficient.

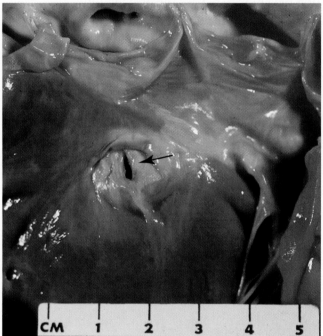

Figure 10-9  Small ventricular septal defect (*arrow*).

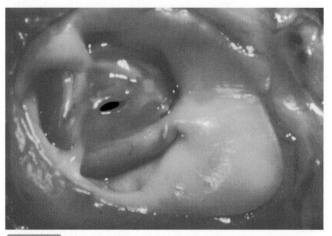

Figure 10-10  Congenital pulmonary stenosis. The valve orifice is reduced to a narrow slit, obstructing outflow from the right ventricle.

## Coarctation of the Aorta

*Coarctation* is a Latin word meaning narrowing, and the term describes a localized narrowing of the proximal aorta that restricts blood flow into the distal aorta. Usually the constriction is located distal to the origin of the large arteries arising from the arch of the aorta. The blood pressure in the aorta and its branches proximal to the coarctation is much higher than normal because the heart has to pump blood at a much higher pressure in order to deliver blood through the narrowed segment of the aorta, but the higher pressure is not adequate to deliver a normal volume of blood through the constriction. The pressure and volume of blood flowing into the aorta distal to the coarctation are both lower than normal, and a collateral circulation develops to bypass the obstruction.

Branches of the subclavian arteries proximal to the coarctation communicate with chest arteries distal to the coarctation (intercostal arteries) to deliver blood into the aorta distal to the obstruction. A subject with a coarctation may appear normal except for high blood pressure identified when measuring pressure in the brachial arteries, but lower-than-normal blood pressure in the arteries of the lower extremities. Often a coarctation is first identified during a medical examination for an unrelated condition in which an unexpected hypertension is detected. Usually the narrowed segment of the aorta is relatively short and can be treated by resecting the constricting segment and reconnecting the aorta so that its caliber is normal throughout its entire length.

## The Tetralogy of Fallot and Transposition of the Great Arteries

Both of these conditions result from abnormal division of a single channel called the truncus arteriosus extending from the developing ventricles that will be divided by a partition to form the aorta and the pulmonary artery. The partition, which is called the aorticopulmonary septum, takes a spiral course as it divides the truncus arteriosus, which is why the aorta and the pulmonary artery spiral around each other as they attach to their respective ventricles. These two abnormalities caused by abnormal division of the truncus arteriosus are relatively common, and both cause intermixing of deoxygenated blood with oxygenated blood, which leads to marked cyanosis.

1. *The tetralogy of Fallot* results if the aorticopulmonary septum divides the truncus unequally. As a result the pulmonary artery is smaller than it should be and the aorta is too large; the upper part of the ventricular septum, which is formed in part from the aorticopulmonary septum, does not connect properly

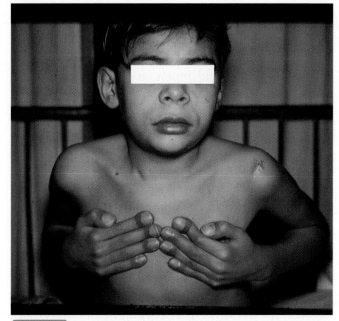

**Figure 10-11** Child with cyanotic congenital heart disease (tetralogy of Fallot) illustrating cyanosis of skin and prominent clubbing of fingers caused by deoxygenated blood mixing with oxygenated blood (right-to-left shunt).

to the aorta and the pulmonary artery that extend from the ventricles. The failed connection results in a large ventricular septal defect that is straddled by the enlarged aorta and receives blood ejected from both ventricles. The four abnormalities comprising the tetralogy are (1) a ventricular septal defect, (2) pulmonary stenosis, (3) an enlarged aorta that overrides the septal defect, and (4) right ventricular hypertrophy that develops as a consequence of the pulmonary stenosis. Marked cyanosis results from shunting large amounts of oxygen-poor arterial blood from the right ventricle through the ventricular septal defect and directly into the aorta. Usually the fingertips and toes become swollen. The condition, which usually is called clubbing, results from overgrowth of connective tissue and blood vessels at the tips of the fingers and toes caused by the low oxygen content of the arterial blood (Figure 10-11). The poorly oxygenated blood also stimulates the bone marrow to increase red cell production (polycythemia) in an attempt to increase oxygen delivery to the tissues that unfortunately has some disadvantages. The heart has to work harder to pump the more viscous blood, and the increased blood viscosity also predisposes to formation of blood clots within the circulation. Treatment consists of enlarging the opening of the narrowed pulmonary artery and closing the septal defect.

2. *Transposition of the great arteries* results if the aorticopulmonary septum divides the truncus arteriosus without following its normal spiral course

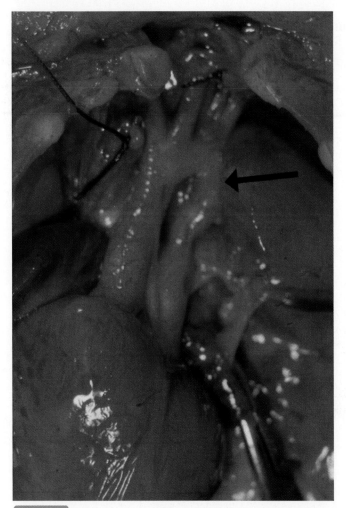

**Figure 10-12** Transposition of the great arteries showing the parallel course of the aorta and pulmonary artery. The aorta is located to the right of the pulmonary artery (*left side* of photograph) and is connected to the right ventricle, and the pulmonary artery is attached to the left ventricle. Some intermixing of blood between the aortic and pulmonary circulations is achieved by the large patent ductus arteriosus (*arrow*), and also by the foramen ovale, which is not demonstrated in the photograph.

as it divides the truncus into the aorta and pulmonary artery. Consequently, the aorta and pulmonary artery develop parallel to each other. The aorta becomes located to the right of the pulmonary artery instead of behind and to the left of the pulmonary artery, which changes the relationship of the arteries to their "correct" ventricles ( Figure 10-12 ). The aorta becomes connected to the right ventricle and the pulmonary artery attaches to the left ventricle, which severely disrupts blood flow in both the pulmonary and systemic circulations. The right ventricle pumps blood into the aorta (instead of the pulmonary artery) to be distributed to the body, and the blood is returned by the superior and inferior vena cava to the right atrium. Consequently the body is supplied by poorly oxygenated blood that is continuously circulated in the systemic circulation. In contrast, the left ventricle pumps oxygenated

blood into the pulmonary artery (instead of the aorta), which returns in the pulmonary veins to the left atrium. The flow of oxygenated blood remains confined to the pulmonary circuit where it serves no useful purpose. After birth the condition is not compatible with life unless there is a communication that permits some intermixing of blood between the pulmonary and systemic circulations such as a patent foramen ovale, atrial septal defect, or ventricular septal defect. Generally, such communications do not provide enough oxygenated blood to supply an infant's needs.

The current treatment of this condition is called the arterial switch operation, which involves cutting across the bases of the aorta and pulmonary artery above their attachments to the ventricles. Then the aorta is connected to the left ventricle and the pulmonary artery is attached to the right ventricle. It is also necessary to reposition the coronary arteries so that they are connected properly to the artery supplying blood to the left ventricle.

 Table 10-2  summarizes the principal features of the congenital cardiovascular malformations described in this section, which are also illustrated in  Figure 10-13 .

## Prevention of Congenital Heart Disease

The only way to prevent congenital heart disease is to attempt to protect the developing fetus from intrauterine injury during the early phases of pregnancy when the fetus is very vulnerable to intrauterine fetal injury, as discussed in Chapter 7.

# Valvular Heart Disease

Rheumatic fever is much less frequent now than formerly. As a result, rheumatic valvular heart disease has also declined, and other conditions that cause valve malfunction have assumed greater importance. These include various degenerative conditions of the aortic valve and an abnormality of the mitral valve that causes it to prolapse into the atrium during ventricular systole.

## Rheumatic Fever and Rheumatic Heart Disease

Rheumatic fever is a complication of infection by the group A beta hemolytic streptococcus, the organism responsible for streptococcal sore throat and scarlet fever. This disease, encountered most commonly in children, is a febrile illness associated with inflammation of connective tissue throughout the body, especially in the heart and joints. Clinically, the affected individual has an acute arthritis affecting multiple

## Table 10-2 Features of Common Congenital Cardiovascular Abnormalities

| Abnormality | Physiologic Disturbance | Complications | Treatment |
|---|---|---|---|
| Patent ductus arteriosus | Aorta to pulmonary artery shunt | Pulmonary hypertension | Ligate or excise ductus |
| Patent foramen ovale | Right-to-left atrial shunt | Usually nonfunctional as long as left atrial pressure exceeds right atrial pressure | Usually no treatment required |
| Atrial, ventricular, and combined septal defects | Left-to-right shunt | Pulmonary hypertension damages lungs. Right ventricular hypertrophy. | Close defect |
| Pulmonary stenosis | Obstructed outflow from right ventricle | Right ventricular hypertrophy | Dilate narrowed valve opening |
| Aortic stenosis | Obstructed outflow from left ventricle | Left ventricular hypertrophy | Dilate narrowed valve opening |
| Aortic coarctation | Obstructed flow into aorta distal to coarctation | Hypertension in arteries supplying head and upper limbs | Excise coarctation and reconnect aorta |
| Tetralogy of Fallot | Right-to-left shunt. Ventricular septal defect straddled by enlarged aorta. Pulmonary stenosis. Right ventricular hypertrophy. | Cyanosis. Polycythemia. Clubbing of fingers and toes. | Enlarge pulmonary artery opening. Close septal defect. |
| Transposition of great arteries | Aorta attached to right ventricle and pulmonary artery attached to left ventricle | Only communication between systemic and pulmonary circulations is through ductus arteriosus and foramen ovale | Reattach aorta and pulmonary artery to proper ventricles. Reposition coronary arteries. |

joints (which is why the disease is called "rheumatic" fever) and evidence of inflammation of the heart.

Rheumatic fever is not a bacterial infection but a type of hypersensitivity reaction induced by various antigens present in the streptococcus. This reaction develops several weeks after the initial streptococcal infection. It is uncertain exactly how the streptococcus induces the development of rheumatic fever. Apparently, some persons form antibody against antigens present in the streptococcus, and the antistreptococcal antibody cross-reacts with similar antigens in the individual's own tissues. The antigen–antibody reaction injures connective tissue and is responsible for the febrile illness. Fortunately, rheumatic fever develops in only a small proportion of persons with group A beta streptococcal infections.

Some patients with acute rheumatic fever die as a result of severe inflammation of the heart and consequent acute heart failure. In most instances, however, the fever and signs of inflammation eventually subside. Healing is often associated with some degree of scarring. In the joints and in many other tissues, scarring causes no difficulties, but scarring of heart valves may produce various deformities that impair function.

Unfortunately, rheumatic fever is likely to recur if the patient develops another streptococcal infection because

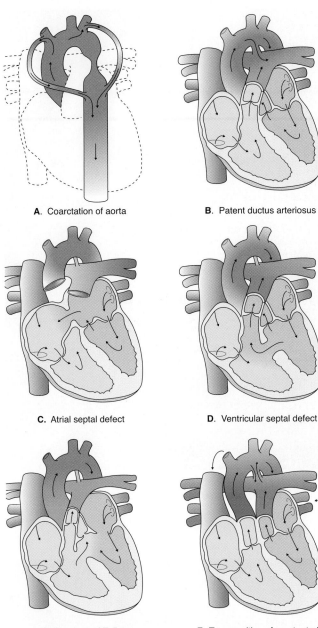

**A.** Coarctation of aorta

**B.** Patent ductus arteriosus

**C.** Atrial septal defect

**D.** Ventricular septal defect

**E.** Tetralogy of Fallot

**F.** Transposition of great arteries

 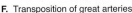

**Figure 10-13** Blood flow patterns in six common congenital abnormalities described in this section. **A,** Aortic coarctation. **B,** Patent ductus arteriosus. **C,** Atrial septal defect. **D,** Ventricular septal defect. **E,** Tetralogy of Fallot. **F,** Transposition of the great arteries.

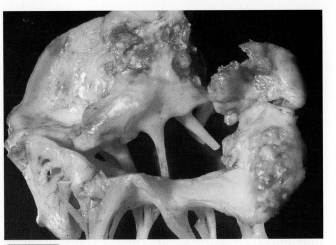

**Figure 10-14** Poorly functioning scarred and calcified mitral valve resulting from valve damage caused by prior rheumatic fever. The valve was excised and replaced by an artificial heart valve.

any subsequent contact with the streptococcus reestablishes the sequence of hypersensitivity and connective tissue damage. Rheumatic heart disease, a complication of rheumatic fever, is caused by scarring of the heart valves subsequent to the healing of a rheumatic inflammation. This complication is relatively common and primarily affects the valves of the left side of the heart; the mitral and aortic valves. If the valve does not close properly, blood refluxes back through it (called regurgitation). Frequently, the damaged valve also does not open properly, and the valve orifice is narrowed. This is called a **valve stenosis**. Valve lesions impair cardiac function. When valvular stenosis is present, the heart must exert more effort than normal to force blood through the narrowed orifice. In regurgitation, a portion of the ventricular output is not expelled normally because some of the blood leaks through the incompetent valve.

An individual with a mild rheumatic valvular deformity that does not seriously interfere with cardiac function may experience little or no disability. However, a severe valve deformity may place a serious strain on the heart, eventually causing heart failure many years after the initial attack of rheumatic fever. When a person is seriously disabled by a rheumatic valvular deformity, it is possible to excise the abnormal, scarred heart valve surgically and replace it with an artificial valve ( Figure 10-14 ).

**Prevention of Rheumatic Heart Disease** Rheumatic heart disease can be largely prevented by treating beta streptococcal infection promptly, thereby forestalling the hypersensitivity state that causes rheumatic fever. Because a person who has once had rheumatic fever is susceptible to recurrent attacks after beta streptococcal infections, many physicians recommend that persons who have had rheumatic fever receive prophylactic penicillin therapy throughout childhood and young adulthood. Penicillin treatment prevents streptococcal infections and reduces the risk of recurrent rheumatic fever and further heart valve damage.

## Nonrheumatic Aortic Stenosis

In about 2 percent of all people, the aortic valve has two rather than the usual three cusps. This abnormality is called a congenital bicuspid aortic valve. The valve functions satisfactorily for a time but is subjected

**valve stenosis**
(sten-ō′sis) Impaired flow of blood through a heart valve that does not open properly.

to unusual stress during opening and closing because of its bicuspid configuration. As a result, the valve gradually becomes thickened and may eventually become calcified after many years, leading to marked rigidity of the valve when a person reaches middle age ( Figure 10-15 ). This condition is called aortic stenosis secondary to bicuspid aortic valve.

Fibrosis and calcification of the valve leaflets of a normal three-cusp aortic valve may also occur in older persons, and sometimes the valve becomes so rigid that it is unable to open properly. This entity is called calcific aortic stenosis ( Figure 10-16 ). Mild degrees of aortic stenosis may not greatly compromise cardiac function, but severe aortic stenosis places a great strain on the left ventricle, which must expel blood through the greatly narrowed and rigid valve orifice. This leads to marked left ventricular hypertrophy and eventual heart failure. Treatment of severe aortic stenosis consists of surgically replacing the stenotic valve with an artificial heart valve.

Aortic stenosis often is considered to be caused by degenerative changes in valve leaflet connective tissue, a consequence of the stresses placed on the valve resulting from the repeated opening and closing of the valve leaflets over many years, followed by calcification that restricts valve mobility. More recent studies, however, have demonstrated deposits of lipids and accumulation of macrophages in the valve leaflets similar to the changes found in coronary atherosclerosis. On the basis of these studies, it now appears that the same risk factors that predispose to coronary artery disease, such as high cholesterol, diabetes, and hypertension, also may contribute to the valve changes leading to aortic stenosis. As our population ages, aortic stenosis

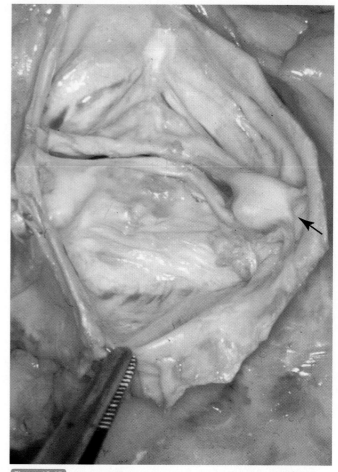

**Figure 10-15** A congenital bicuspid aortic valve viewed from above. Beginning scarring is seen at the right margin of the valve (*arrow*).

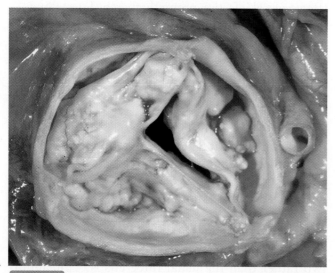

A

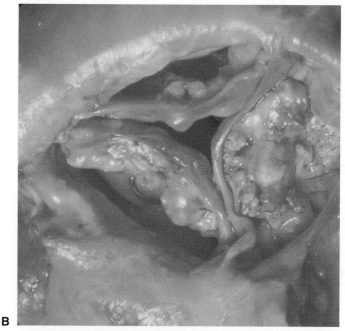

B

**Figure 10-16** Aortic valves viewed from above illustrating marked thickening and nodularity of valve leaflets. **A**, Partial fusion of valve cusps (*left side* of photograph). A normal coronary artery is seen in cross section at right of aortic valve. **B**, Severe calcific aortic stenosis. Extensive calcium deposits within cusps severely limit valve mobility.

is becoming one of the most common types of valvular heart disease. Case 10-1 describes a common clinical presentation of aortic stenosis and also illustrates the management of a patient with this condition.

## Case Study 10-1

During a routine physical examination, a 73-year-old man was found to have a systolic murmur. He was in good health and had not had any serious illnesses in the past, and there was no history of previous rheumatic fever.

Physical examination was completely normal except for the heart murmur. Temperature, pulse, and blood pressure were all within normal limits. Routine laboratory tests and an electrocardiogram were all normal.

An echocardiogram was performed in order to determine the cause of the murmur and revealed that he had mild aortic stenosis. The aortic valve was calcified, and there was a mild-to-moderate restriction of the aortic valve opening. The aortic valve opening was calculated to be 1.2 square centimeters, in contrast to a normal valve opening that should be 3 to 4 square centimeters when fully open. The mean pressure gradient across the aortic valve was 17 mm Hg, indicating that the pressure within the left ventricle during systole was higher than that in the aorta because outflow of blood from the left ventricle was impeded by the valve stenosis.

The patient was told that he had a mild degree of aortic stenosis that was likely to progress over time and that he probably would eventually require a valve replacement. He did not need to restrict his activities, but he was advised to take prophylactic antibiotics before any dental procedures or surgical procedures that could cause transient entry of bacteria into his circulation in order to reduce his risk of endocarditis. He was also advised to take one 81-mg aspirin tablet daily (a "baby aspirin" tablet) both to reduce his risk of coronary heart disease and also to prevent platelets from adhering to the roughened surface of the stenotic aortic valve. He was also advised to have the echocardiogram repeated in 2 years to evaluate possible progression of the stenosis.

## Mitral Valve Prolapse

Mitral valve prolapse is a common condition, and only a very small percentage of persons ever develop any problems related to the prolapse. In this condition, one or both mitral leaflets are enlarged and redundant and prolapse into the left atrium during ventricular systole. Sometimes the prolapsing free margins of the valve leaflets don't fit together tightly, which allows some blood to leak across the closed mitral valve into the atrium, which is called mitral regurgitation. The extent of the prolapse is quite variable, and the amount of blood that leaks into the left atrium through the prolapsing valve depends on how tightly the free margins of the prolapsing valve leaflets come together during ventricular systole ( Figure 10-17 ). The mitral valve leaflets, like other cardiac valve leaflets, are attached to a ring of dense connective tissue called the mitral annulus, which circumscribes the valve opening. The annulus is part of the fibrous framework of the heart to which the valves and cardiac muscle bundles are attached. When one listens to the heart sounds with a stethoscope, one first hears a "click" sound during systole when the leaflets come together, which is often followed by a faint systolic murmur caused by reflux of blood between the closed valve leaflets into the left atrium.

In some cases, the prolapse appears to be caused by degenerative changes in the connective tissue of the valve leaflets, which permits the affected valve leaflets to gradually stretch as a result of the degeneration of the valve connective tissue. Eventually, one or both leaflets may become enlarged and redundant. When this occurs, the stretched prolapsing mitral valve, held at

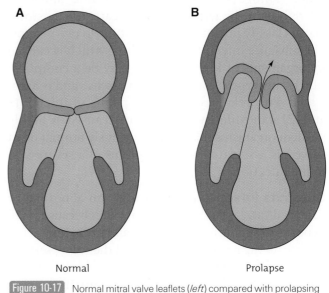

Normal                    Prolapse

Figure 10-17   Normal mitral valve leaflets (*left*) compared with prolapsing mitral leaflets associated with mild mitral insufficiency (*right*).

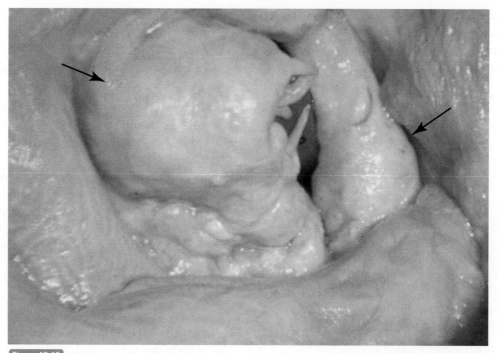

**Figure 10-18** The interior of the left atrium viewed from above, illustrating prolapsing mitral valve leaflets ballooning into the left atrium (*arrows*). Prolapse was complicated by a rupture of mitral valve chordae tendineae.

its margin by the chordae, somewhat resembles an open parachute (Figure 10-18), and a significant amount of blood may reflux into the left atrium. The prolapsing valve may also produce excessive strain on the chordae and papillary muscles, which may provoke bouts of ventricular arrhythmia. Sometimes the excessive stress causes one of the chordae to rupture.

## Infective Endocarditis

Infective endocarditis is an infection of a heart valve, usually caused by bacteria but occasionally caused by other pathogens. In most cases, the infection is in the valves in the left side of the heart. It is customary to classify infective endocarditis into two groups: (1) subacute infective endocarditis, which is caused by organisms of low virulence, may be a complication of any type of valvular heart disease and is associated with relatively mild symptoms of infection; and (2) acute infective endocarditis, caused by highly virulent organisms that infect previously normal heart valves, is associated with symptoms of a severe systemic infection.

**Subacute Infective Endocarditis** An abnormal or damaged valve is susceptible to infection because small deposits of agglutinated platelets and fibrin may accumulate on the roughened surface of the valve, serving as a site for implantation of bacteria. Transient bacteremias occasionally develop from superficial skin infections, after tooth extractions, and in association with various minor infections. In normal persons, transient bacteremia causes no problems because the organisms are normally destroyed by the body's defenses. However, an individual with a damaged valve runs the risk that bacteria may become implanted on the valve and incite an inflammation (Figure 10-19). Frequently, thrombi form at the site of the valve infection, and bits of thrombus may be dislodged and carried as emboli to other parts of the body, producing infarcts in various organs.

**Antibiotic Prophylaxis to Prevent Endocarditis** Infective (bacterial) endocarditis is relatively uncommon, but is a very serious disease. Persons with damaged heart valves or other cardiac abnormalities are at increased risk. Some surgical procedures and many dental procedures, such as cleaning and removal of dental plaque, tooth extractions, and root canal treatment, may cause a shower of bacteria to be discharged into the bloodstream. Because of the hazards of bacterial endocarditis in persons with damaged heart valves, prophylactic antibiotics are recommended for susceptible persons with damaged heart valves. The American Heart Association provides guidelines regarding who should receive antibiotics. Recently these guidelines were liberalized because of the low risk of bacterial endocarditis in most persons with heart murmurs. Now prophylactic antibiotics are only recommended for dental patients who are at high risk of endocarditis. This latter group includes:

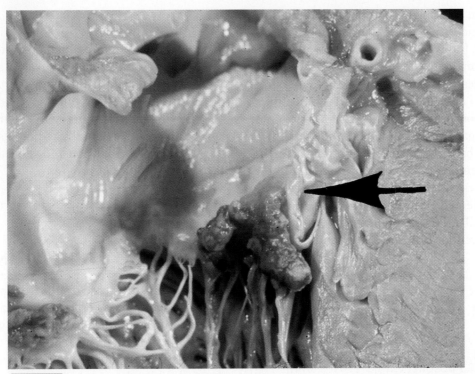

**Figure 10-19** Bacterial endocarditis illustrating vegetations on mitral valve leaflet (*arrow*). Normal coronary artery is seen in cross section (*upper right*).

1. Persons with heart valve damage who have been treated previously for endocarditis.
2. Persons in whom a diseased valve has been replaced by an artificial heart valve.
3. Most persons who have had surgically treated congenital heart disease.

**Acute Infective Endocarditis** Acute infective endocarditis results when highly pathogenic organisms spread into the bloodstream from an infection elsewhere in the body and infect a previously normal heart valve. Virulent staphylococci are a common cause of acute endocarditis and may cause considerable destruction of the affected valve ( Figure 10-20 ). Another group at high risk are intravenous drug abusers; in this group, the infection may involve the tricuspid valve rather than the valves on the left side of the heart. Infection results from using unsterile materials to dissolve and

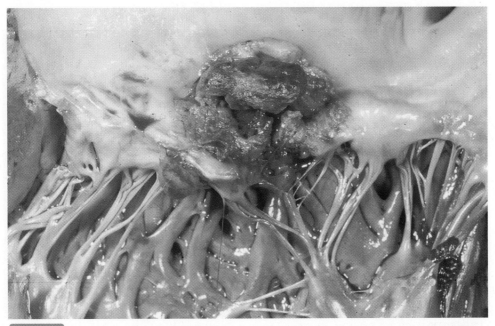

**Figure 10-20** Severe bacterial endocarditis caused by staphylococcal infection of normal mitral valve. Infection has caused extensive destruction and perforation of valve leaflet.

inject the drug. In addition to bacterial contamination, small particles and other debris may contaminate the injected material. Intravenous injection carries the contaminated solution directly to the right side of the heart, where the particles and debris abrade the surface of the tricuspid valve. Platelets adhere to the site of injury and form thrombi, providing a favorable site for the injected microorganisms to implant and start an infection. Often, large bacteria-laden vegetations form on the valve. Pieces often break loose and are swept into the pulmonary arteries where they lodge in the lungs, causing multiple infected pulmonary infarcts and lung abscesses. Case 10-2 illustrates some of the clinical features of an acute endocarditis in a drug abuser.

### Case Study 10-2

A 32-year-old hospital employee was admitted to the hospital because of chills and fever of about 2 weeks' duration. She was an intravenous cocaine user. Physical examination revealed numerous needle marks on the extremities and neck. Laboratory studies revealed increased numbers of polymorphonuclear leukocytes in the blood, suggesting an infection, and blood culture revealed *Staphylococcus aureus*. Special cardiac studies (echocardiograms) demonstrated a large vegetation on the tricuspid valve, and chest x-ray revealed multiple densities throughout both lungs, suggesting pulmonary infarcts secondary to emboli from the infected tricuspid valve. She eventually required surgical removal of the tricuspid valve and entered a drug treatment program.

## Coronary Heart Disease

Coronary heart disease results from arteriosclerosis of the large coronary arteries. The arteries narrow owing to accumulation of fatty materials within the vessel walls. The lipid deposits, consisting of neutral fat and cholesterol, accumulate in the arteries by diffusion from the bloodstream. The initial event may be an injury to the endothelium of the vessel, which is followed by proliferation of cells within the inner layer of the arterial wall (called the intima) and accumulation of cholesterol and other lipids within their cytoplasm ( Figure 10-21 ). Some of the cells accumulate so much cholesterol that it precipitates as crystals within the cytoplasm, disrupting the cells and causing cell necrosis. Cholesterol crystals, debris, and enzymes escape from the disrupted cells, inducing secondary fibrosis, calcification, and other degenerative changes

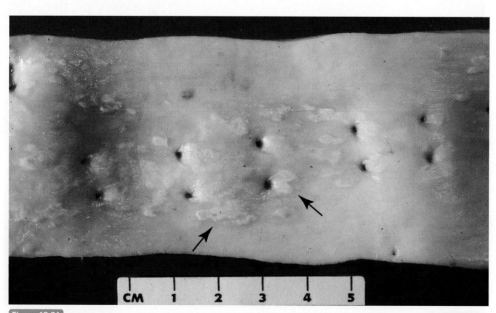

Figure 10-21 Interior of aorta illustrating early atheromatous plaque formation. Two plaques are indicated by *arrows*. Circular openings are orifices of intercostal arteries.

in the arterial wall. The end result is an irregular mass of yellow, mushy debris that encroaches on the lumen of the artery and extends more deeply into the muscular and elastic tissue of the arterial wall. Often the smooth internal lining of the vessel becomes ulcerated over the surface of the fatty deposits, leaving a roughened surface that predisposes to thrombus formation. A collection of fatty material and debris is called an atheromatous plaque or **atheroma** (*athere* = mush); the term for this type of arteriosclerosis is **atherosclerosis** ( Figure 10-22 ). The initial stage in the development of atherosclerosis is reversible, and the newly formed plaques are called unstable plaques. The later stages, characterized by crystallization of cholesterol and secondary degenerative changes, are irreversible. The plaques, which become surrounded by fibrous tissue, are called stable plaques, and the vessel becomes permanently narrowed ( Figure 10-23 ).

## Risk Factors

A number of factors are known to increase the risk of developing coronary heart disease and its associated complications. The four most important of these are (1) elevated blood lipids, (2) high blood pressure, (3) cigarette smoking, and (4) diabetes. If one risk factor is present, the likelihood of coronary heart disease and heart attacks is twice that of an individual lacking risk factors. If two risk factors are present, the risk increases fourfold, and if three factors are present, the risk of heart attack is seven times that of an individual with none. Obesity also increases the risk, probably because an obese person usually has high blood lipids and elevated blood pressure.

## Manifestations

If atherosclerotic plaques narrow the coronary arteries by 50 percent or more, the arteries may still be able to supply enough blood to the heart muscle if the individual is not very active and no excessive demands are placed on the heart. However, blood supply may become inadequate if the subject exerts himself or herself and the heart requires more blood to satisfy the increased demands. *Myocardial ischemia* is the term commonly used to describe a reduced blood supply to the heart muscle caused by narrowing or obstruction of the coronary arteries, and the term *ischemic heart disease* is frequently used interchangeably with coronary heart disease. Although the flow rate through a tube falls as the tube narrows, the decrease is related not directly to the tube diameter but to the fourth power of the diameter. Consequently, a moderate decrease in the caliber of a coronary artery causes a disproportionately large reduction in its flow rate ( Figure 10-24 ).

**atheroma**
(ah-ther-ō′muh) A mass of lipids and debris that accumulates in the intima lining of an artery and narrows its lumen.

**atherosclerosis** A thickening of the lining (*intima*) of blood vessels caused by accumulation of lipids, with secondary scarring and calcification.

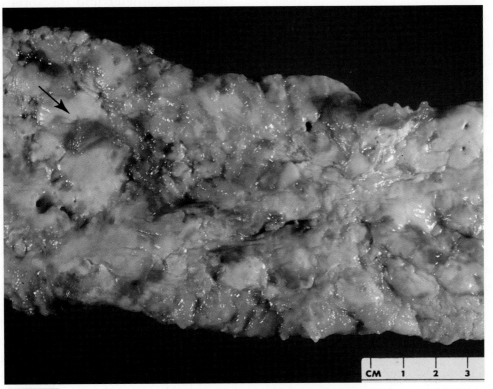

Figure 10-22    Advanced atherosclerosis of aorta. Many plaques are ulcerated and are covered by thrombus material (*arrow*).

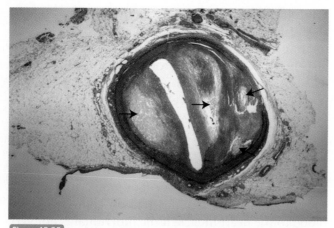

Figure 10-23 Low magnification photomicrograph of coronary artery in cross section illustrating several stable atheromatous plaques (*arrows*) surrounded by dense fibrous tissue.

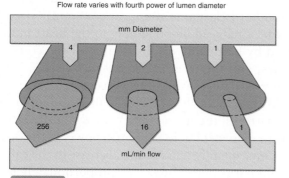

Flow rate varies with fourth power of lumen diameter

mm Diameter

4    2    1

256    16    1

mL/min flow

Figure 10-24 Relation of caliber of artery to flow rate, illustrating how a small reduction in diameter causes a disproportionately large drop in flow rate.

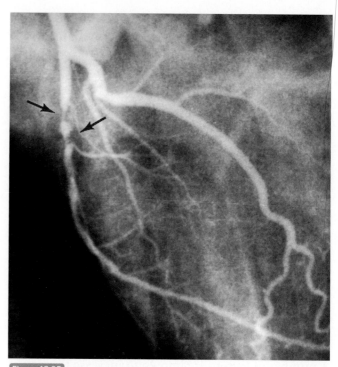

Figure 10-25 A coronary angiogram illustrating segmental narrowing (*arrows*).

The clinical manifestations of coronary heart disease are quite variable. Although many individuals are free of symptoms, some experience bouts of oppressive chest pain that may radiate into the neck or arms. The pain, which is caused by myocardial ischemia, is called **angina pectoris**, which means literally "pain of the chest." The usual type of angina is a midsternal pressure discomfort that occurs on exertion and subsides when the person rests or takes a nitroglycerin tablet, which dilates the coronary arteries and increases blood flow to the heart muscle. This kind of angina is often called stable angina to distinguish it from unstable angina, which is a manifestation of more severe and progressive narrowing of the coronary arteries. Unstable angina is characterized by episodes of pain that occur more frequently, last longer, and are less completely relieved by nitroglycerin.

Although angina is a common manifestation of coronary artery disease, it is not invariably present even though the coronary arteries are severely narrowed.

**angina pectoris**
(an-jī′nuh pek′tōr-is)
Precordial pain experienced on exertion owing to inadequate blood supply to the heart muscle.

## Diagnosis of Coronary Artery Disease

Physicians can now evaluate the extent of coronary artery disease as well as the exact sites where the coronary arteries are obstructed. This is accomplished by passing a catheter into the aorta and injecting a radiopaque dye directly into the orifices of the coronary arteries. The filling of the coronary arteries can be observed, along with the location and degree of arterial obstruction ( Figure 10-25 ). This procedure is called a coronary angiogram (Chapter 1).

## Coronary Disease Manifestations with Apparently Normal Coronary Arteries

Sometimes patients have symptoms of coronary artery disease, but coronary arteriograms reveal apparently normal coronary arteries or only evidence of small arteriosclerotic plaques that do not narrow the coronary arteries significantly. There are three possible reasons for the discrepancies between clinical manifestations and the apparently normal coronary angiograms.

1. *There is arteriosclerosis of the coronary arteries, but the angiogram can't detect it.* For example, a coronary artery may be involved diffusely and uniformly by arteriosclerosis rather than forming discrete plaques that lead to localized narrowing of the artery, and the artery may appear to have a small lumen without evidence of disease. In other cases, isolated plaques may expand outward rather

than extending into the lumen of the vessel and may escape detection.

2. *The coronary arteries are normal, but marked sympathetic nervous system vasoconstrictor impulses may reduce myocardial blood flow by causing coronary artery spasm.* Examples include stress-induced coronary artery vasoconstriction, which may actually lead to myocardial damage, as documented in a recent study of 19 women without coronary artery disease. In these women, severe emotional stress caused coronary artery vasospasm and myocardial injury as demonstrated by abnormal electrocardiograms, elevated cardiac enzymes, and impaired left ventricular function.

3. *The coronary arteries are normal, but the function of the coronary arterioles is not.* Normal coronary arterioles regulate blood flow to the heart muscle in response to myocardial oxygen requirements. When the arterioles are completely dilated, they can increase myocardial blood flow up to five times over basal levels when heart muscle needs more blood during exercise or exertion. In some persons, however, studies have demonstrated that the coronary arterioles are unable to dilate sufficiently to provide adequate blood to the heart muscle during exertion, which leads to symptoms of myocardial ischemia.

## Treatment of Coronary Artery Disease

**Medical Treatment**  Medical treatment of coronary heart disease consists of administering drugs that reduce myocardial oxygen consumption and improve coronary circulation (antianginal drugs). If the patient exhibits cardiac irregularities, drugs that reduce myocardial irritability also are prescribed (antiarrhythmial drugs). Factors that potentiate coronary artery disease also are controlled or eliminated as follows whenever possible ( Figure 10-26 ):

1. Cessation of smoking, which has an adverse effect on the coronary circulation

2. Control of hypertension, which increases myocardial work and accelerates development of atherosclerosis

3. An "anti-coronary diet," which lowers levels of cholesterol and fat in the blood. If a change in diet is not sufficient to lower cholesterol, drugs are added (usually called statins) that block an enzyme required for synthesis of cholesterol and lipoproteins.

4. Weight reduction

5. A program of graduated exercises, which seems to improve myocardial performance

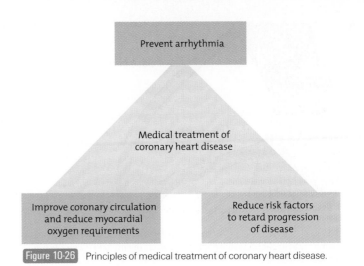

Figure 10-26   Principles of medical treatment of coronary heart disease.

**Surgical Treatment**  Several surgical approaches, called myocardial revascularization procedures, have been devised to improve blood supply to the heart muscle. Surgery is often recommended for patients who do not respond satisfactorily to medical treatment. The usual surgical method is to bypass the obstructions in the coronary arteries by means of segments of saphenous vein obtained from the patient's legs. The proximal ends of the grafts are sutured to small openings made in the aorta above the normal openings of the coronary arteries, and the distal ends are sutured into the coronary arteries beyond the areas of narrowing ( Figure 10-27 ). Myocardial revascularization operations are generally reserved for patients with severe sclerosis of all three major coronary arteries, and usually grafts are used to bypass all three arteries. The operation alleviates or greatly improves symptoms of angina and may also improve survival in some groups of patients. The internal thoracic arteries, which are more often called by their older name of internal mammary arteries, also can be used to bypass obstructed coronary arteries. The internal mammary arteries are paired arteries that arise from the aorta and descend along the undersurface of the thoracic cavity just lateral to the sternum. They can be dissected from their normal location and connected to the coronary arteries, thereby delivering blood directly from the aorta to the coronary arteries beyond the narrowed or blocked areas. In some patients, both vein grafts and internal mammary arteries are used to restore adequate blood flow to the myocardium.

**Coronary Angioplasty**  In some patients, it is possible to dilate areas of narrowing within coronary arteries instead of bypassing them, thereby avoiding major surgery. The procedure is called *coronary angioplasty* (*angio* = vessel + *plasty* = molding) and is illustrated in

**A**

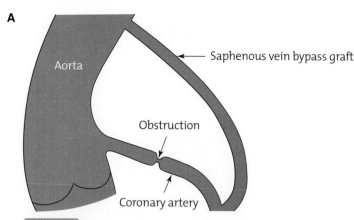

Aorta

Saphenous vein bypass graft →

Obstruction

Coronary artery

**Figure 10-27** **A,** Principles of surgical treatment of coronary heart disease by means of saphenous vein grafts that bypass obstruction in coronary arteries. **B,** Vein graft extending from aorta above the origin of the coronary arteries to the anterior interventricular (anterior descending) coronary artery distal to the site of the arterial narrowing.

**Figure 10-28** . By means of a technique similar to that used to perform a coronary arteriogram (Chapter 1), a guiding catheter is introduced through the skin and into a large artery in the arm or leg, threaded under fluoroscopic control into the narrowed coronary artery, and positioned at the site of narrowing. Then a balloon catheter is threaded through the guide catheter until the balloon lies within the narrowed area. After the balloon is properly positioned, it is inflated briefly under very high pressure, which smashes the plaque and pushes it into the arterial wall, enlarging the lumen of the artery and improving blood flow to the myocardium. Usually a short, expandable metal mesh tube called a **stent** is placed over the balloon catheter with the metal mesh collapsed. The stent expands as the balloon is inflated to enlarge the lumen of the artery and functions as a rigid support to help keep the vessel open (Figure 10-28). This procedure is usually supplemented by administration of drugs that prevent accumulation of platelets at the site where the stent was placed. At first, the procedure was used to treat patients who had only a single narrowed artery, but it is now used to treat patients who have multiple obstructing plaques in their coronary arteries. Successful dilatation of a narrowed coronary artery greatly improves blood flow through the artery.

Although use of stents has been helpful, sometimes ingrowth of tissue from the wall of the stented artery extending between the meshes of the stent may narrow the lumen of the stented artery. In an attempt to avoid this problem, stents have been produced that are coated with drugs (called drug-releasing stents) that suppress the cell proliferation responsible for narrowing the stented artery.

**stent**
An expandable metal hollow tubular device placed within the lumen of a structure such as a blood vessel, often used to expand the lumen of the vessel, where it functions as a support to prevent narrowing of the dilated vessel.

**B**

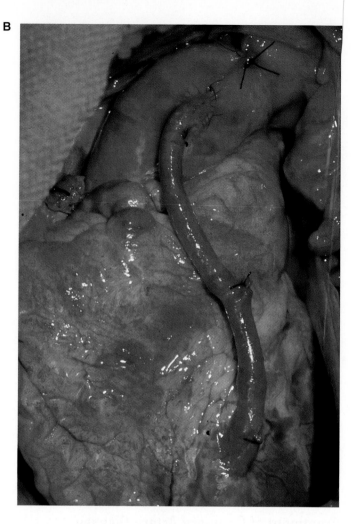

# Severe Myocardial Ischemia and Its Complications: A "Heart Attack"

Severe and prolonged myocardial ischemia may precipitate an acute episode called a "heart attack" ( **Figure 10-29** ). This event may be manifested as either cessation of normal cardiac contractions, called a cardiac arrest, or an actual necrosis of heart muscle, which is termed a *myocardial infarction*. Any one of four basic mechanisms may trigger a heart attack in a patient with coronary artery disease.

1. *Sudden blockage of a coronary artery.* Usually this is caused by a blood clot that forms on the roughened surface of an ulcerated atheromatous plaque ( **Figure 10-30** ). This is called a coronary thrombosis. A less common cause of blockage is an obstruction of the lumen by atheromatous debris. This sometimes occurs if a break develops in the endothelium and

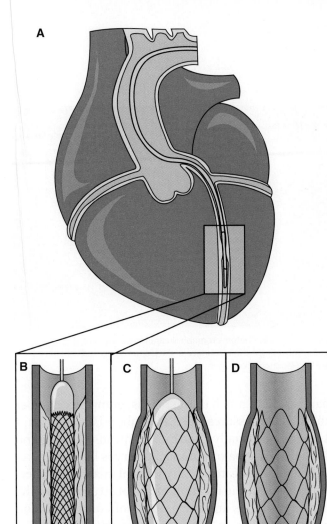

A

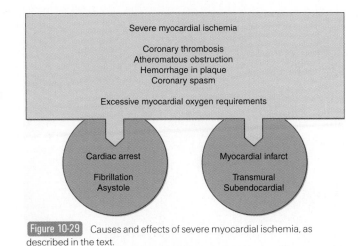

**Figure 10-29** Causes and effects of severe myocardial ischemia, as described in the text.

**Figure 10-28** Principle of coronary angioplasty to reestablish flow through a thrombosed coronary artery (percutaneous coronary intervention) or to enlarge the lumen of an artery narrowed by atheromatous plaques. **A,** An overview illustrating the positioning of the guide catheter at the site of narrowing or obstruction of a coronary artery. **B,** A balloon catheter covered by an unexpanded stent is advanced through the guide catheter and pushed through occluding thrombus and atheromatous material, or positioned within a narrowed segment of an artery partially blocked by atheromatous plaques. **C,** Balloon-inflated expanding stent and opening artery. **D,** Balloon catheter withdrawn, leaving expanded stent that forms a rigid support to help keep the artery open.

fibrous tissue covering a plaque, allowing the contents of the plaque to be extruded and block the lumen.

2. *Hemorrhage into an atheromatous plaque.* Bleeding into a plaque usually results from rupture of a small blood vessel in the arterial wall adjacent to the plaque. The blood seeping into the plaque causes it to enlarge, which further narrows or obstructs the lumen of the coronary artery.

3. *Arterial spasm.* A spasm of a coronary artery has been shown to occur adjacent to atheromatous plaques. This may be the mechanism that precipitates arterial obstruction in some patients with heart attacks.

4. *Sudden greatly increased myocardial oxygen requirements.* Vigorous activity such as running, snow shoveling, or tennis abruptly increases cardiac output, which in turn raises myocardial oxygen consumption. However, the sclerotic coronary arteries are incapable of delivering an adequate blood supply to the heart muscle, and severe myocardial ischemia develops.

## Cardiac Arrest

Myocardial ischemia increases myocardial irritability, which may lead to disturbances of cardiac rhythm called cardiac arrhythmias. A cardiac arrest occurs when an arrhythmia induced by prolonged or severe myocardial ischemia disrupts the pumping of the ventricles. The most devastating arrhythmia is an uncoordinated quivering of the ventricles that is called ventricular fibrillation. It is the most common cause of cardiac arrest and sudden death in patients with coronary heart disease. Ventricular fibrillation is rapidly fatal because the normal pumping action of the ventricles ceases. If the condition is recognized promptly, it is often possible to stop the fibrillation by delivering an electric shock to the heart by means of electrodes applied to the chest. This procedure frequently causes the ventricles to resume normal contractions, but in many cases, ventricular fibrillation occurs without warning, and the patient dies before medical attention can be obtained. A less common cause of cardiac arrest is complete cessation of cardiac contractions, which is called an asystole (*a* = without + systole).

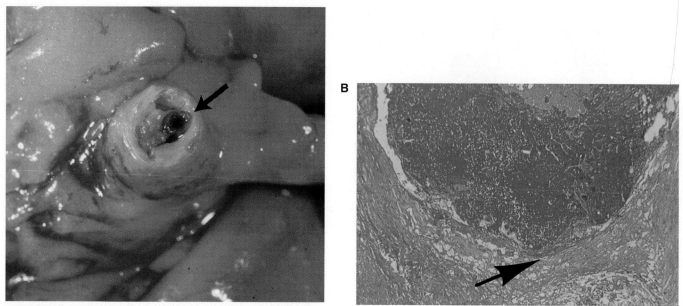

**Figure 10-30** **A,** Marked atherosclerosis of coronary artery with thrombus blocking artery (*arrow*). **B,** Photomicrograph illustrating thrombosis of coronary artery at the site of a ruptured unstable atheromatous plaque. Note absence of fibrous tissue covering the inner surface of the plaque compared with the appearance of the stable plaque illustrated in Figure 10-33. The clusters of pale cells are lipid-laden macrophages.

# Myocardial Infarction

A **myocardial infarct** is a necrosis of heart muscle resulting from severe ischemia. Muscle necrosis occurs when blood flow through one of the coronary arteries is insufficient to sustain the heart muscle and when collateral blood flow into the ischemic muscle from other coronary arteries is inadequate. The infarction is associated with severe chest pain and often with shock and collapse.

An infarct may involve the full thickness of the muscular wall or only part of the wall. A full-thickness infarct extending from endocardium to epicardium is called a transmural infarct (*trans* = across + *muris* = wall) and is usually the result of thrombosis of a major coronary artery. If only a part of the muscle in the wall undergoes necrosis, the term *subendocardial infarct* is often used.

## Location of Myocardial Infarcts

Myocardial infarcts involve the muscle of the left ventricle and septum almost exclusively. Only rarely are the walls of the atria or right ventricle involved. This is because the left ventricle is much more vulnerable to interruption of its blood supply than are other parts of the heart. The left ventricular wall is much thicker than the walls of the other chambers, and it works much harder because it must pump blood at high pressure into the systemic circulation. Consequently, it requires a very rich blood supply. In contrast, the other chambers have much thinner walls, pump blood under much lower pressures, need a less abundant blood supply, and can usually "get by" by means of collateral blood flow if a major coronary artery is blocked.

The size and location of myocardial infarcts are determined by both the location of the obstructions in the coronary arteries and the amount of collateral blood flow. Generally, an obstruction of the left anterior descending artery leads to an infarct of the anterior wall and often of the adjacent anterior part of the interventricular septum. If the circumflex artery is blocked, it is usually the lateral wall that is damaged. Occlusion of the right coronary artery generally causes an infarction of the back wall of the left ventricle and may also involve the adjacent posterior part of the interventricular septum. A block of the main left coronary artery, which fortunately is quite uncommon, causes an extensive infarction of both the anterior and the lateral walls of the left ventricle and is frequently fatal.

## Major Complications of Myocardial Infarcts

Patients who sustain a myocardial infarction are subject to a number of complications. The most important are:

1. Disturbances of cardiac rhythm (arrhythmias)
2. Heart failure
3. Intracardiac thrombi
4. Cardiac rupture

Complications are not inevitable, and prompt restoration of blood flow through the blocked artery can reduce the damage sustained by the heart muscle and improve the patient's prognosis.

**myocardial infarction** (mī-o-kar'dī-ul in-färk'shun) Necrosis of heart muscle as a result of interruption of its blood supply. May affect full thickness of muscle wall (*transmural infarct*) or only part of the wall (*subendocardial infarct*).

**Arrhythmias** Disturbances of cardiac rhythm are common subsequent to a myocardial infarct. The arrhythmias result from the extreme irritability of the ischemic heart muscle adjacent to the infarct and can frequently be controlled by drugs that reduce myocardial irritability. The most serious arrhythmia is ventricular fibrillation, which leads to cessation of the circulation. Another type of disturbance of cardiac rhythm occurs if the conduction system of the heart is damaged by the infarct. Conduction of impulses from the atria to the ventricles may be disturbed, which is called a **heart block**. The conduction disturbance may subside spontaneously as the infarct heals, but sometimes it is necessary to insert various types of electrodes directly into the heart in order to stimulate the ventricles to contract properly. A device of this type is called a cardiac pacemaker, which stimulates the ventricles at a predetermined rate and causes them to contract at a faster, more normal rate.

**Heart Failure** The ventricle may be so badly damaged that it is unable to maintain normal cardiac function, and the heart fails ( Figure 10-31 ). Heart failure may develop abruptly (acute heart failure) or more slowly (chronic heart failure), as described in a subsequent section, and may be difficult to treat.

**Intracardial Thrombi** If the infarct extends to involve the endocardium, thrombi may form on the interior of the ventricular wall and cover the damaged endocardial surface. This is called a mural thrombus ( Figure 10-32 ). Bits of the thrombus may break loose and be carried as emboli into the systemic circulation, causing infarctions in the brain, kidneys, spleen, or other organs. Some physicians attempt to forestall this complication by administering anticoagulants when a patient has sustained a severe infarction.

**Cardiac Rupture** If a patient sustains a transmural infarct, a perforation may occur through the necrotic muscle ( Figure 10-33 ). This permits blood to leak through the rupture into the pericardial sac, and as the blood accumulates, it compresses the heart so the ventricles cannot fill in diastole. The circulation ceases because the heart is no longer able to pump blood.

## Survival After Myocardial Infarction

The survival rate of patients who have had a myocardial infarct depends on many factors, the more important being (1) the size of the infarct, (2) the patient's age, (3) the development of complications, and (4) the presence of other diseases that would adversely affect the patient's survival. Mortality rates vary from about 6 percent in patients who have had small infarcts and who do not develop heart failure to more than

50 percent in patients with large infarcts who develop severe heart failure. Major causes of death after myocardial infarction are fatal arrhythmia, heart failure, and cardiac rupture. If we consider all hospitalized patients as a group, about 90 percent survive and are able to leave the hospital. The data on survival, however, relate only to patients with myocardial infarction who are admitted to the hospital. They do not include patients with severe heart attacks who die suddenly or within a few hours. This is a significant number of patients because it is estimated that one-third of all deaths from heart attacks occur outside the hospital. On the other hand, the survival data also do not include patients with small infarcts that may not be detected clinically. Many small myocardial infarcts cause relatively mild symptoms and heal without complications. The patients may ascribe the chest discomfort associated with the infarction to indigestion or other causes and never seek medical attention. Some studies indicate that as many as 25 percent of all patients with myocardial infarcts have very few symptoms and do not consult a physician.

> **heart block** Delay or complete interruption of impulse transmission from the atria to the ventricles.

## Diagnosis of Myocardial Infarction

Diagnosis of myocardial infarction rests on evaluation and interpretation of the medical history, physical examination, and laboratory data. The clinical history may at times be inconclusive because severe angina may be quite similar to the pain of a myocardial infarction. Conversely, many patients who develop small myocardial infarcts may have minimal symptoms. Physical examination will usually not be abnormal unless the subject exhibits evidence of shock or heart failure. Consequently, the physician must rely on specialized diagnostic studies to demonstrate infarction of heart muscle. The most helpful diagnostic aids are the electrocardiogram and determination of blood levels of various enzymes that leak from damaged heart muscle.

**The Electrocardiogram** The electrocardiogram (ECG), which measures the transmission of electrical impulses associated with cardiac contraction, reveals rather characteristic abnormalities when blood flow to heart muscle is inadequate, and when heart muscle becomes infarcted ( Figure 10-34 ). By means of the ECG the physician can often determine the location and approximate size of an infarct. The process of healing also can be followed by means of serial cardiograms. The ECG can also detect arrhythmias and various disturbances in the transmission of impulses through the cardiac conduction system.

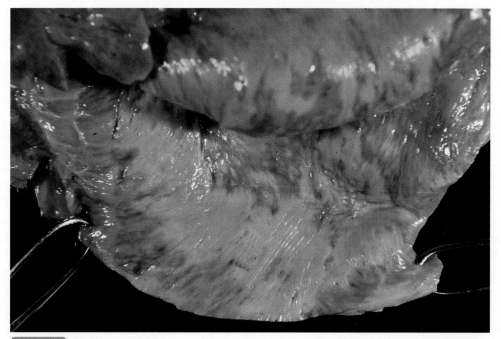

**Figure 10-31** Longitudinal section through infarcted heart muscle, illustrating the pale zone of necrotic muscle that has been infiltrated by inflammatory cells.

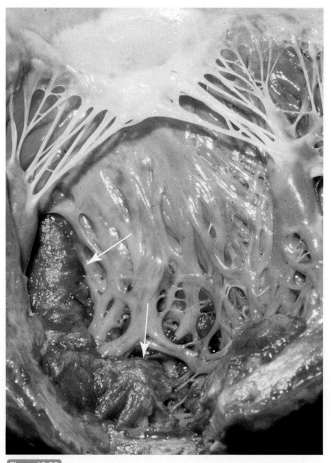

**Figure 10-32** Interior of left ventricle, illustrating mural thrombus (*arrows*) adherent to endocardium adjacent to myocardial infarct. Normal mitral valve leaflets and chordae are seen at *top* of photograph.

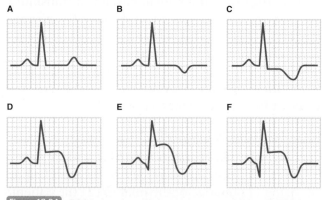

**Figure 10-33** Rupture of heart (*arrow*) through large transmural myocardial infarct.

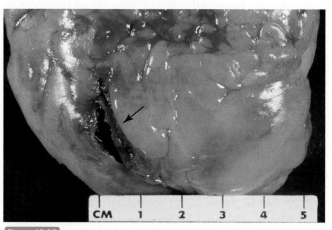

**Figure 10-34** ECG ischemia and infarction patterns. **A,** Normal ECG for comparison. **B,** Mild ischemia demonstrated by inverted T wave. **C,** Moderate ischemia demonstrated by slight ST-segment depression and inverted T wave. **D,** and **E,** ST-segment elevation myocardial infarction. **F,** ST-segment myocardial infarction with prominent Q wave indicating more severe myocardial damage. (Slightly modified from Garcia, T. B., and N. E. Holtz, 2003. *Introduction to 12-Lead ECG.* Sudbury, MA: Jones and Bartlett.)

## Blood Tests to Identify Cardiac Muscle Necrosis

Heart muscle is rich in enzymes that regulate the metabolic activities of the cells and also contains other important proteins concerned with muscle functions. These proteins include proteins concerned with muscle contraction called troponin T and troponin I, and an enzyme called creatine kinase (CK) that is found in cardiac muscle but in some other tissues as well. However, a laboratory test can identify the specific type (isoenzyme) of CK characteristic of heart muscle necrosis that is called CK–MB.

If heart muscle becomes infarcted, these components leak from the necrotic cells into the circulation. The two troponins found in cardiac muscle are not detectable in the blood of healthy normal persons. Even slight damage to heart muscle fibers causes blood levels of cardiac troponins to rise, beginning within a few hours after the muscle damage, peaking at about 24 hours, and remaining elevated for 10 to 14 days. Because troponin tests are so sensitive and specific, the tests can identify minor myocardial damage, which is not sufficient to cause a rise in creatine kinase. The creatine kinase isoenzyme test (CK–MB) is a very popular diagnostic test, which is less sensitive than the troponin tests and does not rise unless there has been significant myocardial damage. The enzyme level starts to rise within a few hours after a major myocardial infarct, reaches a peak in about 24 hours, and returns to normal within a few days.

In general, the larger the infarct, the longer it takes for the elevated enzyme levels to return to normal. The pattern of rapid rise followed by a fall over the succeeding several days is characteristic of a myocardial infarct. These tests help the clinician make a diagnosis of a myocardial infarct and assess the extent of myocardial damage.

## Evaluation and Treatment of Patients with Suspected Myocardial Infarction: The Acute Coronary Syndrome Classification

Patients with chest pain who are suspected of having acute symptoms related to coronary artery disease fall into three major groups that differ in their prognosis and treatment: (1) those with a major myocardial infarction, (2) those with minor myocardial damage, and (3) those with severe unstable angina. These patients are grouped together under the general category of **acute coronary syndromes**. The use of the troponin and CK–MB tests, in conjunction with the clinical assessment of the patient and the interpretation of the electrocardiogram, allows the physician to diagnose the nature of the patient's coronary disease, assess prognosis, and determine the appropriate treatment ( Table 10-3 ).

1. *ST-segment elevation myocardial infarction.* Complete obstruction of a major coronary artery by a thrombus leads to a large transmural infarction. The extensive myocardial injury causes a characteristic elevation of the ST segment in the ECG, and is also associated with marked elevation of cardiac muscle enzymes that leak from the damaged muscle and can be detected in the bloodstream by laboratory tests. This type of myocardial infarct usually is named after its characteristic ECG pattern as a *ST-segment elevation myocardial infarction*, which sometimes is called by its acronym STEMI.

   A ST elevation myocardial infarction is a medical emergency and it is essential to unblock the artery as soon as possible. The faster the blood flow can be restored through the blocked artery, the less severe the heart muscle damage and the better the prognosis. Treatment consists of either performing an angioplasty procedure to open the blocked artery or attempting to dissolve the clot with a clot-dissolving drug (thrombolytic therapy).

2. *Non-ST-segment elevation myocardial infarction.* Incomplete obstruction of a coronary artery causes less damage. The blood clot may not completely block the artery, or the atheromatous debris contained within a ruptured plaque may be extruded into the lumen and carried distally (downstream) to plug small arterioles and capillaries in the distribution of the ruptured plaque instead of completely occluding the artery. Some blood still flows to the damaged myocardium, which leads to a more favorable prognosis than a large transmural infarct. The ECG may show minor abnormalities but does not reveal the ST-segment elevation of a large infarct, and the rise of cardiac enzymes is less pronounced. The very sensitive troponin test result is elevated, but the less sensitive CK test result is normal. This type of myocardial injury is called a *non-ST elevation myocardial infarct* (non-STEMI). Treatment consists of antiplatelet and anticoagulant drugs to prevent further blockage of the artery. If these measures are unsuccessful, an angioplasty procedure may be required.

3. *Unstable angina without evidence of muscle necrosis.* Sometimes a patient with a history of stable angina begins to experience more severe chest pain, and it may be difficult clinically to determine whether the patient has unstable angina or is having a myocardial

**acute coronary syndrome** A general term for the three most serious manifestations of coronary artery disease: unstable angina, non-ST-segment elevation myocardial infarction, and ST-segment elevation myocardial infarction.

## Table 10-3 Acute Coronary Syndrome (ACS) Classification of Coronary Heart Disease

| Condition | ECG | Enzymes | Evaluation and Treatment |
|---|---|---|---|
| Unstable angina | ST depression during angina returns to normal when angina subsides | Not elevated | Treat angina. May progress to minor myocardial damage. Consider adding antiplatelet and anticoagulant drugs. Minimize cardiovascular risk factors. |
| Non-ST-segment elevation myocardial infarction | ST-segment depression | Troponin elevated. Creatine kinase not elevated. | Minor myocardial damage caused by atheromatous debris from ruptured coronary plaque blocking distal branches of artery, or artery partially blocked by thrombus. Treat with anticoagulant and antiplatelet drugs to keep artery open. Consider angioplasty (percutaneous coronary intervention) if anticoagulant–antiplatelet treatment is not successful. |
| ST-segment elevation myocardial infarction | ST-segment elevation | Troponin and creatine kinase both elevated. | Artery completely blocked. Identify site of block by arteriogram and open blocked coronary artery preferably by angioplasty (percutaneous coronary intervention) as quickly as possible to salvage as much cardiac muscle as possible. If facilities not available for angioplasty, attempt to dissolve clot by thrombolytic drugs. |

infarction. The ECG and enzyme tests will help make the distinction. The ECG may show minor abnormalities but does not show the ST elevation pattern of a large infarct, and cardiac enzyme tests indicating muscle necrosis are not elevated. These features favor the diagnosis of unstable angina without evidence of muscle necrosis. The patient requires treatment with anti-angina drugs, but also drugs to prevent aggregation of platelets that may initiate a coronary thrombosis.

## Restoring Blood Flow Through a Thrombosed Coronary Artery

There are two methods that can be used to restore blood flow through a thrombosed coronary artery. One method uses clot-dissolving drugs to dissolve the clot, which is called **thrombolytic therapy**. The second is an angioplasty procedure used to open the blocked artery and place a short expandable metal mesh tube (stent) at the site of the obstruction to keep the artery open, as was illustrated previously in Figure 10-28. When used to open a blocked coronary artery, the procedure is usually called **percutaneous coronary intervention** (often abbreviated PCI).

**Thrombolytic (Clot-Dissolving) Treatment** Dissolving the clot reestablishes the flow through the artery and salvages at least some of the heart muscle supplied by the blocked artery before the muscle becomes completely necrotic. The thrombus must be dissolved very soon after the vessel has become occluded and before the myocardium has sustained extensive and irreparable damage. Several different thrombolytic drugs are available that are administered intravenously. Excellent results are obtained, and mortality is reduced greatly if the clot can be dissolved within 1 hour after the patient experiences the first symptoms of a heart attack. The benefit of thrombolytic therapy decreases progressively as the time interval between coronary thrombosis and clot lysis lengthens. After about 6 hours, administration of a thrombolytic drug is of no benefit because by this time the heart muscle has progressed from ischemia to complete infarction, and it can no longer be salvaged by restoring blood flow through the occluded vessel.

Although thrombolytic therapy improves survival and salvages myocardium, it also tampers with the body's coagulation mechanisms, and treatment may be complicated by serious bleeding. Consequently, patients who are at greater than normal risk of hemorrhagic complications are not suitable candidates for thrombolytic therapy.

### Percutaneous Coronary Intervention (PCI)

In medical centers where facilities are available, many physicians favor restoring coronary blood flow by an angioplasty procedure to open a blocked coronary artery, which is the preferred method of treatment if the procedures can be performed promptly by an experienced physician (within 12 hours after onset of symptoms and within 90 minutes after the patient reaches the hospital or coronary care unit where PCI is to be performed). The procedure is quite similar to the angioplasty procedure used to dilate stenotic coronary arteries described previously and illustrated in Figure 10-28. A coronary angiogram determines the location of the blocked artery, and a guide wire is inserted through the thrombus and atheromatous material blocking the artery. Then a balloon catheter covered by a collapsed expandable stent is directed over the guide wire, and pushed through the clot and atheromatous debris obstructing blood flow through the artery. Then the balloon is inflated, which opens the artery and expands the stent to keep the artery open. Aspirin, heparin, and drugs that block platelet function are also given so that another thrombus will not form at the site of the reopened artery.

Although angioplasty is more successful than thrombolytic therapy for reestablishing blood flow through a blocked artery, the procedure may dislodge small bits of thrombus and atherosclerotic plaque debris from the arterial wall when the artery is opened, which is carried downstream to block small arterioles and capillaries. Consequently, blood flow to the heart muscle is reduced somewhat even though the flow through the artery has been restored. In order to avoid release of debris when opening a blocked artery some physicians prefer to first suction out the clot and then insert a stent without using a balloon to dilate the artery, which may provide better results.

### Subsequent Treatment of Myocardial Infarction

After as much myocardium as possible has been salvaged by restoring flow through the occluded artery, further treatment of myocardial infarction consists of bed rest initially, gradually progressing to limited activity, and then to full activity. Sometimes the injured heart is quite irritable and prone to abnormal rhythms. Therefore, various drugs are often given to decrease the irritability of the heart muscle. Development of heart block may require insertion of a cardiac pacemaker. The patient who has sustained a myocardial infarction may develop a thrombus within the ventricle at the site where the endocardium has been damaged by the infarct, or may develop thrombi in leg veins as a result of reduced activity. Therefore, some physicians also administer anticoagulant drugs to reduce the coagulability of the blood and thereby decrease the likelihood of thromboses and emboli. If the patient shows evidence of heart failure, various drugs are administered to sustain the failing heart.

Patients recovering from a myocardial infarct are at increased risk of sudden death from a fatal arrhythmia or another infarct, and the risk is greatest within the first 6 months after the infarct. Many physicians treat postinfarct patients for at least 2 years with drugs that reduce myocardial irritability (called betablockers) because this seems to reduce the incidence of these complications and improves survival. Ingesting a small amount of aspirin daily also is beneficial. Aspirin inhibits platelet function, making platelets less likely to adhere to roughened atheromatous plaques and initiate a thrombosis in the coronary artery.

**thrombolytic therapy** (throm-bo-lit′-tik) Intravenous administration of clot-dissolving drugs to dissolve a blood clot in an artery blocked by a thrombus in an attempt to reestablish blood flow through the artery.

**percutaneous coronary intervention** (per cue tāy′ne yus) An angioplasty procedure in which a balloon catheter covered by a stent is inserted into the site of a severely narrowed or blocked coronary artery, followed by expansion of the balloon, which enlarges the lumen of the artery and simultaneously expands the stent to keep the artery open.

# Case Studies

The following three cases illustrate some of the clinical features and complications of myocardial infarctions.

### Case Study 10-3

A 74-year-old man was admitted to the emergency room because of severe oppressive chest pain of about 5 hours' duration. For the previous 2 weeks, he had also experienced episodes of less severe chest pain when he walked rapidly, but the pain soon subsided when he rested.

Physical examination revealed an older man in no acute distress. Heart sounds were normal. Lungs were clear. Blood pressure was 190/110 (normal is about 120/80). Electrocardiogram showed the pattern of acute myocardial infarction involving the anterior wall of the left ventricle.

Laboratory studies obtained soon after admission revealed elevated levels of cardiac enzymes creatine kinase CK–MB). Repeat studies the following morning revealed a further elevation of these enzymes.

Despite intensive treatment, his blood pressure fell precipitously as a result of the severe myocardial damage, and the cardiac monitor recorded ventricular fibrillation. Resuscitative measures were unsuccessful.

An autopsy revealed severe arteriosclerosis of all coronary arteries. The left anterior descending coronary artery was occluded by a thrombus, and there was a large transmural anterior and lateral wall myocardial infarction complicated by rupture of the heart muscle. Blood filled the pericardial sac and compressed the heart so that the ventricles were unable to function.

## Case Study 10-4

A 57-year-old man was admitted to the hospital from his place of employment. While at work he complained of a sweaty feeling and then lost consciousness. When he regained consciousness, he noted a constant, oppressive, substernal pain. In the preceding month, he had experienced similar episodes of substernal pain that would last for several minutes and disappear spontaneously. The pain was associated with a feeling of numbness in the arms. The patient had sustained a myocardial infarction 2 years earlier.

Physical examination and blood pressure were normal. An electrocardiogram showed changes of acute myocardial infarction involving the anterior wall and interventricular septum.

Shortly after admission his blood pressure fell precipitously to shock levels caused by severe myocardial damage and could not be restored to normal. Soon afterward the cardiac monitor recorded ventricular fibrillation and resuscitative measures were unsuccessful, and the patient died.

The autopsy revealed old scarring in the posterior wall and the posterior portion of the interventricular septum in the distribution of the right coronary artery. There was a recent area of infarction in the anterior and lateral wall and in the anterior portion of the interventricular septum in the distribution of the anterior descending left coronary artery. The coronary arteries showed a variable degree of arteriosclerosis. The main left and circumflex arteries showed from 35 to 50 percent narrowing. The anterior descending left artery was 85 to 90 percent narrowed but was not occluded. The right coronary artery was occluded by old thrombus material that extended within the vessel for a distance of 7 to 8 centimeters. Lungs exhibited marked pulmonary edema.

## Case Study 10-5

A 52-year-old man experienced an episode of severe precordial pain associated with nausea and vomiting. He attributed this to indigestion and did not consult a physician. He remained at home on restricted activity but felt quite weak and experienced periodic episodes of sweating and chest pain. Eventually he was able to be up and about around the house and felt somewhat better. While eating supper 2 weeks later, he experienced a sudden onset of weakness in the right arm and difficulty with speech. When he attempted to get up from the table, his right leg did not support him and he fell to the floor.

On admission to the hospital, he exhibited a paralysis of the right side of the body. His blood pressure was elevated (210/110). The remainder of the physical examination was normal.

The electrocardiogram showed the pattern of a recent anterior-wall myocardial infarction. Serum cardiac enzyme studies on admission, at 24 hours, and at 48 hours, were all within normal limits because the myocardial infarct had occurred 2 weeks earlier. The elevated levels of enzyme activity had returned to normal by the time the patient entered the hospital.

The patient's disorder was treated as a recent myocardial infarction. A mural thrombus had apparently formed in the left ventricle at the site of the infarct. A piece of the clot had broken loose and had been carried as an embolus to the brain, where it had obstructed a cerebral artery and caused the paralysis. He made a satisfactory recovery but was left with some residual weakness and speech difficulty.

# Taking Aspirin to Reduce the Risk of Cardiovascular Disease

Aspirin is now widely used in clinical medicine to reduce the risk of heart attacks and strokes. Aspirin works by interfering with platelet function (Chapter 9). Aspirin permanently inactivates (acetylates) a platelet enzyme needed to produce a chemical compound called thromboxane A2 that is released by platelets when they adhere to a roughened surface, which causes platelets to clump together and start the clotting process. Blocking platelet function by taking aspirin reduces the likelihood that platelets will adhere to the roughened surface of an atherosclerotic plaque in a coronary or cerebral artery and cause a blood clot to plug the artery.

Aspirin is rapidly absorbed from the stomach and small intestine. Peak levels are obtained in the blood within about 20 minutes after aspirin is ingested, and some inhibition of platelet function can be detected within an hour after the drug is taken. As little as 30 mg per day (less than one-half a baby aspirin) inactivates thromboxane A2 production, which persists for the entire 10-day life span of the platelets. Because about 10 percent of the circulating platelets are replaced every 24 hours, after about 10 days almost no functionally normal platelets are present in the circulation.

Although taking aspirin to inactivate platelet function reduces the risk of cardiovascular disease as well

as strokes caused by blood clots in cerebral blood vessels, aspirin use to reduce the risk of heart attacks slightly increases the risk of bleeding in the brain if the person does have a stroke.

# Cocaine-Induced Arrhythmias and Myocardial Infarcts

Cocaine has very powerful effects on the cardiovascular system, and as the recreational use of cocaine has increased in recent years, so has the number of cocaine-related cardiac deaths. The drug prolongs and intensifies the effects of sympathetic nerve impulses that regulate the heart and blood vessels. As a result, the heart beats faster and more forcefully, thereby increasing myocardial oxygen requirements. The heart muscle becomes more irritable, which predisposes to arrhythmias, and the peripheral arterioles constrict, which raises the blood pressure. Cocaine also constricts the coronary arteries and may induce coronary artery spasm, which leads to severe myocardial ischemia and may be followed by a myocardial infarction. Cocaine-related fatal arrhythmias and myocardial infarcts may occur in persons with normal coronary arteries, and cocaine users who already have some degree of coronary atherosclerosis are at even greater risk.

# Blood Lipids and Coronary Artery Disease

The level of lipids in the blood has been shown to be an important factor in the pathogenesis of coronary atherosclerosis. The lipids of clinical importance are neutral fat (triglyceride) and cholesterol.

## Neutral Fat

Chemically, fat is composed of three molecules of fatty acid combined with one molecule of glycerol. Glycerol is a three-carbon alcohol containing a hydroxyl group (OH) attached to each carbon atom. A fatty acid is a long, straight-chain carbon compound containing a terminal carboxyl group (COOH); this constitutes the acid group of organic molecules. The carboxyl groups of the fatty acids are linked to the hydroxyl groups of glycerol, with loss of a molecule of water, in a linkage called an ester ( Figure 10-35A ).

A neutral fat may be classified as saturated or unsaturated. In a saturated fat each carbon atom in the chain

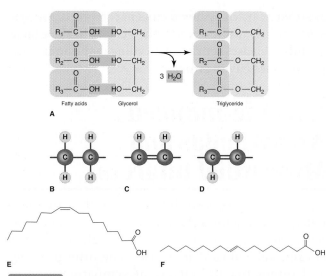

**Figure 10-35** **A,** Structure of a triglyceride composed of three long fatty acid molecules ($R_1$, $R_2$, and $R_3$) each containing 16 to 18 carbon atoms. The carboxyl groups of the fatty acids are joined to glycerol with loss of water molecules to form the triglyceride. **B,** Single bonds join carbon atoms in the triglyceride molecules of a saturated fat. **C,** Double bond in an unsaturated fat in which the hydrogen atoms are on the same side of the chain (cis configuration). **D,** Double bond in an unsaturated fat in which the hydrogen atoms are on opposite sides of the chain (trans configuration). **E,** Representation of the bent fatty acid chain at the site of a cis position double bond. **F,** Representation of the straight fatty acid chain structure caused by the trans-position double bond, which is similar to the chains in a saturated fat.

is joined to the two adjacent carbon atoms, each by a single covalent bond ( Figure 10-35B ). The three fatty acids form long, straight, symmetrical molecules packed closely together parallel to one another. The configuration gives rise to a relatively dense compact molecule. Most animal fats are saturated fats. Most vegetable oils and fats found in fish and poultry are unsaturated fats in which at least one of the fatty acids in the molecule has a double bond between two adjacent carbon atoms and each of the two carbon atoms flanking the double bond has only a single attached hydrogen atom. Each hydrogen atom adjacent to the double bond is attached on the same side of the carbon chain, which is called a cis configuration ( Figure 10-35C ). This arrangement unbalances the chain and causes the chain to bend sharply at the double bond, which requires the chain to occupy more space in the triglyceride molecule ( Figure 10-35E ). In contrast, a trans fat is an unsaturated fat in which the hydrogen atoms flanking the double bond are on opposite sides of the chain, which is called a trans configuration and causes the carbon chain to maintain a more straight-line configuration similar to that of a saturated fat ( Figure 10-35D and Figure 10-35F ). Almost all trans fats are produced artificially by partial hydrogenation of vegetable oils (cis configuration), which converts them to straight-chain trans-configuration molecules. As a result the fatty acid molecules now resemble those of a saturated fat,

and are changed from an oil to a semisolid fat. We know now that trans fats are "bad fats" because of their harmful effects on blood lipids. They are much more atherogenic (promoting atherosclerosis) than saturated fats and should be avoided as much as possible in our diets.

High levels of fat (along with cholesterol) in the blood promote atherosclerosis. Carbohydrate is converted readily into fat in the body, and much of the blood triglyceride is derived not from ingested fat but from ingested carbohydrate. In clinical medicine, most examples of high blood triglycerides can be traced to diets excessively high in carbohydrate. Sugar has been found to be more potent in elevating blood triglycerides than the more complex carbohydrates derived from cereals and other starches.

## Cholesterol

Cholesterol is a complex carbon compound containing several ring structures and is classified as a sterol. Most cholesterol is present in the body in combination with fatty acids as cholesterol esters. Cholesterol is synthesized in the body and is also present in many foods. Normally, cholesterol is also excreted in the bile into the gastrointestinal tract.

Much evidence indicates that a high dietary intake of cholesterol leads to high levels of blood cholesterol and premature atherosclerosis. The level of blood cholesterol is influenced not only by the amount of cholesterol in the diet, but also by the type of dietary fat. Saturated fats, the type found in meats and dairy products, tend to raise blood cholesterol, whereas unsaturated fats, which are found in fish, poultry, and most vegetable oils, tend to lower blood cholesterol. Cholesterol and saturated fat are found together in many foods. In general, foods high in cholesterol also have a high content of saturated fats, whereas foods low in cholesterol contain unsaturated fats rather than saturated fats.

## Transport of Cholesterol by Lipoproteins

Cholesterol is carried in the blood plasma combined with proteins and other lipids as complexes called lipoproteins. There are two different cholesterol-carrying lipoproteins. They have different functions and are classified by their weight (density) into low-density lipoprotein (LDL) and high-density lipoprotein (HDL). About 80 percent of the circulating cholesterol is carried bound to LDL, and the remaining 20 percent is transported by HDL.

The function of LDL is to transport cholesterol from the bloodstream into the cells, whereas the HDL apparently removes cholesterol from the cells and carries it

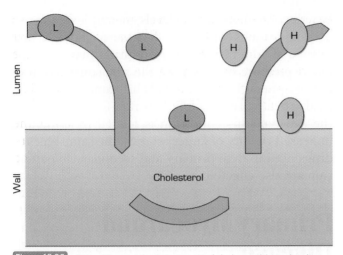

**Figure 10-36** Role of lipoproteins in transport of cholesterol. Low-density lipoprotein (L) promotes atherosclerosis by transporting cholesterol into arterial wall. High-density lipoprotein (H) protects against atherosclerosis by transporting cholesterol to liver for excretion.

to the liver for excretion in the bile. High-density lipoprotein may also "tie up" cholesterol so that it cannot infiltrate the arterial wall (Figure 10-36). This has led to the concept that there is "bad cholesterol" and "good cholesterol." The "bad cholesterol" is the fraction bound to LDL, which can infiltrate the arterial wall and is correlated with atherosclerosis. The "good cholesterol" is the cholesterol fraction carried attached to HDL, and elevations of this cholesterol fraction actually protect against coronary heart disease. Several factors are known to raise HDL cholesterol and thereby reduce risk of coronary heart disease. These factors include regular exercise, cessation of cigarette smoking, and (surprisingly) a modest regular intake of alcoholic beverages.

## Alteration of Blood Lipids by Change in Diet

Various studies have demonstrated that the levels of both cholesterol and triglycerides in the blood can be lowered by dietary change. These studies have also demonstrated that individuals maintained on a modified diet have a lower incidence of coronary artery disease than a comparable group subsisting on an average American diet. The diet (often called an "anticoronary" diet) is modified by decreasing the amount of cholesterol and saturated fat and substituting foods containing polyunsaturated fats. This involves restricting the intake of animal fat and substituting fish and poultry. Carbohydrates are derived primarily from starches and cereals. The consumption of sugar and foods rich in sugar (pies, cakes, candies) is reduced. Alcohol consumption is restricted but not forbidden because of its favorable effect on HDL levels, which seems to protect against coronary heart disease. Modifying the typical American diet is difficult because it requires breaking

old dietary habits. However, some change in diet is desirable because it will significantly reduce the incidence of coronary artery disease. An "anti-coronary" diet is essential for individuals who have high levels of blood lipids because they run a greatly increased risk of death or disability from coronary artery disease.

It should be emphasized that the factors influencing the development of atherosclerosis are complex; an elevated level of blood lipids is only one of many factors concerned with atherogenesis. A number of other conditions, among them obesity, hypertension, cigarette smoking, and genetic factors, also predispose individuals to atherosclerosis.

# Hypertension and Hypertensive Cardiovascular Disease

## Primary Hypertension

The ideal normal blood pressure should be below 120/80. A pressure higher than 140/90 is called **hypertension**, and the higher the pressure, the greater are its harmful effects. Most cases of hypertension result from excessive vasoconstriction of the small arterioles throughout the body, which raises the diastolic pressure. Because of the high peripheral resistance, the heart needs to pump more forcefully in order to overcome the resistance created by the constricted arterioles and supply adequate blood to the tissues, which leads to a compensatory rise in systolic blood pressure. We don't really understand all of the factors responsible for this condition, which is called primary hypertension or essential hypertension, but we know that severe hypertension exerts injurious effects not only on the heart, but also on the blood vessels and kidneys.

**hypertension**
High blood pressure.

**Cardiac Effects** The heart responds to the increased workload resulting from the high peripheral resistance by becoming enlarged. Although the enlarged heart may be able to function effectively for many years, the cardiac pump is being forced to work beyond its "rated capacity." Eventually, the heart can no longer maintain adequate blood flow, and the patient develops symptoms of cardiac failure.

**Vascular Effects** Because the blood vessels are not designed to carry blood at such a high pressure, the vessels wear out prematurely. Hypertension accelerates the development of atherosclerosis in the larger arteries.

The arterioles also are injured; they thicken and undergo degenerative changes, and their lumens become narrowed. This process is termed **arteriolosclerosis**. Sometimes the walls of the small arterioles become completely necrotic owing to the effects of the sustained high blood pressure. Weakened arterioles may rupture, leading to hemorrhage. The brain is particularly vulnerable, and a cerebral hemorrhage is a relatively common complication of severe hypertension.

**Renal Effects**   The narrowing of the renal arterioles decreases the blood supply to the kidneys, which, in turn, leads to injury and degenerative changes in the glomeruli and renal tubules. Severe hypertension may cause severe derangement of renal function and eventually leads to renal failure.

## Secondary Hypertension

In a small proportion of patients, the hypertension results from a known disease or condition such as chronic kidney disease (Chapter 15), endocrine gland dysfunction such as a pituitary or an adrenal tumor, or a hyperactive thyroid gland (Chapter 20). The high blood pressure associated with these conditions is called secondary hypertension because the cause of the hypertension is known. In many cases, successful treatment of the underlying condition cures the hypertension.

## Isolated Systolic Hypertension

As the name implies, isolated systolic hypertension is characterized by a mild to moderately elevated systolic pressure with a normal or even lower than normal diastolic pressure. This condition occurs primarily in older adults because the aorta and major arteries become less flexible with age. Consequently, when blood is ejected into the aorta during ventricular systole, the more rigid arteries are less able to stretch and absorb some of the force of the ejected blood. As a result, the systolic pressure is higher than it would be if the vessels were more flexible. The diastolic pressure remains normal because there is no excessive arteriolar vasoconstriction. Previously this condition was considered to be less serious than hypertension in which both pressures were higher than normal, but unfortunately, more recent studies have demonstrated that isolated systolic hypertension causes the same harmful effects on the heart and blood vessels as primary and secondary hypertension.

**arteriolosclerosis**
(är-tēr-ē-ólo-skler-ō′-sis)
One type of arteriosclerosis characterized by thickening and degeneration of small arterioles.

## Treatment of Hypertension

Although the reason for the hypertension cannot be determined in most instances, the blood pressure can be reduced to more normal levels, thereby lowering risk of complications of high blood pressure. This is accomplished by administering various drugs that lower the blood pressure by lessening the vasoconstriction of the peripheral blood vessels. This same approach is used to treat isolated systolic hypertension. Even though the cause of this condition is related to aging and increased rigidity of larger arteries, the same types of drugs used to treat primary and secondary hypertension are also effective.

# Primary Myocardial Disease

In a small number of patients, heart disease results not from valvular or coronary disease, or hypertension, but from primary disease of the heart muscle itself. There are two major types of primary myocardial disease. One type results from inflammation of heart muscle and is called myocarditis. The second type, in which there is no evidence of inflammation, is designated by the noncommittal term *cardiomyopathy* (*cardio* = heart + *myo* = muscle + pathy = disease).

## Myocarditis

Myocarditis is characterized by an active inflammation in the heart muscle associated with injury and necrosis of individual muscle fibers. In the United States, most cases are caused by viruses. A few are caused by parasites, such as *Trichinella* (Chapter 5), that lodge in the myocardium and cause an inflammation. Occasionally other pathogens such as *Histoplasma* are responsible, especially in immunocompromised patients. Some cases are the result of a hypersensitivity reaction, such as the myocarditis occurring in acute rheumatic fever.

The onset of myocarditis is usually abrupt and may lead to acute heart failure. Fortunately, in most cases, the inflammation subsides completely and the patient recovers without any permanent heart damage. There is no specific treatment other than treating the underlying condition that caused the myocarditis and decreasing cardiac work by bed rest and limited activity while the inflammation subsides.

## Cardiomyopathy

The general term *cardiomyopathy* encompasses two different conditions: dilated cardiomyopathy and hypertrophic cardiomyopathy. Dilated cardiomyopathy is characterized by enlargement of the heart and dilatation of its chambers. The pumping action of the ventricles is greatly impaired, which leads to chronic heart failure. Its cause is uncertain, and there is no specific treatment.

Hypertrophic cardiomyopathy is hereditary and transmitted as a dominant trait. The condition is characterized by disarray of muscle fibers that intersect at odd angles with no apparent organized pattern and marked hypertrophy of heart muscle to such an extent that the thick-walled chambers become greatly reduced in size and do not dilate readily in diastole. Frequently, the muscle of the septum is hypertrophied to a greater extent than the rest of the myocardium and hinders outflow of the blood from the ventricle into the aorta. At times, the thick septum may actually impinge on the anterior mitral valve leaflet, intermittently completely blocking the outflow of blood from the left ventricle ( Figure 10-37 ). This type of cardiomyopathy is often called idiopathic hypertrophic subaortic stenosis, usually abbreviated IHSS. The term indicates that the obstruction (stenosis) is located below the aortic valve (subaortic), resulting from myocardial hypertrophy (hypertrophic) of unknown cause (idiopathic).

Patients with IHSS frequently exhibit manifestations related to inadequate cardiac output, such as episodes of excessive fatigue and lightheadedness related to exertion. The characteristic myocardial hypertrophy with greatly thickened septum can be identified by echocardiography (Chapter 1). Treatment consists of administering drugs that slow the heart (allowing more time for ventricular filling) and reduce the force of ventricular contraction (which tends to reduce the degree of obstruction caused by the hypertrophied septum).

# Heart Failure

Heart failure exists whenever the heart is no longer able to pump adequate amounts of blood to the tissues. It may result from any type of heart disease. Rapid failing of the heart, as when a large portion of muscle undergoes infarction, is called acute heart failure. In most cases, however, cardiac failure develops slowly and insidiously; this is called chronic heart failure. Because the most prominent feature in chronic heart failure is congestion of the tissues as a result of engorgement by blood, the physician often uses the term *congestive heart failure* when referring to chronic heart failure and its attendant clinical manifestations. Although the term indicates that the heart is failing, it does not necessarily indicate a severe life-threatening condition. Although chronic heart failure is a slowly progressing condition, many patients respond well to effective treatment and can live comfortably in reasonably good health for many years.

## Pathophysiology and Treatment of Heart Failure

Sometimes the terms *forward failure* and *backward failure* are used to describe the mechanisms leading to the development of heart failure. In forward failure, the

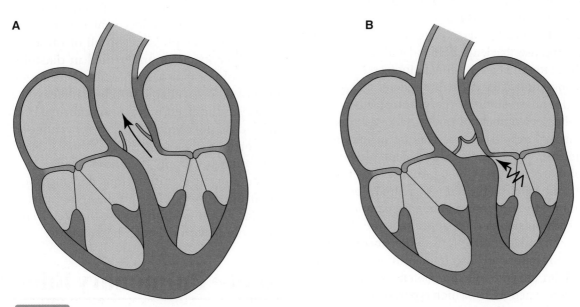

Figure 10-37   A comparison of normal cardiac function with malfunction characteristic of hypertrophic cardiomyopathy. **A,** Normal heart, illustrating unobstructed flow of blood from left ventricle into aorta during ventricular systole. **B,** Hypertrophic cardiomyopathy, illustrating obstruction to outflow of blood from left ventricle by hypertrophied septum, which impinges on anterior leaflet of mitral valve.

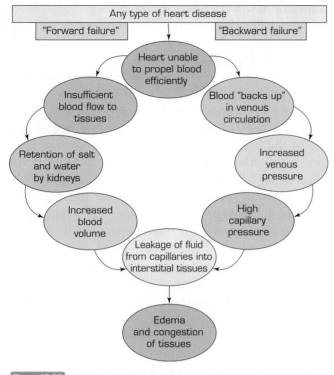

**Figure 10-38** Mechanisms in the pathogenesis of congestive heart failure.

initial effect of inadequate cardiac output is considered to be insufficient blood flow to the tissues. The inadequate renal blood flow results in retention of salt and water by the kidneys. (This effect is mediated indirectly through the adrenal glands.) Fluid retention, in turn, leads to an increased blood volume, and this is soon followed by a rise in venous pressure. The high venous pressure and high capillary pressure cause excessive transudation of fluid from the capillaries, leading to edema of the tissues.

In backward failure, the inadequate output of blood is considered to cause "back up" of blood within the veins draining back to the heart, leading to increased venous pressure, congestion of the viscera, and edema. Figure 10-38 illustrates the interrelation of the various factors concerned in the development of cardiac failure. Probably both forward failure and backward failure are present to some degree in every patient with heart failure. Treatment consists of diuretic drugs, which promote excretion of excess salt and water by the kidneys, thereby lowering blood volume. In addition, digitalis preparations are sometimes administered. They act to increase the efficiency of ventricular contractions. Other medications called ACE inhibitors are also frequently used. These drugs block an enzyme called angiotensin-converting enzyme (abbreviated ACE), which is part of a renal regulatory mechanism called the renin–angiotensin-aldosterone system (Chapter 15) that promotes retention of salt and water by the kidneys and raises blood pressure.

Both of these effects are undesirable in heart failure patients, and blocking this mechanism by an ACE inhibitor has been shown to improve survival of patients in congestive heart failure.

## Comparison of Systolic and Diastolic Dysfunction in Heart Failure

The efficiency of ventricular function in heart failure patients can be measured, which allows the physician to determine whether the heart failure results primarily from inadequate ejection of blood from the ventricles in systole or from inadequate filling of the ventricles in diastole. In most patients with heart failure, the failing ventricles are distended with blood but are unable to expel a normal volume of blood during systole. Consequently, the left ventricular ejection fraction is significantly reduced and may fall from a normal value of about 60 percent to as low as 20 percent. The failing heart is not able to eject sufficient blood from the ventricle during systole, and this condition is called systolic heart failure.

In contrast, the main problem in some heart failure patients is not with the impaired ejection of blood in systole but with inadequate filling of the ventricles during diastole. This condition is called diastolic heart failure. The condition may occur in persons with marked hypertension in whom the thick hypertrophied left ventricular wall can't relax enough in diastole to allow the left ventricular chamber to expand normally. Consequently, less blood can flow into the ventricle and the pressure of the blood within the ventricle is elevated. Some other less common conditions in which the ventricles are unable to relax normally in diastole may also reduce ventricular filling and raise intraventricular pressure. In all of these conditions, the left ventricle is underfilled in diastole, and the stroke volume is also low because there is a smaller volume of blood available in the chamber to be ejected. However, the ejection fraction is normal because both the end-diastolic volume and stroke volume are reduced proportionately. Nevertheless, the cardiac output is inadequate to supply the body's needs.

The clinical manifestations and methods of treatment of both systolic and diastolic heart failure are similar, although diuretics are the preferred treatment for patients with diastolic heart failure.

# Acute Pulmonary Edema

Acute pulmonary edema is a manifestation of acute heart failure and is a very serious life-threatening condition. It is caused by a temporary disproportion in the output of blood from the ventricles. If the output of blood from the left ventricle is temporarily reduced more than the output from the right ventricle, the "right heart" will pump blood into the lungs faster than the "left heart" can deliver the blood to the peripheral tissues. This rapidly engorges the lungs with blood and raises the pulmonary capillary pressure, which leads to outflow of fluid into the pulmonary alveoli. The patient becomes extremely short of breath because fluid accumulates within the alveoli, and oxygenation of the blood circulating through the lungs is impaired. The edema fluid becomes mixed with inspired air, forming a frothy mixture that "overflows" into the bronchi and trachea, filling the patient's upper-respiratory passages.

Treatment consists of supplementary oxygen to get more oxygen into the edematous pulmonary alveoli, intravenous diuretics and other medications to improve cardiac function by reducing circulating blood volume, morphine to relieve anxiety, and measures directed toward correcting the underlying condition that precipitated the acute heart failure.

# Aneurysms

An **aneurysm** is a dilatation of the wall of an artery or an outpouching of a portion of the wall. Most aneurysms are acquired as a result of arteriosclerosis, which causes weakening of the vessel wall. One type of aneurysm involving the cerebral arteries is the result of a congenital abnormality of the vessel wall and is considered in conjunction with the nervous system (Chapter 21).

> **aneurysm**
> (an′ūr-izm) A dilatation of a structure, such as the aorta, a cerebral artery, or a part of the ventricular wall.

## Arteriosclerotic Aneurysm

A small artery that undergoes arteriosclerotic change becomes narrowed and may eventually become thrombosed. A large artery such as the aorta has a diameter so large that complete obstruction is uncommon. However, atheromatous deposits tend to damage the wall of the aorta, reducing its elasticity and weakening the wall (Figure 10-39). The aortic wall tends to balloon out under the stress of the high pressure within the vessel. Aortic aneurysms usually develop in the distal part of the abdominal aorta, where the pressure is highest and the atheromatous change is most severe (Figure 10-40 and Figure 10-41). Usually the interior of the aneurysm becomes covered with a layer of thrombus material, and the wall often becomes partially calcified.

As the name implies, arteriosclerosis is the major cause of arteriosclerotic aneurysms, but there appears to be some genetic predisposition as well, as 15 to 20 percent of patients with an aneurysm also have another affected family member. An aortic aneurysm usually enlarges slowly and does not produce symptoms initially. Because a small aneurysm is difficult to detect by physical examination, current guidelines recommend a routine ultrasound screening examination to identify an asymptomatic aneurysm in any adult over

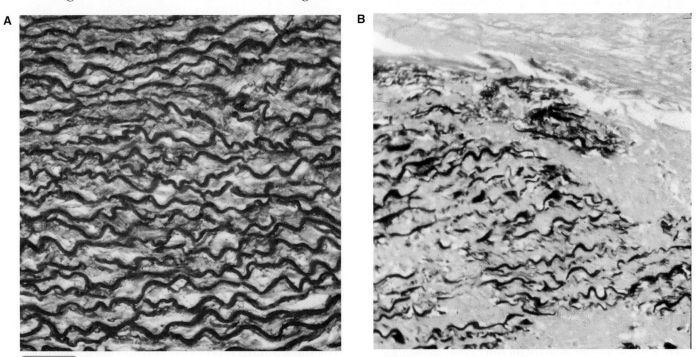

**A**

**B**

Figure 10-39   **A,** Photomicrograph of normal aortic wall stained for elastic tissue. Elastic fibers appear as dark wavy bands. **B,** Aortic wall from a patient with severe aortic atherosclerosis, illustrating marked fragmentation and destruction of elastic fibers, which weakens wall and predisposes to aneurysm (original magnification × 400).

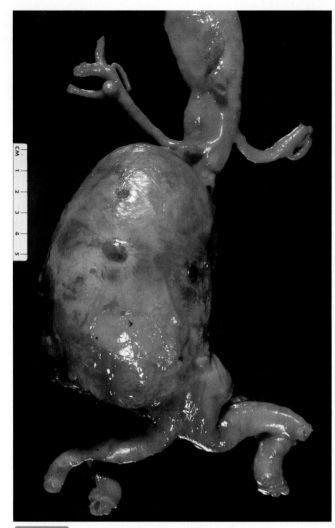

Figure 10-40 Large arteriosclerotic aneurysm extending from renal arteries (*above*) to iliac arteries (*below*).

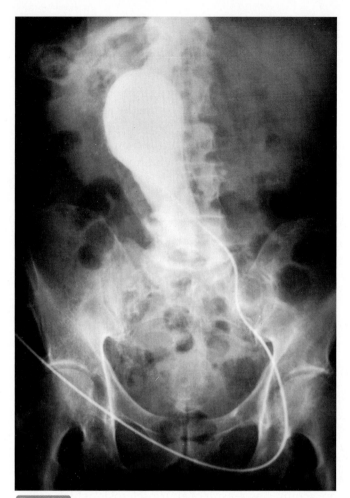

Figure 10-41 Aortic aneurysm demonstrated on x-ray by injection of contrast material into aorta.

age 65 who has risk factors that predispose to arteriosclerosis or who has a family history of an aortic aneurysm.

Aortic aneurysms are dangerous because they may rupture, leading to massive and often fatal hemorrhage. The normal cross-section diameter of the abdominal aorta is about 2 centimeters. An aneurysm exceeding about 5 centimeters in diameter may rupture and should be repaired. In general, the larger the aneurysm, the greater the likelihood of rupture ( Figure 10-42 ).

The standard open surgical aneurysm repair procedure consists of opening the aneurysm and sewing a nylon or Dacron graft into the aorta above and below the aneurysmal segment so that the blood flowing through the aorta flows through the graft rather than through the aneurysm ( Figure 10-43 ). It is not necessary to excise the aneurysm that has been bypassed by the graft, and usually the walls of the aneurysm are wrapped around the graft. This procedure is a well-established, reliable, and highly successful method of treatment, but

it is a major surgical procedure and poses some risks to older patients who may have coronary artery disease and other medical problems.

In selected patients, an alternative method of treatment is available called endovascular aneurysm repair (*endo* = within + *vascular* = blood vessel). Two small incisions are made in the groins to expose the femoral arteries. A specially designed stent graft is inserted through the femoral arteries using specially designed equipment to place the graft within the aneurysm under x-ray guidance. Then a balloon expands the stent graft, which has hooks or similar attachment devices to fix the graft to the aorta proximally, and to the aorta or iliac arteries distally ( Figure 10-44 ). When properly fixed in position, blood flows through the graft instead of through the aneurysm.

## Dissecting Aneurysm of the Aorta

The thick middle layer of the aorta is called the media. It is composed of multiple layers of elastic tissue and muscle bonded together by fibrous connective tissue.

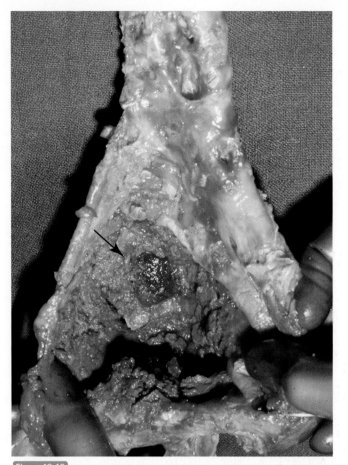

Figure 10-42 Interior of arteriosclerotic aneurysm, illustrating marked degenerative change in wall. Extremely thin area in wall (*arrow*) predisposes to rupture.

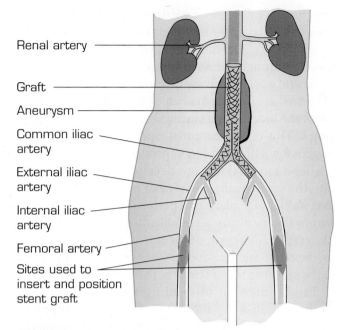

Renal artery

Graft

Aneurysm

Common iliac artery

External iliac artery

Internal iliac artery

Femoral artery

Sites used to insert and position stent graft

Figure 10-44 Endovascular graft to treat abdominal aortic aneurysm. The graft expands within the aorta, and the stent attachments fix graft to aorta proximally and iliac arteries distally.

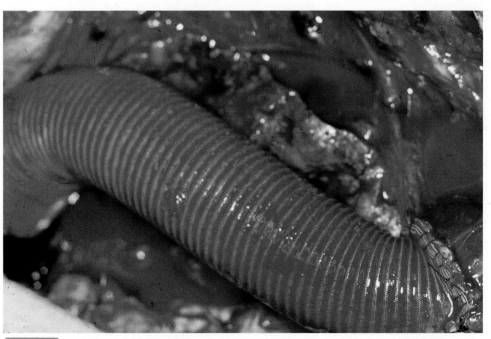

Figure 10-43 Repair of aortic aneurysm by means of tubular Dacron graft.

Degenerative changes sometimes occur in the media, causing the layers to lose their cohesiveness and separate ( Figure 10-45 ). Then the pulsatile force of the blood flowing through the aorta may cause the inner half of the aortic wall to pull away from the outer half in the region where the media has degenerated, and sometimes the inner lining (intima) tears as the media separates. This complication is especially likely to occur in persons with high blood pressure.

After an intimal tear has developed, blood is forced into the aortic wall. The area of medial degeneration forms a cleavage plane that permits the blood to dissect within the media for a variable distance. This event, **a dissecting aneurysm of the aorta**, is associated with severe chest and back pain. The term *dissecting* refers to the splitting (dissection) of the media by the blood, and the somewhat misleading term *aneurysm* was applied because the affected part of the aorta appears wider than normal. The widening results from the hemorrhage within the aortic wall, but the lumen of the aorta is not dilated.

The intimal tear that starts the dissection is usually either in the ascending aorta just above the aortic valve or in the descending aorta just beyond the origin of the large arteries that arise from the aortic arch ( Figure 10-46 ). If the tear is in the ascending aorta, the blood often

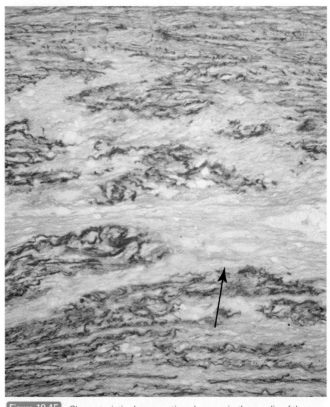

**Figure 10-45** Characteristic degenerative changes in the media of the aortic wall (called cystic medial necrosis) illustrated in the *center* of the photograph (*arrow*), which leads to loss of cohesion between the inner and outer layers of the aortic wall and predisposes to aortic dissection.

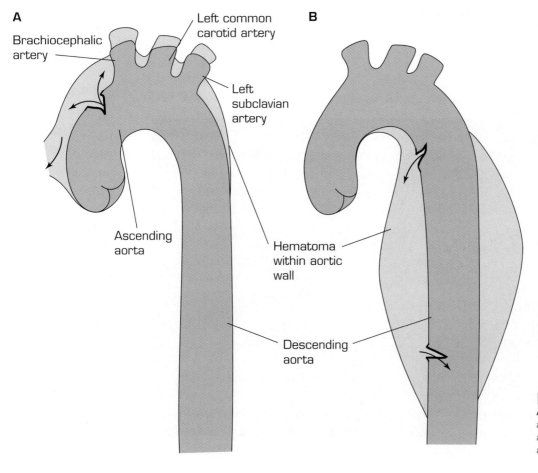

**A**

Brachiocephalic artery

Left common carotid artery

Left subclavian artery

Ascending aorta

**B**

Hematoma within aortic wall

Descending aorta

**Figure 10-46** Sites of aortic dissection. A, Tear in ascending aorta causes both proximal and distal dissection. B, Tear in descending aorta may cause extensive distal dissection and may rupture back into lumen of aorta.

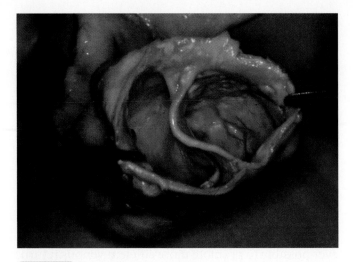

**Figure 10-47** Cross section of aorta illustrating two channels ("double-barreled aorta") caused by dissecting aneurysm. The channel on the *right* of the photograph is true lumen of aorta. The channel on the *left* is the channel in the aortic wall created by the dissection.

dissects proximally as well as distally within the aortic wall, extending into the base of the aorta where the aortic valve attaches and the coronary arteries arise. The dissection may separate the aortic valve from its attachment to the deeper aortic wall so that it no longer functions properly, and severe aortic regurgitation develops. The origins of the coronary arteries may also be compressed by the hemorrhage in the wall, which compromises the blood supply to the heart muscle. A dissection in the ascending aorta is often fatal because the blood frequently ruptures through the outer wall of the aorta at the base of the heart, leading to extensive hemorrhage into the mediastinum or pericardial sac.

If the intimal tear is in the descending aorta, the blood dissects distally and may extend the entire length of the aorta. The blood in the aortic wall may also compress the origins of the large arteries that arise from the aorta, leading to impairment of blood flow to the kidneys, the intestines, or other vital organs. Sometimes the dissection may rupture back into the lumen of the aorta. If this occurs, blood flows not only through the lumen of the aorta, but also through the channel in the aortic wall created by the dissection, which communicates with the lumen of the aorta both proximally and distally ( Figure 10-47 ). Various surgical procedures have been devised to correct this condition.

# Diseases of the Veins

The main diseases of veins are (1) venous thrombosis, (2) inflammation of veins, and (3) excessive dilatation and tortuosity of veins.

Venous thromboses occur most commonly in leg veins, but sometimes clots form within veins elsewhere in the body. Inflammation of a vein is called phlebitis (*phleb* = vein + *itis* = inflammation). If there is an associated thrombosis of the affected vein, the term *thrombophlebitis* is used. Dilated tortuous veins are called varices or varicose veins. (*Varix* is a Latin word meaning dilated vessel; the plural term is *varices*.) Varicosities occur most often in leg veins but may occur in other veins as well.

## Venous Thrombosis and Thrombophlebitis

Thrombus formation in deep leg veins is a frequent problem in postoperative patients and in those confined to bed, and it may be complicated by a pulmonary embolism, as described in Chapter 9. The risk of leg vein thromboses in susceptible patients can be minimized by encouraging active leg exercises to improve venous blood flow and prevent venous stasis, and by early ambulation.

Venous thrombosis and thrombophlebitis are treated by elevation of the leg, heat, and anticoagulant drugs. The anticoagulant stops the progression of the intravascular clotting process while the body's normal protective mechanisms remove the clot. The clot is dissolved by activation of the fibrinolytic mechanism and by ingrowth of connective tissue from the vein wall at the site where the clot adheres to the vein wall. Damage to the vein wall and its valves after thrombophlebitis may disturb venous return and predispose to later development of varicose veins.

## Varicose Veins of the Lower Extremities

Two main groups of veins return blood from the lower limbs: the deep veins and the superficial veins. The deep veins carry most of the venous return. They accompany the major arteries and drain into the iliac veins, which in turn empty into the inferior vena cava. The superficial veins form a network of intercommunicating channels that travel just beneath the skin in the subcutaneous tissue and eventually drain into the deep veins. The largest superficial vein is the great saphenous vein, which extends up the medial surface of the leg from the ankle to the groin and drains into the more deeply placed femoral vein just below the groin. A second large superficial vein called the small saphenous vein ascends the back of the leg and drains into the deep venous system at the back of the knee. Both the superficial and deep veins contain cup-shaped valves, fashioned somewhat like the semilunar valves in the heart, which are interposed along the course of the veins. The arrangement of the valves is such that blood can flow upward in the veins but cannot flow in the reverse direction. The superficial and deep venous systems are also interconnected by short communicating branches that contain valves arranged so that blood normally flows only from superficial to deep veins and not in the reverse direction.

Blood is propelled upward within the deep veins by contraction of the leg and thigh muscles, which intermittently compress the veins and force the blood upward within the veins against gravity. The valves within the veins prevent retrograde flow. In contrast, the superficial veins are relatively unsupported, and venous return is much less efficient. Nevertheless, venous return through the superficial veins is normal provided that the veins do not become excessively dilated and the valves function properly to prevent retrograde flow and venous stasis.

Varicose veins result if the saphenous veins become dilated and their valves become incompetent. As a result, the blood tends to stagnate in the veins instead of flowing back normally to the heart, causing the veins to become elongated and tortuous. The condition tends to run in families, suggesting that the basic cause is a congenital weakness of the vein wall or its valves, which predisposes to the varicosities.

Varicose veins of the saphenous system may also develop if the deeper veins become blocked or if their valves become damaged by previous thrombophlebitis. As a result of damage to the deep veins, more of the venous return is shifted to the unsupported superficial veins, which are unable to cope with the increased flow and become varicose.

**Complications of Varicose Veins** Complications result from stasis of blood in the veins, with poor nutrition of the tissues caused by chronic venous engorgement. The skin of the distal leg and ankle becomes thin and atrophic and quite susceptible to infection. Skin ulcers may develop and heal poorly. The dilated veins are easily injured and may rupture, leading to extravasation of blood and chronic discoloration of the skin. Stasis of blood in the veins also predisposes to repeated bouts of thrombophlebitis.

**Treatment of Varicose Veins** Varicosities of the saphenous veins are treated by elastic stockings to support the veins and elevation of the legs whenever possible to promote more efficient venous return. Sometimes surgical removal of the varicose veins may be required. This is usually performed in conjunction with ligation of the communicating veins that interconnect the superficial and deep venous systems.

**Varicose Veins in Other Locations** Dilated veins around the rectum are called hemorrhoids and are described in Chapter 17 in conjunction with disorders of the gastrointestinal tract. Varicose veins of the esophagus often occur in patients with a disease called cirrhosis of the liver. Esophageal varices may rupture and cause profuse life-threatening hemorrhage. Their pathogenesis and treatment are considered in Chapter 16. Varicose veins of the spermatic cord appear as a mass of vessels in the scrotum above the testicle. The condition is called a **varicocele** (*varix* = vein + *cele* = swelling). The varicosities usually do not cause symptoms but at times may cause mild scrotal discomfort. Rarely, they may impair fertility in some men. Usually no treatment is required.

# CHAPTER REVIEW

## Summary

The normal structure and function of the heart (the cardiac pump) and blood vessels are described as a framework for comparing the various types of heart disease to malfunctions of a mechanical pump. Congenital heart disease is related to faulty pump construction. The fetal channels that bypass blood flow to the non-functional fetal lungs are the foramen ovale, which shunts right atrial blood into the left atrium, and the ductus arteriosus, which delivers pulmonary artery blood directly into the aorta. Sometimes the bypass channels do not close normally, which may be a problem if the ductus arteriosus remains patent. Abnormal communications between cardiac chambers may compromise cardiac function. Communications that allow deoxygenated blood to mix with oxygenated blood lead to cyanosis with resulting poor oxygen delivery to tissues and related complications. Communications that allow oxygenated blood to mix with deoxygenated blood traveling to the lungs do not impair oxygen delivery to the tissues but place an additional workload on the heart. Many congenital malformations can be treated successfully.

Valvular heart disease corresponds to a faulty valve system in a mechanical pump. Valve damage resulting from rheumatic fever is less common now, but aortic valve stenosis is becoming more frequent in our aging population. Mitral valve prolapse is also relatively common. Persons with an abnormal valve are at risk of infective endocarditis, and persons at high risk receive prophylactic antibiotics before dental procedures. Infective endocarditis is treated with appropriate antibiotics. A severely damaged valve can be replaced by an artificial valve if necessary.

Coronary heart disease results from accumulation of cholesterol and other lipids within the major coronary arteries, as well as other large arteries, which narrows their lumens and restricts blood flow to the tissues supplied by the narrowed arteries. This condition corresponds to a narrowed or obstructed fuel line in a mechanical pump. Both medical and surgical treatments can be used to improve blood flow to the heart muscle. Complete obstruction of a major coronary artery can lead to serious complications, including cardiac arrest, ventricular fibrillation, and myocardial infarction, which can cause severe damage to heart muscle. Diagnosis is established by ECG and cardiac enzyme tests. The sooner a blocked coronary artery can be opened, the better the ultimate outcome. Treatment consists of either dissolving the clot or opening the artery by an angioplasty procedure called percutaneous coronary intervention (PCI). The acute coronary syndrome classification provides guidelines for diagnosis and treatment of coronary artery disease. The roles of blood lipids and lipoproteins are considered in relation to coronary artery disease, as well as the harmful effects of trans fats.

A higher than normal blood pressure damages the cardiovascular system and is classified as primary hypertension if the cause is unknown, or secondary hypertension if the elevated pressure is caused by another disease, such as kidney disease. Effective treatment is available. Isolated systolic hypertension results from an increased rigidity of the large arteries that do not stretch normally to absorb the force of systolic contractions. Treatment is directed at reducing the elevated blood pressure, whatever its cause.

Primary myocardial disease is less common than other types of heart disease. Myocarditis is usually caused by a virus and generally resolves without permanent cardiac damage. Cardiomyopathy is more serious, and no specific treatment is available. One type is a hereditary disease characterized by disorganized muscle fibers and a greatly enlarged heart. Often the thickened ventricular septum may restrict outflow from the left ventricle. Treatment consists of drugs to improve cardiac function by slowing the heart and reducing the force of ventricular contraction.

Any type of heart disease can lead to chronic heart failure, which is the inability of the heart to supply the body's requirements. Systolic heart failure is the inability of the heart to eject enough blood during systole; diastolic heart failure results when the thickened hypertrophied left ventricle can't relax enough to allow adequate filling of the chamber in diastole, which reduces the volume of blood that can be ejected from the inadequately filled ventricle. Acute heart failure is a serious condition that can lead to acute pulmonary edema, and requires immediate intensive treatment.

Marked arteriosclerosis of the aorta weakens the wall and causes dilation of the distal aorta where the aortic pressure is highest. This is called an arteriosclerotic aneurysm that may enlarge slowly and is likely to rupture if not recognized and treated. Several effective treatment methods are available. A dissecting aneurysm results from degeneration of the aortic wall that may eventually lead to a tear in the inner lining (intima) of the aorta; consequently, blood dissects into the aortic wall to the site of the wall degeneration, causing a number of very serious complications. This is more difficult to treat than an arteriosclerotic aneurysm.

Dilated veins are called varicose veins and may occur in several locations. They are prone to occur in the long superficial leg veins returning blood to the heart against gravity (saphenous veins) and can be treated effectively. They also occur in other locations, such as in the esophagus (esophageal varices), in the rectum (hemorrhoids), and in the scrotum (called a varicocele).

## Questions for Review

1. How do the heart valves function to provide unidirectional blood flow? What factors determine the level of the systolic and diastolic blood pressure?
2. What are the major causes of heart disease? What is the difference between rheumatic fever and rheumatic heart disease?
3. What is infective endocarditis? How does it arise? How is it prevented? How is it treated?
4. What is coronary heart disease? What are its manifestations? What is the difference between angina pectoris and myocardial infarction?
5. What is the effect of high blood pressure on the heart and the blood vessels?
6. What is heart failure? What is meant by the following terms: *forward failure, backward failure, acute heart failure, chronic heart failure, systolic heart failure, diastolic heart failure*, and *acute pulmonary edema*?

7. What is the usual cause of an aortic aneurysm? How is an aneurysm treated?
8. What is the difference between an arteriosclerotic aneurysm of the aorta and a dissecting aneurysm of the aorta?
9. What are the possible complications of a large myocardial infarction?
10. What is meant by the following terms: *mitral valve prolapse, calcific aortic stenosis*, and *ventricular fibrillation*?
11. What factors predispose to thrombus formation in leg veins? What are the major complications of venous thrombi?
12. What are varicose veins? What veins are commonly affected? What are the clinical manifestations?

## Supplementary Reading

Beckett, N. S., Peters, R., Fletcher, A. E., et al. 2008. Treatment of hypertension in patients 80 years of age or older. *New England Journal of Medicine* 358:1887–98.
     Reducing elevated blood pressure reduces the risk of strokes and also reduces the death rate from cardiovascular disease even in very elderly patients.

Feldman, T., and Leon, M. B. 2007. Prospects for percutaneous valve therapies. *Circulation* 116:2866–77.
     A comprehensive discussion of percutaneous methods available or under active investigation that can be used to treat patients with valvular heart disease who are not good candidates for a standard surgical method of valve replacement. The percutaneous methodology is a "work in progress," as the valves and their methods of insertion are improved continuously based on clinical experience with the current percutaneous valves and their methods of replacement.

Ford, E. S., Adjoin, U. A., Croft, J., et al. 2007. Explaining the decrease in U.S. deaths from coronary disease, 1980–2000. *New England Journal of Medicine* 356: 2388–98.
     Although coronary heart disease and its complications are a leading cause of death in the United States, great progress has been made in reducing mortality, which has declined about 50 percent in the last two decades. About half the mortality reduction resulted from better control of risk factors that promote coronary heart disease, such as lowering blood lipids, better control of hypertension, reduced smoking, and increased physical activity. The other half of the mortality reduction was related to improved methods for diagnosing and treating coronary heart disease and its complications.

Hochman, J. S., and Steg, P. G. 2007. Does preventive PCI work? *New England Journal of Medicine* 365:1572–74.

Percutaneous cornary intervention (PCI) is effective in reducing angina in patients with coronary artery disease, and reduces mortality in patients who have an acute myocardial infarction or high-risk acute coronary syndromes accompanied by myocardial damage. These favorable outcomes have led to more widespread use of PCI to supplement medical therapy in an attempt to improve the long-term prognosis in patients with stable coronary artery disease. PCI offers no additional advantage over standard medical therapy for most patients with stable coronary artery disease.

Shah, S. J., and Gheorghiade, M. 2008. Heart failure with preserved ejection fraction. Treat now by treating comorbidities. *Journal of the American Medical Association* 300:431–733.

Half the patients with heart failure have a normal ejection fraction and standard treatment for heart failure has had limited success. Most of these patients have other conditions that contribute to the heart failure, primarily coronary artery disease and hypertension.

Svilaas, T., Vlaar, P. J., van der Horst, I. C., et al. 2008. Thrombus aspiration during primary percutaneous coronary intervention. *New England Journal of Medicine* 358:557–67.

Primary percutaneous coronary intervention (PCI) is effective in opening an infarct-related artery in patients with a ST-elevation myocardial infarction, but embolization of atheromatous debris and thrombus material plugs distal arterioles and reduces myocardial perfusion. Thrombus aspiration can be performed on most patients with ST-segment elevation myocardial infarction, which results in better reperfusion and better clinical outcomes than conventional percutaneous coronary intervention.

## Interactive Activities

### Matching

Match the cardiovascular disease or condition in the left column with its manifestations in the right column.

| | |
|---|---|
| 1. Bicuspid aortic valve | A. Narrow segment of proximal aorta obstructs blood flow into distal aorta |
| 2. Coarctation of aorta | B. Predisposes to development of aortic stenosis |
| 3. Patent ductus arteriosus | C. Cyanosis results from mixing of low oxygen content arterial blood with normally oxygenated arterial blood |
| 4. Atrial septal defect | D. Blood ejected into the aorta mixes with blood in the pulmonary artery |
| 5. Tetralogy of Fallot | E. Blood in the left atrium mixes with blood in the right atrium |

### Multiple Choice

1. Which of the following conditions is NOT a characteristic feature of the metabolic syndrome?
   A. hypertension
   B. cyanosis
   C. impaired carbohydrate tolerance
   D. obesity
   E. elevated blood lipids

2. A patient complains of chest pain and a myocardial infarction is suspected. Which of the following tests or procedures would not provide information to support the diagnosis of a myocardial infarction?
   A. elevation of the ST segment in the electrocardiogram
   B. elevated blood pressure
   C. blood test indicating elevated creatine kinase (CK–MB)
   D. blood test indicating elevated blood troponin

3. An angiogram performed on a patient with chest pain reveals a recent thrombus blocking a large coronary artery. Assuming that the patient has access to a completely staffed coronary care facility, what would be the most effective way to treat this condition?
   A. bed rest and sedation to alleviate the patient's discomfort
   B. prescribe a low-fat anti-coronary diet
   C. attempt to dissolve the thrombus by thrombolytic therapy
   D. perform a procedure (percutaneous coronary intervention) to remove the thrombus and insert a stent to keep the artery open

4. The main function of the foramen ovale in the fetus is
   A. shunting blood from the left to the right atrium
   B. shunting blood from the right to the left atrium
   C. shunting blood from the pulmonary artery into the aorta
   D. shunting blood from the aorta into the pulmonary artery

5. The main function of the ductus arteriosus is
   A. shunting blood from the left to the right atrium
   B. shunting blood from the right to the left atrium
   C. shunting blood from the pulmonary artery into the aorta
   D. shunting blood from the aorta into the pulmonary artery

## Critical Thinking

1. Peter Smith, a 15-year-old high school student, consulted a physician because of a back injury following a fall. As a routine part of his evaluation his blood pressure was taken, which was 170/110. Peter does not take any medications that could raise his blood pressure and there is no family history of cardiovascular disease. He doesn't understand why his blood pressure is so high. He wants to know what conditions could cause hypertension and what he should do about it. What would you tell him?

2. Sarah Meyers's 64-year-old father was told by his doctor that he has a heart murmur. He was surprised because the murmur had not been detected during routine medical examinations in previous years. He considers himself to be in good health and he asks you what could cause a new-onset murmur, what further studies he needs, and whether he can play golf as he has in the past. What would you tell him?

3. Arnold Reinhart is a 52-year-old man who has recently recovered from a serious heart attack (myocardial infarction). He asks you what he could do to reduce his risk of another heart attack. What would you tell him?

4. Sally Stevenson, a 22-year-old college student, has had a heart murmur for as long as she can remember. Recently she had a medical examination to qualify for joining a basketball team and was told that she should have a further evaluation to determine the cause of the murmur, and its possible effects on her cardiovascular system. She asks you what could cause her murmur and what are the possible effects on her health. What would you tell her?

# The Hematopoietic and Lymphatic Systems

1. Describe the composition of the blood, and enumerate its functions. Explain the functions of the lymphatic system.

2. Explain the principles by which anemias are classified and treated.

3. List and describe the usual causes of hypochromic microcytic anemia and macrocytic anemia. Explain how these anemias are treated.

4. List the usual causes of anemia as a result of bone marrow damage and anemia caused by accelerated blood destruction. Explain their treatment.

5. Describe the causes and effects of polycythemia and thrombocytopenia.

6. Describe the cause and clinical manifestations of infectious mononucleosis.

7. List the common causes of lymph node enlargement.

8. Explain the role of the spleen in protecting the body against infection. Describe the effects of a splenectomy on the body's defenses, and relate them to the management of the patient who has had a splenectomy.

## The Hematopoietic System

### Composition and Function of Human Blood

Blood is essential to transporting oxygen and nutrients to the tissues; carbon dioxide and other waste products of cell metabolism to the excretory organs; and leukocytes, hormones, and antibodies to various locations in the body. The volume of blood, which varies with the size of the individual, is about 5 quarts in the average man. Almost half of the blood consists of cellular elements: red cells, white cells (leukocytes), and platelets suspended in a viscous fluid called blood plasma ( Figure 11-1 ). All blood cells arise

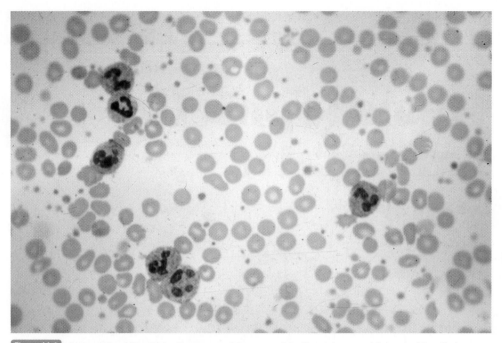

**Figure 11-1** Stained blood film. Red cells appear as biconcave disks. Several neutrophils can be identified near the *center* of the photograph. Small dark structures are platelets (original magnification × 1000).

from precursor cells within the bone marrow called stem cells, which undergo further differentiation to form the red cells, white cells, and platelets circulating in the bloodstream. The numbers of circulating red cells, white cells, and platelets are so great that their numbers are expressed as the number per microliter of blood (1 mL = 1000 microliters). This same quantity can also be expressed as the number per cubic millimeter ($mm^3$) of blood. The terms are equivalent because 1 microliter is the same as 1 cubic millimeter.

Red cells, which are concerned primarily with oxygen transport, are the most numerous cells, averaging about 5 million per microliter of blood. A mature red cell is an extremely flexible biconcave disk measuring about 7 micrometers (microns) in cross-section diameter. Its biconcave configuration is responsible for its characteristic central pallor and more intensely stained periphery, as seen in a stained blood smear. The biconcave configuration also provides the red cell with a large surface area relative to its volume, which facilitates rapid uptake of oxygen as blood flows through the pulmonary capillaries, and a rapid release of oxygen to body cells as blood is delivered to the tissues. The red cell shape also contributes to its extreme flexibility, which allows red cells to squeeze through small blood capillaries less than half the diameter of the red cells. Red cells normally survive for about 4 months in the circulation.

Leukocytes are much less numerous, averaging about 7000 per microliter. The following types of leukocytes are recognized:

1. Neutrophils
2. Eosinophils
3. Basophils
4. Monocytes
5. Lymphocytes

Although lymphocytes are produced chiefly in the lymph nodes and spleen, they are also manufactured in the bone marrow and elsewhere throughout the body where lymphoid tissue is present. Under normal circumstances, production of the other types of white cells is confined to the bone marrow. In contrast with the relatively long survival of red cells, most white cells have a short survival time within the circulation, varying from several hours to several days, and they must be replenished continually. Lymphocytes are an exception. Two populations of lymphocytes are present in the circulation, one surviving about the same length of time as most of the other leukocytes and another surviving for several years.

The proportions of the various leukocytes vary with the age of the individual. The most numerous in the adult are the neutrophils, constituting about 70 percent of the total circulating white cells. Neutrophils are actively phagocytic and predominate in acute inflammatory reactions. Lymphocytes are the next most common type of white cells in adults and are the predominant leukocytes in the blood of children. The lymphocytes in the peripheral blood constitute only a small fraction of the total lymphocytes, most being located in the lymph nodes, spleen, and other lymphoid tissues. Lymphocytes continually recirculate from the bloodstream into lymphoid tissues. Eventually, they leave the lymphoid tissue through the lymphatic channels and the thoracic duct, returning to the circulation and later becoming reestablished for a time in a different site of lymphoid tissue. Lymphocytes take part in cell-mediated and humoral defense reactions.

Small numbers of eosinophils, basophils, and monocytes also are normally present in the blood. **Eosinophils** are related in some manner to allergy. One of their functions appears to be phagocytosis and digestion of antigen–antibody complexes. Eosinophils increase in allergic diseases, in the presence of worm or other animal–parasite infections, and in a few other conditions. **Basophils** are similar to mast cells. Their granules contain histamine and an anticoagulant called heparin. **Monocytes** are actively phagocytic and increase in certain types of chronic infections. A monocyte–lymphocyte interaction is necessary in the initial phase of response to a foreign antigen; it also plays a role in the cell-mediated immune reaction.

Blood platelets, which are essential for normal blood coagulation, are much smaller than leukocytes. They represent bits of the cytoplasm of **megakaryocytes**, large precursor cells present in the bone marrow. Platelets have a short survival, comparable to that of most leukocytes.

# Normal Hematopoiesis

The bone marrow can be compared to a large manufacturing plant. It replenishes the blood cells that are continually being worn out and removed from the circulation. As with any manufacturing process, adequate quantities of raw materials are required. Moreover, the factory must be able to process these raw materials efficiently into finished products (the blood cells). The major raw materials necessary for hematopoiesis are protein, vitamin $B_{12}$, folic acid (one of the vitamin B group), and iron. Inadequate supplies of these substances will handicap the production of blood cells.

## Development, Maturation, and Survival of Red Cells

Red cells develop from large precursor cells in the bone marrow called **erythroblasts** (*erythro* = red + *blast* = a

primitive cell). **Hemoglobin**, the oxygen-carrying protein that is formed by the developing red cells, is composed of four separate pieces called *subunits*, which in turn fit together to form a much larger aggregate called a *tetramer* (*tetra* = four). Each subunit consists of two parts: *heme* and *globin*.

Heme is a complex nitrogen-containing ring structure (called a *porphyrin ring*) containing an iron atom. Globin, which forms the largest part of each hemoglobin subunit, is a short, coiled protein (*polypeptide*) chain. Several types of globin chains, differing in their amino acid composition, are formed at varying times and in differing proportions in the fetus and in the adult. The chains are designated by Greek letters: alpha ($\alpha$), beta ($\beta$), gamma ($\gamma$), delta ($\delta$), and epsilon ($\varepsilon$).

The hemoglobin in the red cells of the normal adult is called *hemoglobin A* or *adult hemoglobin*. Two subunits of the tetramer contain alpha chains and two contain beta chains. The hemoglobin can also be designated by the shorthand notation $\alpha_2\beta_2$. (The chain is designated by the Greek letter and the number of subunits by the subscript.)

In the embryo and fetus, hemoglobin containing different globin chains is produced at various times in the course of prenatal development. Beta chain production does not occur until relatively late in prenatal development. Consequently, the predominant hemoglobin in the fetus is a tetramer of alpha and gamma chains that is termed **fetal hemoglobin** (hemoglobin F). Fetal hemoglobin is able to take up and release oxygen more efficiently than adult hemoglobin when the oxygen partial pressure ($PO_2$) of the blood is low, an ability that is advantageous to the fetus because the $PO_2$ in fetal blood is lower than the $PO_2$ of adult blood. Late in pregnancy, fetal production of beta chains replaces gamma chains, and adult hemoglobin (hemoglobin A) begins to replace fetal hemoglobin in the red cells as the fetus prepares for life outside of the uterus.

The hemoglobin of a newborn infant contains both adult and fetal hemoglobin in approximately equal proportions. Normally, no significant fetal hemoglobin synthesis occurs after birth. As new red cells are

**eosinophil** (ē-ō-sin′o-fil) A cell whose cytoplasm is filled with large, uniform granules that stain intensely red with acid dyes. See also *basophil*.

**basophil** A cell that contains numerous variable-sized granules that stain intensely purple with basic dyes. See also *eosinophil*.

**monocyte** (mon′ō-sī-t) A leukocyte having a kidney-shaped nucleus and light blue cytoplasm; a phagocytic cell that forms part of the reticuloendothelial system.

**megakaryocyte** (mega-carry′o-site) A very large bone marrow cell having abundant granular cytoplasm and multilobed nucleus that forms the platelets circulating in the bloodstream.

**erythroblast** (e-rith′rō-blast) A precursor cell in the bone marrow that gives rise to red blood cells.

**hemoglobin** An oxygen transport protein within red cells composed of an iron-porphyrin complex (heme) combined with a protein chain (globin).

**fetal hemoglobin** A type of hemoglobin containing two alpha and two gamma chains, which is able to take up and release oxygen at much lower $PO_2$ (oxygen partial pressures) than in adult hemoglobin.

**reticulocyte**
(rē-tik´ū-lō-sīt) A young red cell that can be identified by special staining procedures.

**erythropoietin** (er-ith-rō-poy´e-tin) A humoral substance made by the kidneys that regulates hematopoiesis.

**anemia** (an-ē´mē-uh) A decrease in hemoglobin or red cells or both.

produced by the infant to replace those containing fetal hemoglobin that have reached the end of their life span, the new "replacement" red cells contain essentially only hemoglobin A. Consequently, the concentration of hemoglobin A rises in the infant's blood as hemoglobin F falls. By about 6 months of age, the hemoglobin is almost entirely hemoglobin A, which functions normally in the circulation.

The developing red cell accumulates increasing amounts of hemoglobin as it matures. When about 80 percent of its total hemoglobin has been synthesized, the nucleus is extruded. The cell is then discharged from the bone marrow into the circulation, where it completes its maturation and hemoglobin synthesis over the succeeding 24 hours. A newly formed red cell, which lacks a nucleus but still retains its mitochondria and other organelles for a short time, is called a **reticulocyte**. The name comes from its special staining characteristics. Certain stains precipitate the organelles within the cell cytoplasm, causing them to appear as a network (reticulum) of dark blue strands and granules. A reticulocyte is slightly larger than a mature red cell, and it also has a faint blue color because it contains less red-staining hemoglobin than a mature cell. These distinguishing features, which differentiate a reticulocyte from a mature red cell, are soon lost as the cell matures within the circulation.

The red cell, which derives its energy from the enzymatic breakdown of glucose, possesses enzyme systems that permit the cell to perform the diverse metabolic functions necessary for survival. Because the cell lacks a nucleus, it cannot synthesize new enzyme molecules to replace those that gradually wear out. As the cell ages, its enzyme systems gradually become depleted until eventually, after about 4 months, the cell is no longer able to function. The worn-out red cell is then removed by the mononuclear phagocyte system (reticuloendothelial system), primarily in the spleen, and its hemoglobin is degraded. The globin chains are broken down, and their component amino acids are used to make other proteins. The iron is extracted and saved to make new hemoglobin. The porphyrin ring, however, cannot be salvaged. It is degraded and is excreted by the liver as bile pigment.

## Regulation of Hematopoiesis

Red cell production is regulated by the oxygen content of the arterial blood. Decreased oxygen supply to the tissues stimulates erythropoiesis. However, low oxygen tension does not act directly on the bone marrow. The effect is mediated by the kidneys. Certain specialized cells in the kidneys elaborate a hormonelike erythrocyte-stimulating material called **erythropoietin**.

The factors regulating the production of white blood cells and their delivery into the circulation are not well understood. Products of cell necrosis may cause the number of white blood cells in the peripheral blood to increase. Hormone secretion by the adrenals and some other endocrine glands also influences white cell production.

# Anemia

**Anemia** literally means "without blood." Specifically, the term is used to refer to a decrease in red cells or to subnormal hemoglobin levels. Many classifications of anemia have been proposed, and two different methods of classification are widely used. One system, based on the factor responsible for the anemia, is an etiologic classification. A second system, based on the shape and appearance of the red blood cells (as determined by microscopic examination of a stained blood smear), is a morphologic classification.

## Etiologic Classification of Anemia

One simple classification of the anemias is based on the "bone marrow factory" concept ( Figure 11-2 ). Anemia is classified as being caused by either inadequate production of red cells or an excessive loss of cells. Inadequate production, in turn, may result from an insufficiency of raw materials or from factors that render the factory inoperative and no longer able to deliver enough finished products into the circulation. Examples of the latter would be marrow damage or replacement of marrow by abnormal cells. Excessive loss of red cells may be caused either by external blood loss or by accelerated destruction of the cells (and hence shortened survival) in the circulation. Table 11-1 presents a classification of the various causes of anemia.

## Morphologic Classification of Anemia

An anemia in which the cells are normal in size and appearance is called a normocytic anemia. If the cells are larger than normal, the anemia is called a macrocytic anemia. If the cells are smaller than normal, the anemia is called a microcytic anemia. Many times, microcytic cells also have a reduced hemoglobin content, appearing quite pale when examined under the microscope; here, the term *hypochromic anemia* is used. Often the latter two terms are combined, and the anemia is called a *hypochromic microcytic anemia*. Classification of anemia on the basis of red cell appearance

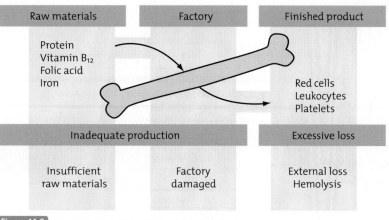

**Figure 11-2** Classification of anemia based on the "bone marrow factory" concept.

| Table 11-1 | Etiologic Classification of Anemia |
| --- | --- |

**Inadequate Production of Red Cells**

Caused by inadequate "raw materials"
  Iron deficiency
  Vitamin B$_{12}$ deficiency
  Folic acid deficiency

Caused by impaired function of bone marrow factory
  Anemia of chronic disease
  Bone marrow damaged or destroyed (aplastic anemia)
  Bone marrow replaced by foreign or abnormal cells
  (bone marrow replacement anemia)

**Excessive Loss of Red Cells**

Caused by external blood loss (hemorrhage)

Caused by shortened survival of red cells in the circulation
  Defective red cells (hereditary hemolytic anemia)
    Abnormal red cell shape
    Abnormal hemoglobin within red cells
    Defective hemoglobin synthesis within red cells
    Deficient red cell enzymes
  "Hostile environment"
    Anti-red cell antibodies
    Mechanical trauma to circulating red cells

is useful because the appearance of the cells provides a clue to the etiology. Iron deficiency anemia is a hypochromic microcytic anemia. Anemia caused by vitamin B$_{12}$ or folic acid deficiency is a macrocytic anemia. Most other types of anemia are normocytic.

## Iron Metabolism and Hematopoiesis

The body contains about 4 grams of iron, of which about 75 percent is contained in hemoglobin. Most of the rest is a reserve supply that is stored in the liver, bone marrow, and spleen combined with an iron-binding protein called apoferritin to form an iron–protein complex called ferritin. A small amount of iron also circulates in the blood bound to a protein called transferrin, which is the iron being transported from place to place in the body.

The usual diet of an adult contains from about 10 to 20 mg of iron, but men absorb merely 1 mg per day, and only slightly more iron is absorbed by women and children. Women need more iron to make up for menstrual losses because 1 mL of blood contains about 0.5 mg of iron. Additional iron is also required during pregnancy to supply the needs of the developing fetus. Children require greater amounts of iron in order to synthesize more hemoglobin during periods of growth when the blood volume is increasing. Iron is absorbed with difficulty from the gastrointestinal tract, and iron stores within the body are carefully conserved.

Figure 11-3 summarizes how iron is handled in the body. Iron is absorbed chiefly in the duodenum, and the amount absorbed depends on the iron content of the duodenal epithelial cells, which in turn is determined by the amount of iron stored as ferritin in the liver, bone marrow, and other iron storage sites. If iron stores are abundant, so also is the iron content of the intestinal epithelial cells, and less dietary iron is absorbed. On the other hand, if body iron stores are depleted, the iron content of the duodenal cells is also reduced, and more iron can be absorbed into the cells for eventual transport to storage sites in order to replenish ferritin stores.

From the duodenal mucosa the iron is transported by transferrin to the bone marrow for hemoglobin synthesis and to the liver and other storage sites where it is available for later use.

As red cells wear out and are destroyed, the iron from the hemoglobin is recycled, transported by transferrin back to the bone marrow, and used to make new hemoglobin. If sufficient recycled iron is not available

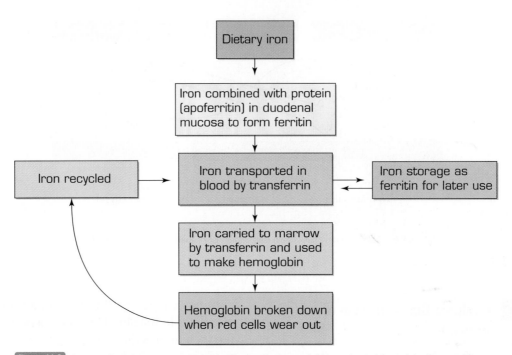

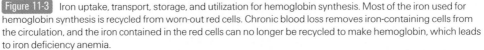

**Figure 11-3** Iron uptake, transport, storage, and utilization for hemoglobin synthesis. Most of the iron used for hemoglobin synthesis is recycled from worn-out red cells. Chronic blood loss removes iron-containing cells from the circulation, and the iron contained in the red cells can no longer be recycled to make hemoglobin, which leads to iron deficiency anemia.

for hemoglobin synthesis, additional iron is mobilized from storage sites.

## Iron Deficiency Anemia

Iron deficiency anemia is the most common anemia encountered in clinical practice. Iron forms an essential part of the hemoglobin molecule, and normal synthesis of hemoglobin requires adequate supplies of iron.

When red blood cells, which have a normal life span of about 4 months, become "senile," they are removed from the circulation. The iron from the destroyed cells is transported back to the bone marrow and is reused by the bone marrow to be incorporated into newly formed red cells. Iron deficiency anemia may result from either (1) insufficient intake of iron in the diet, or (2) inadequate reutilization of the iron present in worn-out red cells, which normally is recycled to make new hemoglobin. Chronic blood loss depletes body iron stores because the iron in the hemoglobin is also lost along with the red cell, and is no longer available to be recycled for red cell production.

Iron deficiency caused by inadequate dietary intake may occur in infants during periods of rapid growth. A normal, full-term infant has been provided with a reserve supply of iron that was transferred to the fetus from the mother during the last part of pregnancy. Consequently, the newborn infant generally has an adequate short-term supply of iron available for hematopoiesis during the neonatal period when the

production of red cells accelerates to supply the needs of an increasing blood volume. Premature infants, however, may not get their full component of iron stores, and may not have enough reserve to supply their postnatal needs. Even in full-term infants, the reserve supply of iron for hematopoiesis is limited and must be supplemented by iron from the diet. Breast milk contains very little iron, although the amount available is well absorbed. If the diet is not supplemented by cereals, fruits, vegetables, other foods containing iron, or some type of iron supplement, iron stores will become rapidly exhausted, and iron deficiency anemia will develop in the first year of life. For this reason, many physicians gradually add supplementary foods containing additional sources of iron to infants' diets. Occasionally, adolescents subsisting on an inadequate or poorly balanced diet develop iron deficiency anemia.

Most cases of iron deficiency anemia in adults result from a failure to recapture the iron present in red cells for hemoglobin synthesis. This failure is a result of chronic blood loss. The iron contained in red cells that is lost from the circulation by bleeding is no longer available to the body for the production of new red cells. Because each milliliter of blood contains 0.5 mg of iron, a loss of 500 mL of blood represents a loss of 250 mg of iron, which is equivalent to one-fourth of the body's entire iron reserves. Unless dietary intake of iron is extremely liberal, iron stores soon become exhausted, and iron deficiency anemia develops.

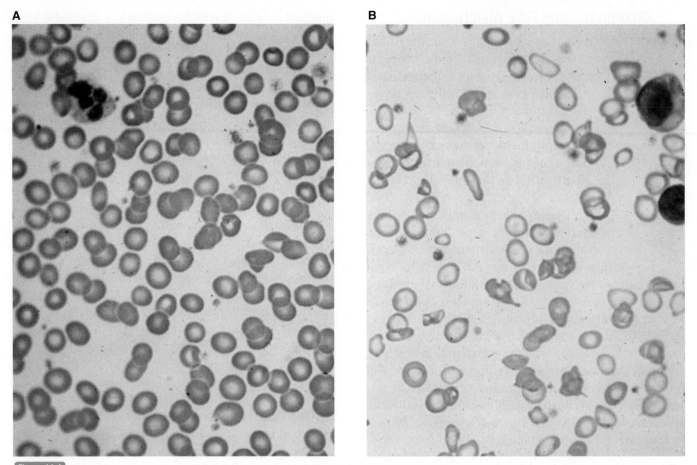

**A**

**B**

Comparison of normal red cells **A**, with those of hypochromic microcytic anemia **B**, caused by chronic iron deficiency (original magnification × 400).

Iron deficiency anemia is a hypochromic microcytic anemia (**Figure 11-4**). The cells are pale because they contain less hemoglobin than normal. The cells are also abnormally small because the body apparently attempts to "scale down" the size of the cell to conform to the reduced hemoglobin content.

**Laboratory Tests to Evaluate Iron Metabolism in Iron Deficiency Anemia** Various laboratory tests that measure iron stores, iron transport, and iron metabolism can be used as diagnostic tests in patients with suspected iron deficiency anemia. These include measurements of serum ferritin, serum iron, and serum iron-binding capacity.

In iron deficiency anemia, body iron stores are depleted and serum ferritin is low. Serum iron is also much lower than normal, but the amount of iron transport protein in the serum is much higher than normal, apparently reflecting the body's attempt to capture the meager iron available and transport it more efficiently. Consequently, the characteristic laboratory profile of iron-deficiency anemia is low serum ferritin and serum iron, but a much higher than normal serum iron-binding

protein with a much lower than normal percent of iron saturation.

**Evaluation and Treatment of Iron Deficiency Anemia** A physician treating a patient with iron deficiency anemia is primarily concerned with learning the cause of the anemia and then directing therapy toward the cause rather than the symptoms. In an infant with a history of a very poor diet, the cause may be obvious. In an adult, the anemia is usually a result of blood loss, and the physician must always be aware of this possibility and investigate to determine the reason for the blood loss. Chronic blood loss, for example, may be caused by a bleeding ulcer or an ulcerated carcinoma of the colon. In women, excessive menstrual bleeding is a common cause of iron deficiency anemia. Another sometimes overlooked cause of iron deficiency anemia in otherwise healthy young adults is too frequent blood donations. When the cause of the blood loss has been determined, proper treatment of the underlying cause can be instituted. In addition, the patient is given supplementary iron to replenish the body's depleted iron stores.

# Vitamin B$_{12}$ and Folic Acid Deficiency

**megaloblast**
(meg'al-ō-blast)
An abnormal red cell precursor resulting from vitamin B$_{12}$ or folic acid deficiency.

**leukopenia** (lōō-kō-pē'ni-uh) An abnormally small number of leukocytes in the peripheral blood.

**thrombocytopenia**
(throm'bō-sī-tō-pē'ny-yuh) A deficiency of platelets.

Vitamin B$_{12}$ is found in meat, liver, and other foods rich in animal protein. Folic acid is widely distributed in nature, being found in abundance in green leafy vegetables as well as many foods of animal origin.

Vitamin B$_{12}$ and folic acid are required not only for normal hematopoiesis, but also for normal maturation of many other types of cells. In the absence of either vitamin B$_{12}$ or folic acid, DNA synthesis is impaired and the developing red cells in the bone marrow exhibit a characteristic disturbance of cell maturation. The developing red cells, which are larger than normal, are called **megaloblasts** (*megalos =* large). The abnormal red cell maturation is called *megaloblastic erythropoiesis*. The mature red cells derived from the abnormal maturation also are larger than normal. Therefore, the anemia is classified morphologically as a macrocytic anemia. The development of white cell precursors and megakaryocytes is also abnormal. Consequently, patients with megaloblastic anemia usually also have **leukopenia** and **thrombocytopenia** as well as a macrocytic anemia. Vitamin B$_{12}$, but not folic acid, is required to maintain the structural and functional integrity of the nervous system; thus, a deficiency of this vitamin also may be associated with pronounced neurologic disturbances.

**Anemia as a Result of Folic Acid Deficiency** The body has very limited stores of folic acid, which rapidly become depleted if not replenished continually. As a result, folic acid–deficiency anemia is relatively common and may result from reduced dietary intake, impaired absorption, or increased folic acid requirements.

Deficiency caused by inadequate dietary intake is found in persons subsisting on inadequate diets and is encountered frequently in persons consuming excessive amounts of alcohol because of their typically deficient diet (Chapter 18), and possibly also impaired absorption of folic acid compared with nondrinkers. Persons with chronic intestinal diseases may become folic acid deficient because of impaired ability to absorb the vitamin. Pregnant women also are at risk because pregnancy greatly increases folic acid requirements. Folic acid–deficiency anemia in pregnancy is uncommon because physicians routinely prescribe folic acid supplements to pregnant women.

**Anemia as a Result of Vitamin B$_{12}$ Deficiency** Efficient absorption of vitamin B$_{12}$ ingested in food requires a substance called intrinsic factor that is secreted by gastric mucosal cells along with hydrochloric acid and digestive enzymes. The intrinsic factor combines with the vitamin B$_{12}$, and the B$_{12}$–intrinsic factor complex is absorbed from the distal small intestine. The absorbed vitamin is stored in the liver and made available to the bone marrow and other tissues as required for cell growth and maturation.

A common cause of vitamin B$_{12}$ deficiency is pernicious anemia. The basic defect in pernicious anemia is atrophy of the gastric mucosa, which sometimes develops in middle-age and older individuals and is often associated with autoantibodies directed against gastric mucosal cells and intrinsic factor. The atrophic mucosa fails to secrete intrinsic factor as well as gastric acid and digestive enzymes, and consequently, vitamin B$_{12}$ is not absorbed. The vitamin B$_{12}$ deficiency causes impaired hematopoiesis as well as various neurologic disturbances.

Pernicious anemia is not the only cause of vitamin B$_{12}$ deficiency. Persons who have had most of their stomach surgically removed because of ulcer or gastric cancer or who have had a gastric bypass procedure to control obesity may not be able to secrete enough intrinsic factor. Persons who have had a small bowel resection of the distal ilium, where the vitamin B$_{12}$–intrinsic factor complex is absorbed, may not be able to absorb enough vitamin to supply their needs, and an individual with chronic intestinal disease affecting the vitamin B$_{12}$–absorbing area in the distal ileum (such as Crohn disease, described in Chapter 17) also may be unable to absorb the vitamin adequately.

Pernicious anemia and other vitamin B$_{12}$ deficiencies are treated with intramuscular administration of vitamin B$_{12}$. Parenteral administration avoids the problem of poor absorption of the vitamin.

**Bone Marrow Suppression, Damage, or Infiltration**
Many conditions can depress bone marrow function. Chronic diseases of all types may impair hematopoiesis and lead to mild or moderate anemia, which is called *the anemia of chronic disease*. In this condition, iron and other "raw materials" supplied to the bone marrow are adequate, but they are not utilized efficiently to make red cells. White blood cell and platelet production are usually not disturbed. The most common cause of this type of anemia is chronic infection, but other chronic diseases and some malignant tumors also may be responsible.

The anemia of chronic disease usually causes only a relatively mild suppression of bone marrow function and improves when the disease that caused it is identified and treated. Chronic infections may respond to treatment, but unfortunately, it is often not possible to "cure" many of the other chronic diseases that lead to this type of anemia.

In contrast to the anemia of chronic disease, much more serious and sometimes irreversible damage to the bone marrow factory results from destruction of the bone marrow stem cells from which mature blood cells and platelets arise. This type of anemia is called **aplastic anemia** (*a* = without + *plasia* = growth), although this term is not strictly accurate because the stem cell damage leads to leukopenia and thrombocytopenia as well as anemia. The anemia is classified as a normocytic anemia because the red cells are normal in size and shape although inadequate in number. Many agents can cause aplastic anemia. Radiation, anticancer chemotherapy drugs, and various toxic chemicals may cause severe marrow damage. Other drugs, including some antibiotics, anti-inflammatory drugs, and anticonvulsant drugs, may damage marrow stem cells in susceptible individuals. In many cases, however, it is the body's own immune system that is responsible for the aplastic anemia, a manifestation of an autoimmune disease in which the body's own cytotoxic T lymphocytes attack and destroy the marrow stem cells.

Aplastic anemia is treated initially by blood and platelet transfusions to maintain an adequate volume of circulating blood cells while the cause of the bone marrow failure is being investigated. If the marrow damage is caused by a toxic drug or chemical and is not too severe, marrow function may recover; however, it is unlikely in severe aplastic anemia, and other methods of treatment are required to restore marrow function. Many patients respond to immunosuppressive agents that act against the destructive (cytotoxic) T lymphocytes responsible for stem cell destruction. Bone marrow transplantation is also effective and can be performed in highly selected patients using the same methods used to treat patients with leukemia (Chapter 8).

An anemia similar to aplastic anemia involving white cells and platelets as well as red cells may also occur if bone marrow stem cells are crowded out and replaced by abnormal cells, such as leukemic cells or metastatic carcinoma. The term *bone marrow replacement anemia* is sometimes used to denote this type of anemia. Unfortunately, it may be difficult to restore marrow function after the marrow has been heavily infiltrated by leukemic cells or cancer cells, although adequate levels of hemoglobin and red cells can be maintained by blood transfusions.

## Acute Blood Loss

A normocytic anemia may result from an episode of acute blood loss, as from a massive hemorrhage from the uterus or gastrointestinal tract. Provided that iron stores are adequate, the lost blood is rapidly replaced by the bone marrow, and the newly formed red cells are normal. This is in contrast with the anemia of chronic blood loss, in which the red cells are hypochromic and microcytic because prolonged bleeding has depleted the body's iron stores.

## Accelerated Blood Destruction

Normal red cells survive for about 4 months. Sometimes, however, their survival is considerably shortened, and anemia results because the regenerative capacity of the marrow is not sufficient to keep up with the accelerated destruction. This type of anemia is called a **hemolytic anemia** and may be a result of either defective red cells or a "hostile environment." Hemolytic anemias caused by defective red cells are called hereditary hemolytic anemias. Those resulting from damage to normal red cells by antibodies or other injurious agents are called acquired hemolytic anemias.

**Hereditary Hemolytic Anemias**   The genetically determined abnormalities of red cells that may shorten their survival fall into four major groups ( Table 11-2 ):

1. Abnormally shaped cells
2. Abnormal hemoglobins
3. Defective hemoglobin synthesis
4. Enzyme deficiencies

*Abnormally Shaped Cells*   The most common abnormality of shape is called **hereditary spherocytosis**. In hereditary spherocytosis, the structural framework (cytoskeleton) of the red cell membrane is defective, which reduces its stability and flexibility. New red cells produced by the bone marrow and released into the circulation have a normal biconcave disk configuration, but bits of their unstable cell membranes become detached from the cells as the red cells squeeze through extremely small capillaries during their travel through the bloodstream, which progressively reduces the surface area of the red cell membranes. The red cells adapt to their reduced surface area relative to their cell volume by gradually changing from biconcave disks to spherical cells, which is the only way that the smaller cell membrane can surround the comparatively large volume of the red cell ( Figure 11-5 ). Unfortunately, the spherical shape puts the red cells at a disadvantage that greatly shortens their survival in the bloodstream. As blood flows through the spleen, normal flexible

**aplastic anemia**
(ā-plas′tik) An anemia caused by bone marrow failure.

**hemolytic anemia**   An anemia caused by increased blood destruction.

**hereditary spherocytosis**   A hereditary anemia caused by a defect affecting the red cell membrane that causes the biconcave disk-shaped red cells to change into small spherical cells that do not survive normally in the circulation.

## Table 11-2  Inheritance and Manifestations of Some Hereditary Hemolytic Anemias

| Anemia | Inheritance | Characteristics of Red Cells | Manifestations |
|---|---|---|---|
| *Hereditary spherocytosis* | Dominant or recessive | Spherocytic | Mild to moderate chronic hemolytic anemia |
| *Hereditary ovalocytosis* | Dominant | Oval | Usually asymptomatic; may have mild anemia |
| *Sickle cell anemia* | Codominant | Normocytic; cells sickle under reduced oxygen tension | Marked anemia |
| *Hemoglobin C disease* | Codominant | Normocytic | Mild to moderate anemia |
| *Sickle cell–hemoglobin C disease* | Codominant | Normocytic; cells sickle under reduced oxygen tension | Moderate anemia |
| *Thalassemia minor* | Dominant (heterozygous) | Hypochromic-microcytic; total number of red cells usually increased | Mild anemia |
| *Thalassemia major* | Dominant (homozygous) | Hypochromic-microcytic | Severe anemia; usually fatal in childhood |
| *Glucose-6-phosphate dehydrogenase deficiency* | X-linked recessive | Normocytic; enzyme-deficient cells | Episodes of acute hemolytic anemia precipitated by drugs or infections |

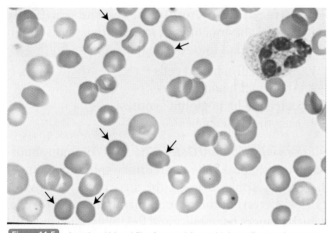

Figure 11-5  A stained blood film from subject with hereditary spherocytosis. The many small dark cells with little or no central pallor are spherocytes (*arrows*). The larger, more normal-appearing red cells are young red cells that have the same cell membrane defect but have not been circulating long enough to acquire a spherical shape. The relative large, faintly blue-staining red cell in the center of the field is a reticulocyte (original magnification × 400).

disk-shaped red cells can "work their way" through the splenic pulp and into the thin-walled veins (sinusoids) that carry the blood out of the spleen, but spherocytes are not thin enough or flexible enough to get through the spleen. They become trapped in the spleen where they are destroyed by the phagocytic cells in the splenic pulp. The bone marrow increases red cell production to compensate for the shortened survival of the spherocytes, resulting in a chronic hemolytic anemia.

Splenectomy cures the anemia by removing the main site of red cell destruction but has no effect on the basic red cell defect.

***Abnormal Hemoglobins***  The arrangement of amino acids in the globin chains of hemoglobin is controlled by genes. If the gene is abnormal, the amino acids forming the globin chains will be altered, leading to the formation of an abnormal hemoglobin. Genes directing the synthesis of the various types of hemoglobin are codominant. If an abnormal gene is present, the abnormal hemoglobin appears in the red cells. Many different abnormal hemoglobins can be identified and characterized by various laboratory tests. Some of the abnormal hemoglobins function normally, but others have unusual properties that impair their function. Hemoglobin S (sickle hemoglobin) is one of the more important abnormal hemoglobins. Its formation results from a change in only a single amino acid in the beta chain of hemoglobin. When the oxygen content (partial pressure) of the blood falls, as in venous blood, the hemoglobin S molecules aggregate and form rigid fibers, a process somewhat like crystallization ( Figure 11-6 ). The "crystallization" is largely reversible, and the hemoglobin becomes soluble again when the oxygen tension rises as the blood is oxygenated in the lungs. About 8 percent of the black population are heterozygous carriers of the sickle cell gene. Their

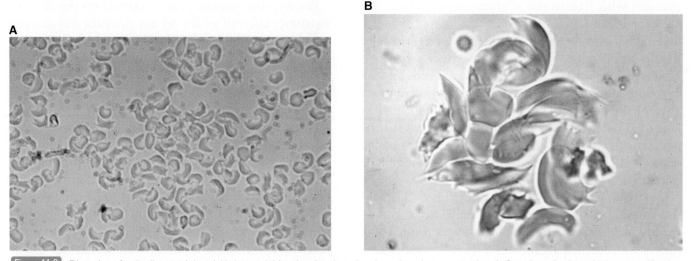

**Figure 11-6** Distortion of red cells containing sickle hemoglobin when incubated under reduced oxygen tension. **A,** Overview of cells under low magnification (× 100). **B,** Higher magnification view (× 400) of red cell distortion caused by sickle hemoglobin.

erythrocytes contain both hemoglobin S and hemoglobin A. This condition is called *sickle cell trait*, and the hemoglobin S in their red cells can be demonstrated easily by a simple blood test. Persons with sickle cell trait normally do not experience any problems related to the sickle hemoglobin in their red cells unless they engage in vigorous activities at high altitude and the oxygen content of their blood falls to a very low level.

The homozygous state is called **sickle cell anemia** and is a serious disease that results when both parents have the sickle cell trait and each transmits the sickle cell gene to the infant. The cells of affected individuals contain no hemoglobin A and become sickled within the capillaries where the oxygen partial pressure is lower than in arterial blood. The clumps of sickled red cells plug blood vessels, which obstruct blood flow, causing progressive damage to the heart, kidneys, spleen, and other organs resulting from the impaired circulation. Anemia develops because the sickle-hemoglobin–containing cells have a shortened survival in the circulation. Consequently, the bone marrow must increase greatly its production of red cells, as demonstrated by an elevated peripheral blood reticulocyte count, in order to compensate for the shortened red cell survival.

Newborn infants with sickle cell anemia do not have problems initially because their red cells also contain a large amount of fetal hemoglobin, which "dilutes" the concentration of sickle hemoglobin in the red cells so that they function more like the red cells of a person with sickle cell trait. Symptoms usually don't appear until the infant is about 6 months old, when the red cells containing both fetal and sickle hemoglobin have been replaced by red cells containing almost entirely sickle hemoglobin.

Although there is no cure for sickle cell anemia, advances in treatment have improved survival, and many affected persons now live 40 to 50 years. They are quite susceptible to infections and should receive pneumococcal vaccine and other immunizing agents to reduce their infection risk. The hyperactive bone marrow requires abundant folic acid to promote red cell production, and folic acid supplements are recommended to ensure that supplies are adequate. A drug called hydroxyurea can be used to stimulate the bone marrow to produce fetal hemoglobin, thereby lowering the proportion of sickle hemoglobin in the red cells, but its long-term safety has not been determined.

Simple, readily available tests can detect sickle cell trait in affected individuals, and genetic counseling is recommended for couples who are at risk of having a child with sickle cell anemia. DNA analysis of fetal cells obtained by amniocentesis can determine whether the fetus carries the sickle cell gene and, if present, whether the fetus is homozygous or heterozygous for the gene.

*Defective Hemoglobin Synthesis* Sometimes the globin chains of hemoglobin are normal, but their synthesis is defective. This genetically determined condition is called **thalassemia** and is transmitted as a Mendelian-dominant trait. Usually the defective synthesis involves the beta chains (*beta thalassemia*). This genetic abnormality is relatively common in persons of Greek and Italian ancestry. (The term *thalassemia* comes from the Greek word *thalassa*, meaning sea, and derives from the high incidence of the condition in

**sickle cell anemia** A hereditary anemia characterized by formation of an abnormal hemoglobin that causes the red cells to become sickle shaped when the oxygen content of the blood is reduced.

**thalassemia** (thal-uh-seem'-mia) A hereditary anemia characterized by defective production of globin chains required to produce normal hemoglobin, leading to a hypochronic microcytic anemia.

persons who live in the regions surrounding the Mediterranean Sea.)

In beta thalassemia, the production of beta chains required to produce hemoglobin is reduced. Because hemoglobin synthesis is reduced, the red cells appear hypochromic and microcytic, somewhat like the appearance of the cells in iron deficiency anemia. In thalassemia, however, the hypochromia is the result of deficient hemoglobin production because of inadequate beta chain synthesis, rather than deficient production caused by iron deficiency.

If a person is heterozygous for the thalassemia gene, the anemia is mild and the condition is called *thalassemia minor*. The red cells are hypochromic and microcytic, and usually there is a compensatory overproduction of red cells; consequently, their numbers are greater than normal. The homozygous condition, which is called *thalassemia major*, occurs if both parents have thalassemia minor and each transmits the abnormal gene. The affected homozygous individual has a severe chronic hemolytic anemia that is usually fatal in childhood.

**Red Cell Enzyme Deficiencies** Red cells derive energy by metabolizing glucose by a series of chemical reactions that are catalyzed by various enzyme systems. These same energy-producing reactions also indirectly help prevent oxidation of the hemoglobin, thereby protecting the hemoglobin from the potentially harmful effects of oxidizing drugs or other agents that can damage it. This protective function is compromised if certain red cell enzymes are deficient. Under such circumstances, exposing the red cells to an oxidizing agent causes denaturation and precipitation of the protein chains of hemoglobin, as well as the cell-membrane proteins.

One of the most common red cell enzyme defects is a deficiency of an enzyme called *glucose-6-phosphate dehydrogenase*. In this condition, which is transmitted as an X-linked recessive trait, the enzyme is unstable and does not function normally. About 10 percent of black men are affected, and 30 percent of black women carry the abnormal gene on one of their X chromosomes. The abnormal gene occurs with high frequency in some white populations as well. The enzyme-deficient cells are highly susceptible to injury by drugs that do not affect normal red cells, and to various bacterial and viral infections. More than 40 drugs are known to induce an acute hemolytic anemia in susceptible subjects. Hemolysis begins soon after exposure to the drug or infectious agent and continues for about a week. Considerable red cell destruction results, followed by red cell regeneration and return of red cell levels to normal in about 4 or 5 weeks.

Because the mutant gene is carried on the X chromosome, affected males do not produce any normal enzyme, and all of their red cells are subject to hemolysis. Females who carry the mutant gene on one of their X chromosomes are also at risk of drug-induced hemolysis. However, because of random inactivation of one of the X chromosomes in the female, as described in Chapter 2, the red cells of the female contain two populations of red cells. Some are derived from red cell precursors in which the X chromosome containing the mutant gene is inactivated, and these cells will contain the normal enzyme. Other red cells will be derived from percursor cells in which the X chromosome containing the normal gene is inactivated, and these cells will contain a defective enzyme and will be susceptible to hemolysis. Usually the normal red cells and the enzyme-deficient red cells are present in approximately equal proportions; therefore, drug-induced hemolysis is less intense in a female carrier than in an affected male, as would be expected, because the proportion of hemolysis-susceptible red cells in the female carrier is always less than that of an affected male, in whom all the red cells contain the defective enzyme.

**Acquired Hemolytic Anemia** Sometimes the red cells are normally formed but are unable to survive normally because they are released into a "hostile environment." For example, antibodies that attack and destroy the red cells may be present in the circulation. Some of the autoimmune diseases, such as lupus erythematosus (Chapter 4), and some diseases of the lymphatic system may be associated with a hemolytic anemia caused by autoantibodies. Some drugs also cause a hemolytic anemia by inducing formation of antibodies that damage red cells.

## Diagnostic Evaluation of Anemia

After it is determined that a patient is anemic, the physician's function is to determine the cause so that proper, effective treatment can be instituted. A careful medical history and physical examination may provide important clues to the most likely cause. A complete blood count is essential in order to assess the degree of anemia and to determine whether leukopenia and thrombocytopenia also are present. Careful microscopic examination of a blood smear allows the physician to determine whether the anemia is hypochromic microcytic, normocytic, or macrocytic. This information helps identify the probable cause of the anemia. The rate of production of new red cells can be estimated by determining the percentage of reticulocytes in the circulation. This is called a reticulocyte count. An increased percentage of reticulocytes indicates rapid regeneration of red cells, as would be encountered after acute blood loss or hemolysis. In some patients, tests that measure iron stores, iron transport, and iron metabolism may be useful. In selected patients, examining the bone marrow provides very useful information. In this procedure, a small amount of bone marrow is removed from the pelvic bone, sternum, or other site and examined microscopically. Characteristic abnormalities in the maturation of the marrow cells are seen in pernicious anemia and in anemia caused by folic acid deficiency. Bone marrow examination also detects interference with bone marrow functions secondary to infiltration by leukemic cells or metastatic tumor. Aplastic anemia can generally be recognized by studying the bone marrow. Certain other tests are used when chronic blood loss from the gastrointestinal tract is suspected. Stools are examined for blood, and x-ray studies of the gastrointestinal tract are frequently performed to localize a site of bleeding. Other diagnostic procedures are performed in special circumstances.

# Polycythemia

An increase of red cells and hemoglobin above normal levels is called **polycythemia**. Polycythemia may be secondary to an underlying disease that leads to decreased arterial oxygen saturation (secondary polycythemia), or it may be a manifestation of a leukemia-like overproduction of red cells for no apparent reason (primary polycythemia).

## Secondary Polycythemia

Any condition associated with a reduced amount of oxygen transported in the bloodstream (low arterial $PO_2$) leads to increased erythropoietin production and hence to increased numbers of circulating red cells. The condition may accompany pulmonary emphysema, pulmonary fibrosis, or some other type of chronic lung disease that impairs the oxygenation of the blood. Persons with types of congenital heart disease associated with shunting of deoxygenated blood from the right cardiac chambers into the systemic circulation also develop secondary polycythemia, as illustrated by the subject with the tetralogy of Fallot described in the previous chapter (Figure 10-11). In these individuals, the amount of oxygen transported in the systemic circulation to supply the tissues is reduced (low arterial $PO_2$) by the admixture of shunted deoxygenated blood, which leads to cyanosis and a compensatory increase in red cell production.

## Primary Polycythemia

Primary polycythemia, also called *polycythemia vera* (true polycythemia), is a manifestation of a diffuse hyperplasia of the bone marrow of unknown etiology. It is characterized by overproduction not only of red cells, but also of white blood cells and platelets. The disease has many features of a neoplastic process, and some patients with polycythemia vera eventually develop granulocytic leukemia.

**polycythemia** (päl-ē-sī-thē′mē–yuh) Increased number of red cells. May be caused by some types of chronic heart or lung disease (*secondary polycythemia*) or by marrow erythroid hyperplasia of unknown causes (*primary polycythemia*).

**hemochromatosis** (hemo-crow-mah-toe′-sis) A genetic disease characterized by excessive iron absorption, leading to accumulation of excessive amounts of iron in the body, causing organ damage.

## Complications and Treatment of Polycythemia

The symptoms of polycythemia are related to the increased blood volume and increased blood viscosity. Many patients with polycythemia develop thromboses because of the increased blood viscosity and elevated platelet levels. Polycythemia vera is usually treated by drugs that suppress the bone marrow overactivity. Secondary polycythemia is sometimes treated by periodic removal of excess blood.

# Iron Overload: Hemochromatosis

Although iron is essential for normal hematopoiesis and has other essential functions in the body, an excess of iron in the body is harmful.

Iron is absorbed with difficulty and excreted with difficulty. Iron uptake is very closely controlled by the body, and there are no normal pathways that allow for excretion of iron in excess of the body's needs. Men excrete only about 1 mg of iron per day, which reflects primarily small losses of iron contained in the cells that are being lost from the skin, intestinal tract, and other sites that are replaced by new cells. Premenopausal women excrete slightly more because of menstrual losses, as each milliliter of red cells contains about 0.5 mg of iron.

Because iron excretory pathways are lacking, any excess iron entering the body can't be eliminated, and the body becomes overloaded with iron, which accumulates in the body's tissues and organs. Eventually this leads to organ damage followed by scarring, leading to permanent derangement in the functions of the affected organs.

The usual cause of iron overload is a genetic disease called **hemochromatosis**, which is transmitted as an autosomal recessive trait. The gene occurs in about 10 percent of the population, but the disease only occurs in homozygous carriers of the gene, who absorb an excessive amount of iron, which leads to excessive accumulation of iron in the body.

Early recognition and treatment prevents progression of the disease and arrests organ damage. Treatment consists of repeated withdrawal of blood (phlebotomy) to remove iron from the body, as each 500 mL of blood withdrawn removes 250 mg of iron. Phlebotomies are repeated until iron stores are depleted, and then periodic phlebotomies are continued for the rest of the patient's life.

The excessive iron absorption and storage characteristic of hemochromatosis can be identified by the same type of laboratory tests used to measure iron storage and transport in subjects with iron deficiency anemia: serum ferritin, serum iron, and serum iron-binding capacity. When the body is overloaded with iron, serum ferritin is very high, reflecting the greatly increased iron stores that can be as much as 15 to 20 grams or more instead of the normal amount of about 1 gram. Serum iron is also much higher than normal and the iron-binding protein transferrin is completely loaded (saturated) with iron. These tests all point to increased uptake and storage of iron.

The following case illustrates the usefulness of screening studies for detecting this disease before irreparable organ damage occurs.

### Case Study 11-1

A 40-year-old healthy woman was seen in consultation by a physician because routine screening laboratory tests had detected elevated serum iron.

Physical examination was normal, as were routine blood and urine tests, but tests measuring iron stores and iron metabolism were all abnormal. Serum iron was much higher than normal (234 mg per 100 mL), and serum iron-binding protein was completely saturated with iron. Serum ferritin was 1335 mg per liter, which is more than 10 times higher than normal. A diagnosis of hemochromatosis was made, and treatment consisting of periodic phlebotomies was begun in order to remove the excess iron from her body.

## Thrombocytopenia

Blood platelets are fragments of the cytoplasm of megakaryocytes that are released into the bloodstream. These small structures serve a hemostatic function, sealing small breaks in capillaries and interacting with plasma factors in the initial stages of blood clotting. A significant reduction in the numbers of platelets in the blood leads to numerous small, pinpoint hemorrhages from capillaries in the skin and mucous membranes, called *petechiae*, and to larger areas of hemorrhage, called *ecchymoses*. This type of skin and mucous membrane bleeding is called **purpura**, and the disease entity is called *thrombocytopenic purpura*. This condition may result either from (1) inadequate production of platelets caused by damage to the bone marrow, or (2) shortened survival of platelets in the circulation caused by antiplatelet autoantibodies.

Thrombocytopenic purpura from bone marrow damage is often caused by drugs, chemicals, or other substances that disrupt platelet production, and may also result if the bone marrow is infiltrated by leukemic cells or metastatic carcinoma that "crowd out" the platelet-producing megakaryocytes. These conditions are called *secondary thrombocytopenic purpura* because the purpura results from an underlying disease of the bone marrow.

In thrombocytopenia caused by shortened platelet survival, the bone marrow produces platelets normally but the antiplatelet autoantibodies in the blood destroy the platelets, and the antibodies can be detected in the blood of the affected person. Cases of this type, in which no underlying bone marrow disease can be detected, are called primary thrombocytopenic purpura. This condition is often encountered in children, sometimes related to a recent viral infection, and subsides spontaneously within a short time. When the disease develops in adults, it tends to be more chronic.

## The Lymphatic System

The lymphatic system consists of the lymph nodes and spleen, together with various organized masses of lymphoid tissue elsewhere throughout the body; these include the tonsils, the adenoids, the thymus, and lymphoid aggregates in the intestinal mucosa, respiratory tract, and bone marrow. The primary function of the lymphatic system is to provide immunologic defenses against foreign material by means of cell-mediated and humoral (antibody-mediated) defense mechanisms. The lymph nodes, which constitute a major part of the system, form an interconnected network linked by lymphatic channels.

Lymph nodes are small, bean-shaped structures that vary from a few millimeters to as much as 2 centimeters in diameter. They are interspersed along the course of lymphatic channels, where they act somewhat like filters. Frequently, they form groups at locations where many lymphatic channels converge, such as around the aorta and inferior vena cava, in the mesentery of the intestine, in the axillae (armpits) and groin, and at the base of the neck. Each node consists of a mass of lymphocytes supported by a meshwork of reticular fibers in which are scattered phagocytic cells of the mononuclear phagocyte system (reticuloendothelial system). As the lymph flows through the nodes, the phagocytic cells filter out and destroy any microorganisms or other foreign materials that have gotten into the lymphatic channels. The lymphocytes and mononuclear phagocytes within the node also interact with the foreign material and initiate an immune response, as described in Chapter 4.

The spleen is specialized to filter blood rather than lymph. Much larger than lymph nodes, it is about the size of a man's fist and is located under the ribs in the left upper part of the abdomen. It consists of compact masses of lymphocytes and a network of sinusoids (capillaries having wide lumens of variable width) within a supporting framework composed of reticular fibers and numerous phagocytic cells. As the blood flows through the spleen, worn-out red cells are removed from the circulation by the phagocytic cells, and the iron that they contain is salvaged for reuse. Abnormal red cells, such as those that are damaged by disease, are abnormal in shape, or contain a large amount of an abnormal hemoglobin, also are destroyed by the splenic phagocytes, which accounts for their shortened survival in the circulation.

The thymus is a bilobed lymphoid organ overlying the base of the heart. It is a large structure during infancy and childhood but gradually undergoes atrophy in adolescence. Only a remnant persists in the adult. The thymus plays an essential role in the prenatal development of the lymphoid system and in the formation of the body's immunologic defense mechanisms.

# Diseases of the Lymphatic System

The principal diseases affecting the lymphatic system are infections and neoplasms.

## Inflammation of the Lymph Nodes (Lymphadenitis)

Lymph nodes draining an area of infection may become enlarged and tender, resulting from spread of infection through the lymphatic channels and acute inflammation in the node. This is called lymphadenitis.

## Infectious Mononucleosis

Infectious mononucleosis is a relatively common viral disease. The virus belongs to the same family as the

herpesvirus that causes fever blisters. The virus has been named the **Epstein-Barr virus** (usually simply called *EB virus*). The disease is encountered most frequently in young adults and is transmitted by close contact, often by kissing. The virus causes an acute, debilitating, febrile illness associated with a diffuse hyperplasia of lymphoid tissue throughout the body. The lymphoid hyperplasia is manifested by a moderate increase of lymphocytes in the peripheral blood, enlargement and tenderness of lymph nodes, and some degree of splenic enlargement. The spleen, which normally weighs about 150 grams and is well protected under the rib cage in the upper abdomen, may double or triple in size and extend several centimeters below the left costal margin. The lymphocytes circulating in the peripheral blood show rather distinctive morphologic abnormalities, and the diagnosis can generally be made by the pathologist from a careful examination of the blood smear. The lymphocytes are larger than normal, with abundant deep blue cytoplasm and an irregularly shaped nucleus ( Figure 11-7 ). Enlargement and ulceration of lymphoid tissue in the throat is responsible for the sore throat often accompanying the disease.

The EB virus infects B lymphocytes, which proliferate actively during the first week of the infection. Then cytotoxic (CD8+) T lymphocytes and antibodies produced by plasma cells against the EB virus destroy the majority of the virus-infected cells, but some evade destruction and persist for life within the lymphatic system of the infected individual. The atypical lymphocytes seen in the blood are the activated cytotoxic T cells attacking the virus-infected cells. Many persons infected with EB virus never develop the clinical

**purpura**
(pur'pura) A condition characterized by hemorrhage in the skin and mucous membranes (petechiae and ecchymoses).
**Epstein-Barr virus** A virus that causes infectious mononucleosis.

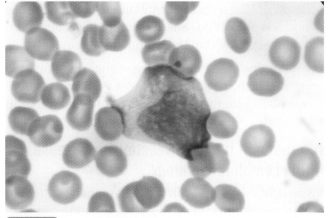

Figure 11-7   Large lymphocyte from subject with infectious mononucleosis, illustrating characteristic morphologic abnormalities, as described in text (original magnification × 1000).

manifestations of infectious mononucleosis because the body's defenses destroy the virus-infected cells. Only a small proportion of infected persons develop the elevated temperature, sore throat, enlarged spleen, and enlarged lymph nodes that are characteristic of the disease.

Generally, the disease is self-limited, and no specific treatment is required; however, it may be several weeks before the patient feels well again. Young adults recovering from infectious mononucleosis should avoid contact sports such as basketball, as long as the spleen remains enlarged and extends below the ribs into the upper abdomen. Any athletic activities that expose the upper abdomen to possible trauma may rupture the enlarged spleen, which is a very serious injury. Individuals with an impaired or suppressed immune system, such as persons with AIDS or persons who have had a bone marrow or organ transplant and are receiving treatment to suppress the immune system, may face another problem. The surviving infected B cells, unrestrained by the nonfunctional immune system, may become activated and proliferate extensively, giving rise to a malignant B cell lymphoma.

## Neoplasms Affecting Lymph Nodes

**Metastatic Tumors** Lymph nodes may be affected by the spread of metastatic tumor from malignant tumors arising in the breast, lung, colon, or other sites. The nodes first affected lie in the immediate drainage area of the tumor. The tumor may then spread to other, more distant lymph nodes through lymphatic channels and may eventually gain access to the circulatory system through the thoracic duct ( Figure 11-8 ).

**Malignant Lymphoma** A lymphoma is a primary malignant neoplasm of lymphoid tissue. The two main types of lymphoma are Hodgkin's disease and non-Hodgkin's lymphoma (Chapter 8). A lymphoma usually begins in a single lymph node or a small group of nodes but often spreads to other nodes; frequently, the disease becomes widespread. The spread of lymphoma to multiple groups of nodes is probably a consequence of the recirculation of lymphocytes within the lymphatic system.

**Lymphocytic Leukemia** Leukemia may develop from lymphoid cells in the bone marrow or from lymphoid tissue elsewhere in the body. Leukemia is covered in Chapter 8.

## Alteration of Immune Reactions in Diseases of the Lymphatic System

Because of the central role of the lymphatic system in immune reactions, many diseases affecting the lymphatic system diffusely, such as leukemias and lymphomas, may be associated with abnormal immune

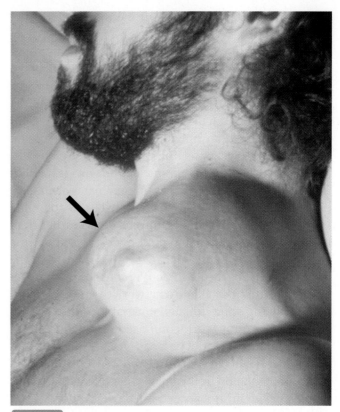

Figure 11-8 Large deposit of metastatic carcinoma in the supraclavicular lymph nodes of a young man with carcinoma of the testicle.

responses. These responses may be manifested either by production of autoantibodies directed against the red cells, white cells, or platelets of the affected individual, or by a loss of normal cell-mediated and humoral defenses that leads to an increased susceptibility to infection.

## The Enlarged Lymph Node as a Diagnostic Problem

The patient who visits a physician because one or more lymph nodes are enlarged may present a difficult diagnostic problem. Lymph node enlargement may be a manifestation of a localized infection in the area drained by the node. It may be caused by a systemic infection with initial manifestations in the node. It may be caused by metastatic tumor in the node, or it may be an early manifestation of leukemia or malignant lymphoma. Often the cause of the lymphadenopathy can be determined by the physician from the clinical evaluation of the patient in conjunction with laboratory studies, including an examination of the peripheral blood. Sometimes the cause cannot be established, however, and the physician must perform a lymph node biopsy to determine the reason for the enlargement. The enlarged lymph node is surgically excised and submitted to the pathologist for microscopic examination and microbiologic studies. In difficult cases, more elaborate and sophisticated studies may be required.

## The Role of the Spleen in Protection Against Systemic Infection

The spleen is an efficient blood-filtration system. Any bacteria or other foreign material that gains access to the bloodstream are promptly removed by the splenic phagocytes as the blood flows through the spleen. In addition, the spleen manufactures antibodies that facilitate prompt elimination of pathogenic organisms.

Sometimes it is necessary to remove the spleen. Splenectomy may be required to prevent fatal hemorrhage if the spleen has been lacerated in an automobile accident or other injury. Splenectomy may be performed on patients with blood diseases characterized by excessive destruction of blood cells within the spleen, such as thrombocytopenic purpura and some types of hereditary hemolytic anemia.

Splenectomized persons are less able to eliminate bacteria that gain access to the bloodstream and do not produce antibodies as well as before removal of the spleen. Consequently, they are more likely to develop serious bloodstream infections caused by pathogenic bacteria. To reduce this risk, splenectomized patients are often immunized with bacterial vaccines because high levels of antibacterial antibodies facilitate removal of bacteria from the circulation, and this can substitute for splenic function to some extent. Many physicians also recommend that a splenectomized patient begin taking antibiotics at the first sign of a respiratory infection or other febrile illness.

# CHAPTER REVIEW

## Questions for Review

1. What types of cells are found in the circulating blood, and what are their major functions?
2. What is anemia? What is the difference between an etiologic and a morphologic classification of anemia? Outline a simple etiologic classification of anemia.
3. What is an iron deficiency anemia? How does it arise? How is it treated? What is the morphologic appearance of the red cells?
4. What is the effect of vitamin $B_{12}$ and folic acid on blood cell maturation? What type of anemia results from deficiency of these vitamins?
5. What is the difference between an aplastic anemia and a hemolytic anemia? What is the difference between polycythemia and thrombocytopenia? What is hemochromatosis? What are its manifestations? How is the condition diagnosed and treated?
6. What is the lymphatic system? How is it organized? What are the major cells of the lymphatic system? What are the major functions of the lymphatic system?
7. What is the EB virus? What is its relationship to infectious mononucleosis? What are the clinical manifestations of infectious mononucleosis? How is the disease treated? What are some possible complications of the infection?
8. A patient has an enlarged lymph node. What types of diseases could produce lymph node enlargement? How does the physician arrive at a diagnosis when the patient presents with enlarged lymph nodes?
9. What types of altered immune reaction are sometimes encountered in diseases of the lymphatic system?
10. What are the functions of the spleen? What are the adverse effects of splenectomy?

## Supplementary Reading

Bain, B. 2005. Diagnosis from the blood smear. *New England Journal of Medicine* 353:498–507.

  Even in the "high-tech" era of medical practice, the blood smear remains a valuable diagnostic tool. Examination of a well-stained blood smear is essential whenever the results of a complete blood count indicate an abnormality. Methods are available to transmit photographs of atypical or abnormal blood smears to consultants for interpretation or second opinions.

Beers, M. H., Fletcher, A. J., Jones, T. V., and Porter, R. 2003. *The Merck Manual of Medical Information; Home Edition.* 2nd ed. New York: Simon & Schuster.

  Good sections on blood coagulation and hematology.

Hoagland, H. C. 1995. Myelodysplastic (preleukemic) syndromes: The bone marrow factory failure problem. *Mayo Clinic Proceedings* 70:673–77.

A review article.

Kark, J. A., Posey, D. M., Schumacher, H. R., and Ruehle, C. J. 1987. Sickle-cell trait as a risk factor for sudden death in physical training. *Journal of the American Medical Association* 317:782–86.

The association between sudden death and exertion is not widely appreciated. The prevalence of sickle cell trait is about 8 percent in the black population, and the incidence of sudden death related to exertion may be about 40 times higher than in the general population.

Likhite, V. V. 1976. Immunologic impairment and susceptibility to infection after splenectomy. *Journal of the American Medical Association* 236:1376–77.

Describes the adverse effects of splenectomy on phagocytosis of bacteria and on antibody formation.

Looker, A. C., Dallman, P. R., Carroll, M. D., et al. 1997. Prevalence of iron deficiency in the United States. *Journal of the American Medical Association* 277:973–76.

Iron deficiency and iron deficiency anemia are still common in toddlers, adolescent girls, and women of childbearing age.

Pagano, J. S. 2002. Viruses and lymphomas. *New England Journal of Medicine* 347:78–9.

A survey of the viruses that cause various types of lymphoid neoplasms, emphasizing the role of EB virus in both B cell and T cell lymphomas.

Pietrangelo, A. 2004. Hereditary hemochromatosis: A new look at an old disease. *New England Journal of Medicine* 350:2383–97.

Several different gene mutations may cause hemochromatosis. The most common cause is a specific mutation of paired HFE genes, and transmission is as an autosomal recessive trait; however, it is not possible to predict how the mutations will be expressed (gene penetrance) in a person homozygous for the mutant gene. Methods for detecting and evaluating hemochromatosis are described. Treatment depends on the manifestations of the disease in an affected person.

## Interactive Activities

### Multiple Choice

1. The usual survival of red cells in the circulation is

   A. 2 weeks
   B. 2 months
   C. 4 weeks
   D. 4 months

2. Which of the following conditions is NOT associated with megaloblastic anemia?

   A. Vitamin $B_{12}$ deficiency
   B. Folic acid deficiency
   C. Iron deficiency

3. A patient has a blood disease characterized by a greatly increased white blood cell count consisting of mature lymphocytes, with anemia and thrombocytopenia. The most likely diagnosis is

   A. Malignant lymphoma
   B. Acute lymphocytic leukemia
   C. Chronic lymphocytic leukemia
   D. Infectious mononucleosis

4. Which of the following statements regarding iron deficiency anemia is NOT true?

   A. May result from bleeding ulcer
   B. May result from excessive blood donations
   C. May result from deficiency of vitamins required for efficient iron absorption
   D. May result from excessive menstrual blood loss

### Critical Thinking

1. Mary Jones is a 23-year-old college student who has a moderate anemia. Her white count and platelets are normal. What possible causes of the anemia appear likely? What tests would you perform to confirm your initial impression?
2. An elderly man consulted his physician because of fatigue and enlarged lymph nodes. What possible conditions would you consider as diagnostic possibilities? What further studies would be helpful to make a diagnosis?

# The Respiratory System

## LEARNING OBJECTIVES

1. Explain the basic anatomic and physiologic principles of ventilation and gas exchange.

2. Describe the causes, clinical effects, complications, and treatment of pneumothorax and atelectasis.

3. Describe the histologic characteristics of a tuberculous infection. Explain the possible outcome of an infection. Describe methods of diagnosis and treatment.

4. Differentiate between bronchitis and bronchiectasis.

5. List the anatomic and physiologic derangements in chronic obstructive lung disease. Explain its

pathogenesis. Describe the clinical manifestations and methods of treatment.

6. Describe the pathogenesis and manifestations of bronchial asthma and respiratory distress syndrome.

7. Explain the causes and effects of pulmonary fibrosis. Describe the special problems associated with asbestosis.

8. List the major types of lung carcinoma. Describe the clinical manifestations of lung carcinoma and explain the principles of treatment.

## Oxygen Delivery: A Cooperative Effort

Normal life processes require that an adequate supply of oxygen be delivered to the tissues and that the waste products of cell metabolism be removed. These functions are carried out by a cooperative effort of the respiratory and circulatory systems. The respiratory system oxygenates the blood and removes carbon dioxide. The circulatory system transports these gases in the bloodstream.

# Structure and Function of the Lungs

The lungs consist of two distinct components: a system of tubes whose chief function is to conduct air into and out of the lungs and the alveoli (singular, alveolus), where oxygen and carbon dioxide are exchanged between air and the pulmonary capillaries. Just as a tree branches progressively and ends in a foliage of leaves, so the conducting tubes branch repeatedly and terminate in clusters of pulmonary alveoli. The lung is divided into several large segments called *lobes*. Each lobe in turn consists of a large number of smaller units called *lobules*. The architecture and structural features of a normal lung can be studied to best advantage when the lung is inflated and air dried (Figure 12-1A). The individual lobes, fissures, and pleural surfaces are well defined. The poorly defined cobblestonelike pattern of the pleural surface defines the location of the individual lung lobules, which frequently are accentuated by carbon pigment deposited in the connective tissue that surrounds and circumscribes the individual lobules. When sections of normal air-dried lung are examined against an illuminated background, one can appreciate the spongelike, fine structure of a normal lung, which is essential for normal gas exchange (Figure 12-1B).

**bronchus**
One of the large subdivisions of the trachea.

**bronchiole** (bron´ke-ōl)
One of the small terminal subdivisions of the branched bronchial tree.

**surfactant** (sur-fak´tant) A lipid material secreted by alveolar lining cells that facilitates respiration by decreasing the surface tension of the fluid lining the pulmonary alveoli.

## Bronchi, Bronchioles, and Alveoli

The largest conducting tubes are called **bronchi** (singular, *bronchus*). Tubes less than about 1 millimeter in diameter are called **bronchioles** (little bronchi), and the smallest bronchioles, which function only for conduction of air, are called *terminal bronchioles*. The tubes distal to the terminal bronchioles are called *respiratory bronchioles* because they have alveoli in their walls and not only transport air, but also participate in gas exchange. Each terminal bronchiole gives rise to several *respiratory bronchioles*, which branch to form alveolar ducts. The *alveolar ducts* in turn subdivide into *alveolar sacs*, and multiple *alveoli* in turn open into each alveolar sac (Figure 12-2A and Figure 12-2B).

Each alveolus is a small air space surrounded by a thin wall, the *alveolar septum*, which consists of thin-walled capillaries supported by a few connective tissue fibers and lined by a layer of epithelial cells (Figure 12-2C). Each alveolus contains a relatively small volume of air surrounded by a large network of capillaries, conditions that promote rapid diffusion of oxygen and carbon dioxide between alveolar air and pulmonary capillaries as the blood flows through the lung. Any condition that enlarges the pulmonary alveoli or reduces the number of pulmonary capillaries impedes the efficiency of pulmonary ventilation.

Two types of cells line the alveoli. Most are flat squamous cells. A few are larger secretory cells that produce a lipid material called **surfactant**, which reduces *surface tension*. Surface tension is the attraction between molecules of a fluid that cause the fluid to aggregate

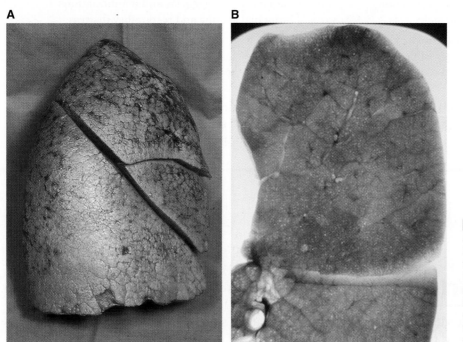

**A**

**B**

Figure 12-1 Normal lung that has been inflated and air dried so that the structure of the lobes and lobules can be visualized and the fine structure of the alveoli can be studied. **A,** External surface illustrating lobes and fissures. The faint cobblestonelike pattern of the pleural surface defines the individual lung lobules. **B,** A backlighted section of lung illustrating the fine, spongelike pattern produced by the respiratory units where gas exchange occurs.

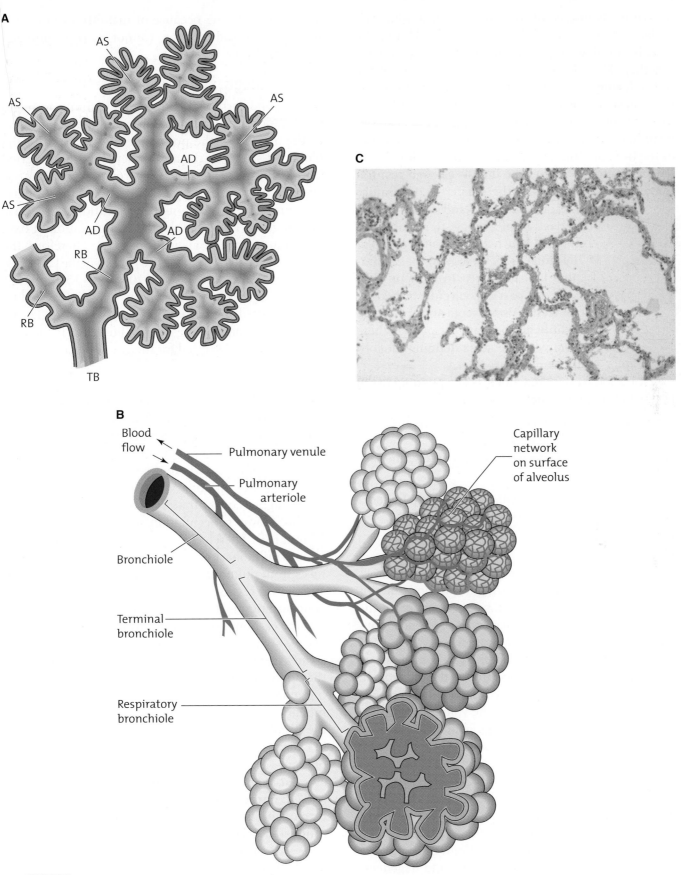

**Figure 12-2** **A,** Structure of a respiratory unit. Representative terminal bronchiole are designated TB. Alveolar ducts are designated AD, and alveolar sacs are designated AS. Multiple alveoli (not labeled) open into each alveolar sac. **B,** Structure of terminal air passages. The interior of one alveolar duct is illustrated in cut-away view. **C,** Histologic structure of the lung illustrating alveoli and thin alveolar septa containing pulmonary capillaries (original magnification × 100).

into droplets instead of spreading as a thin film. The surface tension of the molecules in the fluid lining the alveoli would normally tend to pull the alveolar walls together. This effect would hinder expansion of the lungs during inspiration and would cause the alveoli to collapse during expiration because of the cohesive force of the water molecules. Surfactant acts somewhat like a detergent by lowering the surface tension of the fluid and thereby facilitating respiration.

The functional unit of the lung is called a **respiratory unit**. It is formed by the cluster of respiratory bronchioles, alveolar ducts and sacs, and alveoli derived from a single terminal bronchiole. A *lung lobule* is a small group of terminal bronchioles and the respiratory units that arise from them. Lobules are partially circumscribed by connective tissue septa and are easiest to identify just beneath the pleura where the connective tissue septa defining the lobules can be easily seen (Figure 12-1A).

**respiratory unit** A functional unit of the lung consisting of a cluster of respiratory bronchioles, alveolar ducts, and alveoli derived from a single terminal bronchiole.

Respiration has two functions, corresponding to the two structural components of the lungs:

1. Ventilation, which concerns the movement of air into and out of the lungs
2. Gas exchange between alveolar air and pulmonary capillaries

Both ventilation and gas exchange must function normally if respiration is to be effective.

## Ventilation

Air is moved into and out of the lungs by the bellows action of the *thoracic cage*. During inspiration, the ribs become more horizontal because of the action of the intercostal muscles, and the diaphragm descends. Consequently, the volume of the thoracic cage increases. The lungs expand to fill the larger intrathoracic space, and air is drawn into the lungs through the trachea and bronchi. During expiration, the ribs become more vertical, and the diaphragm rises. The volume of the thoracic cage is reduced. The lungs, which conform to the size of the thorax, also decrease in volume, and air is expelled.

Normal respiratory movements require that respiratory muscles, innervation of the muscles, and mobility of the thoracic cage be normal. Ventilation is impaired if the nerve supply to the respiratory muscles is damaged by disease, as in poliomyelitis, or if the respiratory muscles undergo atrophy and degeneration, as in some uncommon types of muscle disease. Ventilation is also impaired if the thoracic cage is immobile. For example, a person buried in sand up to the neck will suffocate because of inability to move the thoracic cage and therefore cannot move air into and out of the lungs.

## Gas Exchange

Oxygen and carbon dioxide, along with nitrogen and water vapor, are in the atmospheric air that we breathe, in the air within the pulmonary alveoli, and in the blood. At sea level, the atmospheric pressure exerted by the mixture of all the gases is 760 mm Hg. Each gas exerts a proportionate part of the total atmospheric pressure, depending on its concentration in the mixture of gases. For example, the concentration of oxygen in atmospheric air is 20 percent. Therefore, the pressure exerted by oxygen is 20 percent of the total pressure exerted by all the gases ($0.20 \times 760 = 152$ mm Hg). The part of the total atmospheric pressure exerted by a gas is called the partial pressure of the gas. Partial pressure is usually expressed by the letter "P" preceding the chemical symbol for the gas; for example, $PO_2$ 152 mm Hg.

Gases diffuse between blood, tissues, and pulmonary alveoli because of differences in their partial pressures. Venous blood returning from the tissues is low in oxygen ($PO_2$ 40 mm Hg) and high in carbon dioxide ($PCO_2$ 47 mm Hg). This blood is pumped through the pulmonary capillaries, where it comes into contact with the air in the pulmonary alveoli. Alveolar air has a much higher concentration of oxygen ($PO_2$ 105 mm Hg) but a lower concentration of carbon dioxide ($PCO_2$ 35 mm Hg). Therefore, oxygen diffuses from alveolar air into pulmonary capillaries, and carbon dioxide diffuses from pulmonary capillaries into the aveoli. The situation is reversed in the tissues. The tissue oxygen concentration is much lower ($PO_2$ about 20 mm Hg), and the carbon dioxide concentration is much higher ($PCO_2$ about 60 mm Hg); so oxygen diffuses into the tissues from the blood, and carbon dioxide diffuses in the opposite direction.

Exchange of gases between alveolar air and pulmonary capillaries is accomplished by diffusion across the alveolar membrane. Efficient gas exchange requires (1) a large capillary surface area in contact with alveolar air, (2) unimpeded diffusion of gases across the alveolar membrane, (3) normal pulmonary blood flow, and (4) normal pulmonary alveoli. The spongy structure of the lungs, in which each tiny air sac is surrounded by a large network of capillaries, provides the large surface area required for efficient gas exchange (Figure 12-3A). Destruction of alveolar septa leads to coalescence of alveoli and a reduction in the size of the capillary network surrounding the alveoli, resulting in less efficient gas exchange (Figure 12-3B).

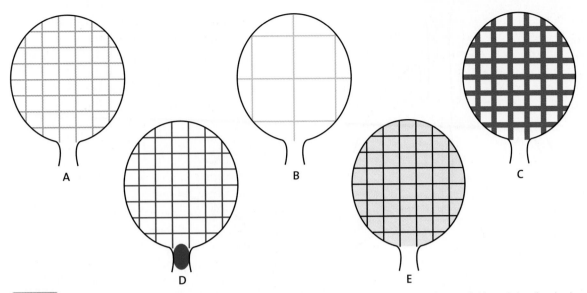

**Figure 12-3** Types of structural and functional abnormalities that adversely affect pulmonary gas exchange. **A,** Normal alveoli and pulmonary blood flow. **B,** Destruction of alveolar septa, leading to coarsening of alveolar structure with corresponding reduction in size of pulmonary capillary bed. **C,** Fibrous thickening *and* scarring of alveolar septa, impeding diffusion of gases across alveolar membrane. **D,** Obstruction of pulmonary blood flow to a part of the lung. **E,** Alveoli filled with fluid or inflammatory exudate.

If the alveolar septa are thickened and scarred, the diffusion of gases across the thickened alveolar membranes is impeded (Figure 12-3C). Gas exchange is also impaired if pulmonary blood flow to a portion of the lung is obstructed, as might be caused by a pulmonary embolus obstructing a large pulmonary artery or by blockage of pulmonary capillaries by fat emboli or foreign material (Figure 12-3D). If the pulmonary alveoli become filled with fluid or inflammatory exudate, inspired air cannot enter the diseased alveoli, and pulmonary gas exchange is impeded (Figure 12-3E).

## Pulmonary Function Tests

Pulmonary function tests can be used to evaluate the efficiency of pulmonary ventilation and pulmonary gas exchange. Pulmonary ventilation is usually tested by measuring the volume of air that can be moved into and out of the lung under standard conditions. Two commonly used measurements are **vital capacity**, which measures the maximum volume of air that can be expelled after a deep inspiration, and the **one-second forced expiratory volume (FEV$_1$)**, which measures the maximum volume of air that can be expelled in 1 second. If the bronchioles are narrowed by inflammation or spasm, impeding the movement of air out of the lungs, FEV$_1$ is often reduced. Specialized tests can measure the total volume of air in the lungs and the volume of air remaining in the lungs after a maximum expiration.

The concentrations of oxygen and carbon dioxide (O$_2$ and CO$_2$) in the patient's arterial blood can also be measured in order to determine the efficiency of gas exchange in the lungs. In chronic pulmonary disease, oxygenation of the blood is inefficient. Oxygen concentration is reduced, and arterial oxygen saturation is decreased correspondingly. Often the arterial PCO$_2$ also is higher than normal because carbon dioxide is inefficiently eliminated by the lungs. Arterial blood for analysis is usually collected by inserting a small needle into the radial artery in the wrist and withdrawing a small amount of blood. One can also determine how effectively the lungs are oxygenating the blood (arterial oxygen saturation) using a device called a *pulse oximeter.* A fingertip is inserted into the device, which measures photoelectrically the changes in light absorption of the hemoglobin in the fingertip capillaries at various wavelengths during systole and diastole. Then the data are used to calculate automatically the oxygen saturation of the arterial blood, and the device promptly displays the result.

## The Pleural Cavity

The lungs are covered by a thin membrane called the **pleura**, which also extends over the internal surface of the chest wall. Because the lungs fill the thoracic cavity, the two pleural surfaces are in contact. The potential space between the lung and chest wall is the *pleural cavity.* Normally, the apposing pleural surfaces move smoothly over one another. In disease, however, the pleural surfaces may become roughened because of inflammation and may become adherent. Inflammatory exudate

**vital capacity**
The maximum volume of air that can be forcefully expelled after a maximum inspiration.

**one-second forced expiratory volume (FEV$_1$)**
The maximum volume of air that can be expelled from the lungs in one second.

**pleura** (plŏŏr′äh) The mesothelial covering of the lung (*visceral pleura*) and chest wall (*parietal pleura*).

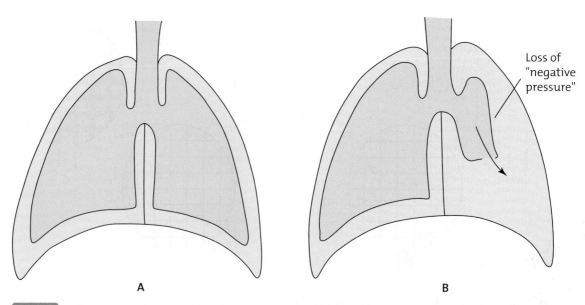

**Figure 12-4** **A,** Normal relation of lung to chest wall. Pleural space is exaggerated, and surfaces are normally in contact. "Negative pressure" is primarily a result of the tendency of the stretched lung to pull away from the chest wall. **B,** Pneumothorax caused by a perforating injury of lung, allowing the air under atmospheric pressure to escape into the pleural cavity.

Loss of "negative pressure"

may accumulate in the pleural cavity and separate the two pleural surfaces.

**Intrapleural and Intrapulmonary Pressures** The lungs are held in an expanded position within the pleural cavity because the pressure within the pleural cavity (*intrapleural pressure*) is less than the pressure of the air within the lungs (*intrapulmonary pressure*). The pressure differences develop when the thoracic cavity enlarges after birth. When respirations are initiated, the size of the thoracic cavity increases. The lungs become filled with air at atmospheric pressure and expand to fill the enlarged thoracic cavity, stretching the elastic tissue within the lungs. The tendency of the stretched lung to pull away from the chest wall and return to its original contracted state creates a slight vacuum within the pleural cavity. Because the intrapleural pressure is slightly less than atmospheric pressure, it is often called "negative pressure."

# Pneumothorax

Because the intrapleural pressure is subatmospheric, air flows into the pleural space if the lung or chest wall is punctured. When this occurs, the subatmospheric ("negative") pressure that holds the lung in the expanded position is lost, and the lung collapses because the elastic tissue within the lung contracts. This condition, which is called a *pneumothorax* (*pneumo* = air), may follow any type of lung injury or pulmonary disease that allows air to escape from the lungs into

the pleural space. It may also result from a stab wound or some other penetrating injury to the chest wall that permits atmospheric air to enter the pleural space (Figure 12-4).

Occasionally, a pneumothorax occurs without apparent cause. This is called spontaneous pneumothorax. Most cases occur in young healthy persons, usually as a result of rupture of a small, air-filled, subpleural bleb at the apex of the lung.

The sudden escape of air into the pleural cavity that is associated with any type of pneumothorax usually causes chest discomfort and often some shortness of breath. The breath sounds, which normally can be heard with a stethoscope when the air moves in and out of the lung during respiration, are diminished on the affected side. A chest x-ray reveals partial or complete collapse of the lung and the presence of air in the pleural cavity (Figure 12-5).

The development of a positive (higher than atmospheric) pressure in the pleural cavity is called a *tension pneumothorax* or alternatively *a positive pressure pneumothorax*. A high intrapleural pressure may accompany any type of pneumothorax. This dangerous complication may occur if the lung has been perforated in such a way that the pleural tear acts as a one-way valve (Figure 12-6). In this circumstance, air flows through the perforation into the pleural cavity as the intrapleural pressure falls on inspiration. On expiration, however, the intrapleural pressure rises and forces the edges of the pleural tear together, trapping the air within the pleural space. With each inspiration,

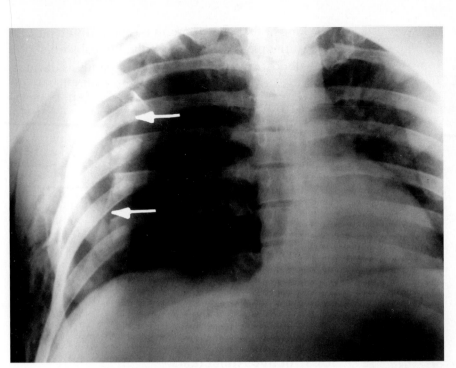

Figure 12-5 X-ray illustrating pneumothorax secondary to multiple rib fractures in which broken ends of fractured ribs have torn through the pleura and torn underlying lung. The *arrows* indicate the surface of lung that is no longer in contact with chest wall.

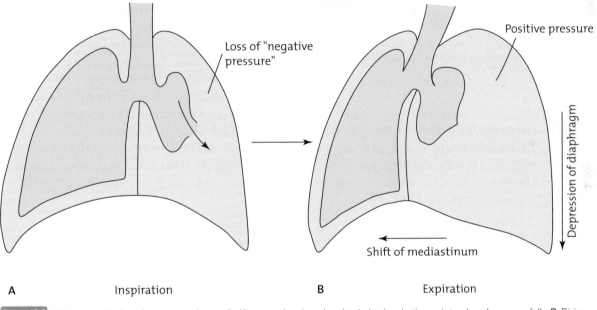

Loss of "negative pressure"

Positive pressure

Depression of diaphragm

Shift of mediastinum

A          Inspiration          B          Expiration

Figure 12-6 Pathogenesis of tension pneumothorax. A, Air enters the pleural cavity during inspiration as intrapleural pressure falls. B, Rising intrapleural pressure on expiration closes the pleural tear, trapping air within the pleural space. The diaphragm on affected side is displaced downward. The trachea and mediastinal structures are shifted away from side of pneumothorax and encroach on opposite pleural cavity.

more air enters the pleural cavity but cannot escape. Eventually, the pleural cavity becomes overdistended with air under pressure, and the affected lung collapses completely. As the pressure builds up in the pleural cavity, the heart and mediastinal structures are displaced away from the side of the pneumothorax and encroach on the opposite pleural cavity, impairing the expansion of the opposite lung (Figure 12-7). A ten-

sion pneumothorax can be fatal if it is not recognized and treated promptly by evacuating the trapped air to relieve the pressure.

A pneumothorax is usually treated by inserting a tube into the pleural cavity through an incision in the chest wall. The tube prevents accumulation of air in the pleural cavity and aids re-expansion of the lung. The tube is connected to an apparatus that permits

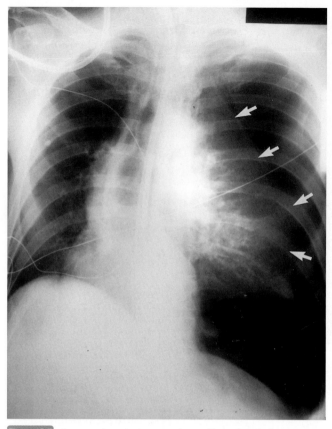

**atelectasis**
(ah-tel-ek´tuh-sis)
Collapse of the lung, either caused by bronchial obstruction (*obstructive atelectasis*) or external compression (*compression atelectasis*).

the lung heals and no more air escapes. Any air remaining in the pleural cavity is gradually reabsorbed into the bloodstream, and the lung re-expands as the air is absorbed. Sometimes a slight vacuum is applied to the tube in order to evacuate the air more rapidly and hasten re-expansion of the lung.

# Atelectasis

**Atelectasis** literally means incomplete expansion of the lung (*ateles* = incomplete + *ectasia* = expansion). It refers to a collapse of parts of the lung. There are two types:

1. Obstructive atelectasis, which results from bronchial obstruction
2. Compression atelectasis, which results from external compression of the lung

## Obstructive Atelectasis

Complete blockage of a bronchus by thick mucous secretions, by a tumor, or by an aspirated foreign object prevents air from entering or leaving the alveoli supplied by the blocked bronchus, and the air already present is gradually absorbed into the blood flowing through the lungs. As a result, the part of the lung supplied by the blocked bronchus gradually collapses as the air is absorbed. The volume of the affected pleural cavity also decreases correspondingly, causing the mediastinal structures to shift toward the side of the atelectasis and the diaphragm to elevate on the affected side (Figure 12-8). If the bronchial obstruction is relieved promptly, the lung re-expands normally. This is

the air to be expelled from the pleural cavity during expiration but prevents the air from being sucked back into the pleural cavity during inspiration. The tube is left in place until the tear in

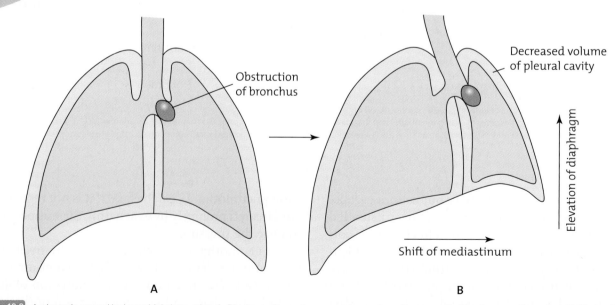

Obstruction of bronchus

Decreased volume of pleural cavity

Elevation of diaphragm

Shift of mediastinum

A

B

**Figure 12-8** Atelectasis caused by bronchial obstruction. **A,** Blockage of bronchus prevents aeration of lung supplied by obstructed bronchus. **B,** Absorption of air causes collapse of the lung and a corresponding reduction in size of the pleural cavity. The diaphragm rises, and the mediastinum shifts toward the affected side.

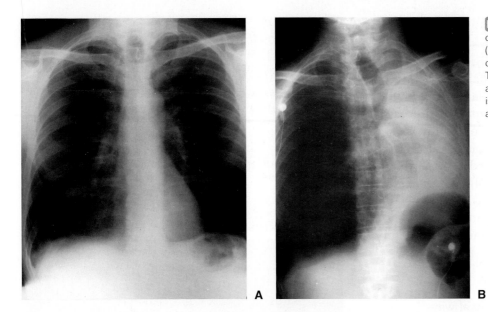

Figure 12-9 Complete atelectasis of the left lung caused by obstruction of left main bronchus (Case 12-1). **A,** Chest x-ray before development of atelectasis. **B,** Atelectasis of entire left lung. The collapsed lung appears dense because the air has been absorbed. The left half of diaphragm is elevated. Trachea and mediastinal structures are shifted toward the side of the collapse.

## Case Study 12-1

A 66-year-old man with a long history of heavy smoking and excessive alcohol consumption consulted his physician because of shortness of breath. He was found to have an atelectasis of the left lung ( Figure 12-9 ). An obstructing carcinoma was suspected, and a bronchoscopic examination was performed. A soft rubber stopper was found obstructing the left main bronchus. The subject had been chewing the stopper and had accidentally inhaled it. The stopper was removed. An x-ray taken the following day revealed that the lung had re-expanded completely.

illustrated by Case 12-1, obstructive atelectasis, which was initially thought to be secondary to an obstructing lung carcinoma.

Atelectasis sometimes develops as a postoperative complication. Because of postoperative pain, the patient does not cough or breathe deeply and mucous secretions accumulate in the bronchi ( Figure 12-10 ). To prevent this problem, the physician encourages the postoperative patient to breathe deeply and cough frequently to keep the respiratory passages clear of secretions.

## Compression Atelectasis

Compression atelectasis results when fluid, blood, or air accumulates in the pleural cavity, reducing its volume and thereby preventing full expansion of the lung.

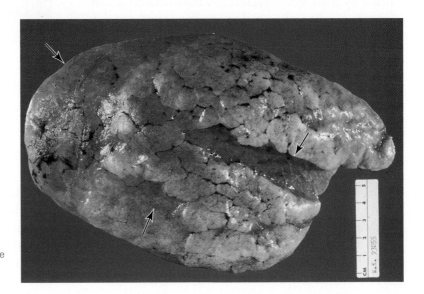

Figure 12-10 Atelectasis of several lung lobules caused by retained mucous secretions. Note the contrast between the pale normally aerated lung and the atelectatic areas (*arrows*), which appear dark and depressed.

# Pneumonia

Pneumonia is an inflammation of the lung characterized by the same type of vascular changes and exudation of fluid and cells as that of inflammation in any other location. However, the inflammatory process is influenced by the spongy character of the lungs. The inflammatory exudate spreads unimpeded through the lung, filling the alveoli, and the affected portions of lung become relatively solid, which is called *consolidation* (Figure 12-11A). The inflammatory exudate may reach the pleural surface in some areas, causing irritation and inflammation of the pleura; sometimes inflammatory exudate accumulates in the pleural space.

## Classification of Pneumonia

Pneumonia may be classified in several ways:

1. By etiology
2. By anatomic distribution of the inflammatory process
3. By predisposing factors that led to its development

The etiologic classification is the most important because it serves as a guide to treatment. Pneumonia may be caused by bacteria, chlamydiae, mycoplasmas, rickettsiae, viruses, or fungi. Whenever possible, the pneumonia is classified in greater detail by designating the exact organism responsible for the infection, such as the pneumococcus, staphylococcus, mycoplasma, or a pathogenic virus.

The anatomic classification describes what part of the lung is involved (Figure 12-11). Lobar pneumonia refers to an infection of an entire lung lobe. Bronchopneumonia describes an infection involving only parts of one or more lobes (lung lobules) adjacent to the bronchi. Lobar pneumonia and bronchopneumonia are infections caused by pathogenic bacteria. A third anatomic classification is called *interstitial pneumonia* or *primary atypical pneumonia* and is usually caused by a virus or mycoplasma (*Mycoplasma pneumoniae*). This type of pulmonary infection involves the pulmonary alveolar septa rather than the alveoli, and the inflammatory cells infiltrating the septa are primarily lymphocytes, monocytes, and plasma cells rather than neutrophils.

Classification of pneumonia by predisposing factors is common. Any condition associated with poor lung ventilation and retention of bronchial secretions predisposes an individual to the development of pneumonia. Postoperative pneumonia is a pulmonary inflammation that develops in the postsurgical patient who is unable to cough or breathe deeply because of pain; the resultant poor ventilation and retention of secretions predisposes to atelectasis of lung lobules, which is

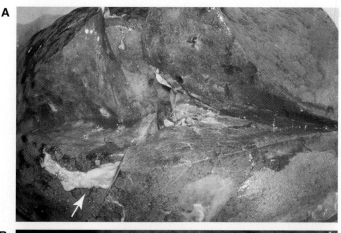

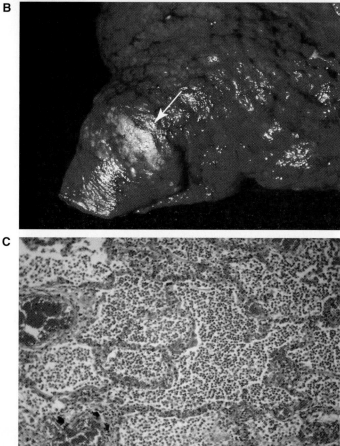

**Figure 12-11** **A,** Consolidation of lung lobe caused by lobar pneumonia. The lung has been incised, and cut surfaces are exposed. An *arrow* indicates a deposit of fibrin on pleura. **B,** Bronchopneumonia. Inflammation involves lung lobules rather than an entire lobe. An *arrow* indicates the most severely involved lobules. **C,** Histologic appearance of pneumonia. Alveoli are filled with neutrophils, and no air can enter the affected alveoli (original magnification × 100).

followed by secondary bacterial invasion leading to bronchopneumonia. Aspiration pneumonia occurs when a foreign body, food, vomit, or other irritating substance is aspirated into the lung. Obstructive pneumonia develops in the lung distal to an area where a bronchus is narrowed or obstructed. Blockage of a bronchus by a tumor or foreign body leads to poor aeration and to retention of bronchial secretions in the obstructed part of the lung, which predisposes to infection.

## Clinical Features of Pneumonia

The signs and symptoms of pneumonia are those of any systemic infection. The patient is ill and has an elevated temperature, and the number of white blood cells in the peripheral blood is frequently higher than normal. Bronchial inflammation is evident, manifested by cough and purulent sputum. If the inflammatory process involves the pleura, the patient experiences pain on respiration because the inflamed pleural surfaces rub against each other. The patient may also have symptoms related to partial loss of lung function caused by consolidation of part of the lung resulting from the accumulation of inflammatory cells within the alveoli. Oxygenation of the blood is impaired, and the patient may become quite short of breath.

Pneumonia is treated by correcting any predisposing factors that contributed to the development of the pulmonary infection and administering appropriate antibiotic therapy.

**Legionnaires' disease** is a type of pneumonia caused by a gram-negative, rod-shaped bacterium called *Legionella pneumophila* that is widely distributed in the environment: in the soil and in freshwater ponds, lakes, and streams. The organism thrives in moist environments such as air conditioning ducts, shower heads, and humidifiers. People become infected by inhaling airborne organisms in aerosolized water droplets. The infection is not transmitted directly from person to person. Clinically, the disease is characterized by the usual symptoms of a pulmonary infection, and the chest x-ray reveals evidence of pneumonia. The infection responds to appropriate antibiotics.

## Pneumocystis Pneumonia

Humans and many animals harbor a protozoan parasite of low pathogenicity named *Pneumocystis jiroveci*, also called by its older name *Pneumocystis carinii*. The parasite is a normal inhabitant of the respiratory passages and does not affect normal persons but may cause serious pulmonary infections in susceptible individuals. Those at risk include adults whose immune defenses have been impaired by disease, such as by AIDS (Chapter 6), or by administration of immunosuppressive drugs, and premature infants in whom immune defenses are poorly developed.

Clinically, pneumocystis pneumonia is characterized by progressive shortness of breath and cough in a person whose immunologic defenses are impaired and who is at high risk of developing the disease. Evidence

of pulmonary consolidation caused by the alveolar exudate can be demonstrated by a chest x-ray. The diagnosis of pneumocystis pneumonia is established by biopsy of lung tissue obtained by bronchoscopy, which reveals large numbers of small round parasites, demonstrable by special stains, intermixed with a protein-rich exudate. Several different antibiotics are available to treat the infection.

# Tuberculosis

Pulmonary tuberculosis is a special type of pneumonia caused by an acid-fast bacterium, the tubercle bacillus *Mycobacterium tuberculosis*. Because the tubercle bacillus has a capsule composed of waxes and fatty substances, it is more resistant to destruction than many other organisms. The body's response to the tubercle bacillus also differs from the usual acute inflammatory reaction. Monocytes accumulate around the bacteria; many of them fuse, forming rather characteristic large multinucleated cells called *giant cells*. Lymphocytes and plasma cells also accumulate, and fibrous tissue proliferates around the central cluster of monocytes and giant cells. The central portion of the cellular aggregation usually becomes necrotic. This characteristic nodular mass of cells with central necrosis is called a *granuloma*, and the inflammatory process is called a *granulomatous inflammation* (Figure 12-12). The granulomatous response to the tubercle bacillus and the necrosis within the granulomas indicate the development of cell-mediated immunity against the organism, which is the primary immune defense against the tubercle bacillus.

**Legionnaires' disease** A type of pneumonia caused by an airborne bacterium called *Legionella pneumophila*.

## Course of a Tuberculous Infection

The initial infection is acquired from organisms inhaled in airborne droplets that have been coughed or sneezed into the air by a person with active tuberculosis who is discharging organisms into the environment. The organisms lodge within the pulmonary alveoli where they proceed to multiply. Initially, the organisms introduced into the lungs do not elicit a marked inflammatory reaction because they do not produce any toxins or destructive enzymes that damage the tissues. Macrophages phagocytose the bacteria but are unable to destroy them; they may even carry the organisms to other parts of the lung and into the regional lymph nodes. After several weeks, however, a cell-mediated immunity develops. Sensitized lymphocytes attract and activate macrophages, which acquire a greatly enhanced phagocytic and destructive capability. The activated macrophages attack and destroy many of the organisms,

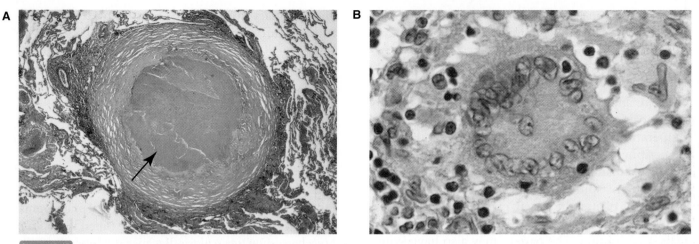

**Figure 12-12** **A,** Granuloma as a result of tuberculosis. The central part (*arrow*) consists of necrotic tissue (original magnification × 40). **B,** Multinucleated giant cell characteristic of tuberculosis infection (original magnification × 400).

forming characteristic granulomas containing areas of necrosis and surrounded by a rim of fibrous tissue. In the majority of cases, the infection is arrested; the granulomas in the lung and regional lymph nodes heal with scarring, often followed by calcification of the granulomas. In most cases, the infection does not cause any symptoms, and the person may be unaware of the infection. Sometimes the granuloma in the lung is large enough to be identified in a chest x-ray, but often the area of infection is too small to be detected in an x-ray. The positive skin test (Mantoux test), which reveals a hypersensitivity to the proteins of the tubercle bacillus, may be the only evidence of recent infection.

Cell-mediated immunity generally controls the infection, and the arrested infection may never cause any further problems. The healed granulomas, however, may contain small numbers of viable organisms, and the infection may become reactivated, leading to progressive pulmonary tuberculosis if the body's cell-mediated immunity declines.

Not all primary infections respond as favorably. If a large number of organisms are inhaled or if the body's defenses are inadequate, the inflammation will progress, causing more extensive destruction of lung tissue (Figure 12-13). Often the granulomatous inflammatory process makes contact with a bronchus, and the necrotic

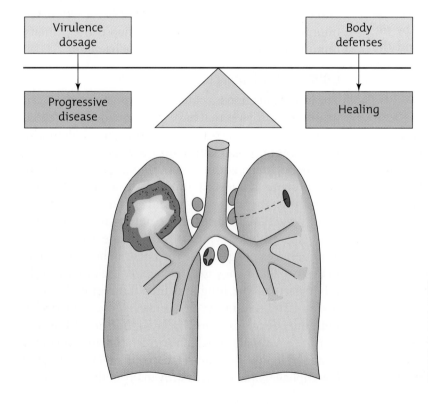

**Figure 12-13** Possible outcome of a tuberculosis infection in relation to virulence and dosage of the organism and resistance of the body. The frequent involvement of the regional lymph nodes is indicated. *Left,* progressive disease with formation of cavity within lung, caused by infection by a large number of organisms or inadequate body defenses. *Right,* healing with scarring as a result of small numbers of organisms or a high degree of resistance to infection.

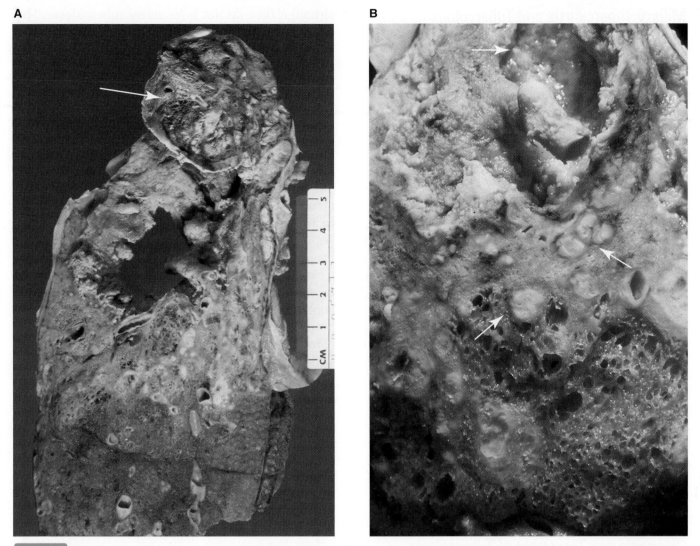

**Figure 12-14** Far-advanced pulmonary tuberculosis. **A,** The upper lobe (*arrow*) has been completely destroyed by tuberculosis, and there is extensive tuberculosis in the lower lobe with a large cavity in the lung that communicates with a bronchus. Only the lower part of the lobe is free of disease (*extreme bottom* of photograph). **B,** A closer view of tuberculosis. A large cavity (*upper arrow*) surrounded by nodular and diffuse granulomatous inflammation. Several discrete granulomas (*lower arrows*) can be seen below the cavity.

inflammatory tissue is discharged into it. A cavity then forms within the lung, surrounded by granulomatous inflammatory tissue containing masses of tubercle bacilli (Figure 12-14). People who have active progressive tuberculosis with a tuberculous cavity can infect others because they discharge large numbers of tubercle bacilli in their sputum. In a tuberculous infection of the lung, organisms are often carried in lymphatic channels from the lung into the peribronchial lymph nodes, leading to a tuberculous inflammation in the regional lymph nodes.

Many cases of active progressive pulmonary tuberculosis do not result from the initial infection. They develop in persons who have been infected at some time in the past and have developed a cell-mediated immunity directed against the organism. In the past,

tuberculosis in previously infected persons was called reinfection tuberculosis because physicians believed that the active tuberculosis was caused by a new infection with the tubercle bacillus in a person who had been infected previously with the organism. Indeed, some cases of tuberculosis in previously infected persons are actually new infections. However, most cases of active tuberculosis in older patients result from a reactivation of an old infection rather than a new infection with the tubercle bacillus. It is well known that old tuberculosis lesions that appear completely healed may harbor tubercle bacilli. If the resistance of the individual is lowered by AIDS or other debilitating diseases, by treatment with adrenal corticosteroids, or by other factors, an apparently healed focus of tuberculosis may flare up and lead to active progressive tuberculosis.

## Miliary Tuberculosis and Tuberculous Pneumonia

Miliary tuberculosis and tuberculous pneumonia are two uncommon but extremely serious forms of tuberculosis. *Miliary tuberculosis* develops if a mass of tuberculous inflammatory tissue erodes into a large blood vessel, disseminating large numbers of organisms throughout the body through the bloodstream. The term *miliary* is derived from the resemblance of the multiple foci of disseminated tuberculosis (present in liver, spleen, kidney, and other tissues) to millet seeds. These foci are small white nodules from about 1 to 2 millimeters in diameter. *Tuberculous pneumonia* is an overwhelming infection characterized by extensive tuberculous consolidation of one or more lobes of the lung. Persons with AIDS and other immunocompromised persons are prone to this type of rapidly progressive infection.

## Extrapulmonary Tuberculosis

Sometimes tuberculosis develops in the kidneys, bone, uterus, fallopian tubes, or other extrapulmonary location. The infection results from hematogenous spread of tubercle bacilli from a focus of tuberculosis in the lung. Sometimes, the secondary focus of infection may progress even though the pulmonary infection has healed, leading to an active extrapulmonary tuberculous infection without clinically apparent pulmonary tuberculosis.

## Diagnosis and Treatment of Tuberculosis

Tuberculous infection is associated with the development of hypersensitivity to proteins in the tubercle bacillus (Chapter 4). A positive skin test (Mantoux test) indicates that the person was at one time infected with the tubercle bacillus; it does not necessarily indicate an active infection. At present, many physicians recommend that people who develop an infection with the tubercle bacillus, as manifested by conversion of a negative into a positive skin test reaction, be treated with antituberculosis drugs. Treatment is also recommended for patients with inactive tuberculosis who have an increased risk of developing a reactivation of an old, apparently healed tuberculosis infection.

Unfortunately, the frequency of tuberculosis, which declined steadily from about 1950 to 1980, began to rise at an alarming rate in the United States, and a number of factors appear to be responsible for the increase. A large number of persons have immigrated to the United States from Asia, Africa, and Latin American countries, where the prevalence of tuberculosis is much higher. Many of these persons have been infected, although they do not have active tuberculosis. This group serves as a reservoir of infected persons in whom active tuberculosis can develop if immunity declines, which in turn may be followed by infection of other persons with whom they are in close contact. Social problems of poverty, drug abuse, alcoholism, and homelessness create conditions favoring transmission of tuberculosis from person to person. Many of these unfortunate persons with active tuberculosis do not receive adequate ongoing medical care; they also may not be motivated to complete the full course of treatment needed to arrest the disease. Failure to complete treatment leads to treatment failure, and premature cessation of treatment also promotes the emergence of drug-resistant strains of the organism. Tuberculosis is treated by a number of different antibiotics and chemotherapeutic agents. Drug-resistant tuberculosis is becoming a major problem, and a significant proportion of tubercle bacilli are now resistant to one or more of the drugs commonly used to treat the infection. Drug-resistant tuberculosis is more difficult to treat. The course of treatment is more prolonged, and the results of treatment are less satisfactory.

Tuberculosis remains a serious problem, and unrecognized cases may expose many susceptible individuals, as illustrated by the following example.

### Case Study 12-2

A 17-year-old female high school student developed a dry cough accompanied by weakness and fatigue, elevated temperature, chills, and a 15-pound weight loss. She had also recently noted that she became short of breath after climbing two flights of stairs. Previously, she had lived for a time with an uncle who had tuberculosis. Examination revealed extensive consolidation in the upper part of both lungs as a result of tuberculosis ( Figure 12-15 ). Smears and cultures of sputum revealed tubercle bacilli. She was hospitalized and received a course of antituberculosis drug therapy. Her school was contacted, and steps were taken to check other students with whom she had had contact for possible tuberculosis infection. The infection slowly responded to therapy, and she was later released from the hospital to continue treatment as an outpatient.

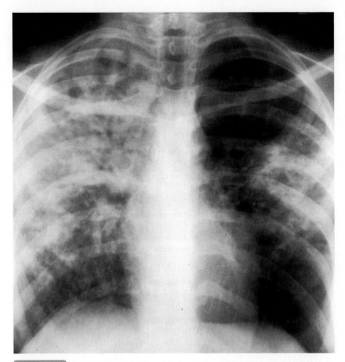

**Figure 12-15** Chest x-ray of high school student with far-advanced pulmonary tuberculosis, illustrating extensive consolidation of both lungs (Case 12-2).

# Bronchitis and Bronchiectasis

Acute inflammation of the tracheobronchial mucosa is common in many upper respiratory infections. The raw throat and cough associated with many respiratory infections are a result of the associated acute bronchitis. Chronic bronchitis also is common; often it results from constant irritation of the respiratory mucosa by smoking cigarettes or breathing air containing large amounts of atmospheric pollution.

Sometimes the bronchial walls in parts of the lung become weakened as a result of severe inflammation or other factors, and the affected bronchi become markedly dilated. This condition is called **bronchiectasis** (*ectasis* = dilation). The distended bronchi tend to retain secretions. Consequently, patients with bronchiectasis frequently have a chronic cough associated with production of large amounts of purulent sputum. Often they suffer repeated bouts of pulmonary infection. The only effective treatment of bronchiectasis is surgical resection of the affected segments of lung.

**bronchiectasis**
(bron-kē′-ek′tuh-sis)
Dilatation of bronchi caused by weakening of their walls as a result of infection.

# Chronic Obstructive Lung Disease

Pulmonary emphysema is a disease in which the air spaces distal to the terminal bronchioles are enlarged and their walls are destroyed. The disease is an important cause of disability and death, and its incidence is increasing at an alarming rate. In emphysema, the normally fine alveolar structure of the lung is destroyed, and large, cystic air spaces form throughout the lung (Figure 12-16). The destructive process usually begins in the upper lobes but eventually may affect all lobes of both lungs. Usually there is an associated chronic inflammation of the terminal bronchioles. Emphysema and chronic bronchitis occur together so frequently that they are usually considered a single entity, designated

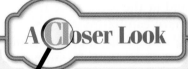

*The development of the first antibiotic effective against tuberculosis was an important contribution to medicine, but was accompanied by much turmoil among the participants.*

The drug was streptomycin, which is an antibiotic agent produced by the mold *Streptomyces griseus*. The person attributed to the discovery was Selman Waksman, who also coined the term *antibiotic*. He was a professor of biochemistry and microbiology at Rutgers University in New Jersey. He had been studying the *Streptomyces* family for many years and had identified many different antibiotics produced by these organisms. He was awarded the Nobel Prize in 1952 for the discovery of streptomycin, the first antibiotic effective against tuberculosis. Streptomycin was patented and the royalties were used in part to fund the Waksman Institute of Microbiology at Rutgers University. Actually, much of the work on the discovery was performed by a graduate student in his department named Albert Schatz, who strongly objected to not being recognized as a co-discoverer and not sharing in the royalties from the discovery. Schatz brought suit against Waksman and Rutgers for being excluded, and also to claim credit for his role in the discovery, and for a share of the royalties. Shatz's requests were granted in an out-of-court settlement.

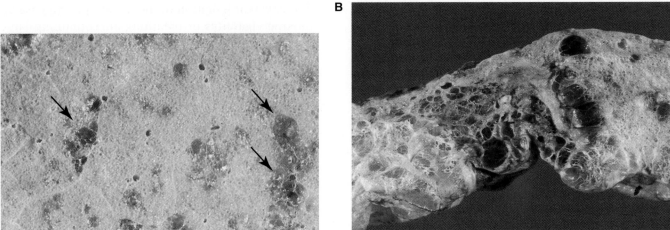

**Figure 12-16** Sections of air-dried lung preparations illustrating the gross appearance of emphysema. **A,** Mild emphysema. Beginning breakdown of lung tissue to form cystic spaces (*arrows*). Most of the alveoli appear normal. **B,** Advanced emphysema with multiple confluent cystic spaces within lung. Very little normal lung tissue remains. The dark color is a result of accumulation of carbon pigment in the emphysematous lung from inhaling "dirty" air.

chronic obstructive pulmonary disease, or simply COPD. The chief clinical manifestations of any type of chronic pulmonary disease are dyspnea and cyanosis. *Dyspnea* is a sensation of shortness of breath. *Cyanosis* is a blue tinge of the skin and mucous membrane that results from an excessive amount of reduced hemoglobin in the blood. Reduced hemoglobin is dark purplish red, in contrast with normally oxygenated blood, which is bright red.

**chronic obstructive pulmonary disease (COPD)** A chronic pulmonary disease characterized by emphysema and coexisting chronic bronchitis.

The three main anatomic derangements in chronic obstructive pulmonary disease are (1) inflammation and narrowing of the terminal bronchioles, (2) dilatation and coalescence of pulmonary air spaces, and (3) loss of lung elasticity. These derangements in turn cause severe disturbances in pulmonary function.

## Derangements of Pulmonary Structure and Function

Chronic inflammation of the bronchioles probably initiates the destructive process. Chronic inflammation causes swelling of the bronchial mucosa, which reduces the caliber of the bronchi and bronchioles and stimulates increased bronchial secretions. Because a tube's resistance to air flow varies with the fourth power of its diameter, a slight reduction in the caliber of the bronchioles greatly restricts the flow of air. Normally, the bronchi and bronchioles dilate slightly during inspiration and become smaller during expiration. Consequently, air can enter the lungs more readily than it can be expelled through the narrowed bronchioles; so air tends to become trapped in the lungs during expiration. The lungs cannot empty completely, and they become chronically overinflated. As a result, the amount of additional air that can be inspired when the subject takes a deep breath is much reduced, and the subject is unable to increase his or her ventilation adequately in response to increased demand.

The bronchiolar obstruction also disturbs pulmonary function by causing unequal air flow to various parts of the lung. Some alveoli are overventilated; others are inadequately supplied, reducing the overall efficiency of pulmonary ventilation. The excess air supplying the overventilated alveoli is "wasted" because more is provided than is needed to oxygenate completely the blood flowing through the surrounding pulmonary capillaries. Conversely, the blood flowing to the poorly ventilated alveoli does not become fully oxygenated. When it mixes with normally oxygenated blood flowing from other parts of the lungs, the oxygen content of the blood delivered to the tissues is reduced. The destruction of the alveolar septa leads to enlargement of the air spaces and at the same time reduces the number of pulmonary capillaries available for gas exchange (Figure 12-17). Normally, there are about 400 million alveoli in both lungs, and the surface area of the pulmonary capillaries supplying the alveoli is about 30 times as great as the surface area of the body. Each alveolus contains a relatively small volume of air surrounded by a rich network of capillaries. This arrangement promotes optimal diffusion of gases between alveolar air and pulmonary capillaries. Diffusion of gases is much less efficient from large cystic spaces because the spaces contain a much larger volume of air than does a normal alveolus and are surrounded by a relatively sparse network of capillaries. Moreover, the movement of air into and out of the enlarged spaces is impeded by the bronchiolar obstruction. Destruction of the alveolar septa also leads to loss

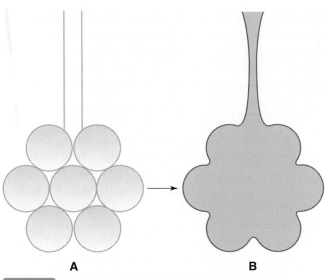

**Figure 12-17** Derangement of pulmonary function resulting from enlargement of air spaces and reduction of pulmonary capillary bed. **A,** Normal structure, illustrating schematically a cluster of alveoli surrounded by a rich capillary bed connected to normal bronchiole. **B,** Emphysema, illustrating coalescence of air spaces to form a large cystic space with greatly reduced capillary bed and narrowed bronchiole.

oxygen consumption. The pressure required to actively force air out of the lungs during expiration also raises the intrapleural pressure and compresses the lungs, which causes further problems with pulmonary ventilation. The bronchi and bronchioles have lost their normal structural support, because of loss of lung elasticity, and tend to collapse during expiration, obstructing the outflow of air and trapping more air within the lungs.

The chief symptom of emphysema is shortness of breath. Initially this is noted only on exertion, but later it may be present even at rest. The patient usually also has a chronic cough with purulent sputum, owing to the associated chronic bronchitis. Eventually, severely affected patients may die because they lack enough functionally normal lung tissue to sustain life or because of a superimposed pulmonary infection. Emphysema is also a frequent cause of respiratory acidosis, one of the common disturbances of acid–base balance. This is discussed in Chapter 19.

## Pathogenesis of Chronic Obstructive Pulmonary Disease

Cigarette smoking and atmospheric air pollution appear to be the major factors responsible for the rising incidence of emphysema. Exactly how they exert their destructive effect on the lung is not completely understood. Figure 12-18 summarizes one concept of the

of the elastic tissue in the septa that forms the structural framework of the lungs, and so the lungs no longer "recoil" normally after they have been stretched during inspiration. Expiration is no longer a passive process. The air must be actively forced out of the lungs by contraction of the intercostal muscles. Breathing requires more effort that in turn requires a greater

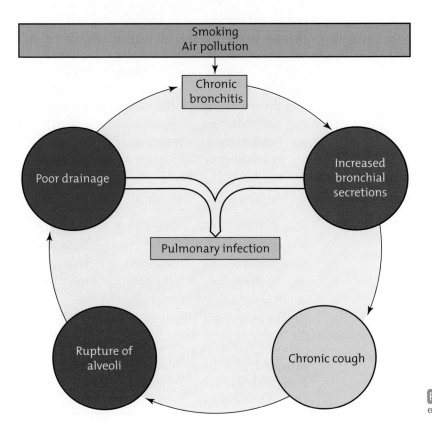

**Figure 12-18** A concept of the pathogenesis of pulmonary emphysema.

pathogenesis of this serious and disabling disease. Smoking and air pollution are considered to expose the bronchial mucosa to chronic irritation, eventually producing chronic bronchitis associated with a chronic cough and increased bronchial secretions. The inflammatory swelling of the mucosa narrows the smaller bronchioles, increasing their resistance to expiration and causing air to be trapped within the lung.

Repeated bouts of coughing, with consequent extreme elevations in intrabronchial pressure, cause the alveolar septa to rupture, gradually converting the alveoli into large, cystic air spaces. The lungs become overdistended and lose their normal elasticity. The patient cannot expel air normally from the overdistended lungs because normal lung elasticity is lost and the bronchioles are obstructed; difficulty expectorating the excessive bronchial secretions also is apparent. Retention of secretions and poor drainage of secretions from the bronchi tend to perpetuate the chronic bronchitis, and a vicious circle is created. The diseased lungs are also more susceptible to infection because of impaired pulmonary ventilation, bronchial inflammation, bronchiolar obstruction, and excessive bronchial secretions. Therefore, patients with emphysema frequently have repeated bouts of pneumonia, further damaging the lung tissue.

## Prevention and Treatment

For the most part, emphysema can be prevented by refraining from smoking and avoiding inhalation of other substances known to be injurious to the lungs. Atmospheric air pollution contributes to the increasing incidence of emphysema, and various measures are being undertaken to control this serious public health problem.

After emphysema has developed, the damaged lungs cannot be restored to normal. However, several measures can be employed to promote the drainage of bronchial secretions, to improve pulmonary ventilation, and to decrease the frequency of superimposed pulmonary infections. These measures, along with cessation of smoking, will retard or arrest further progression of the disease.

Surgical procedures called lung volume reduction surgery have also been investigated. These procedures excise the nonfunctional extremely emphysematous segments of the upper lobes, thereby reducing the size of the overinflated lungs so that the less severely involved lower lobes might be able to function more efficiently. A large U.S. government-sponsored clinical trial involving more than 1000 patients (The National Emphysema Treatment Trial) compared the results of lung volume reduction surgery in one group of patients with medical treatment in a comparable group. In general, the overall mortality rates in both groups were similar, indicating that surgical treatment did not improve survival for most patients. One group, however, did benefit from surgery: patients who had a very limited capacity for exercise caused by the emphysema, in which the emphysema was restricted to the upper lobes of the lungs. On the other hand, patients who did not meet these criteria had a higher mortality rate than medically treated patients and did not get any significant benefit from the surgical procedures. Unfortunately, even the initial benefit of surgery in the group that responded was of short duration, and 2 years later their pulmonary function had declined to the point where it was no better than it had been before surgery.

The following case illustrates the clinical features of a patient with chronic pulmonary emphysema who developed severe respiratory insufficiency that was precipitated by a bout of pneumonia.

### Case Study 12-3

A 70-year-old man entered the hospital because of severe, progressive shortness of breath for the previous 2 weeks. He had had chronic pulmonary emphysema for many years secondary to heavy cigarette smoking and had stopped smoking recently. On physical examination, he was very short of breath, and there was moderate cyanosis of the lips and nailbeds. Lungs appeared overinflated, and respiratory excursions were poor. Laboratory studies revealed a low arterial oxygen content ($PO_2$ 31 mm Hg) and oxygen saturation (53 percent), with elevated carbon dioxide tension ($PCO_2$ 53 mm Hg) and high plasma bicarbonate (40 mEq/L). Blood pH was reduced to 7.29. These changes indicated severe pulmonary emphysema with respiratory acidosis. Chest x-ray revealed pneumonia in the right lower lobe. Treatment consisted of supplementary oxygen, antibiotics, and various other measures to improve pulmonary function. The pneumonia slowly subsided, and the patient left the hospital 2 weeks later.

# Bronchial Asthma

Bronchial asthma is a spasmodic contraction of the smooth muscle in the walls of the smaller bronchi and bronchioles. It is also associated with increased secretions by the bronchial mucous glands. Asthmatic attacks cause shortness of breath, and wheezing respirations occur caused by restricted movement of air through the tightly constricted air passages. The physiologic derangements in asthma result from narrowing of the bronchioles and are similar to those in patients with emphysema. Bronchiolar spasm exerts a greater effect on expiration than on inspiration because the caliber of the bronchioles varies with the phase of respiration. Consequently, air flow is impeded more on expiration than on inspiration, which leads to trapping of air within the lungs and overinflation of the lungs.

Many cases of asthma have an allergic basis. The attacks are precipitated by inhalation of dust, pollens, animal dander, or other allergens, which interact with mast cells coated with IgE antibody. This leads to release of chemical mediators that induce the bronchospasm. Acute attacks are treated by administering drugs such as epinephrine or theophylline, which relax the bronchospasm. Often one can prevent attacks by administering drugs that block the release of mediators from mast cells. (Allergic diseases are considered in Chapter 4.)

# Respiratory Distress Syndrome

## Respiratory Distress Syndrome of Newborn Infants

The condition known as *respiratory distress syndrome of newborn infants* is characterized by progressive respiratory distress that occurs soon after birth, leading to serious problems in oxygenation of the blood. The condition occurs most often in premature infants, infants delivered by cesarean section, and infants born to mothers with diabetes. The basic cause is an inadequate quantity of surfactant in the lungs of the affected infants. As a result, the alveoli do not expand normally during inspiration and tend to collapse during expiration. The permeability of the pulmonary capillaries also is increased, and protein-rich fluid leaks from the pulmonary capillaries. The fluid, which is rich in fibrinogen, tends to clot and form adherent membranes that line the air passages. These membranes contribute to respiratory distress by impeding the diffusion of gases between the air passages and the pulmonary capillaries. The presence of these prominent acellular red-staining membranes lining the alveoli was the basis for the older name, *hyaline membrane disease*, which was given to this condition (Figure 12-19).

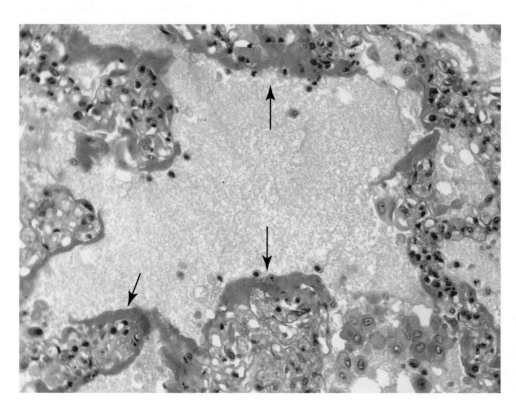

Figure 12-19 Neonatal respiratory distress syndrome. Eosinophilic hyaline membranes (*arrows*) composed of coagulated protein cover alveolar septa, impeding gas exchange between alveoli and pulmonary capillaries.

If delivery of a premature infant with immature lungs cannot be avoided, adrenal corticosteroid hormones administered to the mother within 24 hours of anticipated delivery will stimulate increased production of surfactant by the fetal lungs, thereby reducing the risk of respiratory distress syndrome. Infants who have developed respiratory distress syndrome after delivery are treated with supplementary oxygen and are also treated by instillation of a surfactant-type material that resembles natural surfactant. The material is instilled by means of a tube inserted into the infant's trachea (endotracheal tube) and the surfactant treatments are continued for several days after delivery. Table 12-1 compares the respiratory distress syndrome in infants with a somewhat similar condition in adults, which has a different pathogenesis and method of treatment, although the histologic changes in both conditions are quite similar.

## Adult Respiratory Distress Syndrome

The *adult respiratory distress syndrome* is often called by its initials ARDS, or sometimes by the term *shock lung* because shock is a major manifestation of the syndrome. The conditions causing this syndrome fall into two major groups. The first group contains many different conditions that cause shock with consequent fall in blood pressure and correspondingly reduced blood flow to the lungs. The shock may result from any type of severe injury (traumatic shock) or from a serious systemic infection (septic shock), and the pulmonary capillary and alveolar damage is an indirect result of the impaired pulmonary blood flow. The second group encompasses various conditions that directly damage the pulmonary capillaries and alveolar septa, including such conditions as aspiration of acid gastric contents, inhalation of irritant or toxic gases, or lung damage caused by some virus infections.

Whatever the predisposing cause of the alveolar damage, the pathophysiologic derangements are the same as in the neonatal respiratory distress syndrome: damage to alveolar capillaries and alveolar lining cells, impaired formation of surfactant, leakage of protein-rich fluid from the injured capillaries into the alveolar septa with formation of intraalveolar hyaline membranes, and impaired diffusion of oxygen across the swollen, thickened alveolar septa.

Treatment is directed toward correcting the shock, treating the underlying condition that initiated the respiratory distress, and improving the oxygenation of the blood by means of a ventilator capable of delivering an increased concentration of oxygen to the lungs under slightly increased pressure, thereby facilitating diffusion of oxygen across the swollen alveolar septa.

# Pulmonary Fibrosis

The lungs are continually exposed to a number of injurious substances, such as irritant gases discharged into the atmosphere and many kinds of airborne organic and inorganic particles. Severe pulmonary injury may lead to pulmonary fibrosis. Fibrous thickening of alveolar septa makes the lungs increasingly rigid, restricting normal respiratory excursions. Diffusion of oxygen and carbon dioxide between alveolar air and pulmonary capillaries also is hampered because of the increased thickness of the alveolar septa. Pulmonary fibrosis causes progressive respiratory disability similar to that encountered in pulmonary emphysema.

Some types of collagen diseases, characterized by injury to connective tissue, may have as their major manifestation injury to the connective-tissue framework of the lung, leading to pulmonary fibrosis.

| Table 12-1 | Comparison of Neonatal and Adult Respiratory Distress Syndrome | |
|---|---|---|
| | **Neonatal** | **Adult** |
| Groups affected | Premature infants<br>Delivery by cesarean section*<br>Infant born to diabetic mother** | Adults who have sustained direct or indirect lung damage |
| Pathogenesis | Inadequate surfactant | *Direct damage:* lung trauma, aspiration, irritant or toxic gases<br>*Indirect damage:* reduced pulmonary blood flow caused by shock or sepsis<br>*Associated condition:* surfactant production reduced |
| Treatment | Corticosteroids to mother before delivery<br>Endotracheal surfactant<br>Oxygen | Support circulation and respiration<br>Endotracheal tube and respirator<br>Positive pressure oxygen |

*Labor increases surfactant synthesis, which is lacking in cesarean delivery.

**High insulin blood level in the fetus of a mother with diabetes suppresses surfactant synthesis.

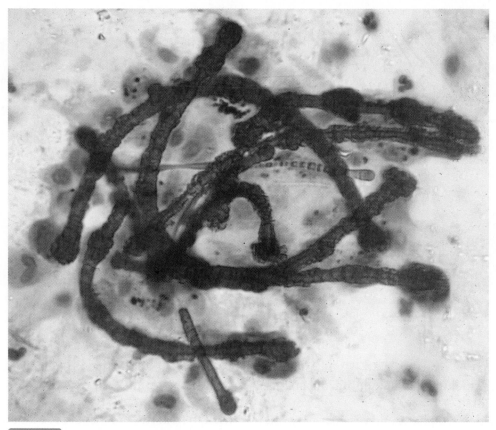

Figure 12-20 Cluster of asbestos bodies in sputum (original magnification × 1,000).

Certain occupational diseases are recognized as being caused by inhalation of injurious substances. The general term **pneumoconiosis** (*pneumo* = lung + *konis* = dust + *osis* = condition) is used to refer to lung injury produced by inhalation of injurious dust or other particulate material. The best known of the pneumoconioses are silicosis and asbestosis. **Silicosis** is a type of progressive nodular pulmonary fibrosis caused by inhalation of rock dust. **Asbestosis** is a diffuse pulmonary fibrosis caused by inhalation of asbestos fibers. Within the body, the fibers become coated with a protein having a high content of iron to form characteristic structures called **asbestos bodies**. Sometimes these can be identified in the sputum of patients with asbestosis (Figure 12-20). Inhalation of coal dust, cotton fibers, certain types of fungus spores, and many other substances attending certain occupations may also cause pulmonary fibrosis.

Patients with asbestosis have other problems as well, because asbestos fibers appear to be carcinogenic. These patients have a higher incidence of lung carcinoma than the general population, and some develop an unusual type of malignant tumor arising from pleural mesothelial cells, called a malignant mesothelioma.

# Lung Carcinoma

Lung carcinoma is another important disease related to cigarette smoking. Lung carcinoma was once uncommon. Now it is a common malignant tumor in men, and the incidence in women has also increased to such an extent that the mortality from lung cancer in women now exceeds that of breast cancer. The tumor is uncommon in nonsmokers. Because the neoplasm usually arises from the bronchial mucosa, the term *bronchogenic carcinoma* is often used when referring to lung cancer. There are several different histologic types. *Squamous cell carcinoma* and *adenocarcinoma* are two of the more common (Figure 12-21). A third type composed of large, bizarre epithelial cells is called by the descriptive term *large-cell carcinoma*. A fourth type is composed of small, irregular dark cells with scanty cytoplasm that look somewhat like lymphocytes. This type is called a small-cell carcinoma and

**pneumoconiosis** (nōō′mō-kō-nēēiō′-sis) An occupational lung disease caused by inhalation of injurious substances such as rock dust.

**silicosis** (sil-ik-ō′sis) A type of occupational lung disease caused by inhalation of rock dust.

**asbestosis** (as-bes-tō′sis) A type of pneumoconiosis caused by inhalation of asbestos fibers.

**asbestos body** (as-bes′tus) An asbestos fiber coated with protein and iron that is found in lungs and sputum of patients with asbestosis.

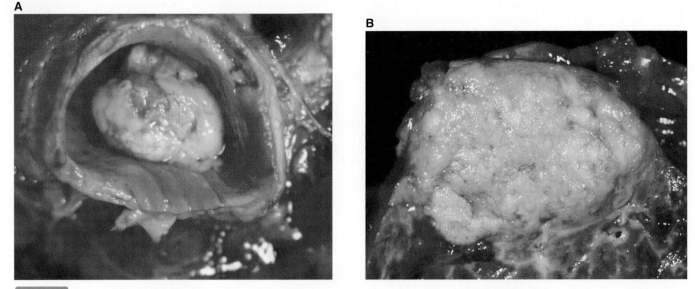

**Figure 12-21** Gross appearance of lung carcinoma. **A,** A squamous cell carcinoma partially obstructing a major bronchus. **B,** An adenocarcinoma arising from smaller bronchus at the periphery of the lung.

carries a very poor prognosis (Figure 12-22). Frequently tumor cells can be identified in the sputum of patients with lung carcinoma.

Because of the rich lymphatic and vascular network in the lung, the neoplasm readily gains access to lymphatic channels and pulmonary blood vessels and soon spreads to regional lymph nodes and distant sites. Treatment usually consists of surgical resection of one or more lobes of the lung. Radiation therapy in combination with anticancer chemotherapy rather than surgery is used to treat small-cell carcinoma and is also used to treat tumors that are too far advanced for surgical resection. Results of treatment are disappointing because the disease is often widespread by the time it is recognized. This tumor could largely be prevented by elimination of cigarette smoking.

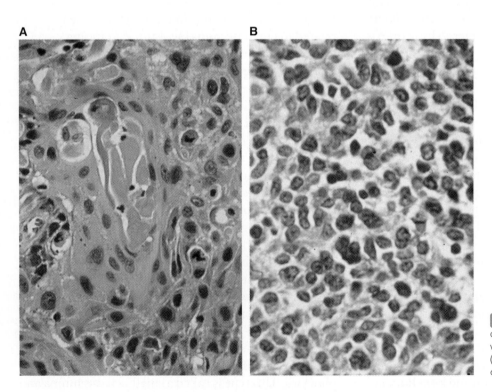

**Figure 12-22** Histologic appearance of two common types of lung carcinoma. **A,** Moderately well-differentiated squamous cell carcinoma (original magnification × 200). **B,** Small-cell carcinoma (original magnification × 200).

# CHAPTER REVIEW

## Summary

The lungs consist of a system of tubes that move air in and out of the lungs (ventilation) communicating with a collection of respiratory units where gas exchange occurs between alveolar air and the pulmonary capillaries (gas exchange). The efficiency of these functions can be evaluated by appropriate pulmonary function tests. When the lungs expand after birth to fill the pleural cavities, the recoil of the stretched lungs creates a slight vacuum in the pleural cavities, which is called a negative intrapleural pressure. Any condition that allows air from the lung to escape into the pleural cavity reduces or eliminates the vacuum (subatmospheric pressure), and the lung collapses, which is called a pneumothorax. In some circumstances a positive pressure may develop within the pleural cavity associated with the pneumothorax, which is a very hazardous complication that can be treated by evacuating the air.

Atelectasis refers to collapse of lung lobes or lobules caused by blockage of the bronchi supplying the involved part of the lung, or may result from accumulation of fluid within the pleural cavity that compresses the lung. Infection of the lung is called pneumonia, and the infection is classified by the organism responsible for the infection, and to some extent also by the amount of lung tissue involved as well as the condition that predisposed to the pneumonia. The etiologic classification is the most important because it helps the physician select an appropriate treatment. Pneumocystis pnenumonia is a relatively uncommon type of pneumonia that only occurs in persons whose immune system is not functioning normally.

Tuberculosis is becoming a problem because many persons coming into this country have been infected, and the disease may become active years later, leading to spread of the infection to persons with whom the infected person has contact. Failure to complete a course of treatment leads to development of resistant strains that are difficult to treat.

Acute bronchitis is self limited and of short duration, but chronic bronchitis is often associated with COPD and is more difficult to treat. Severe chronic inflammation may weaken the bronchial walls, causing them to dilate, which is a condition called bronchiectasis. Chronic obstructive pulmonary disease (COPD) affects many people and causes considerable disability. The condition is characterized by coalescence of alveoli to form air-filled sacs and associated bronchial inflammation that disrupts effective pulmonary ventilation and gas exchange. Treatment can arrest or slow progression of the disease, but cannot repair the damaged lung tissue.

Normal pulmonary ventilation requires surfactant, a detergentlike material made by alveolar cells that reduces the cohesive force of water molecules in the lung and facilitates ventilation. Lack of adequate surfactant in newborn infants may hamper respiration, leading to severe respiratory distress that can be treated by instillation of surfactantlike material into the respiratory tract to improve breathing. A comparable condition in adults follows any type of lung injury or disease that hampers surfactant production by the lung.

*Pneumoconiosis* is a general term for occupation-related lung damage caused by inhalation of hazardous materials such as rock dust (silicosis), coal dust (anthracosis), asbestos fibers (asbestosis), and a number of other materials. Prevention of exposure by use of appropriate safety equipment prevents lung damage.

Lung carcinoma still remains a serious problem, related primarily in smokers who are exposed to the carcinogens in cigarette smoke. Unfortunately the disease has a relatively poor prognosis because it spreads easily into pulmonary blood and lymphatic vessels. Even sophisticated diagnostic procedures that can detect a carcinoma early have provided an earlier diagnosis but have not had much impact on the unfavorable outcome. Treatment is based on the stage of the disease and the type of tumor.

## Questions for Review

1. How do the lungs function? What is the difference between ventilation and gas exchange? How is pulmonary function disturbed if the alveolar septa are thickened and scarred?

2. What is pneumothorax? How does it develop? What is its effect on pulmonary function?

3. What is pneumonia? How is pneumonia classified? What are its major clinical features?

4. How does the tubercle bacillus differ in its staining reaction from other bacteria? What type of inflammatory reaction does it cause? What factors determine the outcome of a tuberculous infection? How does a cavity develop in lungs infected with tuberculosis? Is a person with a tuberculous cavity infectious to other persons? What is miliary tuberculosis?

5. A patient has tuberculosis of the kidney, but no evidence of pulmonary tuberculosis is detected by means of a chest x-ray. How did this happen?

6. What is meant by the term *inactive tuberculosis*? Under what circumstances may an old inactive tuberculous infection become activated? What type of patients are susceptible to reactivation of a tuberculous infection?

7. What is the difference between bronchitis and bronchiectasis?

8. What is pulmonary emphysema? What factors predispose to its development? How may it be prevented? What is the difference between pulmonary emphysema and pulmonary fibrosis?

9. What is the relationship between carcinoma of the lung and cigarette smoking? How is lung carcinoma treated?

## Supplementary Reading

Antonucci, G., Girardi, E., Raviglione, M. C., et al. 1995. Risk factors for tuberculosis in HIV-infected persons. *Journal of the American Medical Association* 274:143–48.

TB is a big problem in HIV-infected persons and may progress rapidly. Methods for monitoring persons at risk are discussed.

Bach, P. B., Jett, J. R., Pastorino, U., et al. 2007. Computed tomography screening and lung cancer outcomes. *Journal of the American Medical Association* 297:953–67.

Screening for lung cancer by computed tomography (CT) may detect cancers earlier but may not reduce the risk of advanced cancer or the lung cancer death rate.

Centers for Disease Control and Prevention. 2003. Update: Outbreak of severe acute respiratory syndrome—worldwide. *Morbidity and Mortality Weekly Report* 52:241–46, 269–72.

Describes the highly communicable atypical pneumonia caused by an unusual coronavirus that infects both humans and animals.

Colditz, G. A., Brewer, T. F., Berkey, C. S., et al. 1994. Efficacy of BCG vaccine in the prevention of tuberculosis. *Journal of the American Medical Association* 271:698–702.

BCG vaccination reduces the risk of tuberculosis by about 50 percent. The term *BCG* is an abbreviation for Bacillus Calmette-Guerin, which is an attenuated strain of the bovine tubercle bacillus (*Mycobacterium bovis*) used to immunize children in countries where there is a high incidence of tuberculosis in the population. The vaccine may reduce the likelihood of a tuberculosis infection in children, and helps prevent spread of tuberculosis to the nervous system or other sites if a child does become infected. BCG is not used in this country, where the incidence of tuberculosis is low.

Daley, C. L., Small, P. M., Schecter, G. F., et al. 1992. An outbreak of tuberculosis with accelerated progression among persons infected with the human immunodeficiency virus. *New England Journal of Medicine* 326:231–35.

HIV infection promotes rapid progression of tuberculosis.

Driver, C. R., Valway, S. E., Morgan, W. M., et al. 1994. Transmission of *Mycobacterium tuberculosis* associated with air travel. *Journal of the American Medical Association* 272:1031–35.

A flight attendant became infected after exposure to a family member who died of tuberculosis. She did not receive prophylactic treatment and developed active tuberculosis 3 years later. She infected other airline crew members and may also have infected passengers before her disease was diagnosed and treated.

Dye, C. 2004. A booster for tuberculosis vaccines. *Journal of the American Medical Association* 291:2127–128.

A large group of Alaska Eskimos who received BCG vaccination were followed for many years, and the vaccine appeared to be effective for as long as 60 years. BCG vaccination does provide some protection against infection.

Holmes, K. V. 2003. SARS-associated coronavirus. *New England Journal of Medicine* 348:1948–51.

> The SARS-associated coronavirus is a previously unknown coronavirus, probably acquired from an animal, that somehow acquired the ability to affect humans. A previous outbreak was controlled and the virus eliminated by quarantine alone, but safe and effective drugs and vaccines need to be developed.

Man, S. F., McAlister, F. A., Anthonisen, N. R., and Sin, D. D. 2003. Contemporary management of chronic obstructive pulmonary disease. *Journal of the American Medical Association* 290:2313–316.

> Early evaluation and treatment are recommended for any patient suspected of having COPD. Principles of diagnosis and treatment are considered.

Markel, H., Gostin, L. O., and Fidler, D. P. 2007. Extensively drug-resistant tuberculosis (XDR-TB). An isolation order, public health powers, and a global crisis. *Journal of the American Medical Association* 298:83–86.

> A very interesting article on XDR-TB and its potential impact, including discussion of legal authority to quarantine in the United States, and on travel restrictions when dealing with XDR-TB. The article describes a subject being treated for TB with standard medications, who was planning to marry and honeymoon in Europe. He was contacted as soon as his sensitivity test results became available, which revealed that he had XDR-TB and should not travel, and also should undergo specialized treatment. Instead he advanced his travel schedule and traveled by airplane to Greece and Rome. While in Rome he was contacted by the Centers for Disease Control and Prevention (CDC) and told that he should not travel by air and should report to Italian health authorities. Instead he flew to Prague, then to Montreal, and then drove into the United States. As a result of his travels, which exposed many people, the Centers for Disease Control and Prevention (CDC) and other health facilities from multiple countries had to attempt to locate the hundreds of airline passengers who may have been exposed to XDR-TB.

National Emphysema Treatment Trial Research Group. 2003. A randomized trial comparing lung-volume-reduction surgery with medical therapy for severe emphysema. *New England Journal of Medicine* 348:2059–73.

> The definitive article analyzing the applications and limitations of this procedure.

Patel, J. D., Bach, P. B., and Kris, M. G. 2004. Lung cancer in U.S. women: A contemporary epidemic. *Journal of the American Medical Association* 291:1763–68.

> As a result of increased smoking by women beginning in about 1930 and continuing to the present, lung cancer in women has increased 600 percent, and lung cancer now causes as many deaths as all breast cancers and all gynecologic cancers combined. Women appear to be more susceptible than men to the carcinogenic properties of cigarette smoke.

Ryu, J. H., Colby, T. V., and Hartman, T. E. 1998. Idiopathic pulmonary fibrosis: Current concepts. *Mayo Clinic Proceedings* 73:1085–101.

> Pulmonary fibrosis results from many different causes, and proper classification allows more reliable prognosis and management.

Voelker, R. 2007. Pattern of U.S. tuberculosis cases shifting. *Journal of the American Medical Association* 297:685.

> Previously reported Centers for Disease Control (CDC) data showed that from 1994 to 2004 TB cases among U.S.-born residents fell by 62 percent, while increasing in foreign-born persons to 54 percent of all U.S. cases. Twenty-four percent of the TB cases were in foreign-born persons who had been living in the United States for more than 5 years, and most of the cases resulted from reactivation of a latent infection that had been acquired in their country of origin many years ago. Tuberculin testing and treating of latent infections in foreign-born persons should be extended to include longer-term foreign-born residents living in the United States.

## Interactive Activities

**Multiple Choice**

Circle the correct statement.

1. Which of the following factors does NOT cause a pneumothorax?
   A. Laceration of the lung and pleura caused by a fractured rib
   B. Cardiac rupture following a myocardial infarction
   C. Stab wound of the chest wall penetrating the lung
   D. Rupture of an emphysematous air-filled cyst into the pleural cavity.

2. The frequency of chronic obstructive pulmonary disease is
   A. Increasing
   B. Decreasing
   C. Remaining unchanged from year to year

3. Which of the following statements does NOT apply to pulmonary emphysema?
    A. Inefficient oxygenation of the blood
    B. Increased blood flow to the lung
    C. Coalescence of alveoli that form cysts in the lungs is associated with reduced number of pulmonary capillaries available for gas exchange
    D. Chronic bronchial inflammation narrows the diameter of the bronchi and bronchioles

4. Which of the following statements does NOT apply to pulmonary tuberculosis?
    A. The incidence of the disease is increasing
    B. Causes a granulomatous inflammation
    C. Cavities may form within the lungs resulting from necrosis of infected lung tissue
    D. Antibiotic-resistant organisms are extremely rare

5. The main cause of the increasing incidence of lung carcinoma in women is
    A. Air pollution
    B. More women are developing COPD
    C. Fewer women are developing breast carcinoma
    D. Cigarette smoking

6. The condition characterized by chronic bronchial inflammation associated with dilation of the bronchi and bronchioles is called
    A. Bronchitis
    B. Bronchiectasis
    C. COPD
    D. Bronchogenic carcinoma

7. Inhalation of a foreign body into the lung may cause
    A. Bronchial and pulmonary infection
    B. Lung carcinoma
    C. Pneumothorax
    D. Pulmonary emphysema

8. A 35-year-old man has chills, fever, chest pain, and purulent sputum. The most likely diagnosis is
    A. Pneumonia
    B. Emphysema
    C. A pulmonary infarct
    D. Lung carcinoma

9. Which of the following conditions does NOT appear to be directly related to cigarette smoking?
    A. Lung carcinoma
    B. COPD
    C. Pulmonary emboli
    D. Carcinoma of the larynx

10. A postoperative patient with a normal temperature has chest pain, shortness of breath, a bloody sputum, and a pulmonary infiltrate demonstrated by a chest x-ray. The most likely diagnosis is
    A. Lobar pneumonia
    B. Pulmonary emphysema
    C. Carcinoma of the lung
    D. Pulmonary infarct

## Fill in the Blanks

1. Movement of air in and out of the lungs is called _____ and movement of oxygen and carbon dioxide between alveoli and pulmonary capillaries is called _____.

2. Escape of air from the lung associated with collapse of the lung is called a _____.

3. Development of a positive (higher than atmospheric) pressure in the pleural cavity associated with collapse of the lung is called a _____ and the condition is treated by _____.

4. Collapse of part of the lung caused by obstruction of bronchi or bronchioles with absorption of the trapped air into the bloodstream is called _____.

5. The cause of the acute respiratory distress syndrome in newborn infants is _____.

6. The usual cause of a pulmonary infarct is _____.

7. The characteristic multinucleated cell associated with the necrosis in tuberculosis is called a _____.

8. The skin test that detects hypersensitivity to the antigens in the tubercle bacillus as an indication of previous exposure to the organism is called the _____ test.

9. Deficiency of surfactant in the lungs of premature infants leads to a condition called _____.

10. The condition characterized by breathing difficulty caused by bronchospasm is called _____.

11. Progressive pulmonary fibrosis caused by inhalation of rock dust is called _____.

12. Pulmonary fibrosis caused by inhalation of asbestos fibers is called _____.

13. The disease caused by exposure to asbestos fibers may predispose a person to development of malignant lung and pleural tumors. The lung tumor is called a _____, and the pleural tumor is called a _____.

14. The disease characterized by chronic bronchitis associated with breakdown of alveolar septa, formation of cystic spaces throughout the lung, and loss of lung elasticity is called _____.

15. _____ is the major factor responsible for the rising incidence of lung carcinoma in women.

## Critical Thinking

1. Peter Jones is a 65-year-old man who has noted progressive shortness of breath on exertion for the past year. He has smoked about two packs of cigarettes daily since he was about 17 years old, but he has cut back on his smoking recently. He wonders what his problem is and what he should do about it. He is planning to see his physician next week but he would like your opinion now.

2. Mary Larson is a 26-year-old student who works part time in a nursing home. She had to have a Mantoux test before she started working at the nursing home and the test was negative. However, the most recent Mantoux test performed 6 months later is positive. She wants to know what this means and what she should do about it. What would you tell her?

# 13

# The Breast and Female Reproductive System

1. Describe the normal structure and physiology of the breast. List and define the common developmental abnormalities.

2. Explain the applications and limitations of mammography in the diagnosis and treatment of breast disease.

3. List the three common breast diseases that present as a lump in the breast, and explain how they are differentiated by the physician.

4. Describe the clinical manifestations of breast carcinoma. Explain the methods of diagnosis and treatment.

5. Explain the role of heredity in the pathogenesis of breast carcinoma.

6. Describe the common infections of the genital tract, and relate them to sexually transmitted diseases.

7. Describe the clinical manifestations and complications of endometriosis.

8. List the common causes of irregular uterine bleeding.

9. Describe the common diseases of the cervix, endometrium, myometrium, and vulva.

10. List the common cysts and tumors of the ovary.

11. Explain the pathogenesis, clinical manifestations, and treatment of toxic shock syndrome.

12. Categorize the common methods of artificial contraception; explain how they prevent conception, and describe their possible side effects.

# The Breast

## Structure and Physiology of the Breast

The female breasts are each composed of about 20 lobes of glandular tissue embedded in fibrous and adipose tissue. Each lobe consists of clusters of glands, called *lobules*, connected by a series of branching ducts that converge to form large ducts that extend to the nipple. The breasts are modified sweat glands that have become specialized to secrete milk. Before puberty, breast tissue in both sexes consists only of branching ducts and fibrous tissue without glandular tissue or fat. In the female, they enlarge at puberty in response to estrogen and progesterone produced by the ovaries, whereas the unstimulated male breasts retain their prepubertal form. Postpubertal changes in the female include proliferation of glandular and fibrous tissue and accumulation of adipose tissue within the breasts. Variations in the size of the postpubertal breasts of nonpregnant women are caused primarily by variations in the amount of fat and fibrous tissue in the breasts rather than to differences in the amount of glandular tissue.

The breasts are fixed to the chest wall by bands of fibrous tissue called suspensory ligaments, which extend from the skin of the breast to the connective tissue covering the muscles of the chest wall.

The breasts have an abundant blood supply and a rich lymphatic drainage. Lymphatic channels drain from each breast into groups of lymph nodes (axillary lymph nodes) located in the armpit (axilla), above the clavicle (supraclavicular lymph nodes), and beneath the sternum (mediastinal lymph nodes).

The breasts are extremely responsive to hormonal stimulation. Mild cyclic hyperplasia followed by involution of breast tissue occurs normally during the menstrual cycle. The glandular and ductal tissues of the breast become markedly hypertrophic under the hormonal stimulus of pregnancy and lactation, and the breast undergoes regression in the postpartum period. After menopause, sex-hormone levels decline, and the breasts gradually decrease in size. Figure 13-1 illustrates the histologic appearance of breast tissue under varying hormonal conditions.

## Mammograms

A *mammogram* is a special type of x-ray examination that allows the physician to visualize the internal structure of the breast and recognize abnormalities that may not be detected by clinical examination. In a mammogram,

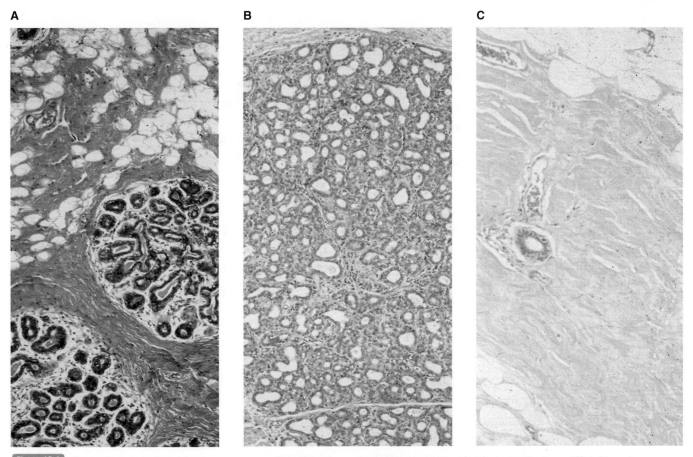

**Figure 13-1** Photomicrographs illustrating the appearance of breasts under varying hormonal conditions (original magnification × 40). **A,** Normal nonpregnant breast. Two lobules of glandular tissue appear in the *lower half* of the photograph. **B,** Glandular hyperplasia in pregnancy. **C,** Postmenopausal atrophy.

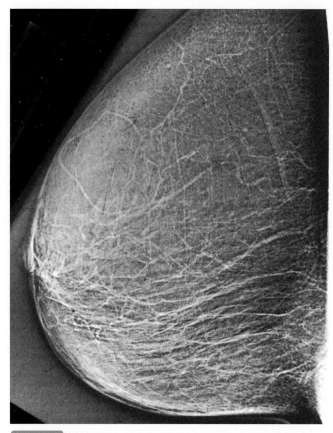

Figure 13-2 A normal mammogram.

the fibrous and glandular tissues of the breast appear as interlacing white strands. The less dense fatty tissue, which transmits x-rays readily, appears dark ( Figure 13-2 ). Cysts and tumors within the breast appear as dense white masses surrounded by the less dense dark tissue of the adjacent normal breast. Cysts and benign tumors appear well circumscribed, whereas malignant tumors often have irregular margins that indicate infiltration of the tumor into the surrounding breast tissue. These same criteria are used to distinguish between benign and malignant tumors on gross examination when a biopsy specimen is examined. Malignant tumors also frequently contain fine flecks of calcium that indicate calcification within the carcinoma. This is another feature suggestive of malignancy when seen on the mammogram.

The mammogram is most useful for examining the breasts of postmenopausal women because they contain more fat and less glandular tissue than the breasts of younger women. A dense tumor within a postmenopausal breast usually contrasts sharply with the less dense fatty tissue and is more easily identified. In contrast, a mammogram is less useful for examining the breasts of younger women, which appear much denser because they contain much more glandular and fibrous tissue. Consequently, it is more difficult to recognize a tumor

in such a breast because there is less contrast between the tumor and the surrounding dense breast tissue.

Periodic mammograms are recommended for all women as a screening procedure. Mammograms can detect early breast cancers much sooner than they could be felt by physical examination of the breasts, and early detection followed by prompt treatment while a tumor is still small greatly increases the woman's chance of survival. Although mammography is an extremely valuable screening procedure for detecting early breast carcinoma, the procedure may not always identify a small carcinoma in the dense breast tissue of younger women, which obscures the tumor.

# Abnormalities of Breast Development

## Accessory Breasts and Nipples

Embryologically, the breasts develop from columns of cells called *mammary ridges*, which extend along the anterior body wall from the armpits to the upper thighs ( Figure 13-3 ). Most of the ridges disappear in the course of prenatal development except for the parts in the

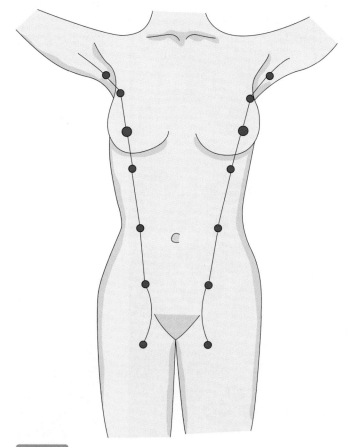

Figure 13-3 Common sites of accessory breasts and nipples, which may form anywhere along the course of the embryonic mammary ridges.

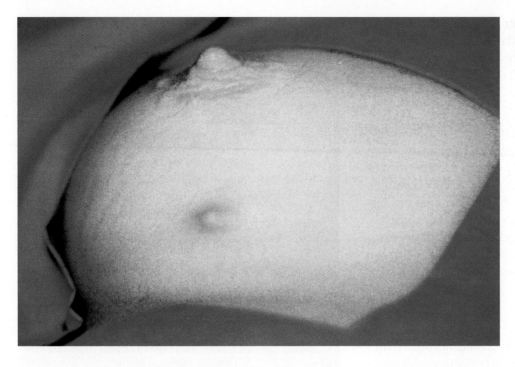

Figure 13-4 An extra nipple below and medial to left breast and nipple. (Photograph courtesy of Dr. Kent Van De Graaff.)

midthoracic region, which give rise to the breasts and nipples. Sometimes, persons have extra breasts or nipples. These are most commonly found in the armpits or on the lower chest below and medial to the normal breasts, but they may appear anywhere along the course of the embryonic mammary ridges (Figure 13-4). Extra nipples and breast tissue may be a source of embarrassment to the subject, but usually they do not cause other problems. Occasionally, however, accessory breast tissue may cause symptoms, as illustrated in Case 13-1.

## Unequal Development of the Breasts

The fully developed breasts are usually similar in size and shape but are not identical. Occasionally, one breast may fail to develop as much as its counterpart and may be significantly smaller than the opposite

### Case Study 13-1

A 22-year-old woman visited a medical clinic for an examination and Pap smear. In the course of the examination, bilateral soft masses of tissue were palpated in both armpits. Each mass measured about 5 centimeters in diameter, and they became quite prominent when the subject raised her arms above her head. On further questioning, she stated the lumps had been present for some time. They often became tender just before the onset of her menstrual period, and the overlying skin sometimes became irritated by rubbing against her clothing. She was advised that the lumps were masses of extra breast tissue and could be removed surgically if they continued to cause problems.

### Case Study 13-2

A 20-year-old woman visited a medical clinic seeking contraceptive pills. Examination revealed that the left breast was much smaller than the right, which the subject masked by padding the left brassiere cup. The rest of the examination was normal. She was advised that contraceptive pills could be prescribed. However, because of the effect of the hormones contained in these pills on the glandular tissues of the breast, slight breast enlargement could result. Such enlargement might accentuate the difference in the size of the two breasts. The client decided not to use contraceptive pills and chose to be fitted with a diaphragm instead.

breast. Moreover, any condition that causes the breasts to enlarge may accentuate the disproportion. This possibility must be considered when prescribing medications, as illustrated by Case 13-2.

## Breast Hypertrophy

Sometimes at puberty the breasts overrespond to hormonal stimulation and may enlarge excessively. True breast hypertrophy is primarily caused by overgrowth of fibrous tissue, not glandular tissue or fat. The subject may experience considerable back and shoulder discomfort caused by the excessive weight of the breasts. If symptoms are severe, the excessive breast tissue may be surgically resected, after which the breasts can be reconstructed so that they have a more normal size and shape.

## Gynecomastia

Occasionally at puberty the ductal and fibrous tissue of the adolescent male breast may begin to proliferate, forming a distinct nodule of breast tissue under the nipple. This condition, which is called *gynecomastia* (*gyne* = woman + *mastos* = breast), may affect one or both breasts. It appears to result from a temporary imbalance of male and female hormones that sometimes occurs in the male at puberty. Normally, the male secretes both male and female hormones, but male hormones predominate and "cancel out" the effects of the female hormones. Gynecomastia results when there is a temporary increase in estrogen relative to male hormones. The condition is not serious, usually subsides spontaneously, and no treatment is require. If the condition persists and causes considerable emotional distress to the affected youth, the excess breast tissue can be removed surgically.

# Benign Cystic Change in the Breast

Benign cystic change in breast tissue, often called benign cystic disease or benign fibrocystic disease, is a very common condition. It is characterized by focal areas of proliferation of glandular and fibrous tissue in the breast associated with localized dilatation of ducts, resulting in the formation of various-sized cysts within the breast. Cystic change appears to be caused by irregularities in the response of the breast tissue to the normal cyclic variations of each menstrual cycle. Clinically, a breast cyst may feel very firm and may appear to be a solid tumor. Ultrasound examination of the breast is often very helpful in distinguishing a cystic from a

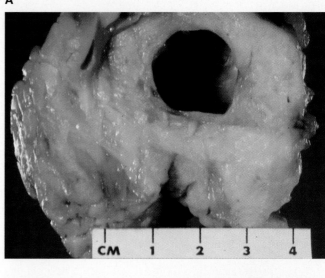

**A**

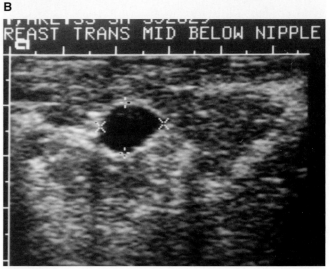

**B**

REAST TRANS MID BELOW NIPPLE

Figure 13-5 A benign cyst of the breast. **A,** A cyst viewed in cross section. Cyst is filled with fluid that escapes when the cyst is incised. **B,** An ultrasound examination of breast, revealing a breast cyst (a dark area near the *center* of the photograph).

solid mass in the breast ( Figure 13-5 ). Often, if the physician believes the mass to be a cyst rather than a solid tumor, an attempt is made to aspirate the cyst. A needle is introduced into the breast under local anesthesia. If a cyst is present, the fluid is aspirated and the mass disappears. If no fluid can be obtained, surgical excision is performed.

# Fibroadenoma

Fibroadenoma is a benign, well-circumscribed tumor of fibrous and glandular breast tissues that is seen most commonly in young women. It is readily cured by simple surgical excision ( Figure 13-6 ).

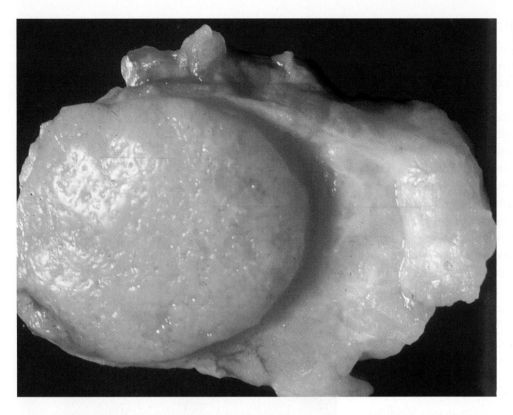

**Figure 13-6** Benign fibroadenoma of breast. The tumor is well circumscribed and readily separates from adjacent normal breast tissue.

# Carcinoma of the Breast

Breast carcinoma occurs in both sexes. It is a rare tumor in men whose breast tissue is not subjected to stimulation by ovarian hormones, but is a very common tumor in women. There is some tendency for breast carcinoma to run in families, and a woman is at higher than normal risk if her mother or sister has had a breast carcinoma. Hormonal factors also influence the risk of breast carcinoma. Women who have never borne children or had their first child after age 30 are at increased risk, as are women who have had early onset of menses (menarche) or late menopause.

## Breast Carcinoma Risk Related to Hormone Treatment

Hormones have been used for many years to treat menopausal symptoms. Treatment consisted of either estrogen or estrogen along with a progestin (a synthetic compound with progesterone activity). Long-term hormone use does increase the risk of breast carcinoma, and the magnitude of the risk depends on what hormones are taken and how long they are used. Estrogen–progestin use poses the greatest risk. The breast carcinoma risk associated with hormone treatment was documented in a large clinical trial dealing with the risks and benefits of hormone therapy in healthy postmenopausal women. The clinical trial also identified an increased risk of cardiovascular disease, venous thrombosis, and pulmonary embolism associated with hormone use. After the results were published, hormone use to treat menopausal symptoms declined 38 percent in the United States and was followed by a 6.7 percent reduction in the incidence of breast carcinoma beginning in 2002, which continued the following year and then stabilized at the new lower level, in contrast to previous years when breast carcinoma had been increasing about 0.5 percent per year.

## Breast Carcinoma Susceptibility Genes

A small proportion of breast carcinomas is hereditary and can be traced to inheritance of mutant breast cancer susceptibility genes. The two most important susceptibility genes have been designated as the *BRCA1* and *BRCA2* genes. The *BRCA1* gene is a very large gene, and a large number of different mutations have been described. A woman who inherits a mutant *BRCA1* gene has an 80 percent chance of developing breast carcinoma during her lifetime and an approximately 20 to 40 percent lifetime risk of ovarian carcinoma as well. A woman who inherits a mutant *BRCA2* gene also has an 80 percent lifetime risk of breast carcinoma, but the lifetime risk of ovarian carcinoma is about 10 to 20 percent, which is significantly lower than the ovarian carcinoma risk associated with a *BRCA1* mutation. (The role of tumor suppressor genes on cell functions and the effects of inherited mutations were considered in Chapter 8.)

## Classification of Breast Carcinoma

Breast cancers are classified according to the site of origin, the presence or absence of invasion, and the degree of differentiation of the tumor cells. More than 90 percent of carcinomas arise from the epithelium of the ducts and are called *ductal carcinomas*. The rest arise from the lobules and are designated *lobular carcinomas*. Initially, a carcinoma remains confined for a time within the duct or lobule in which it arose and is called a *noninfiltrating* or in situ ductal or lobular carcinoma. Eventually, however, the tumor breaks through the ducts or lobules and extends into the adjacent breast tissue, becoming an invasive ductal or lobular carcinoma. Histologically, the degree of differentiation of the tumor also is specified. A well-differentiated carcinoma is composed of cells that resemble the epithelium of the ducts or lobules in which the tumor arose, whereas a poorly differentiated tumor is composed of bizarre cells in haphazard arrangement that appear immature and quite different from normal breast epithelial cells.

## Evolution of Breast Carcinoma

In its early stages, a breast carcinoma is too small to be detected by breast examination but can often be demonstrated by mammography, sometimes as early as 2 years before it becomes large enough to form a palpable lump within the breast. Frequently, focal areas of necrosis occur within the proliferating tumor cells, and calcium salts diffuse from the bloodstream into the areas of necrosis ( Figure 13-7 ). These small focal calcium deposits often can be identified in mammograms, which suggest possible calcium deposits within a ductal carcinoma. Calcium deposits, however, are not conclusive evidence of breast carcinoma, as calcium deposits also can accumulate in some benign breast lesions.

As a breast tumor continues to grow, it infiltrates the breast tissues more extensively, and left untreated, eventually metastasizes to regional lymph nodes and distant sites. Five-year survival rates and the problem of late metastases are discussed in Chapter 8. Early diagnosis allows prompt treatment and improves the cure rate. For this reason, all women are encouraged to examine their breasts and to consult their physicians if an abnormality is detected. Routine screening mammograms also are highly recommended, as noted earlier.

Many breast carcinomas induce fibrosis in the surrounding normal breast tissue that is being invaded by the tumor cells, as though the body were trying to defend itself by laying down fibrous tissue to contain the tumor. Consequently, many breast cancers are very firm and have a puckered, scarred appearance with irregular margins that blend into the surrounding breast tissue. This appearance is caused more by the proliferation of fibrous

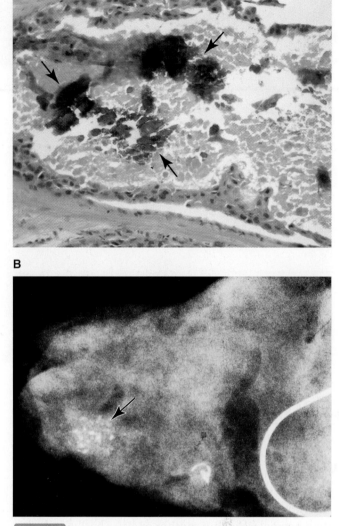

**Figure 13-7**    **A,** Ductal carcinoma of the breast, showing necrosis and calcification (*arrows*) within the tumor. **B,** Characteristic appearance of stippled calcification within the tumor (*arrow*) that can be identified by mammograms.

tissue in response to the tumor than to the tumor cells themselves. Nevertheless, this appearance is quite characteristic of many breast cancers and aids in identifying a carcinoma by mammography ( Figure 13-8 ). Not all breast carcinomas have such a characteristic appearance. In many instances, the mammogram identifies only an abnormal or suspicious area within the breast that could be an early carcinoma but is not conclusive, and a biopsy is necessary to establish the exact diagnosis.

## Clinical Manifestations

The most common initial manifestation of breast carcinoma is a lump in the breast. It is often first detected by the patient herself or by a routine mammogram. Sometimes the carcinoma may also cause secondary changes in the overlying skin or the nipple. The neoplasm may infiltrate the suspensory ligaments, exerting traction on the ligaments and causing them to shorten.

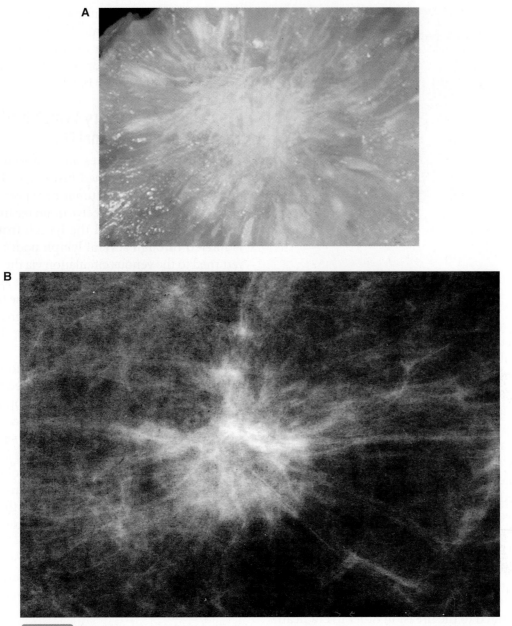

**Figure 13-8** Breast carcinoma. **A,** Cross section of a breast biopsy. The tumor appears as a firm, poorly circumscribed mass that infiltrates the surrounding fatty breast tissue. **B,** The appearance of breast carcinoma in a mammogram. The tumor appears as a white area with infiltrating margins. Note that the same criteria used to identify breast carcinoma on gross examination are used to recognize malignancy in the mammogram.

Because the ligaments attach to the skin of the breast, shortening of the ligaments causes the overlying skin to retract as well. Consequently, skin or nipple retraction generally indicates the presence of an infiltrating carcinoma deeper within the breast.

If the tumor infiltrates and plugs the lymphatic vessels that drain lymph from the skin, the overlying skin will become edematous. (Lymphatic obstruction as a cause of edema is considered in Chapter 9.) Skin edema produces a rather characteristic appearance in which the normal cutaneous hair follicles stand out sharply as multiple small depressions within the edematous skin. The appearance has been compared to the skin of an orange and is usually called the orange-peel sign ( Figure 13-9 ). Unfortunately, this finding indicates an advanced carcinoma that has already invaded lymphatic vessels and has probably also metastasized to regional lymph nodes. The likelihood of curing the cancer is much reduced at this stage.

If the patient delays in consulting her physician and a breast cancer is not treated, the tumor will eventually infiltrate the entire breast and will become fixed to the chest wall. The tumor will also metastasize widely. Although a far-advanced cancer often can be controlled for a time by various methods of treatment, there is no longer a possibility of cure.

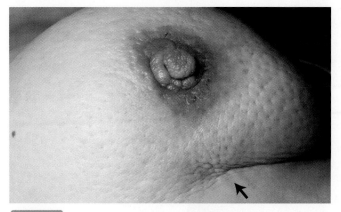

**Figure 13-9** Changes in the breast caused by advanced carcinoma. Skin retraction (*arrow*) and orange-peel appearance of the skin.

## Treatment

There are two ways to treat invasive breast carcinoma, and both methods achieve the same long-term results. One method of treatment is a surgical procedure called modified radical mastectomy or total mastectomy with axillary lymph node dissection. As the names indicate, the procedure consists of resecting the entire breast along with the axillary tissues that contain the lymph nodes draining the breast, but leaving the pectoral muscles overlying the chest wall. The mastectomy can be followed by a breast reconstruction using a saline or silicone-filled implant.

A second method of treatment consists of removing only part of the breast along with the tumor (partial mastectomy) or removing only the tumor along with a small amount of adjacent breast tissue (lumpectomy). In these procedures, axillary lymph nodes also are removed, as in a total mastectomy. A course of radiotherapy is then administered to the breast in order to eradicate any carcinoma remaining within the breast that was not removed by the surgical procedure. This treatment offers the advantage of preserving the breast but has the disadvantage of possible complications related to the radiotherapy.

**sentinel node** The lymph node in a group of lymph nodes that is located closest to a malignant tumor, which is examined to determine whether the tumor has spread to the node. If the sentinel node is not involved, additional lymph node dissection is not required.

Whichever method of treatment is selected, part of the tumor obtained at the time of the surgical procedure is tested for the presence of estrogen and progesterone receptors, and a test is also performed on the tumor cells to detect amplification of a gene called *HER-2*. Determination of the hormone receptor status of the tumor has two purposes:

1. To provide information on prognosis. Tumors containing hormone receptors are better differentiated than those lacking receptors, and patients with tumors containing hormone receptors have a more favorable clinical course.

2. As a guide to further treatment. Tumors containing hormone receptors respond to adjuvant therapy using drugs that block these receptors.

## Examination of Axillary Lymph Nodes: The Role of the Sentinel Node

The axillary lymph nodes are removed primarily so that they can be examined histologically in order to determine whether the tumor has spread beyond the breast. The nodes that receive drainage from the breast are interconnected, and the lymph from the breast is filtered through several lymph nodes before being returned to the venous circulation via the thoracic duct or right lymphatic duct. If one or more axillary lymph nodes contain metastatic carcinoma, the tumor already has spread beyond the breast, and the greater the number of involved axillary lymph nodes, the less favorable the prognosis.

Axillary lymph node dissection performed to guide further treatment may at times be complicated by edema of the arm resulting from disruption of the lymphatic drainage channels in the axilla and may also be associated with temporary limitation of shoulder mobility and axillary discomfort. Sometimes it is possible to avoid an axillary dissection while still obtaining information about the presence or absence or axillary metastases. It is possible to identify the first lymph node in the chain of axillary lymph nodes that receives drainage from the tumor. This node is called the **sentinel node**. If the sentinel node does not contain metastatic tumor, it is very unlikely that any of the other axillary nodes will contain the tumor, and a more extensive axillary dissection is avoided.

## Estrogen and Progesterone Receptors in Breast Carcinoma

A breast carcinoma is derived from cells whose growth and functions are influenced by various hormones: estrogen, progesterone, growth hormone, prolactin, and adrenal corticosteroids. Many breast tumors require these hormones for their continued growth and may undergo temporary regression if the body's hormonal balance is changed. The tumor cells of many breast carcinomas are stimulated by estrogen and progesterone and undergo regression if the hormone receptors on the tumor cells are blocked by drugs (called antiestrogen drugs) that prevent the tumor cells from responding to these hormones. Laboratory tests performed on the tumor cells can determine whether the tumor cells require these hormones by testing the

**Figure 13-10** Action of estrogen receptor. **A,** Estrogen enters cytoplasm and binds to estrogen-receptor protein. **B,** Estrogen-receptor complex enters nucleus. **C,** Complex attaches to nuclear chromosome, activating mRNA synthesis. Messenger RNA directs protein synthesis on ribosomes in cytoplasm.

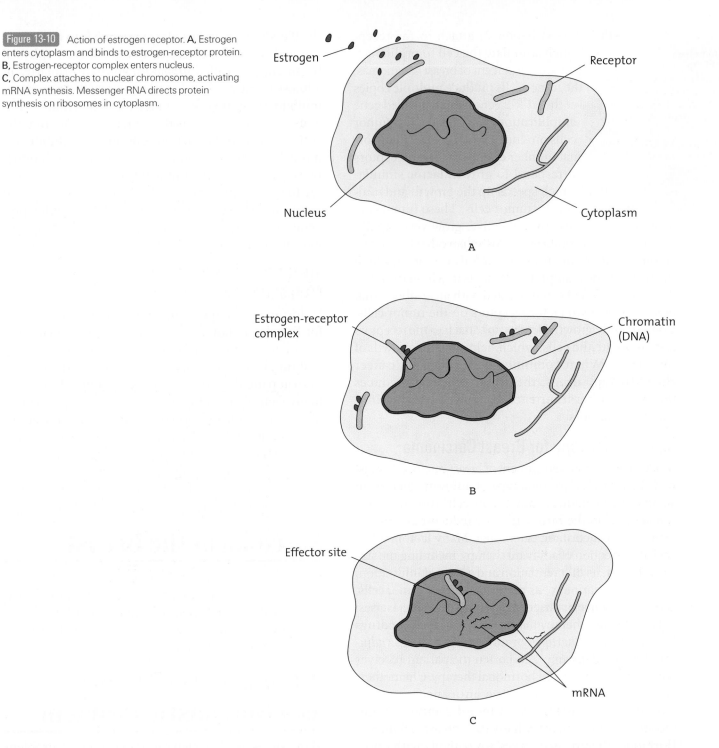

A

B

C

cells for the presence of hormone receptor proteins in the cells. If a receptor binds estrogen, the cell is estrogen-receptor positive; if a receptor binds progesterone, the cell is progesterone-receptor positive. Approximately 60 percent of all breast tumors are estrogen-receptor positive, and most estrogen-receptor-positive tumors are also positive for progesterone receptors. Tumors lacking these receptors do not respond to antiestrogen drugs.

**Figure 13-10** illustrates how estrogen interacts with its receptor protein, and a similar mechanism applies to progesterone as well. In order for a cell to respond to estrogen, the hormone must enter the cell and combine with the estrogen receptors in the cytoplasm. The hormone–protein complex then moves into the nucleus and attaches to the nuclear DNA, which stimulates the growth and other metabolic activities of the cell.

## *HER-2* Gene Amplification in Breast Carcinoma

The *HER-2* gene, located on chromosome 17, directs the production of growth factor receptors on the cell membrane. Soluble growth-promoting substances called

**aromatase inhibitor** (air-ō′-muh-tase) A drug that inhibits the conversion of adrenal androgenic steroids to estrogens, used as post-resection adjuvant therapy to treat post-menopausal women with estrogen-positive breast carcinoma.

*growth factors* (Chapter 2) attach to the receptors, which stimulate the cell to proliferate. In about 25 percent of breast carcinomas, the tumor cells produce multiple copies of the *HER-2* gene, which is called gene amplification. As a result, the tumor cells produce a much greater than normal number of growth factor receptors that respond to growth factor stimulation, which speeds up the growth and multiplication of the tumor cells. These tumors are usually estrogen-receptor negative, grow very rapidly, and have a less favorable prognosis than other breast carcinomas. Laboratory tests can identify tumors in which the *HER-2* gene is amplified. Patients in whom the *HER-2* gene is amplified can be treated with an antibody that blocks the growth factor receptors on the tumor cells. Consequently, growth factors can't attach to the receptors and stimulate the cells, which help slow the growth of the tumor. When combined with other anticancer chemotherapy drugs, the antibody greatly reduces the breast cancer recurrence risk in women with *HER-2*–positive tumors.

## Adjuvant Therapy for Breast Carcinoma

In addition to surgical treatment of breast carcinoma, most patients also receive some type of adjuvant therapy in an attempt to eradicate any tumor cells that may have spread beyond the breast, thereby reducing the risk of recurrent or metastatic carcinoma. Many factors influence the selection of adjuvant therapy, including the size of the tumor, its differentiation and extent of infiltration, the results of various tests performed on the tumor cells, and the presence or absence of lymph node metastases.

The adjuvant therapy may consist of anticancer drugs (*adjuvant chemotherapy*) or antiestrogen drugs (*adjuvant hormonal therapy*), and often the patient receives both chemotherapy and hormonal therapy. Chemotherapy consists of administering anticancer drugs at monthly intervals for 4 to 6 months and is recommended for all women with invasive breast carcinoma. Hormonal therapy is reserved for patients with estrogen-receptor-positive tumors. Two types of drugs are available. One is tamoxifen or a similar drug taken daily for 5 years. Tamoxifen prevents estrogen from stimulating tumor cells by blocking the estrogen receptors to which estrogen must attach in order to stimulate tumor cells. The other estrogen-blocking drugs are called *aromatase inhibitors*, which are also taken daily and are useful for treating postmenopausal women. Although their ovaries no longer produce estrogen, their adrenal glands produce small quantities of androgenic (testosteronelike) steroid hormones that circulate in

the bloodstream and can be converted into estrogens. The androgen-to-estrogen conversion is accomplished by an enzyme called *aromatase* located primarily in adipose tissue but in other tissues as well. **Aromatase-inhibitor** drugs prevent estrogen formation from androgens in postmenopausal women by blocking the conversion step. The action of aromatase inhibitors is quite different from tamoxifen. Aromatase inhibitors prevent estrogen from stimulating tumor cells by blocking the conversion of adrenal androgenic hormones to estrogens in postmenopausal women. Tamoxifen prevents estrogen from stimulating tumor cells by blocking estrogen receptors to which the estrogen must attach.

## Treatment of Recurrent and Metastatic Carcinoma

Unfortunately, a significant number of patients treated for breast carcinoma develop recurrent or metastatic carcinoma that may appear many years after the original tumor had been resected. The methods selected to treat patients with recurrent carcinoma depend on many factors, including the hormone receptor status of the tumor, the location of the metastases, the age of the patient, and the length of time that has elapsed between the initial treatment and the appearance of the metastases. Although the tumor is no longer curable, treatment can control tumor growth, relieve symptoms, and improve the patient's quality of life.

# Sarcoma of the Breast

Sarcoma of the breast is rare in comparison with breast carcinoma. It may arise from the fibrous tissue or blood vessels within the breast. Sarcomas often form large, bulky tumors that may metastasize widely. Treatment is by surgical resection of the involved breast.

# A Lump in the Breast as a Diagnostic Problem

Many times, a physician faces the difficult problem presented by a patient who has a lump in her breast. It may have been detected either by the patient herself or a mammogram, or by the physician in the course of a routine physical examination. The lump could be a benign cyst, a fibroadenoma, a carcinoma, or one of many other less common diseases of the breast. Certain clinical features may suggest to the physician the probability that the breast lesion is benign or malignant, and mammograms of the breast may provide helpful information. However, the only way to be certain is to perform an aspiration biopsy or needle biopsy of the mass,

or to excise the mass completely. The biopsy can be examined by a pathologist, who can make an exact diagnosis. If the lesion is benign, limited conservative treatment is all that is required. If the lesion proves to be malignant, the surgeon can perform a more extensive surgical operation.

# Female Reproductive System

## Infections of the Female Genital Tract

Infections of the genital tract are common. Frequently involved sites are the vagina, the cervix, and the fallopian tubes. In addition, certain virus infections of the genital tract cause highly characteristic lesions called condylomas.

## Vaginitis

Vaginal infections are common. They frequently cause vaginal discharge, together with vulvovaginal itching and irritation. There are three major causes:

1. The fungus *Candida albicans*
2. The protozoan parasite *Trichomonas vaginalis*
3. A small gram-negative bacterium called *Gardnerella (Haemophilus) vaginalis*, in conjunction with various anaerobic vaginal bacteria

Candida vaginitis was considered along with other fungal infections, and the protozoan parasite *Trichomonas vaginalis* was considered with the parasitic infections in Chapter 5. The third common type of vaginitis, often called nonspecific vaginitis, is usually associated with a profuse, foul-smelling vaginal discharge. Highly specific methods of treatment are available for each type of vaginitis.

## Cervicitis

Mild chronic inflammation of endocervical glands is very common in women who have had children. Cervicitis causes few symptoms and is of little clinical significance. More severe cervical inflammation may result from a gonococcal or a chlamydial infection (Chapter 6). Both infections are sexually transmitted and may be followed by the spread of the infection into the fallopian tubes and adjacent tissues.

## Salpingitis and Pelvic Inflammatory Disease

Salpingitis means an inflammation of the fallopian tube (*salpinx* = tube). The more general term *pelvic inflammatory disease*, or simply PID, refers to any infection that affects the fallopian tubes and adjacent tissues. Sometimes the ovaries are infected along with the fallopian tubes. Most cases are secondary to the spread of a cervical gonorrheal or chlamydial infection through the uterus into the fallopian tubes and surrounding tissues. Less commonly, other pathogenic organisms are involved. An acute pelvic infection causes severe lower abdominal pain and tenderness, together with elevated temperature and leukocytosis.

Both gonorrheal and nongonorrheal salpingitis respond to appropriate antibiotic therapy; healing of the inflammation, however, may be associated with scarring and obstruction of the tubal lumen. Sterility may result if the tubal obstruction is bilateral ( Figure 13-11 ). Sometimes, even if the tubes are not completely

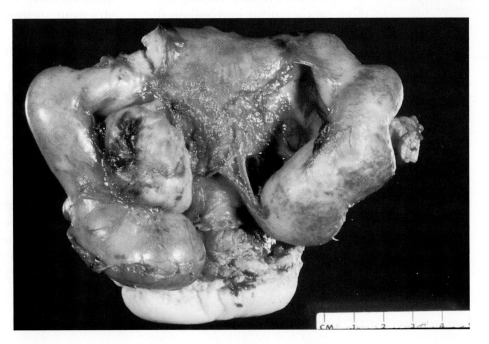

Figure 13-11 Chronic pelvic inflammatory disease. Resected uterus, tubes, and left ovary viewed from behind. Tubes are swollen, and fimbriated ends are occluded. There are numerous adhesions between tubes and uterus.

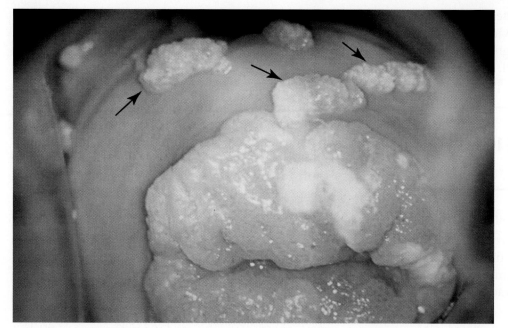

Cervical and vaginal mucosa viewed through vaginal speculum, revealing multiple condylomas (*arrows*) arising from mucosa.

occluded, the scarring may delay the transport of a fertilized ovum through the tube and lead to implantation of the ovum in the fallopian tube rather than in the endometrial cavity. This condition is called an ectopic pregnancy and is considered in Chapter 14.

## Condylomas of the Genital Tract

**Condylomas** are benign warty, tumorlike overgrowths of squamous epithelium caused by a virus called human papillomavirus (HPV) that is spread by sexual contact. They vary in size from a few millimeters to more than 1 centimeter in diameter and are frequently multiple. Condylomas develop most often on the vulvar mucosa, on the mucosa of the cervix and vagina ( Figure 13-12 ), around the vaginal opening, and around the anus. Treatment consists of destroying the lesions, which may be accomplished by applying a strong chemical (podophyllin), by electrocoagulation, by freezing (cryocautery), or by surgical excision.

**condyloma**
(kon-di-lō'ma) A warty tumorlike overgrowth in the squamous epithelium of the anorectal or genital tract, caused by a virus that is spread by sexual contact.

**endometriosis** (en-dō-mē trē-ō'sis) Presence of endometrial tissue in abnormal locations, such as in the ovary or pelvis.

# Endometriosis

The term **endometriosis** refers to the presence of endometrium in any location outside the endometrial cavity ( Figure 13-13 ). Ectopic deposits (*ecto* = outside) of endometrium may occasionally be encountered in the wall of the uterus ( Figure 13-14 ), in the ovary ( Figure 13-15 ), or elsewhere in the pelvis. Sometimes, endometrial tissue is found in the appendix or in the rectum. Endometriosis is a common problem, which occurs in about 10 to 15 percent of women, and much more frequently in infertile women and in women with pelvic pain, irregular menses, or dysmenorrhea. Often the condition appears to occur in families, and a woman is more likely to develop endometriosis if her mother had endometriosis. The reason that endometrial deposits occur in unusual locations is unknown, although many theories have been proposed. Some cases seem to be caused by reflux of bits of shed endometrium along with menstrual blood through the fallopian tubes into the peritoneal cavity during menstruation (retrograde menstruation), which then implant and grow in the pelvis. This does not provide a complete explanation, however, because retrograde menstruation is common, but implantation of menstrual endometrium carried through the tubes into the peritoneal cavity is infrequent.

Endometrial deposits respond to normal hormonal stimuli and therefore undergo cyclic menstrual desquamation and regeneration. Because the misplaced endometrial tissue does not communicate with the endometrial cavity, the "menstruating" tissue is not discharged through the vagina. Old blood and desquamated material are retained in the ectopic sites, leading to considerable scarring and causing crampy pain during menstrual periods. Obstruction of the fallopian tubes by scarring may cause sterility.

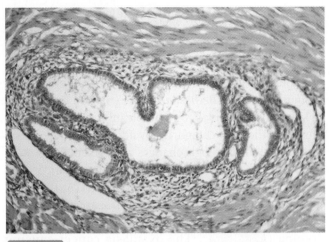

Figure 13-13  A photomicrograph of endometriosis in the uterine wall. Normal endometrial glands and stroma are surrounded by uterine muscle (original magnification × 100).

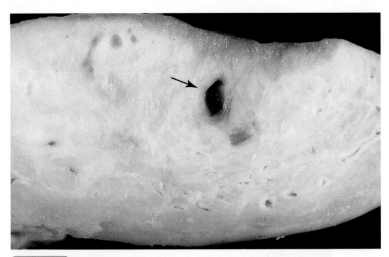

Figure 13-14  A cross section of resected uterus illustrating a cystic deposit of endometriosis filled with old blood located in the uterine wall (*arrow*).

Diagnosis of endometriosis is usually established by visualizing the ectopic deposits within the pelvis with a lighted tubular instrument called a *laparoscope* (Chapter 1). The laparoscope is inserted into the abdominal cavity through a small incision in the umbilicus. Treatment consists of removing or destroying the deposits surgically or impeding the progression of endometriosis by administering drugs or hormones. Three methods of hormone treatment are commonly used:

1. Synthetic hormones having progesterone activity completely suppress the menstrual cycles.

2. Birth-control pills suppress ovulation, so the endometrium becomes thin and atrophic, and menstrual periods are very light. The endometriosis is similarly suppressed, retarding its progression and associated scarring.

3. Drugs are administered that suppress the output of gonadotropins from the pituitary gland. This in turn leads to a decline in ovarian function, similar to that occurring in menopause. The deposits of endometriosis, deprived of cyclic estrogen–progesterone stimulation, undergo regression.

**A**

**B**

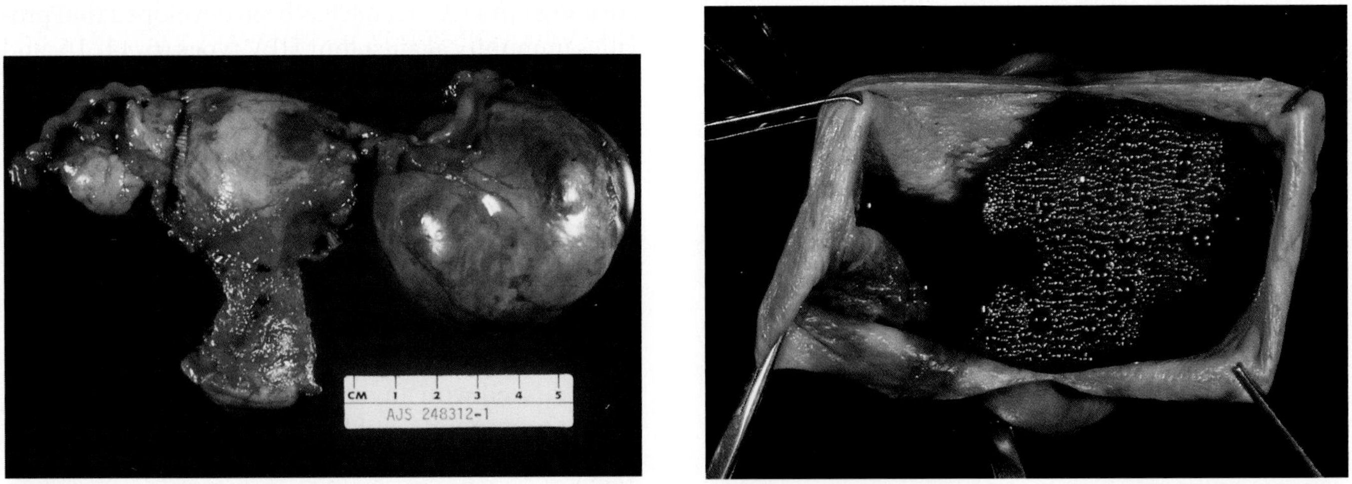

Figure 13-15  **A,** Endometriosis of the ovary. An accumulation of blood and debris within the ovarian endometriosis has led to formation of an endometrium-lined cyst filled with old blood and desquamated endometrial tissue within the right ovary (*right side* of photograph). **B,** Endometrial cyst opened, revealing cyst contents consisting of old blood and debris derived from the endometrium lining the cyst.

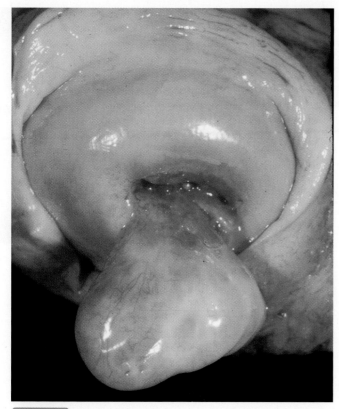

Figure 13-16  Large cervical polyp.

## Cervical Polyps

Occasionally, benign polyps arise from the cervix. Usually, they are small and do not cause symptoms, but some may be quite large ( Figure 13-16 ). Sometimes the tip of the polyp becomes eroded and causes bleeding. Treatment consists of surgically removing the polyp.

## Cervical Dysplasia and Cervical Carcinoma

Abnormal growth and maturation of cervical squamous epithelium is called cervical dysplasia. Dysplastic changes range from mild disturbances of epithelial maturation to severe cellular abnormalities. Mild dysplasia may result from cervical inflammation or other causes and may regress spontaneously. Severe dysplasia usually does not regress and may progress to in situ carcinoma and eventually to invasive carcinoma after a variable period of time. Most physicians regard cervical dysplasia and in situ carcinoma as very closely related, constituting different stages in a progressive spectrum of epithelial abnormalities. Indeed, many physicians classify both dysplasia and in situ carcinoma under the general term *cervical intraepithelial*

*neoplasia*, which is usually abbreviated CIN and is graded I, II, and III. In this terminology, mild dysplasia is called CIN I. Moderate dysplasia is termed CIN II. Severe dysplasia and in situ carcinoma are classified together and are designated CIN III. Another grading system called the *Bethesda system* (named from a city in Maryland) provides comparable information but supplements the CIN categories by adding a detailed classification of the cytologic changes observed in Pap smears together with an assessment of their significance.

Persons infected with some types of HPV, the same virus that causes genital condylomas, are at increased risk of developing cervical dysplasia and cervical carcinoma ( Figure 13-17 ). The dysplasia cancer-causing strains can infect the cervical epithelial cells and become incorporated into the cell's DNA, which induces cell dysfunction leading to cell dysplasia and cervical carcinoma.

There are more than 80 different types of HPV, and about 40 types can infect the genital tract; but only about eight different types (called *high-risk types*) are considered to be carcinogenic (cancer causing). HPV genital tract infections are common. Many young sexually active women become infected, but over 90 percent of the infections resolve spontaneously within 6 to 12 months as the body's immune system responds to the infection and destroys the virus. Some women have repeated infections, and their immune systems eradicate the viruses, leaving no long-term harmful effects. Only the small proportions of women infected with a cancer-causing HPV type who are unable to eliminate the virus are at risk of cervical dysplasia and cervical carcinoma.

**HPV Vaccine**  A vaccine has been developed that provides immunity against four HPV types (6, 11, 16, and 18). Types 16 and 18 are responsible for 70 percent of the cases of cervical dysplasia-carcinoma and types 6 and 11 cause 90 percent of HPV papillomas. Unfortunately the vaccine is not effective against any of the four HPV types to which the subject has already been infected, but can still provide protection from the other viruses covered by the vaccine. The vaccine is recommended primarily for girls 11–12 years old, before they become sexually active, because they are unlikely to have been infected with any of the four HPV types covered by the vaccine and would get the most protection from the vaccine. HPV vaccine should not be considered an all purpose "anticancer vaccine." Regular gynecologic care and Pap smears are still required because other carcinogenic viruses not covered by the vaccine may still cause papillomas, dysplasia, and cervical cancer.

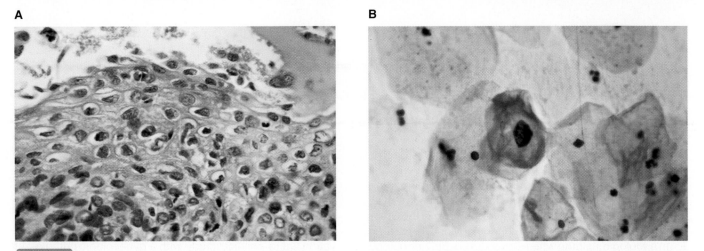

**A**

**B**

Figure 13-17   **A,** Cervical epithelial dysplasia caused by papillomavirus. Compare with normal epithelium in Figures 2-4 and 2-10A. **B,** Dyplastic epithelial cell identified in Papanicolaou smear (original magnification × 400).

## Diagnosis and Treatment

The cellular abnormalities indicative of dysplasia or carcinoma develop first in the cells at the junction between the squamous epithelium covering the exterior of the cervix and the columnar epithelium lining the cervical canal. Abnormal cells indicative of dysplasia or carcinoma can be identified by means of a Pap smear prepared from material obtained from around the external opening in the cervix leading into the endocervical canal (called the external os) and also from the endocervical canal.

An abnormal Pap smear requires further evaluation, which is usually accomplished by means of a binocular magnifying instrument called a **colposcope**. This instrument provides the physician with a greatly magnified view of the cervix and endocervical canal. In cervical dysplasia and carcinoma, one can often identify characteristic abnormalities in the cervical epithelium and underlying blood vessels and can define the location and extent of the abnormal epithelium. Then multiple biopsy specimens are taken from the abnormal-appearing areas, and material is also obtained from the endocervical canal. Treatment depends on the results of the biopsies. Dysplasia and in situ carcinoma are usually treated by destruction of the abnormal epithelium by freezing (cryocautery), by laser light, by surgical excision of the abnormal area, or sometimes by removal of the uterus (hysterectomy). Invasive carcinoma is treated either by radiation or by resection of the uterus, fallopian tubes, ovaries, and adjacent tissues (radical hysterectomy).

Dysplasia and in situ carcinoma can be cured by proper treatment and carry an excellent prognosis. In situ carcinoma may remain localized within the epithelium of the cervix for as long as 10 years before eventually becoming invasive. After invasion has occurred, however, the neoplasm is much harder to treat, and the results are less satisfactory.

# Endometrial Hyperplasia, Polyps, and Carcinoma

Occasionally, the endometrium of the uterus may undergo benign hyperplasia, which is often associated with irregular uterine bleeding ( Figure 13-18 ). Benign polyps in the endometrium are also common ( Figure 13-19 ). Sometimes an endometrial polyp may cause uterine bleeding if the tip becomes inflamed or ulcerated. Endometrial adenocarcinoma has been increasing in frequency. This condition also is manifested by irregular uterine bleeding or postmenopausal bleeding. Endometrial carcinoma is often related to prolonged or excessive stimulation of the endometrium by estrogen.

# Uterine Myomas

Benign smooth muscle tumors called **myomas** arise in the wall of the uterus ( Figure 13-20 ). They are frequently encountered and are said to occur in approximately 30 percent of women over 30 years of age. Occasionally, myomas may be responsible for excessive or irregular uterine bleeding or may produce symptoms related to pressure on the adjacent bladder or rectum ( Figure 13-21 ). Hysterectomy is performed if the myomas are producing symptoms. Other methods of treatment are also available.

**colposcope**
(kol′pos-kōp) A binocular magnifying instrument used to view the cervix and endocervical canal.

**myoma** (mī-ō′muh) A benign smooth muscle tumor such as commonly develops in the uterus.

*A research project on guinea pig ovaries eventually led to the well-known Pap smear.*

The man for whom the smear was named was George Papanicolaou, who was born in Greece in 1883. Although medicine was not his major interest, at the urging of his physician-father he obtained a medical degree in 1904, and later served for a time as a medical officer in the Greek army. However, his interest lay in zoology, and he enrolled in a zoologic institute where he received a PhD in zoology. Later he immigrated to the United States, where he was able to obtain a position in the anatomy department at Cornell University in New York. One of his research projects was studying guinea pig eggs (oocytes) extracted from the ovaries, which he needed to collect just before ovulation. However, the time of ovulation was difficult to determine, so he developed a method for determining the time of ovulation by examining guinea pig vaginal epithelial cells, which varied in response to changes in levels of the ovarian hormones that lead to ovulation. As a result, he was able to determine the preovulatory phase of the guinea pig reproductive cycle by examining stained smears prepared from guinea pig vaginal epithelial cells, which enabled him to collect the guinea pig eggs at the correct time. In further studies on women Papanicolaou also observed similar hormone-related changes in the vaginal epithelial cells during the proliferative and secretory phases of their reproductive (menstrual) cycles. Occasionally he found abnormal-appearing epithelial cells in vaginal smears from women who had uterine cancer. This chance observation led to a clinical study with a gynecologic pathologist Herbert F. Traut to evaluate the potential of vaginal smears as a screening test to detect uterine cancer. The work was published by Papanicolaou and Traut in 1943 in a monograph "Diagnosis of Uterine Cancer by the Vaginal Smear" followed by "Atlas of Exfoliative Cytology" published by Papanicolaou in 1954, which established the value of the Pap smear as a screening test to detect epithelial dysplasia and cancer. Dr. Papanicolaou continued his cytologic studies for the rest of his career until his death in 1962 at age 78. This is a fascinating example of how a research project by a zoologist blossomed into a major advance in clinical medicine.

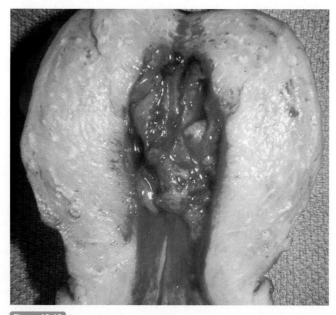

**Figure 13-18** Benign endometrial hyperplasia. The uterus opened to reveal polypoid masses of hyperplastic endometrium filling the endometrial cavity.

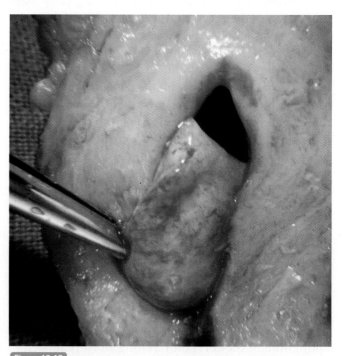

**Figure 13-19** A longitudinal section of resected uterus revealing a large endometrial polyp (*held by forceps*) within the endometrial cavity.

**A**

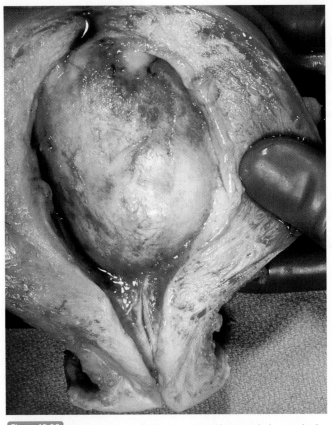

**B**

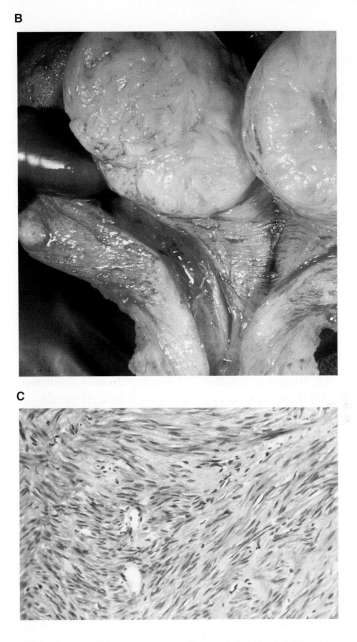

**C**

Figure 13-20 Uterine myoma. **A,** A uterus opened to reveal a large spherical myoma protruding into the endometrial cavity. **B,** A cross section of myoma illustrating a well-circumscribed tumor without evidence of necrosis, features suggesting a benign neoplasm. **C,** Histologic appearance, revealing interlacing bundles of mature smooth muscle cells that resemble the normal muscle cells from which the tumor arose (original magnification × 100).

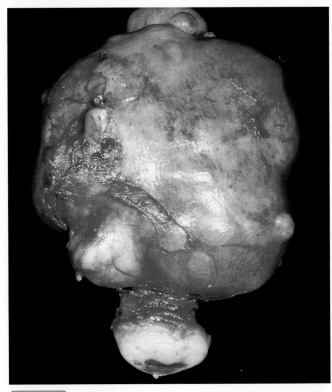

Figure 13-21 Enlarged irregularly shaped uterus containing multiple myomas that bulge from the uterus. The cervix is at *bottom* of photograph.

# Irregular Uterine Bleeding

Excessive or irregular uterine bleeding is a common gynecologic problem. Most cases in younger women result from a disturbance in the normal cyclic interaction of estrogen and progesterone on the endometrium. This is usually called dysfunctional uterine bleeding. In older women, bleeding can be the result of many causes.

## Dysfunctional Uterine Bleeding

Normally, the first half of the menstrual cycle is characterized by proliferation of endometrial glands and stroma under the influence of estrogen produced by the ovarian follicle. At about mid-cycle, ovulation occurs, and the follicle discharges its egg. Then the follicle becomes a corpus luteum, which produces both progesterone and estrogen. Under the influence of progesterone, the endometrium becomes secretory in preparation for receiving a fertilized ovum. If no pregnancy occurs, the corpus luteum begins to decline, and estrogen–progesterone levels begin to drop. The secretory endometrium is deprived of its hormonal support and is shed along with a small amount of blood, constituting the menstrual flow, after which a new cycle begins.

Most cases of dysfunctional uterine bleeding occur because the follicle fails to mature to the point of ovulation and, consequently, no corpus luteum forms. As a result, the endometrium is subjected to continuous estrogen stimulation and responds by shedding in an irregular manner associated with irregular uterine bleeding, instead of shedding all at once as in a normal period. This condition is also called *anovulatory bleeding* (*ana* = without + ovulation). It tends to arise at both extremes of reproductive life: when normal menstrual cycles are being established at puberty and near menopause when ovarian function is declining.

Dysfunctional uterine bleeding is treated by administering hormones to restore the proliferative–secretory sequence in the endometrium that is characteristic of a normal menstrual cycle. In one common treatment, the patient is given a synthetic steroid hormone having progesterone activity. The hormone induces secretory changes in the endometrium and stops the bleeding. The hormone treatment is then stopped, and the endometrium sheds as in a normal period. Frequently, the next cycle is normal, and no further treatment is required.

### Other Causes of Uterine Bleeding

Other conditions that may cause endometrial bleeding include benign endometrial hyperplasia, endometrial and cervical polyps, uterine myomas, and uterine carcinoma.

### Diagnosis and Treatment

Irregular bleeding is always a cause for concern when it occurs in an older woman nearing the end of her reproductive years or after menopause because it may be the result of an endometrial carcinoma. Bleeding in older women is usually treated by dilating the cervix with various metal dilators and then scraping out the lining of the uterus with a long-handled scoop-like instrument called a curette. This procedure is called a dilation and curettage, or simply D and C (usually abbreviated D&C). The tissue removed is examined microscopically by the pathologist. If the endometrial tissue is not malignant, no further treatment is needed. If endometrial carcinoma is detected,

further treatment is required. Usually this consists of hysterectomy, sometimes preceded by a course of radiation therapy.

# Dysmenorrhea

**Dysmenorrhea** means painful menstruation. There are two types: *primary dysmenorrhea*, in which the pelvic organs are normal, and *secondary dysmenorrhea*, which results from various diseases of the pelvic organs, such as endometriosis.

Primary dysmenorrhea is the more common type. The cramplike pain begins just prior to menstruation and lasts for 1 or 2 days after onset of the menstrual flow. Usually, menstrual periods are painless for the first year or two after onset of menses during adolescence because early menstrual cycles are usually anovulatory and primary dysmenorrhea does not occur unless ovulation occurs. Dysmenorrhea does not usually become a problem until regular ovulatory menstrual cycles are established.

Cramplike menstrual pain is caused by a class of compounds called prostaglandins, complex unsaturated fatty-acid derivatives that are synthesized in many locations throughout the body and have many functions. The name derives from the prostate gland, where these substances were first identified. Prostaglandins are synthesized within the endometrium under the influence of progesterone produced by the ovary during the secretory phase of the cycle. When the endometrium breaks down during menstruation, the prostaglandins are released and diffuse into the myometrium, where they cause the spasmodic myometrial contractions that are responsible for the crampy menstrual pain. Dysmenorrhea does not occur if cycles are anovulatory because no corpus luteum forms and no progesterone is produced to stimulate prostaglandin synthesis.

Treatment consists of aspirin or another anti-inflammatory drug, which is administered before the onset of menses. These drugs suppress the synthesis of prostaglandins within the endometrium. Primary dysmenorrhea can also be treated very effectively with oral contraceptive pills, which prevent dysmenorrhea by suppressing ovulation.

# Cysts and Tumors of the Ovary

The ovary gives rise to a wide variety of cysts and tumors, and only the more common ones are considered here. Benign ovarian cysts are common. They arise either from ovarian follicles or from corpora lutea, as

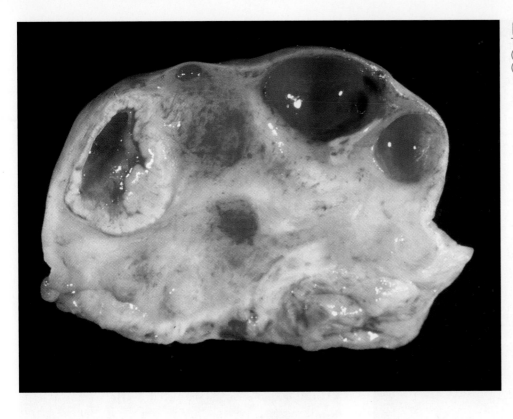

Figure 13-22 Section of normal ovary. There are two follicles beneath the capsule (*right side*) and a corpus luteum (*left side*).

illustrated in Figure 13-22, that have failed to regress normally and instead become converted into fluid-filled cysts. Follicle cysts and corpus luteum cysts are often called *functional cysts* because they represent a derangement of the normal maturation and involution of a follicle or corpus luteum. Functional cysts do not usually become very large, and most regress spontaneously.

Endometrial deposits in the ovary may form cysts lined by endometrium and filled with old blood and debris. These are called **endometrial cysts** (Figure 13-15). True ovarian neoplasms may arise in one or both ovaries. They may be either benign or malignant, cystic or solid. Benign cystic teratomas, often called *dermoid cysts*, commonly develop in the ovary. These tumors arise from unfertilized ova that have undergone neoplastic change. They often contain skin, hair, teeth, bone, parts of gastrointestinal tract, thyroid, and other tissues growing in a jumbled fashion (Figure 13-23). Sometimes teeth and bone contained in dermoid cysts can be detected in x-ray films of the pelvis. A dermoid cyst apparently represents an attempt of an unfertilized ovum to realize its potential by producing diverse tissues like those in a fetus. In contrast with the frequency of benign ovarian teratomas, malignant teratomas of the ovary are quite rare.

Another group of ovarian tumors are those arising from the epithelial cells on the surface of the ovary, and the epithelium of the tumor cells may resemble the epithe-

lium found in other parts of the genital tract. If the tumor epithelium resembles the cells lining the fallopian tube, the tumor is classified as a *serous tumor*. If the tumor epithelium resembles the mucus-secreting epithelium of the endocervix, it is called a *mucinous tumor;* if the tumor epithelium resembles endometrium, it is termed an *endometrioid tumor.* Many of the serous and mucinous tumors are cystic, and the term *serous cystadenoma* or *serous cystadenocarcinoma* is used. In many of these serous tumors, the neoplastic epithelium may extend onto the external surface of the tumor (Figure 13-24). When this occurs, small pieces of the projecting tumor may break off and implant elsewhere in the pelvis, peritoneal cavity, and omentum, where they continue to grow. Tumors manifesting this behavior may be difficult to remove completely.

A mucinous tumor is designated as either a mucinous cystadenoma or a mucinous cystadenocarcinoma. Most of the ovarian tumors with endometriumlike epithelium are malignant and are called endometrioid carcinomas. Another common ovarian tumor arises from the fibrous connective tissue cells of the ovary and is called a fibroma.

Some ovarian tumors may become quite large, as illustrated by the following case.

**endometrial cyst**
(en-dō-mē′trē-ul) An ovarian cyst lined by endometrium and filled with old blood and debris. A manifestation of endometriosis.

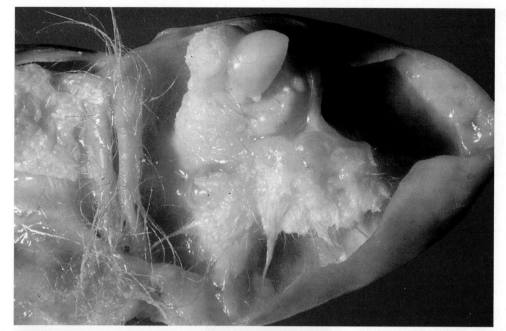

A

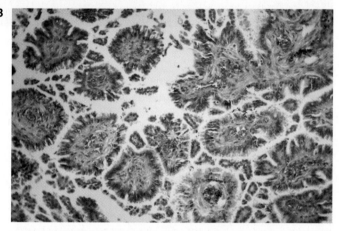
B

**Figure 13-23** Opened dermoid cyst of ovary (benign cystic teratoma) with contents removed. The cyst contains a well-formed jawbone with two teeth (*center*). Note the hair arising from the skin that lines the cyst.

**Figure 13-24** **A,** A resected serous tumor of the ovary measuring 10 centimeters in diameter. Several masses of tumor (*arrows*) project from the surface. **B,** Histologic appearance of the tumor, which forms papillary processes covered by well-differentiated epithelial cells (original magnification × 100).

## Case Study 13-3

A young woman who was 7 months pregnant had noted marked enlargement of the abdomen that she attributed to the pregnancy. Examination by her physician revealed a large cystic mass lying above and posterior to the pregnant uterus. At operation, a large benign cystic tumor of the ovary was encountered. It contained 15 liters of fluid and weighed 35 pounds ( Figure 13-25 ). The day after the operation, the patient went into labor and delivered a premature infant who was transferred to the pediatric intensive care unit. Both mother and infant did well after the operation.

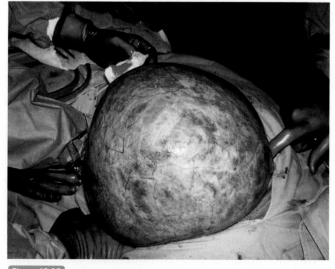

**Figure 13-25** A large benign cystic ovarian tumor removed from a pregnant woman (Case 13-3). The tumor weighed 35 pounds.

# Diseases of the Vulva

## Vulvar Dystrophy

The epithelium of the vulva may exhibit irregular areas of thickening and inflammation that appear as white patches. Histologically, the affected epithelium is heavily keratinized, and the epithelial cells show variable abnormalities of maturation. Clinically, the condition is associated with intense itching and tenderness of the affected areas. The descriptive term *leukoplakia* (*leuko* = white + *plakia* = patch) has often been applied to this lesion but has been discarded in favor of the term *vulvar dystrophy* (*dys* = abnormal + *trophe* = growth). In some cases, vulvar dystrophy progresses gradually over a period of years into in situ carcinoma and eventually into invasive carcinoma. Consequently, many physicians consider vulvar dystrophy a precancerous lesion. Various types of local treatment are frequently effective, but if significant precancerous changes are present in the epithelium, the affected areas are generally removed surgically.

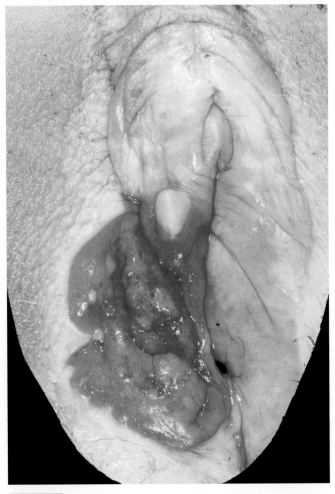

**Figure 13-26** A large carcinoma of the vulva. The white appearance of the skin adjacent to the carcinoma is caused by preexisting vulvar dystrophy.

## Carcinoma of the Vulva

Vulvar carcinoma is occasionally found in both premenopausal and postmenopausal women, frequently arising in areas of vulvar dystrophy ( Figure 13-26 ). Treatment consists of resection of the vulva (vulvectomy) along with the inguinal lymph nodes, which receive lymphatic drainage from the vulva.

# Toxic Shock Syndrome

Toxic shock syndrome (TSS) is a disease that was first recognized about 20 years ago in menstruating women who used high-absorbency tampons, but its frequency has declined as other menstrual products replaced them, although no tampon is entirely free from risk.

Clinically, the disease is characterized by elevated temperature, vomiting and diarrhea, muscular aches and pains, a fall in blood pressure (often to shock levels), and various other systemic manifestations. A characteristic feature of the disease is an erythematous (sunburnlike) skin rash that is followed by flaking and peeling of the affected skin (somewhat like the peeling that occurs after a severe sunburn).

The clinical manifestations of toxic shock syndrome are caused by a toxin produced by *Staphylococcus aureus* that grows in the vagina of the affected patients. The menstrual blood and secretions provide an excellent culture medium that fosters the growth of the staphylococci and the production of toxin.

Treatment of toxic shock syndrome consists of general supportive measures to sustain the patient until the effects of the toxin have worn off. Antibiotics are often prescribed to eradicate the staphylococci, but the antibiotics do not shorten the course of the disease.

Rarely, toxic shock syndrome occurs in nonmenstruating women and in men. These cases are a result of staphylococcal infections in other parts of the body, such as the skin, kidneys, or bone, with liberation of toxins from the infected site into the circulation.

# Contraception

Methods of contraception fall into two major groups: "natural" methods and artificial methods. Natural family planning methods attempt to prevent pregnancy by avoiding intercourse around the time of ovulation when pregnancy is more likely to occur. These methods have no side effects or medical complications but require a high degree of motivation and are generally less effective than artificial methods. In contrast, artificial methods act by preventing the union of sperm and egg, preventing ovulation, or preventing implantation of the fertilized ovum. Many of these methods are highly effective, but some have potentially serious side effects.

Diaphragms and condoms are mechanical devices that are usually used in conjunction with a spermicidal foam or jelly. They function by preventing the union of sperm and egg; they are highly effective when used correctly and have no serious side effects.

Contraceptive pills, a very popular contraceptive method, consist of a synthetic estrogen combined with a compound having progesterone activity (progestin). "The pill" prevents ovulation by suppressing release of the pituitary gonadotropic hormones that regulate ovarian follicle growth, maturation, and ovulation, and also causes changes in the cervical mucus and endometrial lining that also discourage pregnancy. When taken properly, contraceptive pills are almost 100 percent effective, but there are some side effects. The estrogen in the pill promotes increased synthesis of blood coagulation factors, predisposing to formation of blood clots within the circulatory system. Women who smoke cigarettes and women over 35 years of age are at especially high risk. Some women on the pill develop high blood pressure. Women on the pill are closely observed for this complication, and the pill is discontinued if the blood pressure starts to rise.

An intrauterine device (IUD) is a small, flexible plastic structure that is inserted into the uterine cavity by a physician or nurse practitioner. IUDs are less frequently used now by women in the United States and Canada, but worldwide they are widely used as an effective and relatively inexpensive contraceptive method that does not require much attention from the user. A string attached to the device extends through the cervix into the vagina. The string serves two purposes. The woman can assure herself that the device is still within the uterine cavity by feeling the string. It also facilitates removal of the IUD by a physician or other health-care practitioner when it is no longer needed.

Intrauterine devices do not prevent conception but act by preventing implantation of the fertilized ovum.

Most of the devices that were popular previously are no longer marketed because of concerns about lawsuits initiated by women who may have experienced complications from use of the devices.

# Emergency Contraception

Many unintended pregnancies occur each year. Most result from failure to use effective contraception, but some result from failure of the method being used such as a broken condom, or from a sexual assault, and could be prevented by the use of emergency contraception. As described in the next chapter, sperm can survive in a woman's genital tract for as long as 5 or 6 days and still be able to fertilize an ovum. Therefore, intercourse several days before ovulation can still lead to a pregnancy. Even if an ovum is fertilized, it still takes about 1 week for the fertilized ovum to travel through the fallopian tube and implant within the uterus. The likelihood of pregnancy after unprotected intercourse can be greatly reduced by a postcoital (after intercourse) contraceptive. The preferred contraceptive is a single progestin-only pill (1.5-mg levonorgestrel) that should be taken regardless of the cycle day when unprotected intercourse occurred. The progestin in the pills exerts several effects that prevent pregnancy. The progestin may inhibit ovulation, and it also impairs tubal motility, which slows transport of the ovum through the fallopian tube, effects that reduce the likelihood of conception. Finally, the progestin changes the endometrium so that it becomes unsuitable for implantation even if fertilization should occur, and the progestin-mediated change in the endometrium occurs before a fertilized ovum can complete its 7-day journey into the endometrium. The sooner the pill is taken, the better it works. When the pills are taken within 12 hours after unprotected intercourse, the pregnancy risk is less than 1 percent and is about 3 percent when taken within 72 hours, but some protection is still provided for as long as 5 days.

# CHAPTER REVIEW

## Summary

The female breast consists of branching ducts and lobules in fibrous and fatty tissue attached to the chest wall by bands of fibrous tissue called suspensory ligaments. The breast tissue undergoes cyclic change in response to hormonal stimulation. The breasts develop from mammary ridges that extend from the axilla to the groin. Normally only two breasts and nipples develop, but occasionally extra breasts and nipples occur. Breasts are not always the same size, and the disproportion may be accentuated as the breasts enlarge. Temporary enlargement of male breast tissue may occur in males during adolescence, which is called gynecomastia.

Benign cystic change may occur in the breasts, and benign breast tumors called fibroadenomas also occur in young women. They are not hazardous but must be distinguished from breast carcinoma. Hormone treatment of menopausal symptoms increases breast cancer risk and is no longer recommended. Breast cancers may arise from the epithelium of ducts or lobules and various methods of treatment are available, depending on the woman's preference. To guide proper treatment breast cancer tissue is tested for estrogen and progesterone receptors, and for amplification of the *HER-2* gene, which indicates an aggressive tumor requiring special treatment methods. Adjuvant tamoxifen therapy is recommended for women with estrogen receptor-positive (ER-positive) tumors, and aromatase-inhibitor drugs are useful for postmenopausal women with ER-positive tumors. Adjuvant chemotherapy may also be recommended for some patients. Unfortunately, not all cancers are cured by treatment. Chemotherapy, radiation, or various hormones may be used to control metastatic breast cancer. A lump in the breast is always a diagnostic problem, which may be a cyst, a benign tumor, or a carcinoma. A number of diagnostic tests can be applied to distinguish among these conditions so that appropriate treatment can be selected.

Mild vaginal infections are common and easy to treat. Cervical infections caused by the gonococcus or chlamydia are potentially more serious because the infections may spread to the fallopian tubes and pelvic tissues (PID). Endometriosis is characterized by deposits of endometrium outside its normal location, which may cause problems, including dysmenorrhea and impaired fertility related to fibrous tissue proliferation in response to the cyclic desquamation of the ectopic endometrium that is retained within the pelvis. Several methods are available to retard the progression of endometriosis and its adverse effects on fertility.

Cervical dysplasia results from infection by carcinogenic strains of the papillomavirus, which may progress to in situ and eventually invasive carcinoma (CIN). Screening for CIN is by Pap smears supplemented by tests for papillomavirus infection; diagnosis is established by cervical biopsy, and the treatment is eradication of the abnormal epithelium. The HPV vaccine protects against some but not all carcinogenic strains of the papillomavirus, and some physicians are concerned about its limited protection, unknown duration of immunity, possible need for booster injections to maintain immunity, and lack of information about possible adverse long-term effects of the vaccine.

Benign endometrial hyperplasia may lead to irregular uterine bleeding that can be treated successfully but must be differentiated from endometrial carcinoma when irregular bleeding occurs in older women, and especially when occurring in postmenopausal women. Uterine myomas occur frequently, and may require treatment if they cause uterine bleeding or pressure symptoms from pressing on the rectum or bladder.

The term *dysmenorrhea* refers to painful menses. Primary dysmenorrhea refers to cramps that are not related to uterine disease. Many cases are caused by release of prostaglandins produced by secretory endometrium that diffuses into the myometrium and stimulates uncomfortable uterine contractions when the endometrium breaks down during menstruation. The cramps can be prevented by drugs that inhibit prostaglandin synthesis, taken before the onset of menses. Secondary dysmenorrhea is caused by disease of the pelvic organs and is treated by dealing with the disease responsible for the dysmenorrhea.

The ovary may give rise to various cysts and tumors. Benign functional cysts occur frequently and often resolve without treatment. Benign cystic teratomas (dermoid cysts) are also relatively common in young women and require surgical removal. Malignant ovarian tumors may be difficult to identify and results of treatment are less satisfactory. Irregular patches of atypical vulvar epithelium (vulvar dystrophy) often respond to conservative treatment, but some cases may progress to dysplasia or carcinoma and require more aggressive treatment.

Toxic shock, originally described in menstruating women using high-absorbency tampons, results from growth of toxin-producing staphylococci in the vagina, and is treated with antibiotics to eradicate the staphylococci but has no effect on the toxin already produced by the bacteria.

Various methods of contraception are available. Emergency contraception is effective for preventing a pregnancy following a sexual assault or failure of a contraceptive method, such as a broken condom.

## Questions for Review

1. What are the three common diseases of the breast that may be manifested as a lump in the breast? How does a physician distinguish one from another?
2. What is a mammogram? How is it used by a physician?
3. What are estrogen receptors in tumor cells? How is an estrogen receptor analysis used in the management of patients with breast carcinoma?
4. What is gynecomastia?
5. What methods are used to treat breast carcinoma?
6. What is an aromatase inhibitor, and how is it used?
7. What parts of the female genital tract may be affected by gonorrheal infection? How does gonorrhea lead to sterility?
8. What is the difference between in situ and invasive cervical carcinoma? How is the Pap smear used in the diagnosis of carcinoma?
9. A patient consults her physician because of irregular uterine bleeding. What are some of the diseases of the genital tract that can cause this bleeding?
10. What is endometriosis? What symptoms does it produce? What are some complications that may be associated with endometriosis?
11. What is a dermoid cyst?
12. What is toxic shock? How does tampon use predispose to this syndrome? What role do staphylococci play?
13. How do contraceptive pills and IUDs exert their contraceptive effects? What medical problems may be associated with their use?
14. What is vulvar dystrophy? What symptoms does it cause? What are its complications?

## Supplementary Reading

Berg, J. W., and Robbins, G. F. 1966. Factors influencing short- and long-term survival of breast cancer patients. *Surgery, Gynecology, and Obstetrics* 122: 1311–16.

> A classic article on factors influencing prognosis. Information on late recurrences.

Boston Women's Health Book Collective. 2005. *Our Bodies, Ourselves for the New Century*. New York: Simon & Schuster.

> Covers a wide range of subjects dealing with sexual anatomy, physiology, and pathology in a clear and concise manner. A useful reference.

Eisenhauler, E. A. 2001. From the molecule to the clinic: Inhibiting HER-2 to treat breast cancer (Editorial). *New England Journal of Medicine* 344:841–42.

> A summary of the functions of *HER-2*, which is overexpressed in 25 to 30 percent of all breast cancers as a result of gene amplification and a review of the use of a monoclonal antibody to treat the neoplasm.

Fenton, J. J., Taplin, S. H., Carney, P. A., et al. 2007. Influence of computer-aided detection on performance of screening mammography. *New England Journal of Medicine* 356: 1399–409.

> Computer-aided detection does not increase the accuracy of the interpretation of screening mammograms, and leads to increased numbers of biopsies. The detection rate of early invasive breast carcinoma was not improved by computer-aided mammography.

Fletcher, S. W., and Elmore, J. G. 2003. Mammographic screening for breast cancer. *New England Journal of Medicine* 348:1672–80.

> An update on the applications and limitations of mammography, including the problems associated with false-positive results. Many cases of ductal carcinoma in situ will never evolve into invasive breast cancer.

Gann, P. H., and Morrow, M. 2003. Combined hormone therapy and breast cancer: A single-edged sword (Editorial). *Journal of the American Medical Association* 289:3304–06.

> Summary and comments on the Women's Health Initiative Randomized Trial relating to the use of estrogen and progestin on breast cancer and mammography in healthy postmenopausal women. (*Journal of the American Medical Association* 289:3243–53 and 3254–63.)

Gostin, L. O., and DeAngelis, C. D. 2007. Mandatory HPV vaccination. *Journal of the American Medical Association* 297:1921–23.

> An article cautioning against a mandatory HPV vaccination although the vaccine will protect against an infection, but research has not shown how long the protection can last and whether there may be long-term harmful effects.

Greene, M. H. 1997. Genetics of breast cancer. *Mayo Clinic Proceedings* 72:54–65.

> An excellent review article with emphasis on *BRCA 1* and *BRCA2*.

Haber, D. 2002. Prophylactic oophorectomy to reduce the risk of ovarian and breast cancer in carriers of *BRCA* mutations (Editorial). *New England Journal of Medicine* 346:1660–61.

> The risk of ovarian cancer is lower than breast cancer risk in carriers of *BRCA* mutations, but ovarian cancer carries a poor prognosis and is difficult to detect in early stages. Consequently, many physicians recommend prophylactic oophorectomy to reduce ovarian cancer risk in *BRCA* mutation carriers. Oophorectomy also reduces breast cancer risk by reducing estrogen stimulation of breast tissue.

Ho, G. Y. F., Bierman, R., Beardsley, L., et al. 1998. Natural history of cervicovaginal papillomavirus infection in young women. *New England Journal of Medicine* 338:423–28.

> Six hundred and eight college women were examined every 6 months for 3 years by means of cervicovaginal specimens for detection of HPV DNA, and results were correlated with age ethnicity, number of sex partners, and types of sexual activity. The incidence of HPV infections during the period of observation was 43 percent and the median duration of a new HPV infection was 8 months. Persistence of HPV infection for more than 6 months was more likely to occur in older women and those infected with high-risk types were associated with cervical neoplasms. Abnormal Pap smears were more likely to occur in subjects with persisting HPV infections, especially those infected with high-risk types.

Lehman, C. D., Gatsonis, C., Kuhl, C. K., et al. 2007. MRI evaluation of the contralateral breast in women with recently diagnosed breast cancer. *New England Journal of Medicine* 356:1295–303.

> Up to 10 percent of women with breast carcinoma also have an unsuspected carcinoma in the contralateral (opposite) breast. In a group of 969 women with a carcinoma in one breast, in 3 percent of these women an unsuspected carcinoma was detected in the opposite breast that appeared normal by clinical examination and mammography.

Meijers-Heijboer, H., van Geel, B., van Putten, W. L. J., et al. 2001. Breast cancer after prophylactic bilateral mastectomy in women with *BRCA1* and *BRCA2* mutation. *New England Journal of Medicine* 345:159–64.

> Prophylactic mastectomy reduces the incidence of breast carcinoma. None of the 66 mastectomy patients developed cancer, but 8 of 63 patients followed by regular surveillance developed breast cancer.

Munoz, N., Bosch, F. X., de Sanjose, S., et al. 2003. Epidemiologic classification of human papillomavirus types associated with cervical cancer. *New England Journal of Medicine* 348:518–27.

> Cervical cancer is the most common cancer in women worldwide and is caused by the human papillomavirus. More than 80 HPV types have been identified, and about 40 can infect the genital tract. Fifteen HPV types are carcinogenic. Eight different types are responsible for 95 percent of carcinomas, with types 16 and 18 being the major viral carcinogens.

Ravdin, P. M., Cronin, K. A., Howlader, N., et al. 2007. The decrease in breast-cancer incidence in 2003 in the United States. *New England Journal of Medicine* 356:1670–74.

> The age-adjusted incidence of breast carcinoma fell sharply (by 6.7 percent) beginning in 2002 and extending into 2003, and had begun to level off in 2004 as compared with the rate in 2002. The decrease was most marked in women age 50 or older, and was most marked in women with estrogen-receptor-positive tumors. The decrease most likely correlates with the decreased use or hormones to treat menopausal symptoms.

Writing group for the Women's Health Initiative investigators. 2002. Risks and benefits of estrogen plus progestin in healthy postmenopausal women: Principal results from the Women's Health Initiative randomized clinical trial. *Journal of the American Medical Association* 288:321–33.

> Hormone use increases breast carcinoma risk, and also increases risk of cardiovascular disease including

heart attacks and strokes, and risk of leg vein thrombosis and pulmonary embolism.

Rossouw, J. E., Anderson, G. L., Prentice, R. L., et al. 2007. Postmenopausal hormone therapy and risk of cardiovascular disease by age and years since menopause. *Journal of the American Medical Association* 294: 1465–77.

> The timing of beginning hormone therapy may influence its effect on cardiovascular disease. Initiating hormone treatment (HT) soon after onset of menopause reduced coronary heart disease (CHD) risk by retarding the accumulation of atheromatous plaque in coronary arteries. However, the risk increased if treatment was begun several years after onset of menopause, presumably because the women were older, had more years to accumulate plaque, and had more advanced coronary artery disease. However, HT increased the risk of stroke regardless of the years since menopause.

Runowicz, C. D. 2007. Molecular screening for cervical cancer—Time to give up Pap tests (Editorial). *New England Journal of Medicine* 357:1650–52.

> The Pap test has been a very successful screening method for detecting cervical dysplasia and carcinoma. However, the test is not very sensitive because a single smear may fail to detect a cytologic abnormality in almost 50 percent of women in whom cytologic abnormalities are present, so repeat screening tests must be performed at regular intervals in order to detect any cytologic abnormalities that were missed in an earlier examination. Consequently, HPV testing has been proposed as the primary screening test for cervical cancer because it is more sensitive than the Pap test for detecting high-grade cervical dysplasia and carcinoma. However, although the HPV test is more sensitive than the Pap test, it is less specific, which means that the HPV test may produce a significant number of false-positive results in subjects who do not have a HPV infection.

Santen, R. J., and Mansel, R. B. 2005. Benign breast disorders. *New England Journal of Medicine* 353:275–85.

> Describes pathogenesis of fibrocystic changes in breast and the various proliferative changes that increase breast cancer risk, as well as measures to reduce risk.

Shapiro, C. L., and Recht, A. 2001. Side effects of adjuvant treatment of breast cancer. *New England Journal of Medicine* 344:1997–2008.

> Adjuvant chemotherapy, tamoxifen, or both are recommended for women with invasive breast cancers, regardless of whether axillary nodes are involved. Benefits are greatest in women under 50 years of age. Various adverse effects are described, including cardiovascular damage and second tumors related to treatment.

Stoler, M. H. 2002. New Bethesda terminology and evidence-based management guidelines for cervical cytology findings (Editorial). *Journal of the American Medical Association* 287:2140–41.

> Half the women in whom the Pap test reveals atypical squamous cells of uncertain significance may have benign atypical changes in their cervical epithelium but do not have cervical dysplasia, although the other half of this group of women do have cervical dysplasia and require further evaluation and treatment. The HPV test helps separate the women in these two groups.

Westhoff, C. 2003. Emergency contraception. *New England Journal of Medicine* 349:1830–35.

> Sperm can survive in the genital tract for 5 to 6 days and can fertilize an egg when ovulation occurs several days after unprotected intercourse. The preferred "morning-after pill" is a progestin-only formulation (1.5-mg levonorgestrel) that should be taken regardless of the cycle day when unprotected intercourse occurred.

Wright, T. C., and Schiffman, M. 2003. Adding a test for human papillomavirus DNA to cervical cancer screening. *New England Journal of Medicine* 348: 489–90.

> In patients with atypical cells detected in a Pap test, a single test for human papillomavirus (HPV) DNA identified almost all women found to have severe cervical dysplasia and was more effective than a single colposcopic examination or two additional Pap tests.

## Interactive Activities

### Fill in the Blanks

1. Persons with mutations of the tumor suppressor genes *BRCA1* or *BRCA2* have a greatly increased risk of not only breast carcinoma but also carcinoma of the _____.

2. A well-circumscribed benign tumor occurring in the breast of a young woman is called a _____.

3. Breast enlargement in the male breast is called _____.

4. Following treatment of an invasive breast carcinoma, most patients are also treated with drugs or hormones. This type of treatment is called _____.

5. When examining axillary lymph nodes from patients with breast carcinoma, it is possible to identify and examine the first lymph node that receives lymphatic drainage from the axilla. This node is called a _____.

### True or False

Indicate whether the following statements are true or false by writing T or F at the end of the statement.

1. A mutation of either the *BRCA1* or *BRCA2* gene increases the long-term risk of both breast and ovarian carcinoma.____

2. Long-term treatment of postmenopausal patients with estrogen and progestin increases the risk of breast carcinoma.____

3. When treating breast carcinoma, the long-term results of total mastectomy with axillary lymph node dissection are much better than the results of segmental mastectomy or lumpectomy followed by radiation therapy.____

4. An estrogen-receptor-positive breast carcinoma has a better prognosis than a breast carcinoma lacking hormone receptors.____

5. The prognosis of a breast carcinoma in which the *HER-2* gene is amplified is much better than that of a breast carcinoma lacking an amplified *HER-2* gene.____

6. An axillary lymph node containing metastatic carcinoma is called a sentinel lymph node.____

7. An estrogen-receptor-negative breast carcinoma is usually treated with the drug tamoxifen, which blocks estrogen receptors.____

8. Unprotected sexual intercourse several days before ovulation may result in a pregnancy.____

9. Postmenopausal uterine bleeding usually is caused by endometriosis.____

10. The human papillomavirus (HPV) often causes dysmenorrhea.____

11. A chlamydial infection may spread to the fallopian tubes and may cause a tubal infection.____

12. The new HPV vaccine protects against all carcinogenic papillomaviruses.____

13. A functional ovarian cyst frequently develops into an ovarian carcinoma.____

14. Deposits of ectopic endometrium in the pelvis (endometriosis) may cause infertility.____

15. Most smooth muscle tumors of the uterus are malignant.____

### Critical Thinking

1. Sally Richardson is an 18-year-old college student. She felt a small nontender lump in her right breast while taking a shower. She is concerned that it might be cancer, although there is no family history of breast cancer. She asks you what other conditions might cause the lump and what she should do. What would you tell her?

2. George Anderson is a 54-year-old salesman who felt a small 1-centimeter diameter lump beneath the skin of his chest below and medial to the right nipple. He asks you whether it could be cancer, and what other conditions could cause the lump. He asks you what he should do. What would you tell him?

3. Susan Jones is a 27-year-old school teacher who had a routine Pap smear last week as part of a routine pelvic examination. The Pap smear was reported as showing atypical cells. What does this mean and what should she do now?

4. Mary Smith's 67-year-old mother experienced a small amount of vaginal bleeding several days ago that subsided spontaneously. She asked Mary what could be responsible for the bleeding, and what she should do about it. What should Mary tell her mother about the possible cause of the bleeding, and what she should do about it?

# 14 Prenatal Development and Diseases Associated with Pregnancy

## LEARNING OBJECTIVES

1. Explain the processes of fertilization, implantation, and early development of the ovum, including the origin of the decidua, fetal membranes, and the placenta.

2. Describe how amnionic fluid is formed and eliminated. Identify the conditions leading to abnormal amounts of amnionic fluid.

3. Explain the causes and effects of spontaneous abortion and ectopic pregnancy.

4. Describe the mechanism and clinical manifestations of the problems associated with abnormal attachment of the placenta within the uterus.

5. Differentiate between identical and fraternal twins. Describe how zygosity can be determined from examination of the placenta.

6. List the disadvantages of a twin pregnancy.

7. Classify the types of gestational trophoblast disease. Explain their prognoses, and describe the methods of treatment.

8. Explain the pathogenesis, clinical manifestations, diagnostic criteria, and methods used to diagnose, prevent, and treat Rh hemolytic disease, and to diagnose and treat ABO hemolytic disease.

9. Understand the causes and effects of gestational diabetes and pregnancy-associated toxemia.

# Fertilization and Prenatal Development

## Fertilization

The tadpolelike sperm consists of three parts: a head, a middle piece, and a tail ( Figure 14-1A ). The sperm head contains genetic material. It is partially covered by a thin, membranelike structure called the *head cap*, which contains enzymes that enable the sperm head to penetrate the ovum at the time of fertilization. The middle piece contains the enzymes that provide the energy required to propel the sperm, and the tail is the propulsive portion. Sperm can travel several millimeters per minute by their own propulsive efforts, but they are also passively transported by rhythmic contractions of the uterine muscles that aspirate them upward into the uterus and fallopian tubes.

**A**

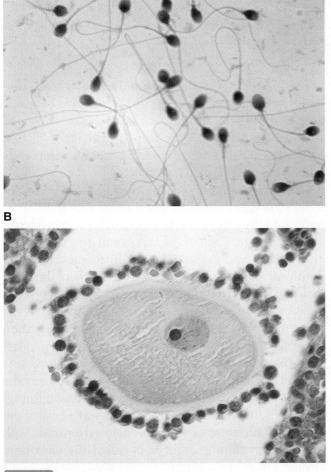

**B**

Figure 14-1    **A,** Normal sperm in vaginal secretions. The darkly staining head containing the genetic material is covered by a lightly staining head cap that contains the enzymes needed to penetrate the ovum during fertilization. The long narrow tail provides propulsion (original magnification × 1000). **B,** Mature ovum with adherent granulosa cells. The nucleus is seen near the center of the cell. The homogeneous band surrounding the ovum is the zona pellucida (original magnification × 400).

The ovum is expelled from the follicle at ovulation. It is surrounded by a thin layer of acellular material called the zona pellucida to which are attached clusters of cells from the follicle that are called granulosa cells ( Figure 14-1B ). The ovum is swept into the fallopian tube by the beating of the cilia covering the tubal epithelium and is propelled down the tube by the peristaltic contractions of the smooth muscle in the tubal wall. Fertilization is possible when intercourse occurs reasonably close to the time of ovulation. However, the likelihood of a successful conception is related primarily to the survival time of the ovum, about 12 to 24 hours, rather than the sperm, which can survive in the genital tract and fertilize an ovum for as long as 6 days. Based on data from a large group of women who were trying to become pregnant and in whom the time of ovulation had been determined precisely, some conceptions occurred when intercourse occurred as early as 6 days before ovulation. The likelihood of a successful conception increased as intercourse occurred closer to the time of ovulation, but no conceptions occurred the day after ovulation ( Table 14-1 ). In many successful conceptions, the sperm were already "lying in wait" for the ovum in the fallopian tube. When the ovum was ovulated and entered the fallopian tube, it was fertilized by the waiting sperm. The enzymes in the head cap of the sperm disperse the cluster of granulosa cells and permit the sperm head to penetrate the zona pellucida. After the sperm has penetrated, the ovum completes its second meiotic division (oogenesis is described in Chapter 2). Sperm penetration causes the zona pellucida to become impermeable to penetration by other sperm, ensuring that only one sperm can enter the egg. Fusion of the sperm head and egg nucleus (each containing 23 chromosomes) restores

| Table 14-1 | Conception Rate Based on Day of Intercourse |
|---|---|
| Day of Intercourse | Percentage of Conceptions |
| 6 days before ovulation | 8 percent |
| 5 days before ovulation | 10 percent |
| 4 days before ovulation | 16 percent |
| 3 days before ovulation | no data |
| 2 days before ovulation | 28 percent |
| 1 day before ovulation | 32 percent |
| day of ovulation | 36 percent |
| day after ovulation | none |

Based on data from Wilcox, A. J. et al. *New England Journal of Medicine* 333:1517–21.

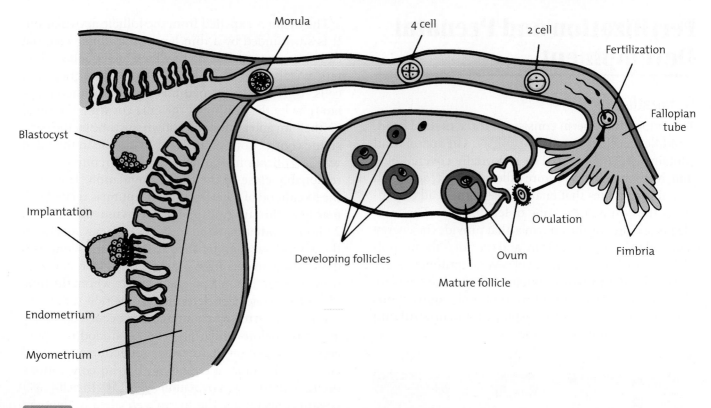

**Figure 14-2** Summary of the maturation of the ovum, fertilization, and early development of the fertilized ovum.

**zygote**
(zi´gōt)
The fertilized ovum.

**morula** A mulberry-shaped solid cluster of cells formed by division of the fertilized ovum.

**blastocyst** A stage of development of the fertilized ovum (*zygote*) in which a central cavity accumulates within the cluster of developing cells.

**inner cell mass** A group of cells that are derived from the fertilized ovum and are destined to form the embryo.

**trophoblast** Cell derived from the fertilized ovum that gives rise to the fetal membranes and contributes to the formation of the placenta.

**germ disk** A three-layered cluster of cells that will eventually give rise to an embryo.

**amnionic sac**
(am-nē-on´ik) The fluid-filled sac surrounding the embryo. One of the fetal membranes.

the genetic component of the cell to 46 chromosomes, and the fertilized ovum is now termed a **zygote**.

## Early Development of the Fertilized Ovum

As the fertilized ovum passes along the fallopian tube, it undergoes a series of mitotic divisions. The first cell division is completed about 30 hours after fertilization. Subsequent divisions occur in rapid succession and convert the zygote into a small, mulberry-shaped ball of cells called a **morula**, which is enclosed within the zona pellucida. The morula reaches the endometrial cavity by about the third day. Soon fluid begins to accumulate in the center of the morula, and a central cavity forms. At this stage of development, the structure is called a **blastocyst**. The cells of the blastocyst begin to differentiate into two different groups of cells: the **inner cell mass**, which will form the embryo, and a peripheral rim of cells, called the **trophoblast**, which will give rise to the fetal membranes and will contribute to the formation of the placenta.

The blastocyst lies free within the endometrial cavity for several days. Then the zona pellucida degenerates, exposing the trophoblast. The blastocyst begins to burrow into the endometrium by the end of the first week after fertilization and soon becomes completely embedded (Figure 14-2).

Soon after implantation, the inner cell mass becomes a flat structure called the **germ disk**, which differentiates into the three germ layers: ectoderm, mesoderm, and endoderm. Each of the layers will give rise to specific tissues and organs. A fluid-filled sac called the **amnionic sac** forms between the ectoderm of the germ disk and the surrounding trophoblast, and a second sac called the **yolk sac** forms on the opposite side of the germ disk. The interior of the blastocyst cavity then becomes lined by a layer of primitive connective-tissue cells (mesoderm) that also covers the external surfaces of the amnionic sac and yolk sac. As soon as the blastocyst cavity acquires a connective-tissue lining, it is called the *chorionic cavity*, and its wall is called the **chorion**. The entire sac with its enclosed amnion, yolk sac, and developing embryo is called the **chorionic vesicle**. Fingerlike columns of cells called **chorionic villi** extend from the chorion and anchor the chorionic vesicle in the endometrium (Figure 14-3).

The chorionic cavity continues to enlarge, and the chorionic vesicle increases in size and complexity. By the end of the second week after fertilization, the small

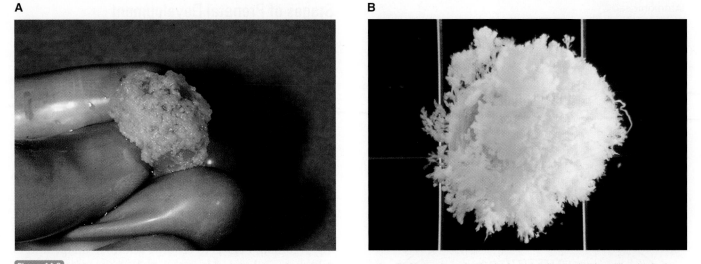

Figure 14-3  **A,** Spontaneously aborted chorionic vesicle about 6 weeks after conception. **B,** Closer view of a chorionic vesicle illustrating frondlike chorionic villi projecting from the chorion.

germ disk with its surrounding amnion and yolk sac projects into the chorionic cavity, suspended from the wall of the chorion by a mass of connective tissue called the **body stalk** ( Figure 14-4 ).

By the fourth week after fertilization, the organ systems begin to form, and the embryo, which had been flat, becomes cylindrical. The central part of the germ disk grows more rapidly than the periphery, owing to the beginning formation of the nervous system. As a result, the germ disk flexes and bulges into the amnionic cavity. The amnionic sac, which is attached to the lateral margins of the germ disk, follows the changing contour of the embryo and is reflected around the embryo.

Part of the yolk sac also becomes enfolded within the embryo when flexion occurs ( Figure 14-5 ). The enclosed part will give rise to the intestinal tract and other important structures. The lateral margins of the germ disk also fuse in the midline to form the ventral (anterior) body wall. The fusion is incomplete in the middle of the body wall where the umbilical cord is attached, and part of the yolk sac that was not included within the embryo protrudes through the defect. It persists for a time but soon degenerates.

**yolk sac**
A sac that is formed adjacent to the germ disk and that will form the gastrointestinal tract and other important structures in the embryo.

**chorion** (kõ′ri-on) The layer of trophoblast and associated mesoderm that surrounds the developing embryo.

**chorionic vesicle** The chorion with its villi and enclosed amnion, yolk sac, and developing embryo.

**chorionic villi** Fingerlike columns of cells extending from the chorion that anchor the chorionic vesicle in the endometrium.

**body stalk** The structure connecting the embryo to the chorion. Eventually develops into the umbilical cord.

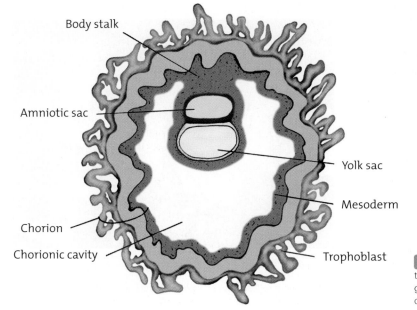

Figure 14-4  Appearance of the chorionic vesicle at the end of the second week after ovulation, illustrating the relation of the germ disk to the amnion, chorion, body stalk, and chorionic cavity.

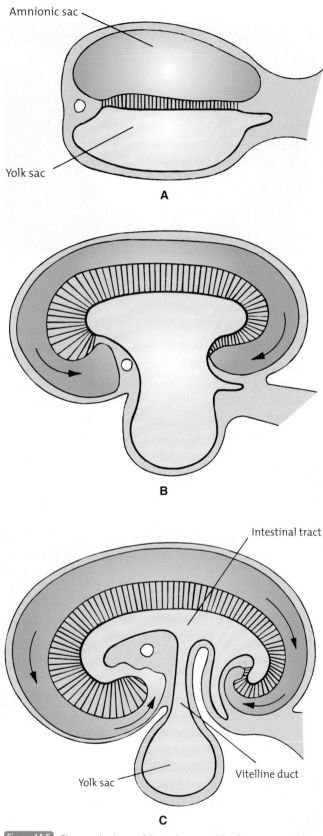

## Stages of Prenatal Development

It is customary to subdivide prenatal development into three main periods:

1. The preembryonic period
2. The embryonic period
3. The fetal period

The first 3 weeks after fertilization are the *preembryonic period*. During this time the blastocyst becomes implanted and the inner cell mass differentiates into the three germ layers that will eventually form specific tissues within the embryo.

The *embryonic period* extends from the third through the seventh week. This is the time when the developing organism begins to assume a human shape and is called an **embryo**. This is also the time when all the organ systems are formed. Consequently, it is a very critical period of development. At this stage, drugs ingested by the mother, radiation, some viral infections, and various other factors may disturb embryonic development and lead to congenital abnormalities, as described in Chapter 7.

The *fetal period* extends from the eighth week until the time of delivery. The developing organism is no longer called an embryo; the term **fetus** is now applied. As the fetus grows, it becomes larger and heavier, but there are no major changes in its basic structure comparable to those in the embryonic period. Initially, the fetal head is disproportionately large, and the body appears quite scrawny because subcutaneous fat has not yet been deposited. Shortly before delivery, subcutaneous fat begins to accumulate and the body begins to fill out. Figure 14-6 illustrates the progressive changes in the size of the fetus in relation to the duration of the gestation.

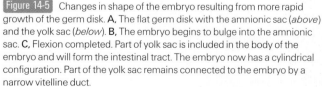

**Figure 14-5** Changes in shape of the embryo resulting from more rapid growth of the germ disk. **A,** The flat germ disk with the amnionic sac (*above*) and the yolk sac (*below*). **B,** The embryo begins to bulge into the amnionic sac. **C,** Flexion completed. Part of yolk sac is included in the body of the embryo and will form the intestinal tract. The embryo now has a cylindrical configuration. Part of the yolk sac remains connected to the embryo by a narrow vitelline duct.

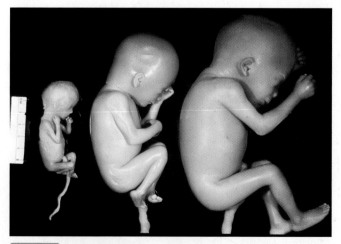

**Figure 14-6** Progressive changes in size of the fetus at various stages of gestation. *Left,* Three and one-half months (32 grams). *Center,* Four and one-half months (230 grams). *Right,* Five and one-half months (420 grams).

## Duration of Pregnancy

The total duration of pregnancy from fertilization to delivery is called the *period of gestation*. This is approximately 38 weeks when dated from the time of ovulation. Usually, however, the actual date of ovulation is not known, and the length of gestation is calculated from the beginning of the last normal menstrual period. Expressed in this way, the duration of pregnancy is 40 weeks because the first day of the calculation is actually about 2 weeks before the date of conception. The gestation calculated in this way may also be expressed as 280 days, as 10 lunar (28-day) months, or 9 calendar (31-day) months. Sometimes the 9 calendar months are subdivided into three periods called *trimesters*, each of 3 months' duration.

# Decidua, Fetal Membranes, and Placenta

Figure 14-7 demonstrates the relationship of the embryo to the surrounding amnionic sac and chorion about 7 weeks after fertilization.

## The Decidua

The endometrium of pregnancy is called the **decidua**. Special names are applied to the parts of the decidua in which the chorionic vesicle is embedded, as indicated in Figure 14-8A. The part beneath the chorionic vesicle is called the *decidua basalis*. The part that is stretched over the vesicle is called the *decidua capsularis*, and the part that lines the rest of the endometrial cavity is called the *decidua parietalis* (*parietes* = wall). As the embryo and its surrounding amnionic sac continue to increase in size, the thin capsular decidua becomes stretched and thinned. Eventually, it fuses with the decidua parietalis on the opposite wall of the uterus (Figure 14-8B).

## The Chorion and Chorionic Villi

At first, the chorionic villi arise from the entire periphery of the chorion, but soon the villi arising from the superficial part of the chorion become compressed by the decidua capsularis and atrophy. This part of the chorion, which is devoid of villi, is called the *chorion*

**embryo** (em'brē-ō) The developing human organism from the third through the seventh weeks of gestation.

**fetus** The unborn offspring after eight weeks' gestation.

**decidua** (de-sid'ū-ah) The endometrium of pregnancy.

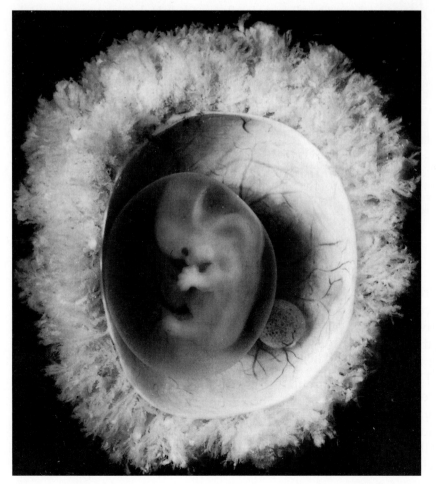

Figure 14-7  Relationship of the embryo to the amnionic sac, yolk sac, and chorionic cavity at about 7 weeks after conception. The chorionic sac has been bisected. At this stage, villi still arise from the entire periphery of the chorion, and the amnionic sac surrounding the embryo does not completely fill the chorionic cavity. The embryo is attached to the chorion by the umbilical cord (not shown in the photograph). The yolk sac is located to the *right* of the amnionic sac, between the amnionic sac and the chorion (photograph courtesy of the Carnegie Institution of Washington).

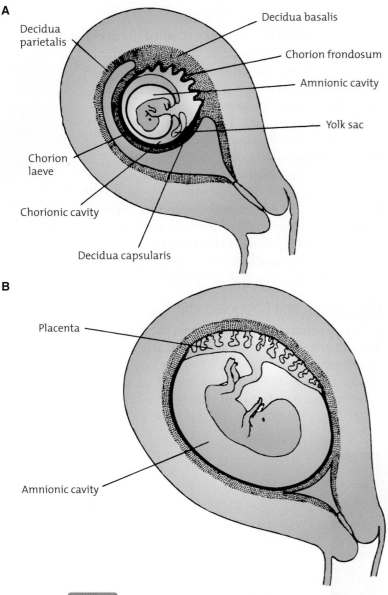

**A**

Decidua
parietalis

Decidua basalis

Chorion frondosum

Amnionic cavity

Yolk sac

Chorion
laeve

Chorionic cavity

Decidua capsularis

**B**

Placenta

Amnionic cavity

**Figure 14-8** **A,** Relationship of the fetus to the decidua, fetal membranes, and chorion in early pregnancy. The part of the yolk sac not incorporated within the fetus lies between the amnionic sac and the chorion. **B,** Relationship in late pregnancy. The amnionic sac envelops the fetus and now completely fills the chorionic cavity. The amnionic membrane lies against the chorion. The decidua capsularis has become adherent to the decidua paretalis on the opposite wall of the uterus.

**cotyledon**
(co-ti-lē'don) A unit of the placenta visible grossly on the maternal surface as an irregularly shaped lobe circumscribed by a depressed area.

*laeve* (*laeve* = smooth). In contrast, the villi arising from the deeper portion of the chorion adjacent to the decidua basalis proliferate actively. This part of the chorion is called the *chorion frondosum* because of the frondlike appearance of the villi. These villi project into the large blood-filled spaces within the decidua basalis through which the maternal blood flows. Blood vessels that form within the villi as they grow become connected with blood vessels that are

forming in the chorion and the body stalk, as well as within the body of the embryo. As soon as the embryo's heart begins to beat, blood begins to flow through this developing network of vessels.

## The Amnionic Sac

The amnionic sac is enclosed within the chorion. At first the sac is much smaller than the chorionic cavity, but the enlarging sac expands into the chorionic cavity. Eventually the amnionic sac completely fills the chorionic cavity and the amnionic membrane lies against the chorion. The sac functions as a buoyant, temperature-controlled environment that protects the fetus throughout pregnancy and assists in opening the cervix during childbirth.

## The Yolk Sac

In the human being, the yolk sac never contains yolk, but it performs other important functions. Part of the yolk sac becomes incorporated into the body of the embryo to form the intestinal tract. The part that is not included within the embryo persists for a time but eventually atrophies.

## The Placenta

The placenta is a flattened, disk-shaped structure weighing about 500 grams. It has a dual origin, both fetal and maternal ( Figure 14-9 ). The chorion and the villi are formed from the trophoblast, which is of fetal origin, and the decidua basalis in which the villi are anchored is derived from the endometrium. Incomplete partitions of decidua extend into the villi and divide them into aggregates called **cotyledons** that impart a vague cobblestone appearance to the maternal surface of the placenta. The amnion and chorion extend from the margins of the placenta to form the fluid-filled sac that encloses the fetus and that ruptures at the time of delivery. The fetus is connected to the placenta by the *umbilical cord*, which contains two arteries and a single vein. The vessels follow a spiral course in the cord and then divide on the surface of the placenta to send branches into the chorionic villi with one arterial branch supplying the villi in each cotyledon. Blood returning from the villi is collected into large veins on the surface of the placenta that join to form the single *umbilical vein* that enters the cord.

**Circulation of Blood in the Placenta** The placenta has a dual circulation of blood ( Figure 14-10 ). The *feto-placental circulation* delivers arterial blood low in oxygen from the fetus to the chorionic villi through the two umbilical arteries. Oxygenated blood is returned from the placenta to the fetus in the single umbilical

**A**

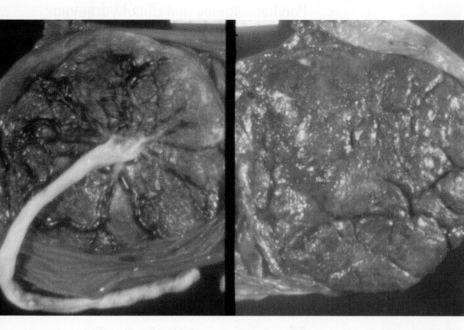

**B**

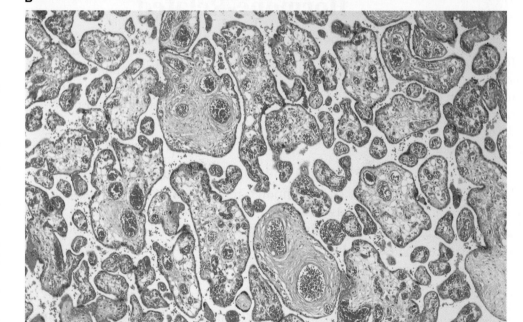

vein. The *uteroplacental circulation* delivers oxygenated arterial blood from the mother into the large placental blood spaces that are located between the villi, which are called the *intervillous spaces*. The blood spurts into the intervillous spaces from the many uterine arteries that penetrate the basal portion of the placenta. It flows back into the maternal circulation through veins that penetrate the basal part of the placenta. The arrangement of the two circulations in the placenta brings the maternal and fetal blood into close approximation. In this way, oxygen and nutrients can be exchanged between the maternal and fetal circulations, but there is no actual intermixing of fetal and maternal blood.

### Endocrine Function of the Placenta

The placenta synthesizes two steroid hormones, *estrogen* and *progesterone*, and two protein hormones called **human placental lactogen (HPL)** and **human chorionic gonadotropin (HCG)**. HPL stimulates maternal metabolic processes, and HCG is quite similar to the gonadotropic hormones produced by the

**human placental lactogen (HPL)** (lak´tō-jen) One of the hormones produced by the placenta that has properties similar to pituitary growth hormone.

**human chorionic gonadotropin (HCG)** (kōr-ē-on´ik gō-na-dō-trō´pin) A hormone made by the placenta in pregnancy having actions similar to pituitary gonadotropins. Same hormone is made by neoplastic cells in some types of malignant testicular tumors.

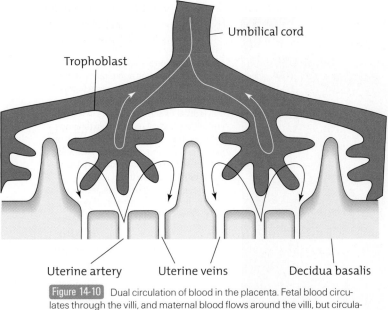

Figure 14-10 Dual circulation of blood in the placenta. Fetal blood circulates through the villi, and maternal blood flows around the villi, but circulations do not intermix.

**Umbilical cord**

**Trophoblast**

**Uterine artery** **Uterine veins** **Decidua basalis**

## Polyhydramnios and Oligohydramnios

**Polyhydramnios** is a condition in which the volume of amnionic fluid is markedly increased. There are two common causes:

1. A congenital maldevelopment of the fetal brain called anencephaly (Chapter 21), which disturbs the normal swallowing mechanism, so that the fetus is unable to swallow amnionic fluid.
2. A congenital obstruction of the fetal upper intestinal tract that blocks the entry of swallowed fluid into the small intestine where it can be absorbed.

**Oligohydramnios** is a marked reduction in the volume of amnionic fluid. It occurs either because the fetal kidneys have failed to develop and no urine is formed, or because a congenital obstruction blocks the urethra so that urine cannot be excreted.

# Hormone-Related Conditions in Pregnancy

Pregnancy affects almost all of the hormones produced by a woman's endocrine glands and by her placenta, which maintain the pregnancy and sustain the fetus, but some have undesirable effects on the pregnant woman.

## Nausea and Vomiting During Early Pregnancy

This condition is related to the rapidly increasing levels of estrogen in early pregnancy; nausea and vomiting often occur in the morning (morning sickness) but may occur at any time, and usually subside by the end of the first trimester (first 3 months of pregnancy).

## Hyperemesis Gravidarum

This term literally means *excessive vomiting of pregnancy*, and probably has the same hormonal basis as morning sickness but is more prolonged and severe. Weight loss and dehydration may require treatment with intravenous fluids.

## Gestational Diabetes

In all pregnancies during the second 3 months (second trimester) the high placental hormone levels cause the body to become less responsive to insulin (called insulin resistance), which tends to raise blood glucose, but usually the pregnant woman compensates by secreting more insulin, and the blood glucose remains normal.

However, some women who were considered nondiabetic before becoming pregnant may not be able to produce enough additional insulin to maintain a normal

**polyhydramnios**
(pä-lē-hī-dram′nē-yus)
An excess of amnionic fluid.

**oligohydramnios**
(ol-ig-ō-hī-dram′nē-yus)
An insufficient quantity of amnionic fluid.

pituitary gland. Tests that detect HCG are called *pregnancy tests*. The newer, very sensitive tests can be performed on blood or urine and become positive as early as 10 to 12 days after fertilization, even before the woman misses her first period.

# Amnionic Fluid

Amnionic fluid is produced both by filtration and by excretion, and its quantity varies with the stage of pregnancy. During the early part of pregnancy, the amnionic fluid is formed chiefly by filtration of fluid into the amnionic sac from maternal blood as it passes through the uterus and from fetal blood passing through the placenta. Additional fluid diffuses directly through the fetal skin and from the fetal respiratory tract. Later, when the fetal kidneys begin to function in the last part of pregnancy, the fetus urinates into the amnionic fluid, and fetal urine becomes the major source of this fluid.

Both filtration and fetal urine continually add to the volume of fluid, but the additions are counterbalanced by losses of amnionic fluid into the fetal gastrointestinal tract. Normally, the fetus swallows as much as several hundred milliliters of fluid per day. This fluid is absorbed from the fetal intestinal tract into the fetal circulation, transferred across the placenta into the mother's circulation, and eventually excreted by the mother in her urine.

glucose concentration during pregnancy because of the insulin resistance caused by the high hormone levels in pregnancy, and a high maternal blood glucose is harmful to the fetus. The condition is called *gestational diabetes* because the blood glucose is likely to return to normal after the pregnancy, although women with gestational diabetes may be at higher risk of developing type 2 diabetes in later years.

Gestational diabetes occurs in about 2 percent of pregnancies, and is much higher in older and obese patients, and in patients from ethnic groups having a high frequency of diabetes. It is important to identify pregnant women with gestational diabetes so that they can be treated by diet and additional insulin if necessary to maintain normal blood glucose during pregnancy, which avoids the hazards of hyperglycemia on her fetus.

Almost all pregnant women are screened for gestational diabetes by performing a screening test that consists of 50 grams of glucose solution given orally without regard to fasting status. Then the concentration of glucose in the patient's blood is determined in a sample collected 1 hour later. If the result exceeds a predetermined concentration, more comprehensive studies are performed to confirm the diagnosis of pregnancy-related diabetes, and a course of treatment is started to regulate her blood glucose, which consists of a diabetic diet supplemented by insulin if needed.

# Spontaneous Abortion ("Miscarriage")

Most spontaneous abortions occur early in pregnancy. The actual incidence is difficult to establish but is estimated to be from 10 to 20 percent of all pregnancies. Many spontaneous abortions are a result of chromosomal abnormalities or maldevelopment of the embryo, conditions that are incompatible with survival. Others result from defective implantation of the fertilized ovum within the endometrial cavity. In many cases, the cause of spontaneous abortion in early pregnancy cannot be determined.

Occasionally, intrauterine fetal death occurs late in pregnancy. This is generally caused by partial detachment of the placenta from the wall of the uterus, which is called **placental abruption**, or by obstruction of the blood supplied through the umbilical cord. Compression of the blood vessels in the umbilical cord, shutting off the blood supply to the fetus, may occur if the cord becomes knotted or wrapped tightly around the infant's neck or limbs ( Figure 14-11 ). If the placenta becomes separated from its uterine attachment or the cord becomes obstructed, the fetus no longer receives oxygen and nutrients from the mother, and the fetus dies. A dead fetus is usually expelled promptly, but occasionally may be retained within the uterine cavity for several weeks or months.

If a dead fetus is retained for some time within the uterine cavity, products of degenerated fetal tissue diffuse into the maternal circulation. This material has thromboplastic activity and may induce a hemorrhagic disease in the mother because of depletion of maternal blood-coagulation factors that occurs when the coagulation mechanism is activated by the thromboplastic material. A retained dead fetus is one cause of the disseminated intravascular coagulation syndrome, which is discussed in the section on blood coagulation in Chapter 9.

Cocaine abuse in pregnancy also has been shown to cause intrauterine fetal death. Cocaine increases

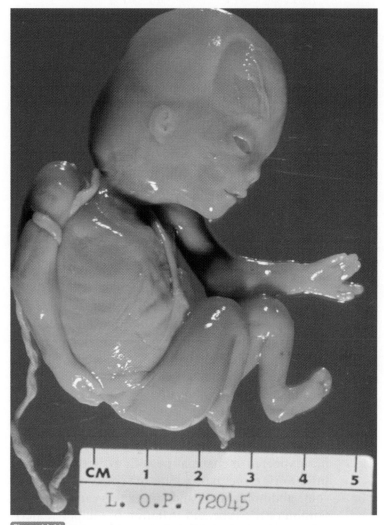

**Figure 14-11** Fetus spontaneously aborted late in pregnancy because of interruption of blood supply through the umbilical cord. The cord extended around back of neck and had become tightly wrapped around upper arm, shutting off circulation and leading to intrauterine death.

maternal heart rate, constricts arterioles, and raises blood pressure. The constriction of uterine arterioles reduces uterine blood flow and impairs oxygen supply to the fetus. In some patients, the high pressure within the uterine arterioles may cause one of the vessels to rupture. As a result, a large hemorrhage forms between the uterine wall and the placenta and partially separates the placenta from the uterus (placental abruption), which severely compromises oxygenation of fetal blood.

# Ectopic Pregnancy

An ectopic pregnancy (*ecto* = outside) is the development of an embryo outside its normal location within the uterine cavity. Most ectopic pregnancies occur in the fallopian tubes, but on rare occasions a fertilized ovum develops in the ovary or abdominal cavity. Normally, fertilization occurs in the fallopian tube and the fertilized ovum then proceeds into the endometrial cavity, where implantation takes place at the end of the first week after fertilization. Implantation may take place in the fallopian tube, however, if transport of the ovum is delayed. Two factors predispose to this complication:

1. A previous infection in the fallopian tubes. Often this is followed by scarring and fusion of tubal folds, which retards the passage of the fertilized egg through the tube.
2. Failure of the muscular contractions of the tubal wall to propel the ovum through the tube.

Frequently, the conditions that predispose to a tubal pregnancy affect both fallopian tubes. Consequently, a woman who has had one tubal pregnancy may develop another ectopic pregnancy in the opposite tube in a subsequent pregnancy.

## Consequences of Tubal Pregnancy

An ectopic pregnancy in the fallopian tube gradually distends the tube. The embryo may develop normally for a time but rarely survives for more than a few months. The invading trophoblast erodes tubal blood vessels, causing bleeding into the lumen and wall of the tube and sometimes into the tissues surrounding it.

A woman with an ectopic pregnancy experiences signs and symptoms of early pregnancy and misses her expected menstrual period, as with a normal intrauterine pregnancy. She may also complain of some abdominal pain and tenderness caused by distention of the tube and irritation of the pelvic peritoneum caused by bleeding in the tube wall and adjacent tissues. She may also experience slight vaginal bleeding if blood leaks from the tubal implantation

site, escapes into the uterus, and is discharged into the vagina.

Rupture of the tube can occur at any time (Figure 14-12). This catastrophe is accompanied by severe abdominal pain and profuse intra-abdominal bleeding caused by disruption of large tubal blood vessels at the site of rupture. If the patient is not treated promptly, tubal rupture may prove fatal because of the severe hemorrhage that occurs.

Because of the potential life-threatening risk of a ruptured tubal pregnancy, a physician always considers the possibility of a tubal pregnancy in any woman of reproductive age who exhibits any symptoms sug-

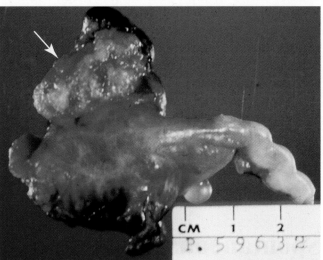

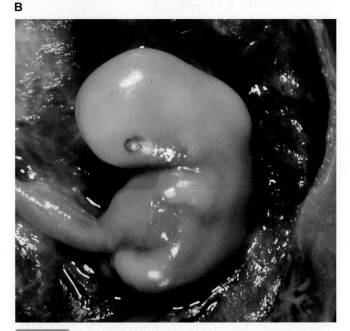

**Figure 14-12** Ectopic pregnancy in right fallopian tube. **A,** A mass of placental tissue protrudes through the wall of a greatly distended fallopian tube (*arrow*). **B,** The embryo contained within the intact amnionic sac.

gesting a tubal pregnancy. A pelvic examination reveals an area of tenderness adjacent to the uterus and may also reveal a mass caused by the swollen tube. A positive pregnancy test confirms the pregnancy, and an ultrasound examination demonstrates that the chorionic vesicle indicative of pregnancy is not within the uterus. If these findings indicate that a tubal pregnancy is likely, a laparoscopic examination is performed, which allows the physician to visualize the fallopian tubes and ovaries and to identify the unruptured pregnancy within the fallopian tube.

The following case illustrates some of the common clinical features encountered in a patient with a ruptured ectopic pregnancy.

## Case Study 14-1

A 34-year-old woman consulted her physician because of recent onset of severe abdominal pain. Her last normal menstrual period had been 10 weeks earlier. For the previous 2 weeks, she had experienced mild abdominal pain and slight intermittent vaginal bleeding. On examination, she exhibited evidence of severe blood loss, and her abdomen was diffusely tender. A diagnosis of ruptured ectopic pregnancy was made, and an operation was performed immediately. A large amount of blood was found within the abdominal cavity caused by bleeding from the tubal blood vessels that were disrupted when the tube ruptured. The ruptured tube was removed, and the severe blood loss was treated by several blood transfusions. The patient made a satisfactory recovery.

# Abnormal Attachment of the Placenta

## Placenta Previa

Normally, the placenta attaches high on the anterior or posterior uterine wall. If the placenta becomes attached in the lower part of the uterus, it may cover the cervix. This is called a **placenta previa** ( Figure 14-13 ). The term literally means a placenta blocking the exit from the uterus (*pre* = before + *via* = pathway). A placenta that completely covers the cervix is called a *central placenta previa*. If only the edge of the placenta encroaches on

the cervix, the abnormality is designated a *partial placenta previa*. The patient with a placenta previa experiences episodes of bleeding during the last part of pregnancy, as a consequence of partial separation of the placenta from the uterine wall. Normally, the lower part of the uterus undergoes gradual dilation during the last part of pregnancy in preparation for childbirth. The abnormally located placenta is unable to stretch to conform to the contour of the expanding lower part of the uterus, and parts of the placenta therefore tear loose. The tearing disrupts the large uterine vessels that penetrate the basal part of the placenta to supply the intervillous spaces (see Figure 14-10). Placenta previa is hazardous to the mother. She may bleed to death if a large part of the placenta is torn from the uterine wall. Large areas of placental disruption may also prevent proper oxygenation of fetal blood passing through the placenta, leading to the death of the fetus.

Because the placenta blocks the cervix, vaginal delivery is not possible without the risk of severe hemorrhage and injury to the cervix. Delivery is generally accomplished by cesarean section.

# Twins and Multiple Pregnancies

Normally, about 1 percent of all pregnancies are twins (approximately 1 in 100). Twins may be either identical (*monozygotic*) or fraternal (*dizygotic*). Approximately 0.01 percent of pregnancies (approximately 1 in 10,000) are triplets. Quadruplets, quintuplets, and sextuplets are very rare. The incidence of all types of multiple pregnancies is much higher than normal when ovulation is induced by administration of gonadotropic hormones or similar drugs that often induce ovulation of several ova instead of a single ovum, or when a large number of previously fertilized eggs are implanted in the uterus, as occurred in the recently reported case of a woman who delivered eight very premature infants.

## Fraternal Twins

Seventy percent of twins are fraternal and result from fertilization of two separate ova by two different sperm. Fraternal twins are no more alike than brothers and sisters, but they share a family resemblance because they are born of the same parents. Each fertilized ovum implants separately, and each twin forms its own placenta and fetal membranes. Frequently, the margins of the two placentas grow together and fuse, but each fetus remains enclosed

**placenta previa** (prē′vē-yuh) Attachment of the placenta in the uterus such that it partially or completely covers the cervix.

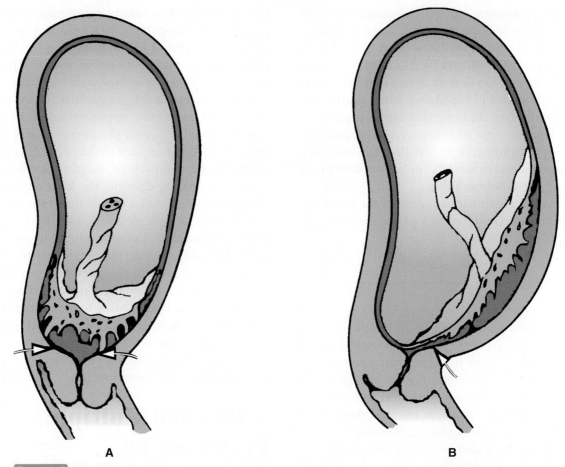

**Figure 14-13** Types of placenta previa. **A,** Central placenta previa. **B,** Partial placenta previa. The *arrows* indicate the usual locations where the placenta tears from its attachment to the lower part of the uterus late in pregnancy.

within its own amnion and chorion. A fused placenta of this type is called a *diamnionic dichorionic placenta.*

## Identical Twins

Thirty percent of twins are identical and result from the splitting of a single fertilized ovum. Splitting may occur at various times after fertilization, as illustrated in [Figure 14-14]. In about 30 percent of monozygotic twin pregnancies, the fertilized ovum splits before the inner cell mass forms. Each half of the zygote implants separately, forms a complete embryo, and develops its own placenta. The two placentas may remain separate or may become fused to form a diamnionic dichorionic placenta in the same manner as that for fraternal twins.

More commonly (in almost 70 percent of monozygotic twin pregnancies), the inner cell mass divides after the blastocyst has formed but before implantation takes place. In this instance, each half of the inner cell mass forms a complete embryo and develops its own amnion and yolk sac, but both develop within a single chorionic cavity. This gives rise to a placenta called a *diamnionic monochorionic placenta.*

Rarely, the inner cell mass divides after the amnionic sac has already formed. When this occurs, the two embryos develop within a single amnionic cavity and form a *monoamnionic monochorionic placenta.* If the division of the inner cell mass is incomplete, conjoined (Siamese) twins are formed.

## Determination of Zygosity of Twins from Examination of Placenta

It is often desirable to know at the time of birth whether the twins are identical or fraternal. If they are of different sexes, they must be fraternal, but if they are the same sex, they could be either fraternal or identical. Sometimes the zygosity of the twins can be determined by examining the placenta. If there are two separate placentas, the twins must have implanted separately. A single placenta with two amnionic sacs, however, could be either a *monochorionic placenta* or a *dichorionic placenta.* It is possible to distinguish between these two types of placentas by gross and microscopic examination of the partition between the two amnionic sacs because the structure of the partition indicates how it

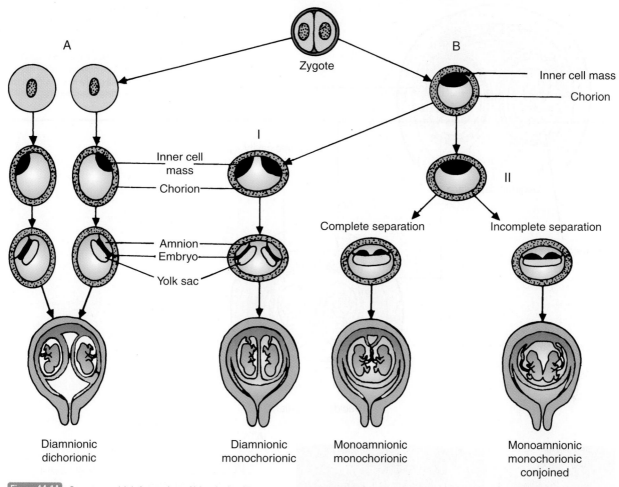

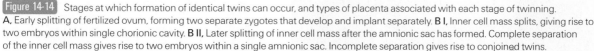 Stages at which formation of identical twins can occur, and types of placenta associated with each stage of twinning. A, Early splitting of fertilized ovum, forming two separate zygotes that develop and implant separately. B I, Inner cell mass splits, giving rise to two embryos within single chorionic cavity. B II, Later splitting of inner cell mass after the amnionic sac has formed. Complete separation of the inner cell mass gives rise to two embryos within a single amnionic sac. Incomplete separation gives rise to conjoined twins.

was formed. Figure 14-15 compares the arrangement of fetal membranes of twins implanted separately (dichorionic placenta) with that of twins developing within a single chorionic cavity (monochorionic placenta). As the amnionic sacs gradually enlarge, the membranes eventually establish contact and form a midline partition between the two sacs (Figure 14-16). If the placenta is monochorionic, the dividing septum consists only of two amnions without intervening chorions; in a dichorionic placenta, four separate membranes can be identified in the partition: two outer amnions and two inner chorions (Figure 14-17). A diamnionic monochorionic placenta always indicates identical twins, as does the rare monoamnionic monochorionic placenta. If the placenta is diamnionic dichorionic or if there are two separate placentas, the twins could be either identical or fraternal. All fraternal twins have a diamnionic dichorionic placenta or separate placentas, but so do 30 percent of identical twins.

## Twin Transfusion Syndrome

The placental circulations of identical twins are frequently joined by multiple *vascular anastomoses* (interconnecting blood vessels), and consequently, there is normally some intermixing of blood from the two fetuses in the placentas (Figure 14-18). Sometimes the placental anastomoses are such that an excess of blood from the fetoplacental circulation from one infant (called the *donor twin*) flows into the circulation of the second twin (called the *recipient*). If this occurs, the donor twin may become anemic and the recipient twin may become overloaded with blood (*polycythemic*). Some degree of twin-to-twin transfusion is relatively common and is reported in about 15 percent of all twin births. Minor differences in the blood volumes of the two twins can be tolerated, but large disproportions are harmful to both twins (Figure 14-19). The severe anemia may be fatal to the donor twin, and the circulation of the recipient twin may become so overloaded

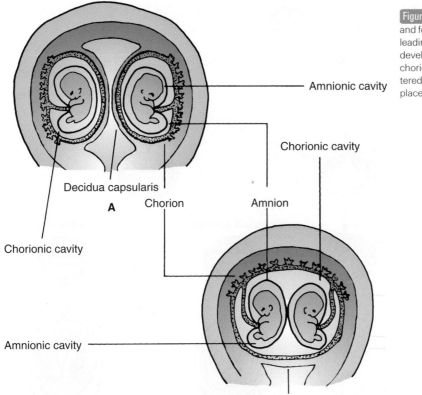

Figure 14-15 A comparison of the formation of the placentas and fetal membranes in twins. **A,** Separate implantations leading to the formation of a dichorionic placenta. **B,** Twins developing in a single chorionic cavity and forming a monochorionic placenta. A dichorionic placenta can be encountered in either fraternal or identical twins. A monochorionic placenta occurs only in identical twins.

Amnionic cavity

Chorionic cavity

Decidua capsularis

Chorion

Amnion

Chorionic cavity

Amnionic cavity

**A**

Amnionic cavity

Decidua capsularis

**B**

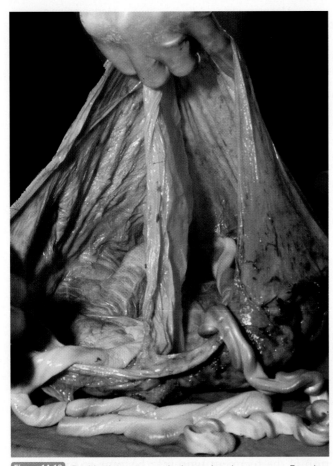

Figure 14-16 Partition between amnionic sacs in twin pregnancy. Examination of the partition may indicate the zygosity of the twins.

**A**

**B**

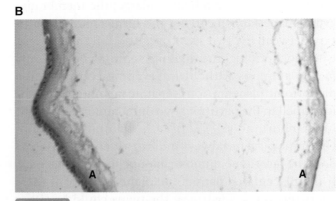

Figure 14-17 Comparison of histologic appearance of partition between amnionic sacs in twin pregnancies. **A,** Diamnionic dichorionic placenta, illustrating four layers, two outer layers of amnion (**A**) and two inner layers of chorion (**C**). **B,** Diamnionic monochorionic pregnancy of identical twins, illustrating only two layers of amnion (**A**) without chorions interposed between the two amnions.

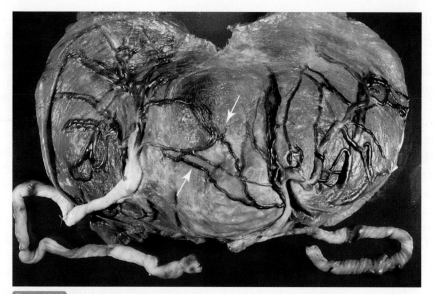

Figure 14-18 Placenta of identical twins with amnions removed revealing interconnecting blood vessels (*arrows*).

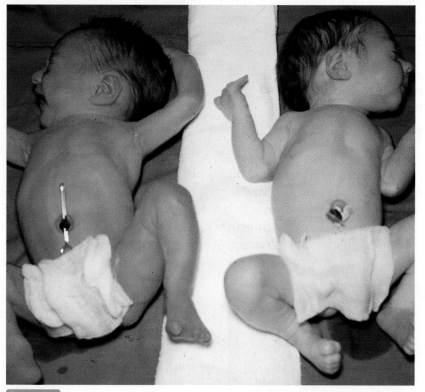

Figure 14-19 Identical twins exhibiting twin transfusion syndrome. The twin on the *right* in the photograph is pale and anemic. The twin on the *left* appears ruddy and contains an excess of blood. Both twins survived.

by the great excess of blood that the polycythemic twin dies of heart failure.

In selected cases, when the twin-to-twin connections between the placental circulations are putting the fetuses at risk of intrauterine death, it is sometimes possible to visualize the placenta using a device called an endoscope that is inserted into the uterus to visualize the placenta.

Then the twin-to-twin blood vessel connections are coagulated to stop the blood transfer between the twins.

## Vanishing Twins and Blighted Twins

Sometimes one twin of a twin pregnancy fails to develop and dies early in pregnancy. The actual incidence of twin pregnancies is significantly higher than indicated from data based on the delivery of two infants at term. Ultrasound studies of first trimester pregnancies reveal that many more pregnancies start out as twins than survive to term. The other twin that fails to survive may be a vanishing twin that is completely absorbed, leaving no trace, or may persist as a blighted twin, which is a degenerated embryo or fetus that is retained within the uterus until the surviving fetus is delivered at term. Figure 14-20 illustrates a blighted fetus associated with a triplet pregnancy as described in Case 14-2.

**preeclampsia**
(pre ek-lamp′-sē-ă) A pregnancy-related complication characterized by hypertension and proteinuria, which usually occurs after the twentieth week of gestation, thought to be caused by placental dysfunction.

**eclampsia** (ek-lamp′-sē-ă) One or more convulsions in a pregnant woman with preeclampsia.

## Conjoined Twins

Incomplete separation of the inner cell mass leads to a variable degree of union between two conjoined twins. The twins may be joined at the head, thorax, abdomen, or pelvis, the union being face to face, side to side, or back to back. The extent of union is variable but often considerable, and often the twins share common internal organs to such a degree that it is not possible to separate them surgically. The conjoined twins are generally equal in size and are often well formed except for their failure to separate.

## Disadvantages of Twin Pregnancies

Twins are at a disadvantage compared with singletons. Because they are overcrowded within the uterus, a twin is always smaller than a single infant at a comparable stage of gestation. Overdistention of the uterus frequently promotes premature onset of labor, leading to delivery of premature infants having a reduced chance of survival. Congenital malformations occur twice as

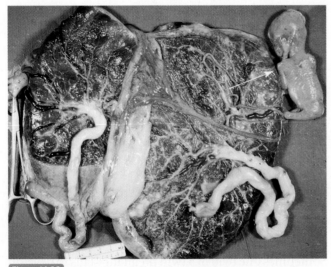

Figure 14-20 Triplet placenta. Two infants were born prematurely. The third fetus (*arrow*) died early in pregnancy and was retained within the uterus until delivery of the surviving twins (Case 14-2).

### Case Study 14-2

A 30-year-old woman delivered normal, well-formed female twins prematurely at 36 weeks' gestation. Examination of the placenta after delivery revealed a third amnionic sac containing a compressed degenerated fetus measuring 13 centimeters in length (Figure 14-20). The partition between the amnionic sacs consisted of double amnions and double chorions. In this triplet pregnancy, one fetus died at about 17 weeks' gestation and was retained within the uterus until the delivery of the two remaining infants at 36 weeks. Each fetus was enclosed within its own amnion and chorion. Consequently, the zygosity of the surviving twins could not be determined from examination of the placenta because a diamnionic dichorionic placenta can be associated with either identical or fraternal twins.

often in twins as in singletons, and vascular anastomoses within the placental circulation may lead to a twin transfusion syndrome.

## Preeclampsia and Eclampsia: Toxemia of Pregnancy

**Preeclampsia** is a pregnancy-associated elevated blood pressure exceeding 140/90 accompanied by protein in the urine, which has its onset anytime from the 20th week of gestation to the end of the pregnancy. It is more common in young girls and older women, in twin pregnancies, and in women who have had preeclampsia in a previous pregnancy. In severe cases blood pressure exceeds 160/110 and may be associated with convulsions, which is called **eclampsia**. The two conditions are grouped under the general term *toxemia of pregnancy*, and appear to be caused by inadequate blood flow to the placenta. The placental dysfunction leads to releases of substances that constrict blood vessels, raise blood pressure, promote clumping of platelets with formation of intravascular thrombi in the kidneys (leading to proteinuria), in the placenta, and in other tissues. Extremely severe cases can lead to partial separation of the placenta from the uterine wall, and also may be complicated by a disseminated intravascular coagulation syndrome, as described in Chapter 9.

Mild cases can be managed by bed rest and close observation, delaying premature delivery as long as possible without endangering the mother's health. Severe cases are hazardous to both mother and fetus. Treatment consists of trying to control the hypertension and vascular damage until the fetus is mature enough to be delivered prematurely, even as early as 20-weeks' gestation but preferably delaying until 24-weeks' gestation if possible. A number of drugs are used to control the hypertension and hopefully prevent convulsions. The condition usually relents when the placenta (which appears to be the cause of the problem) is expelled after delivery.

# Hydatidiform Mole and Choriocarcinoma

Sometimes, when a pregnancy does not develop normally, the embryo either fails to form or dies and is absorbed, the trophoblastic cells covering the villi continue to grow at an excessive rate, and the proliferating trophoblast produces a much greater amount of chorionic gonadotropin hormone than is encountered in a normal pregnancy. Masses of abnormal proliferating trophoblastic tissue may invade the uterus, spread into the vagina, and even metastasize to distant sites. Three different degrees of abnormal trophoblastic activity are recognized, and the general term **gestational trophoblast disease** is used to encompass all three types:

1. The most common type, which occurs in about 80 percent of affected patients, is a relatively benign trophoblast proliferation called a **hydatidiform mole**.
2. A more aggressive and destructive proliferative process, which occurs in about 15 percent of patients, is called an **invasive mole**.
3. A malignant growth of trophoblastic tissue, which affects only a small percentage of patients, is called a **choriocarcinoma**. This aggressive trophoblastic neoplasm can metastasize widely and kill the patient unless controlled by proper treatment.

## Benign Hydatidiform Mole

In a benign hydatidiform mole, the villi that are covered by proliferating trophoblast become converted into large cystic structures resembling masses of grapes (Figure 14-21). The unusual name given to this condition is derived from its gross appearance. A hydatid is a fluid-filled vesicle, and a mole is a shapeless mass of tissue.

A hydatidiform mole is a relatively uncommon complication of pregnancy that occurs about once in 1500 pregnancies in the United States and Canada, but is encountered 10 times more frequently in women from the Far East and Southeast Asia. Because of the increased

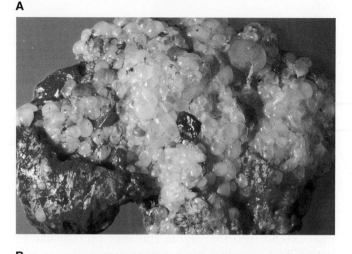

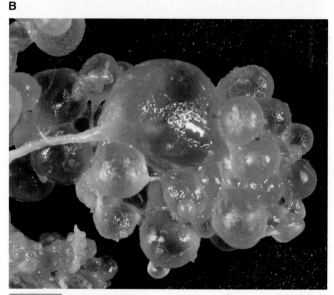

Figure 14-21 Hydatidiform mole. **A,** Placenta converted into a large mass of cystic villi. **B,** Closer view of cystic villi.

volume of the placenta caused by the multiple cystic villi, the patient with a mole experiences an enlargement of the uterus that is much greater than would be expected in relationship to the duration of the pregnancy. Erosion of maternal blood vessels by the mole may cause irregular uterine bleeding. The overdistension of the uterus caused by the mole may precipitate uterine contractions leading to expulsion of pieces of the mole. Diagnosis of a mole is based on the clinical features of the pregnancy, by identifying cystic villi covered by proliferating trophoblast that have been expelled from the uterus, or by ultrasound examination that reveals a characteristic appearance caused by the cystic villi that fill the uterine cavity.

**gestational trophoblast disease** (jes-tay´-shun-ul tro´-fo-blast) A general term for all diseases characterized by abnormal trophoblast proliferation. Includes both hydatidiform mole and choriocarcinoma.

**hydatidiform mole** (hī-da-tid´i-form mōl) A neoplastic proliferation of trophoblast associated with formation of large cystic villi.

**invasive mole** An aggressive hydatidiform mole that invades the uterine wall.

**choriocarcinoma** (kōr´rē-ō-kär-sin-ō´muh) A malignant proliferation of trophoblastic tissue.

## Invasive Mole

An invasive mole resembles a complete hydatidiform mole but exhibits a much more marked trophoblastic proliferation and a much more aggressive behavior. The trophoblastic tissue may invade deeply into the uterine wall and cause considerable bleeding, but does not metastasize.

## Choriocarcinoma

This is the most aggressive form of gestational trophoblast disease and behaves like a malignant tumor. Masses of abnormal actively proliferating trophoblast may extend into the vagina and may metastasize to the lungs, brain, and other distant sites. Unless vigorously treated, the tumor may eventually kill the patient.

## Treatment of Gestational Trophoblast Disease

Treatment of a mole consists of evacuating the uterus by curettage and then performing periodic determinations of the level of chorionic gonadotropins in the patient's blood to be certain all the abnormal tissue has been removed. After successful treatment, the chorionic gonadotropin level in the patient's blood should gradually fall to undetectable levels within about 8 weeks. If the level does not fall or if it starts to rise again after an initial fall, this means that the mole was incompletely removed and has recurred or has become invasive, and further treatment is needed. Generally, the treatment consists of anticancer chemotherapy, although sometimes a hysterectomy is performed if the patient does not wish to have further pregnancies. A choriocarcinoma is usually treated vigorously by several courses of anticancer chemotherapy, and most patients can be cured by adequate treatment as illustrated by the metastatic choriocarcinoma ( Figure 14-22 )

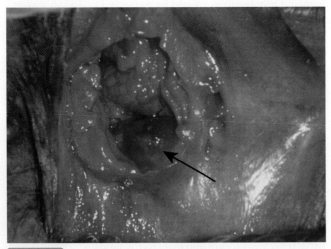

Figure 14-22 Metastatic choriocarcinoma in the posterior wall of the vagina (*arrow*). The patient had an excellent response to chemotherapy and later had a normal pregnancy and delivery.

in a woman who was cured by chemotherapy. Later she had a normal pregnancy and delivered a normal healthy infant.

A woman who has had a mole removed should always have periodic follow-up examinations because some moles can be quite aggressive and may recur, and choriocarcinoma may arise after incomplete removal of an invasive or incompletely removed mole. If a woman has had a mole removed and is being followed by periodic measurements of chorionic gonadotropins, she should not become pregnant for 1 year after the mole has been removed. The reason is because a pregnancy would complicate the interpretation of follow-up chorionic gonadotropin tests. The physician would be unable to determine whether the elevated chorionic gonadotropin was caused by recurrent gestational trophoblast disease, which requires anticancer chemotherapy, or a normal pregnancy.

# Hemolytic Disease of the Newborn (Erythroblastosis Fetalis)

Hemolytic disease of the newborn is a hemolytic anemia in the newborn infant resulting from sensitization of the mother to a "foreign" blood group antigen present in the red cells of the fetus but lacking in the maternal cells. Many different blood group antigens are known to cause hemolytic disease. The best known is the Rh antigen. Normally hemolytic disease does not occur in the first blood group-incompatible pregnancy because no significant numbers of sensitizing fetal red cells enter the mother's circulation until the placenta separates from the uterus after delivery. However, once the mother's immune system has been sensitized to the foreign blood group antigen, she will form antibodies in any subsequent pregnancy with a fetus having the same blood group antigen that induced the initial maternal sensitization; the antibody-mediated red cell destruction will lead to hemolytic anemia and jaundice in the affected infant. The term jaundice refers to the yellow skin discoloration resulting from bilirubin in the fetal blood. Bilirubin is a yellow–brown breakdown product derived from the hemoglobin that is released from antibody-damaged fetal red cells.

## Changes in Hemoglobin and Bilirubin After Delivery

Figure 14-23 illustrates the typical changes in hemoglobin and bilirubin levels after delivery of an infant with hemolytic disease. The infant always becomes more anemic after

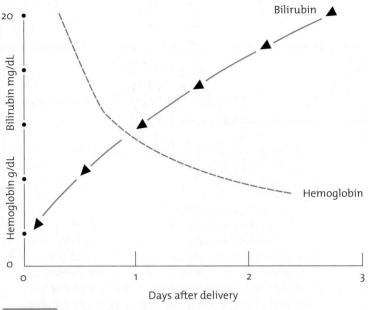

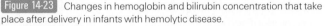

birth, and the level of bilirubin also rises rapidly. The anemia increases after delivery because red cell production declines as soon as the infant starts to breathe room air, which raises the oxygen content of the infant's blood. However, the antibodies already in the infant's blood continue to destroy the red cells until the antibodies eventually are eliminated from the infant's blood.

The rising bilirubin results from the continuing antibody-mediated red cell destruction. Before the fetus is born, much of the bilirubin in the fetal blood crosses the placenta into the maternal circulation where it is processed (conjugated) in the mother's liver and excreted in the mother's bile. After birth the infant has to process and excrete the large amount of bilirubin formerly handled by the mother, but the liver of the newborn infant is relatively inefficient at conjugating and excreting bilirubin. As a result the level of unconjugated bilirubin in the infant's blood rises rapidly. This condition is called *hyperbilirubinemia* (*hyper* = elevated + bilirubin + *heme* = blood) and is hazardous to the infant. A high level of unconjugated bilirubin is toxic to the nervous system, where it causes bile staining and degeneration of parts of the brain called the basal ganglia (basal nuclei), and damages other parts of the brain as well. This condition is called kernicterus (*kern* = kernel, referring to brain basal ganglia + *icterus* = jaundice), also called bilirubin encephalopathy.

## Rh Hemolytic Disease

The features characteristic of any maternal-fetal blood group incompatibility also apply to Rh hemolytic dis-

ease resulting from Rh antibodies formed by an Rh-negative mother directed against the red cells of her Rh-positive fetus.

The Rh system is a relatively complex blood group system consisting of a series of allelic genes that determine multiple Rh antigens on the red cells. The most important Rh antigen is named the *D antigen* in one terminology and the *Rh_o antigen* in another terminology. The subscript "o" refers to original, meaning that it was the first Rh antigen recognized, and also the most important. The presence of the D (Rh_o) antigen is considered to be determined by the allelic genes *D* and *d*, giving three possible genotypes: *DD*, *Dd*, and *dd*. For clinical purposes, persons whose red cells possess the D (Rh_o) antigen are considered Rh positive, regardless of the presence or absence of other Rh antigens, and persons lacking the D antigen (genotype *dd*) are considered Rh negative. An Rh-positive person may be either homozygous (*DD*) or heterozygous (*Dd*). Consequently, two heterozygous Rh-positive parents may have an Rh-negative child if each parent passes a *d* gene to the offspring. It is also possible for a heterozygous Rh-positive father and Rh-negative mother to have an Rh-negative child.

The first Rh-positive infant born to an Rh-negative mother is usually normal. However, after the mother has been sensitized to Rh-positive fetal cells by a previous pregnancy with an Rh-positive fetus, Rh hemolytic disease will develop in any subsequent pregnancy in which the fetus is Rh positive.

Now Rh hemolytic disease occurs infrequently because usually we can prevent the formation of Rh antibodies by an Rh-negative woman pregnant with an Rh-positive fetus, and we also have effective ways to treat any unfortunate newborn infants who have hemolytic disease. Although Rh hemolytic disease occurs infrequently, knowing about the disease and its effects on the fetus emphasizes how important it is to prevent the disease in susceptible Rh-positive infants born to Rh-negative mothers.

## Diagnosis of Hemolytic Disease in the Newborn Infant

From knowledge of the pathogenesis of the disease, it follows that the diagnosis of hemolytic disease can be made when the following features are demonstrated.

1. The mother is Rh negative and the infant is Rh positive.
2. The mother's blood contains Rh antibodies.

> **bilirubin**
> (bil-i-rū′bin) One of the bile pigments derived from breakdown of hemoglobin.

*The investigation of a severe transfusion reaction in a postpartum patient established the cause of neonatal hemolytic disease and identified the antibody responsible for most cases.*

Hemolytic disease of newborn infants was recognized by midwives as far back as the 1700s but its cause was unknown. Nothing was known about blood group systems until the ABO groups were identified by Landsteiner in 1901, which improved the safety of blood transfusions. However, sometimes transfusion reactions still occurred despite matching ABO blood groups between donor and recipient. Then followed a period when investigators tried to identify other blood groups by injecting animals with red blood cells to produce an antibody that could be used to test human red cells, and hopefully identify new red cell antigens. The big breakthrough came in about 1940 when investigators injected rabbits with red blood cells from a rhesus monkey and found that the rhesus antibody reacted with the red cells of about 85 percent of white persons and about 95 percent of black persons in the New York City area. The persons who reacted were called rhesus posi-

tive, which was shortened to Rh positive, and the nonreactors were called Rh negative. At about the same time a woman delivered an infant with hemolytic disease in a difficult delivery with significant blood loss and required a blood transfusion. As was the practice at that time, blood transfusions were given as direct transfusions from one person to another, and the woman's ABO compatible husband was selected as the donor. The woman had a severe transfusion reaction when the blood was given, which must have been caused by an antibody not related to an ABO blood group incompatibility between the mother and her husband. Some of the newly produced anti-Rh antibody was obtained to test the blood cells of the woman (who was determined to be Rh negative) and her husband (who tested as Rh positive), and the maternal antibody that caused the transfusion reaction was identified as anti-Rh antibody. The cause of neonatal hemolytic disease was determined and the antibody responsible for most cases was identified. Soon methods were developed to treat affected infants; later a method was developed to prevent sensitization of an Rh-negative mother to the Rh-positive cells of her infant.

3. The antibodies are attached to the infant's red cells, which can be demonstrated by a relatively simple laboratory test (direct Coombs test).
4. The antibody damages the infant's red cells, as demonstrated by anemia and elevated blood bilirubin, which reflect the severity of the hemolytic anemia.

In routine clinical practice, this information can be obtained promptly without great difficulty. Generally, blood typing of the mother and tests to determine the presence of antibodies are performed routinely during pregnancy by the physician, who generally knows before delivery whether the mother has been sensitized and is likely to deliver an affected infant. When the infant is born, a sample of blood from the umbilical cord (which is the infant's blood) is sent to the laboratory to confirm that the baby is Rh positive and that the baby's red cells are coated with antibody. Tests to determine the hemoglobin and bilirubin concentration in the baby's blood indicate the severity of the hemolytic disease. Normally the concentration of unconjugated bilirubin normally rises after delivery even in normal infants, usually reaching a peak of about 6 mg/dL or sometimes even higher within the first few days after delivery and then falls toward normal. In hemolytic disease, unconjugated bilirubin lev-

els rise faster, and are often much higher than in a normal newborn infant. Levels exceeding 20 mg/dL are potentially hazardous, put the infant at risk of kernicterus, and require treatment to lower the bilirubin concentration ( Table 14-2 ).

## Treatment of Hemolytic Disease

When hemolytic disease caused by Rh incompatibility was a more common problem than it is now, a commonly used treatment was **exchange transfusion**, a complicated procedure that gradually replaced the infant's Rh-positive blood with Rh-negative blood. The

| Table 14-2 | Diagnosis of Hemolytic Disease |
| --- | --- |

| Characteristic Feature | Means of Recognition |
| --- | --- |
| Production of antigenic fetal cells | Maternal–fetal blood group differences; mother lacks antigen present in fetal cells |
| Maternal sensitization | Mother's blood contains antibody against antigenic cells |
| Transplacental passage of maternal antibody | Positive direct Coombs test on cord blood |
| Increased blood destruction in newborn infant | Decreased hemoglobin in cord blood; elevated bilirubin |

infant with hemolytic disease is in jeopardy because the infant's body is saturated with passively transferred maternal antibody. The antibody is the cause of the hemolytic anemia and jaundice, and several months are required before the antibody can be completely eliminated from the infant's circulation. The rationale of exchange transfusion is to provide the infant with a population of cells that will not be destroyed by the antibody. At the same time, exchange transfusion provides the infant with bilirubin-free plasma to replace the jaundiced plasma, thereby helping to prevent severe elevation of potentially toxic, unconjugated bilirubin. The exchange transfusion has no effect on the infant's own blood type. The transfused Rh-negative cells will be gradually eliminated and replaced by the infant's own Rh-positive cells. The purpose of the exchange transfusion is to tide the infant over in an acute situation. This is accomplished by decreasing the rate of red cell destruction through transfusion of cells not subject to hemolysis and by lowering the concentration of potentially toxic unconjugated bilirubin in the infant's plasma.

## Fluorescent Light Therapy for Hyperbilirubinemia

The elevated level of unconjugated bilirubin that causes kernicterus can be reduced by exposing the unclothed jaundiced infant to fluorescent lights continuously for several days. The infant is turned frequently so that the skin receives maximum exposure to the fluorescent light. The eyes are covered to protect them from the bright light. The light exposure acts by converting the toxic unconjugated bilirubin into less toxic compounds that are not as hazardous to the infant. This procedure, called **phototherapy**, has reduced the need for exchange transfusions.

## Prevention of Rh Hemolytic Disease with Rh-Immune Globulin

**Postpartum Administration** As previously stated, the first Rh-positive infant born to an Rh-negative mother is usually normal because Rh antibodies are rarely formed during the first pregnancy. Although a few Rh-positive cells may periodically enter the mother's circulation during pregnancy, their numbers are not sufficient to induce sensitization. The greater numbers of Rh-positive cells required to sensitize the mother usually do not enter the maternal circulation until after delivery. When the placenta begins to separate from the uterus and is eventually expelled, the barrier separating the maternal and fetal circulations is disrupted, and some of the Rh-positive fetal cells within the villi may be expressed into the uterine blood vessels and may enter the mother's circulation ( Figure 14-24 ). In general, the larger the volume of fetal blood entering the mother's circulation, the greater the likelihood of sensitization to Rh antigen, and after sensitization has occurred, Rh hemolytic disease will develop in any subsequent pregnancy in which the fetus is Rh positive.

Rh-immune globulin is a gamma globulin containing a high concentration of Rh antibody. When administered to an unsensitized Rh-negative mother within 72 hours after delivery of an Rh-positive fetus, it is extremely effective in preventing the formation of Rh antibody. The Rh antibody in the immune globulin coats the Rh antigen sites on the surface of any fetal

**exchange transfusion** Partial replacement of blood of infant with hemolytic disease by blood lacking the antigen responsible for hemolytic disease, as when transfusing Rh-negative blood to an Rh-positive infant. Performed to reduce intensity of hemolytic jaundice.

**phototherapy** Fluorescent light treatment of jaundiced babies to reduce the concentration of unconjugated bilirubin in their blood.

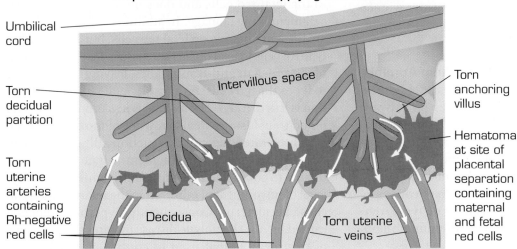

**Rh-positive fetal red cells supplying chorionic villi**

Umbilical cord

Torn decidual partition

Torn uterine arteries containing Rh-negative red cells

Intervillous space

Decidua

Torn anchoring villus

Hematoma at site of placental separation containing maternal and fetal red cells

Torn uterine veins

**Rh-negative maternal red cells in decidua supplying intervillous spaces**

Figure 14-24 Transfer of fetal Rh-positive red cells into maternal circulation during postpartum placental separation. Separation of the placenta disrupts maternal decidua containing maternal blood vessels that supply blood to the intervillous spaces, and also disrupts blood vessels in villi anchoring placenta to basal decidua. Fetal and maternal blood cells escaping from torn blood vessels form a collection of blood (hematoma) between the placenta and basal decidua. Uterine contractions that expel placenta compress the hematoma and may force blood from the hematoma (containing fetal red cells) into maternal circulation. The *arrows* indicate direction of blood flow.

red cells that have entered the mother's circulation, leading to rapid removal of the antibody-coated red cells so that they do not persist long enough to induce sensitization. Rh-immune globulin is recommended for all Rh-negative mothers who have not already formed Rh antibodies and who have given birth to an Rh-positive infant. It is of no value if the mother has already formed antibodies. Unsensitized Rh-negative patients should also receive Rh-immune globulin after an abortion or ectopic pregnancy because these conditions may also induce sensitization. The risk is low, however, if the gestation is fewer than 12 weeks.

The standard dose of Rh-immune globulin is sufficient to "neutralize" and eliminate about 1 ounce of fetal blood. In the very uncommon situation in which a larger volume of fetal blood enters the maternal circulation, more Rh-immune globulin is required. Special laboratory tests can detect and determine the volume of fetal blood in the mother's circulation, enabling the physician to determine how much additional Rh-immune globulin to administer.

The incidence of Rh hemolytic disease has been greatly reduced by the routine use of Rh-immune globulin, but the disease has not been completely eliminated. There are two reasons why the disease persists:

1. A very small number of Rh-negative women form Rh antibody in their first pregnancy, apparently because of prior contact with Rh antigen from an unrecognized abortion, transfusion of Rh-positive blood, or other cause.
2. Rh-immune globulin is not 100-percent effective. About 1.5 percent of Rh-negative women will form antibodies in a subsequent Rh-positive pregnancy despite postpartum administration of Rh-immune globulin. (About 15 percent of Rh-negative women would be expected to form antibodies if no treatment were administered.)

**Combined Antepartum and Postpartum Administration** One of the reasons why postpartum administration of Rh-immune globulin does not always prevent Rh sensitization is that small numbers of fetal Rh-positive red cells sufficient to induce sensitization occasionally enter the mother's circulation late in pregnancy through small breaks in the placental villi. When this occurs, the antigenic fetal cells may cause the mother to become sensitized prior to delivery, rendering postpartum administration of Rh-immune globulin ineffective.

In an effort to further reduce the failure rate of Rh-immune globulin, many physicians recommend that an injection of Rh-immune globulin be given at about 28 weeks' gestation, in addition to the postpartum injection. Combined antepartum and postpartum administration reduces the incidence of sensitization to about 0.5 percent compared with a 1.5-percent incidence when only postpartum administration is employed. When Rh-immune globulin is used prior to delivery, it is given to all Rh-negative mothers, many of whom are carrying an Rh-negative fetus and do not need it. However, the Rh-immune globulin injection is not harmful to the mother, even though it would not be necessary if the infant were Rh negative (a fact that could not be determined until after the baby was born). Only mothers with Rh-positive babies would need to receive the postpartum injection.

## ABO Hemolytic Disease

With the decline in the frequency of Rh hemolytic disease, now most cases of hemolytic disease result from ABO blood group differences between the mother and infant. In this condition, called **ABO hemolytic disease**, the mother is group O (and has anti-A and anti-B antibodies in her serum), and the infant is either group A or group B. In most women, the A or B fetal antigens stimulate the maternal ABO antibodies, increasing their concentration and changing their character so that they are able to cross the placenta into the fetal circulation and attach to fetal cells. ABO hemolytic disease occurs in a first ABO-incompatible pregnancy because it is caused by preexisting anti-A and anti-B antibodies.

Generally, ABO hemolytic disease is a much less severe disease than Rh hemolytic disease because A and B antigens on fetal cells are not as well developed as on adult cells, so the antibody does not fix as firmly to the fetal red cells and does not cause as much red cell membrane damage. In addition, A and B antigens are present not only on fetal red cells, but also on other types of cells in fetal organs and tissues that absorb much of the anti-A or anti-B antibodies, leaving less available to fix to the red cells. As a result, fetal red cell destruction is less marked. The anemia is less pronounced, and blood transfusions are usually not required. However, the accelerated red cell destruction still generates an excessive amount of bile pigment, which the infant is unable to conjugate and excrete efficiently, and a high level of unconjugated bilirubin in the infant's blood can cause kernicterus. Consequently, hyperbilirubinemia caused by ABO hemolytic disease requires the same type of treatment as that used to control elevated serum bilirubin in Rh hemolytic disease. Generally, the elevated bilirubin responds well to fluorescent light phototherapy, and exchange transfusion usually is not required.

The following two cases illustrate hemolytic disease caused by ABO incompatibility with two different outcomes, which illustrate the importance of prompt and vigorous treatment of affected infants.

## Case Study 14-3

An ABO-incompatible pregnancy in which the hyperbilirubinemia was recognized promptly after the infant had left the hospital and responded well to fluorescent light therapy.

A normal full-term, 8-pound male infant was born without complications to a group O Rh-positive mother. The mother and baby did well after delivery and were discharged 2 days later. After returning home, the parents noted that the infant appeared jaundiced and brought him back to the hospital for further evaluation and treatment. When examined at the hospital, the baby did not appear ill but was moderately jaundiced, and the serum bilirubin was elevated. Laboratory tests revealed that the baby was group A Rh positive, and the Coombs test was positive, indicating that maternal anti-A antibodies were attached to the infant's red cells. Fluorescent light treatment was started, and serum bilirubin concentrations were monitored periodically. Bilirubin levels fluctuated from a maximum of 17.8 mg/dL to a low of 11.2 mg/dL in response to fluorescent light treatment. The infant was discharged after 4 days of fluorescent light treatment and had no further difficulties.

## Case Study 14-4

An ABO-incompatible pregnancy reported in the medical literature in which recognition and treatment of hyperbilirubinemia were delayed and kernicterus developed despite fluorescent light treatment and exchange transfusions.

A normal 6-pound male group A Rh-positive infant was delivered normally without complications to a group O Rh-positive mother and was discharged about 20 hours after delivery. A 2-week follow-up appointment was scheduled with a pediatric clinic. Nine days later the parents called the clinic because the infant appeared very jaundiced, was lethargic, and was not eating well. A return appointment was scheduled, which revealed that the infant was very jaundiced, had lost weight, and was dehydrated. Serum bilirubin was 41.5 mg/dL, which was well above the maximum "safe" level of 20 mg/dL. Despite fluorescent light treatment and exchange transfusions, the infant developed severe permanent neurologic dysfunction characteristic of kernicterus.

# CHAPTER REVIEW

## Summary

This chapter begins with a review of fertilization, conception, prenatal development, the various structures that support the pregnancy, and the structure and function of the placenta. The abnormalities affecting the amnionic fluid include too much amnionic fluid (polyhydramnios) and not enough fluid (oligohydramnios), both of which lead to problems. The various hormone-related conditions include nausea and vomiting (morning sickness), severe vomiting, and gestational diabetes, which is caused by insulin resistance related to high placental hormone levels. The condition requires treatment by a diet supplemented by insulin if necessary. The diabetes relents postpartum, but carries an increased risk of diabetes later in life.

Spontaneous abortion occurs in from 10 to 20 percent of all pregnancies. In early pregnancy the condition results from chromosome abnormalities or defective implantation of the conception. Later abortions are caused by detachment of the placenta (placental abruption) or obstructed blood flow through the umbilical cord. Cocaine is potentially hazardous to a pregnancy because it causes abruption and impairs placental blood flow.

Most ectopic pregnancies occur in the distal part of the fallopian tube. Prompt diagnosis and treatment are essential to prevent tube rupture and severe life-threatening hemorrhage. Various treatment methods are available that may allow termination of the pregnancy without sacrificing the fallopian tube.

The term *placenta previa* refers to implantation of the placenta that completely or partially covers the uterine cervix, and requires treatment by cesarean section. Twins and other multiple pregnancies have more problems than singleton pregnancies. The type of twin pregnancy (fraternal or identical) often can be determined from examination of the partition between the two amnionic sacs. Sometimes the blood vessels in the placenta of identical twins are interconnected, leading to differences in the blood supply to the twins. One twin may receive too much blood, and the other may not receive enough (twin transfusion syndrome); the condition may be extremely hazardous to both twins. The most effective treatment is a laparoscopic procedure to close the connections between the two circulations.

Gestational trophoblastic disease is an abnormal pregnancy characterized by an excessive and abnormal overgrowth of trophoblastic tissue that can be very aggressive and potentially life threatening, but can be treated effectively.

Preeclampsia and eclampsia, grouped together under the general term of *pregnancy toxemia*. result from an insufficient blood flow to the placenta that leads to the release of substances that constrict blood vessels, raise blood pressure, and cause problems related to activation of the blood-clotting mechanism. Severe preeclampsia can be hazardous to both the mother and the fetus, which may require premature delivery of the fetus and the placenta (which is the cause of the problem).

Blood group differences between mother and fetus can lead to hemolytic disease in the infant. Rh hemolytic disease is less common than in previous years because Rh-negative mothers who have given birth to Rh-positive infants are treated with Rh-immune globulin to eliminate any Rh-positive fetal cells that have entered the maternal circulation when the placenta separates from the uterus. Elimination of the fetal cells prevents later development of hemolytic disease in a subsequent pregnancy with an Rh-positive fetus. ABO hemolytic disease is a milder disease affecting group A or B infants carried by a group O mother, in which the maternal anti-A and anti-B antibodies cross the placenta and damage fetal cells. In hemolytic disease a high concentration of the hemoglobin breakdown product bilirubin resulting from the hemolysis can cause brain damage (kernicterus), but its concentration can usually be controlled by fluorescent light treatment that converts the bilirubin to a less harmful substance.

## Questions for Review

1. Why do spontaneous abortions occur? What are the consequences of prolonged retention of a dead fetus within the uterine cavity?

2. What is an ectopic pregnancy? What factors predispose to development of an ectopic pregnancy in the fallopian tube? What are the consequences of a tubal pregnancy?

3. What is the difference between a hydatidiform mole and a choriocarcinoma?

4. What is hemolytic disease of the newborn? How does it affect the infant? How does it affect the mother?

5. In infants with hemolytic disease, why does jaundice increase after delivery? Why does anemia become more severe after delivery?

6. How does the physician make a diagnosis of hemolytic disease? How is the disease treated?

7. How does ABO hemolytic disease differ from Rh hemolytic disease?

8. What structures contribute to the formation of the placenta? What are the main functions of the placenta?

9. Describe the effect of a placenta previa on the pregnancy and delivery of the infant.

10. What is the source of amnionic fluid? What factors regulate the total volume of amnionic fluid?

11. Why does a pregnancy test become positive? When does it become positive?

12. What are the possible causes and the significance of polyhydramnios? of oligohydramnios?

## Supplementary Reading

Centers for Disease Control and Prevention. 2004. Availability of revised guidelines for identifying and managing jaundice in newborns. *Journal of the American Medical Association* 292:1678.

Assess all infants before discharge from birth hospital. Measure serum bilirubin. Schedule a follow-up visit within 3 to 5 days after birth when the bilirubin level is likely to be highest. Encourage breastfeeding at least 8 to 12 times per day (to promote rapid passage of bilirubin through the bowel to avoid reuptake of excreted bilirubin from bowel contents, which can greatly reduce risk of hyperbilirubinemia). Provide parents with written and oral information about the risks associated with hyperbilirubinemia.

Dennery, P. A., Seidman, D. S., Steverson, D. K., and Stevenson, D. K. 2001. Neonatal hyperbilirubinemia. *New England Journal of Medicine* 344:581–90.

Discusses pathogenesis and treatment. A good diagram illustrating the pathways of heme breakdown and the formation of bilirubin. Newborn infants become jaundiced because the liver enzyme that conjugates bilirubin is less efficient, no bacterial flora have yet colonized the intestinal tract, which can break down excreted bilirubin into other compounds within the bowel, and intestinal peristalsis is less active, which allows the bilirubin to remain within the bowel instead of being excreted rapidly.

Heffner, L. J. 2004. Advanced maternal age: How old is too old? *New England Journal of Medicine* 351:1927–29.

Many women are having their first child at a much older age than in previous years. The number of first births in women ages 35 to 39 increased by 36 percent when compared with data 10 years previously and increased 70 percent in women ages 40 to 44. In 2002, 263 births were reported in women ages 50 to 55. Delaying conception creates problems. Fertility declines progressively after age 30, and older women have more difficulty becoming pregnant. They also have more difficulty in carrying the pregnancy to term because the frequency of spontaneous abortions rises as the woman ages, as does the incidence of chromosomal abnormalities in infants who survive to term. Older women are also more prone to develop hypertension and other pregnancy-related complications than younger women. The American Society for Reproductive Medicine is attempting to make women more aware of the risks related to delaying childbearing.

Quintero, R. A., Dickinson, J. E., Morales, W. J., et al. 2003. Stage-based treatment of twin–twin transfusion syndrome. *American Journal of Obstetrics and Gynecology* 188:1333–40.

Treatment should be based on stage of gestation and the changes resulting from the twin–twin transfusion. Endoscopic laser coagulation of artery to vein communications offers advantages over serial amniocentesis.

Senat, M. V., Deprest, J., Boulvain, M., et al. 2004. Endoscopic laser surgery versus serial amnioreduction for severe twin-to-twin transfusion syndrome. *New England Journal of Medicine* 341:136–44.

Endoscopic laser coagulation of twin-to-twin anastomoses is more effective treatment than repeated amniocentesis to prevent hydramnios in the recipient twin.

Solomon, C. G., and Seely, E. W. 2004. Preeclampsia—Searching for a cause. *New England Journal of Medicine* 350:641–42.

A discussion of current concepts based on placental vascular insufficiency leading to systemic manifestations. Accurate classification is important in order not to misinterpret chronic hypertension without proteinuria in a pregnant woman as preeclampsia.

Wilcox, A. J., Weinberg, C. R., and Baird, D. D. 1995. Timing of sexual intercourse in relation to ovulation. *New England Journal of Medicine* 333:1517–21.

In a carefully studied group of women who were planning to become pregnant, the likelihood of conception from a single intercourse increased from 8 percent 6 days before ovulation to 36 percent on the day of ovulation. There were no pregnancies from intercourse on the day after ovulation or more than 6 days before ovulation.

Williams, W. W., Ecker, J. L., Thadhani, R. I., and Rahemtulla, A. 2005. Case 38-2005: A 29-year-old pregnant woman with nephrotic syndrome and hypertension. *New England Journal of Medicine* 353:2590–600.

A discussion of the management of preeclampsia. Treatment of preeclampsia is to deliver the infant and the placenta, which is the cause of the preeclampsia. Delivery can be accomplished as early as 22 to 24 weeks' gestation; extremely premature infants have many problems and complications but early delivery may be necessary to protect the mother's health. Delaying delivery to 24 weeks is preferable if possible without undue risk to the mother.

Woods, J. R., Plessinger, M. A., and Clark, K. E. 1987. Effects of cocaine on uterine blood flow and fetal oxygenation. *Journal of the American Medical Association* 257:957–61.

Cocaine alters fetal oxygenation by reducing uterine blood flow and impairing oxygen transfer to the fetus.

## Interactive Questions

**Multiple Choice**

Select the correct answer.

1. Which of the following statements regarding a hydatidiform mole is INCORRECT?
   A. Occurs less frequently in American and Canadian women than in women living in the Far East and Southeast Asia.
   B. Incomplete removal of a mole may be followed by development of a choriocarcinoma.
   C. A woman who has had a mole evacuated by curettage (D&C) may attempt another pregnancy as soon as normal menstrual periods resume after the curettage.
   D. Some moles may exhibit aggressive behavior and invade the uterine wall.

2. A 22-year-old woman has missed her last menstrual period and her pregnancy test is positive. She has begun to experience some irregular vaginal bleeding. Which of the following conditions is the most likely cause?
   A. A spontaneous abortion
   B. Polyhydramnios
   C. Endometrial carcinoma
   D. Uterine leiomyoma

3. A 27-year-old pregnant woman is in the first trimester of her pregnancy but her uterus is much larger than it should be at this stage of her pregnancy. Which of the following conditions is the *least likely* cause?
   A. Endometriosis
   B. Hydatidiform mole
   C. A twin pregnancy
   D. Polyhydramnios

4. Which of the following statements regarding an ectopic pregnancy is INCORRECT?
   A. Often associated with a missed menstrual period
   B. Most likely to occur in women using contraceptive pills
   C. A woman who has had a previous ectopic pregnancy has a greater than normal risk of having another ectopic pregnancy
   D. Usually associated with a positive pregnancy test

5. A previously healthy woman is pregnant and a screening blood test reveals an elevated blood glucose. What does this mean?
   A. The result may be disregarded because many pregnant women may have a higher than normal blood glucose.
   B. This may be a false-positive test because her blood glucose test was probably normal before she became pregnant.
   C. She may have gestational diabetes. She needs further evaluation and possible treatment.
   D. Further evaluation can be deferred until after she has delivered her baby.

## True or False
Indicate whether the following statements are true or false by writing T or F at the end of the statement.

1. An Rh-negative infant may be born to two Rh-positive parents._____
2. A placenta previa is a placenta that blocks the exit of the fetus from the uterus._____
3. Polyhydramnios occurs when the fetus is unable to urinate into the amnionic sac._____
4. Contraceptive pills predispose to an ectopic pregnancy._____
5. The yolk sac nourishes the fetus during the early part of pregnancy before the placenta starts to function._____
6. Postmenopausal vaginal bleeding is always abnormal and requires further investigation to determine its cause._____

7. Identical twins result when sperm fertilize two separate ova, each implanting separately within the endometrium._____
8. A twin transfusion syndrome results when the blood vessels of the twins carrying blood to the placenta are interconnected._____
9. ABO hemolytic disease may occur in a group A infant of a group O mother._____
10. Preeclampsia is hazardous to both the fetus and the mother._____

## Critical Thinking

1. Maria Robles is Rh negative and plans to become pregnant, and she is concerned about the possibility of having a baby who will develop Rh hemolytic disease. What would you tell her?
2. Last year Jane Smith had an ectopic pregnancy that ruptured and caused a serious hemorrhage. She asks you why she had the ectopic pregnancy and whether she could have another ectopic pregnancy. Are there any measures that she could take to reduce her risk? What would you tell her?
3. Maryann Larson wants to defer a pregnancy until she completes her college education. She has heard that contraceptive pills are effective but doesn't understand how they function to prevent a pregnancy. She has also heard of pills that can be taken after intercourse to prevent pregnancy, but she doesn't understand how they differ from regular contraceptive pills. How would you answer her questions?

# 15 The Urinary and Male Reproductive Systems

## LEARNING OBJECTIVES

1. Describe the normal structures of the kidneys and their functions.

2. Explain the pathogenesis of glomerulonephritis, nephrosis, nephrosclerosis, and glomerulosclerosis. Describe the clinical manifestations of each of these disorders.

3. Describe the clinical manifestations and complications of urinary tract infections.

4. List the causes of renal tubular injury. Describe the manifestations of tubular injury and the treatments for each disorder.

5. Differentiate between benign prostatic hyperplasia and prostatic carcinoma. Describe clinical manifestations and methods of treatment.

6. List the three most common types of testicular cancer. Describe their manifestations, and explain the methods of treatment.

7. Name the anatomic structures of the male reproductive system. Describe their functions as they relate to the diseases affecting them.

8. Explain the mechanisms responsible for formation of urinary tract calculi. Describe the complications of stone formation. Explain the manifestations of urinary tract obstruction.

9. Differentiate the major forms of cystic disease of the kidney and their prognoses. Name the more common kinds of tumors affecting the urinary tract.

10. Describe the causes, clinical manifestations, and treatment of renal failure. Describe the principles of hemodialysis.

# Structure and Function of the Urinary System

The urinary system (Figure 15-1A) consists of

1. The kidneys that produce the urine
2. An excretory duct system (renal calyces, renal pelves, and ureters) that transports the urine
3. The bladder, where the urine is stored
4. The urethra, which conveys the urine from the bladder for excretion

## The Kidneys

The kidneys are paired, bean-shaped organs located along the back body wall below the diaphragm and adjacent to the vertebral column. Their structure is illustrated in Figure 15-1A. The region where the blood vessels enter and leave and where the ureter exits to descend to the bladder is called the *hilus of the kidney*. The expanded upper end of the ureter is the *renal pelvis* (plural, *pelves*). The pelvis divides into several large branches called the *major calyces* (singular, *calyx*), and these in turn subdivide to form the minor calyces. The renal substance is divided into an outer *cortex* and an inner *medulla*. The cone-shaped masses of renal tissue in the medulla that project into the minor calyces are called the *renal pyramids*, and

the tip of each pyramid is called the *renal papilla*. Columns of cortical tissue that extend into the medulla between the pyramids are called the *renal columns* (Figure 15-1B).

The calyces and pelves convey the urine into the ureters, which extend downward to enter the posterior wall of the bladder near its base. Each ureter enters the bladder at an angle so that, when the bladder contracts, its muscular wall compresses the ureters as they run obliquely through it, somewhat like a one-way valve. This prevents backflow of urine into the ureters during voiding (urination). The ureteral openings in the bladder are also partially covered by folds of mucosa that help prevent retrograde flow of urine.

## The Ureters

The ureters are muscular tubes that propel the urine into the bladder by wavelike contractions of their muscular walls (peristalsis). Urine is discharged into the bladder in spurts. It does not drain by gravity.

## The Bladder and Urethra

The *urinary bladder* is the distensible reservoir for urine. It is lined by transitional epithelium continuous with that which lines the remainder of the urinary tract. The opening of the urethra is located at the base of the bladder, and the ureteral openings are located

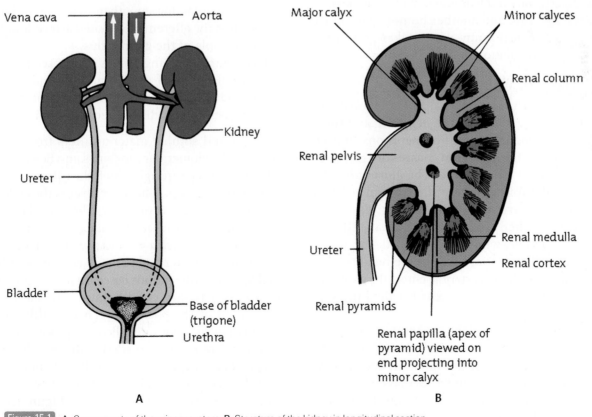

**A**

**B**

**A,** Components of the urinary system. **B,** Structure of the kidney in longitudinal section.

on either side and behind the urethral opening. The triangular area at the base of the bladder bounded by the two ureteral orifices posteriorly, and the urethral orifice anteriorly, is called the trigone of the *bladder* (*tri* = three).

# Function of the Kidneys

The kidneys are important excretory organs, functioning along with the lungs in excreting the waste products of food metabolism. Carbon dioxide and water are end-products of carbohydrate and fat metabolism. Protein metabolism produces urea, as well as various acids, which only the kidneys can excrete. The kidneys also play an important role in regulating mineral and water balance by excreting minerals and water that have been ingested in excess of the body's requirements and conserving minerals and water as required. It has been said that the internal environment of the body is determined not by what a person ingests but rather by what the kidneys retain.

The kidneys serve an endocrine function as well. Specialized cells in the kidneys elaborate a hormone called erythropoietin, which regulates red blood cell production in the bone marrow, and another humoral substance called **renin**, which takes part in the regulation of the blood pressure.

## The Nephron

The basic structural and functional unit of the kidney is the **nephron**, and there are about one million nephrons in each kidney. Each nephron consists of a glomerulus and a renal tubule. The *glomerulus* is a tuft of capillaries supplied by an *afferent glomerular arteriole*. The capillaries of the glomerulus then recombine into an *efferent glomerular arteriole*, which in turn breaks up into a network of capillaries that supplies the renal tubule. The site where the afferent arteriole enters the glomerulus and the efferent arteriole exits is called the vascular pole of the glomerulus.

The histologic structure of the glomerulus and related structures is illustrated schematically in Figure 15-2 . The expanded proximal end of the tubule is called **Bowman's capsule**. The tuft of capillaries that make up the glomerulus is pushed into Bowman's capsule much as one would push a fist into a balloon. The layer of Bowman's capsule cells, which is pushed in (invaginated), becomes closely applied to the capillaries of the glomerulus. The cells of this layer have long, footlike cytoplasmic processes and are usually called podocytes (*podos* = foot). The outer layer of Bowman's capsule is the *capsular epithelium*. The space between the two layers, into which the urine filters, is called *Bowman's space*.

The capillary tuft is held together and supported by groups of highly specialized cells embedded in a basement membranelike material. The cells are located between the capillaries and are concentrated at the vascular pole of the glomerulus. Because of their location between the capillaries, they are called **mesangial cells** (*meso* = middle + *angio* = vessel). In addition to their support function, they are contractile cells that play a role in regulating glomerular filtration by varying the caliber of the capillaries, and they also function as phagocytic cells. Also located at the vascular pole is a specialized cluster of cells called the **juxtaglomerular apparatus** (*juxta* = near to), which regulates blood flow through the glomerulus, and plays a role in regulating blood pressure by producing renin, as described in a later section. The juxtaglomerular apparatus consists of three parts:

1. The macula densa, a condensation of cells in the distal part of the renal tubule, where it is in contact with the vascular pole of the glomerulus.
2. The juxtaglomerular cells, which are specialized renin-containing smooth muscle cells located in the wall of the afferent glomerular arteriole at the vascular pole of the glomerulus.
3. A group of mesangial cells interposed between the vascular pole of the glomerulus and the macula densa (Figure 15-2B). They are continuous with the mesangial cells between the capillaries.

Water and soluble material filters from the blood through the glomerular capillaries into Bowman's space. The membrane through which the filtrate passes consists of three layers. The *inner layer* is the *endothelium* of the glomerular capillaries. The cytoplasm is very thin and is perforated by many small holes called *fenestrations* (*fenestra* = window). This layer is freely permeable to water and to many large molecules. The *middle layer* is the porous *basement membrane* that supports the capillary endothelium. The *outer layer* is composed of the *podocytes*. Their highly branched cytoplasmic processes are called foot processes, and their terminal branches are called pedicels ("little feet"). The pedicels are attached to the basement membrane, and the pedicels of one cell interdigitate with others from the same cell or adjacent cells (Figure 15-2). The narrow spaces between adjacent interdigitating pedicels

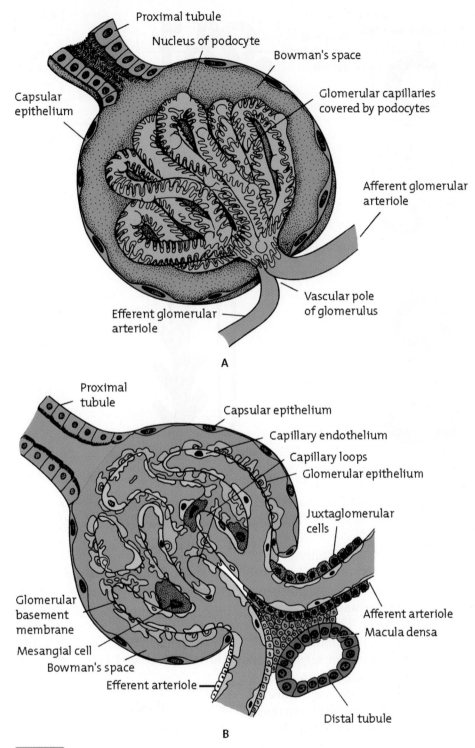

**Figure 15-2** The structure of the glomerulus and Bowman's capsule. **A,** Anterior half of Bowman's capsule removed to reveal capillary tuft covered by podocytes (schematic). **B,** Cross-section through glomerulus to reveal structure of glomerular filter and juxtaglomerular apparatus.

are called filtration slits. Each slit is covered by a thin membrane called a filtration membrane. The filtration membranes are less porous than the other layers of the glomerular filter and perform much of the filtration.

The renal tubules are long tubes that measure as much as 4 centimeters in length. The proximal end of

the tubule is invaginated by the glomerulus, and its distal end empties into a collecting tubule. The tubule is divided into three parts ( Figure 15-3 ):

1. The proximal convoluted tubule
2. The loop of Henle
3. The distal convoluted tubule

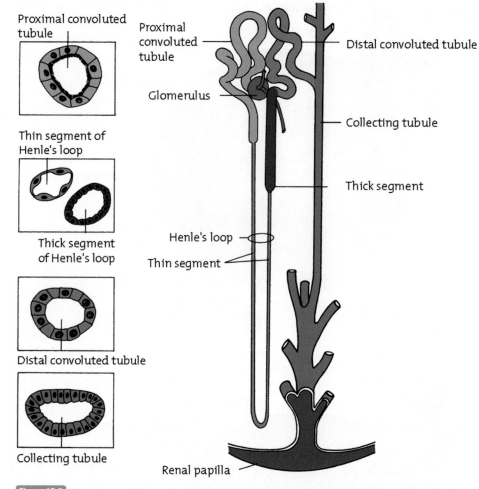

**Figure 15-3** The structure of the renal tubule, illustrating its relationship to the glomerulus and the collecting tubule. The epithelia characteristic of each part of the renal tubule and the collecting tubule are also illustrated.

The *proximal convoluted tubule* is the greatly coiled first part of the tubule. Its convolutions are located very close to the glomerulus. The *loop of Henle* is a U-shaped segment composed of descending and ascending limbs joined by a short segment. The descending limb and proximal half of the ascending limb are lined by flat epithelial cells, forming the *thin segment of Henle's loop*. The distal part of the ascending limb, called the *thick segment of Henle's loop*, is lined by tall columnar epithelium similar to that lining the distal tubule. The loop descends from the cortex into the medulla and then bends back sharply, returning to the cortex close to the vascular pole of its own glomerulus, where it becomes continuous with the distal convoluted tubule. The *distal convoluted tubule* is much shorter than the proximal tubule. It empties into a *collecting tubule*, which passes through the medulla to drain into one of the minor calyces at the apex of a renal pyramid (renal papilla).

**angiotensinogen**
(an-jee-o-ten-sin′-o-gen) A blood protein converted to angiotensin I by renin secreted by the kidneys. Part of the renin-angiotensin-aldosterone system.

**angiotensin-converting enzyme** An enzyme that converts angiotensin I to angiotensin II.

The renal tubules selectively reabsorb water, minerals, and other substances that are to be conserved and excrete unwanted materials that are eliminated. Urine is the glomerular filtrate that remains after most of the water and important constituents have been reabsorbed by the renal tubules, and other substances excreted by the renal tubules have been added.

## Renal Regulation of Blood Pressure and Blood Volume

The kidneys play a major role in regulating both the blood pressure and blood volume by secreting renin, which is released into the bloodstream from the juxtaglomerular cells in the walls of the afferent glomerular arterioles. Renin is an enzyme that interacts with a blood protein called **angiotensinogen** and splits off a short peptide fragment called angiotensin I. Then, as the blood flows through the lungs, the newly formed angiotensin I is almost immediately converted to angiotensin II by an enzyme called **angiotensin-converting enzyme** (ACE) that is present in the endothelium of the pulmonary capillaries.

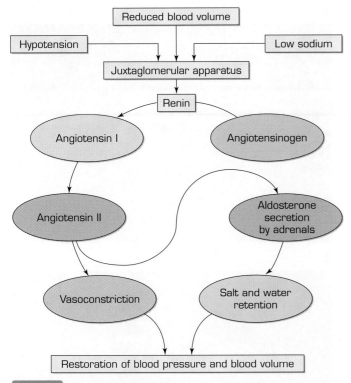

**Figure 15-4** The role of the kidneys in regulation of blood pressure and blood volume, as described in the text.

Angiotensin II is a powerful vasoconstrictor that raises the blood pressure by causing the peripheral arterioles to constrict. Angiotensin II also stimulates the adrenal cortex to secrete a steroid hormone called **aldosterone**, which increases reabsorption of sodium chloride and water by the kidneys. As a result, the blood volume is increased by the greater volume of salt and water entering the circulation, and the blood pressure rises because there is more fluid within the vascular system. Thus, renin regulates blood pressure both by controlling the degree of arteriolar vasoconstriction and by regulating the volume of fluid within the circulation. The system is self-regulating because renin secretion declines as blood pressure, volume, and sodium concentration are restored to normal (Figure 15-4).

## Requirements for Normal Renal Function

The functions of the two kidneys reflect the sum of the functions of their individual nephrons. For a nephron to function normally, the following conditions must be satisfied:

1. There must be free flow of blood through the glomerular capillaries.
2. The glomerular filter must function normally. An adequate volume of filtrate must be produced, but the filter must restrict passage of blood cells and proteins.

3. The tubules must be able to selectively reabsorb important substances from the filtrate and to excrete other constituents into the filtrate.
4. The urine formed by the nephron must be able to flow freely from the kidney into the bladder and out of the urethra.

Derangement of any of these functions results in kidney disease.

# Developmental Disturbances

The urinary system develops from several different components. The kidneys form from masses of primitive connective tissue (mesoderm) located along the back body wall of the embryo. The bladder develops as an offshoot of the lower end of the intestinal tract. The ureters, renal pelves, renal calyces (the urinary drainage system), and the renal collecting tubules derive from paired tubular structures called ureteric buds. Each bud grows upward from the developing bladder and connects with the kidney that is forming on the corresponding side. The kidneys begin their development within the pelvis. Later, as the embryo grows, the kidneys and their excretory ducts come to occupy a higher location, until eventually they ascend to reach their final positions in the upper lumbar region.

Sometimes this developmental process is disturbed, and congenital malformations result. Two of the more common developmental abnormalities are

**aldosterone**
A steroid hormone produced by the adrenal cortex that regulates the rate of sodium absorption from the renal tubules.

1. Failure of one or both kidneys to develop, which is called renal agenesis
2. Malpositions of one or both kidneys, which is often associated with fusion of the two kidneys

Renal agenesis (*a* = without + *genesis* = formation) may affect one or both kidneys. Bilateral renal agenesis is uncommon. It often accompanies other congenital malformations and is incompatible with postnatal life. In contrast, unilateral renal agenesis is a relatively common condition that has an incidence of about 1 in 1000 persons, about the same frequency as cleft palate. When one kidney is absent, the other kidney enlarges and is able to carry out the functions of the missing kidney; so the affected person is usually not inconvenienced by the abnormality. The recognition of this condition, however, is of great importance to the clinician who is treating an individual with kidney disease because one can never assume that the patient has two kidneys. Before a surgeon performs a kidney operation, diagnostic studies must always be performed first in order to ascertain that the patient has two kidneys. Such precautions are essential to prevent inadvertent removal of a solitary kidney.

Abnormalities of position and fusion of the kidneys may occur if both kidneys remain in the pelvis where they began their development or if they ascend only part way. Kidneys that fail to ascend normally are in very close approximation as they develop and may become fused. One of the more common fusion abnormalities is a union of the lower poles of the two kidneys to form a U-shaped mass of renal tissue called a horseshoe kidney.

# Glomerulonephritis

**Glomerulonephritis** is an inflammation of the glomeruli caused by an antigen–antibody reaction within the glomerular capillaries. The interaction of antigen and antibody activates complement and liberates mediators that attract polymorphonuclear leukocytes. The actual glomerular injury is caused by destructive lysosomal enzymes that are released from the leukocytes that have accumulated within the glomeruli.

**glomerulonephritis**
(glo-mär′ū-lō-nef-rī′tis)
An inflammation of the glomeruli caused by either antigen-antibody complexes trapped in the glomeruli, or by antiglomerular basement membrane antibodies.

**immune complex** An aggregate consisting of an antigen combined with a specific antibody to which complement may also be fixed, which is often associated with autoimmune diseases.

The antigen–antibody reaction within the glomeruli may take place in two ways. In most cases, the antigen and antibody interact within the circulation, forming small clumps called **immune complexes** that are deposited in the walls of the glomerular capillaries as the blood filters through the glomeruli. Glomerulonephritis that occurs in this way is called immune-complex glomerulonephritis. Less commonly, the glomerular inflammation is caused by an autoantibody directed against the basement membranes of the glomerular capillaries. This type of glomerulonephritis is called antiglomerular basement membrane (anti-GBM) glomerulonephritis. Figure 15-5 illustrates the histologic appearance of these two types of glomerulonephritis compared with the appearance of a normal glomerulus.

## Immune-Complex Glomerulonephritis

Immune-complex glomerulonephritis may develop as a complication about 2 weeks after infection by certain beta streptococci, the same type of organism that causes the familiar streptococcal sore throat. However, glomerular inflammation occurs only in a small percentage of patients with streptococcal infections. In affected subjects, the body responds to the streptococcal

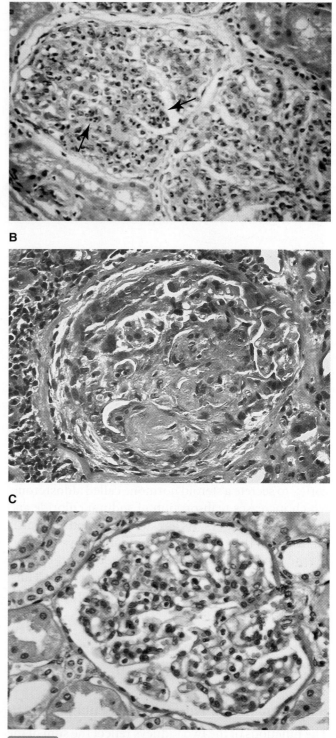

Figure 15-5 **A,** Immune-complex glomerulonephritis. Two glomeruli in the photograph contain large numbers of neutrophils (*arrows*). **B,** Anti-GBM glomerulonephritis, revealing severe glomerular injury and scarring. **C,** Normal glomerulus for comparison (original magnifications × 400).

infection by forming antistreptococcal antibodies that interact in the bloodstream with soluble antigens from the streptococci to form immune complexes. Some of the antigen–antibody complexes are small enough to pass completely through the walls of the glomerular capillaries and be excreted in the urine. Larger complexes, however, pass through the endothelium and basement membranes of the glomerular capillaries but become trapped between the filtration slits of the glomerular epithelial cells, where they induce an inflammatory reaction.

Acute glomerulonephritis may at times follow other bacterial infections or viral infections. The mechanism of glomerular injury is similar to that of poststreptococcal glomerulonephritis. Immune complexes composed of a bacterial or viral antigen and its corresponding antibody interact in the circulation and are trapped in the glomeruli, where they produce inflammation and injury by activating complement and attracting leukocytes (Figure 15-5A).

The signs and symptoms of glomerulonephritis are related to the changes within the glomeruli. Many glomeruli are completely blocked by inflammation, and thus, less blood is filtered and less urine is excreted. As urinary output is reduced, waste products are retained and accumulate in the blood. Other glomeruli, damaged by lysosomal enzymes, are no longer able to function as efficient filters. Protein and red cells leak through the damaged glomerular capillary walls and are excreted in the urine. Frequently, masses of red cells and protein accumulate within the tubules and become molded to the shape of the renal tubules before finally being excreted. These structures, which are called urinary casts, are an important indication of glomerular injury.

In most cases, glomerulonephritis subsides spontaneously and the patient recovers completely without residual kidney damage, but sometimes the inflammation is quite severe, and in some patients the glomerulonephritis never heals completely. The disease becomes chronic, progresses slowly, and eventually causes renal failure.

Immune-complex glomerulonephritis may also occur in association with autoimmune diseases in which autoantibody-containing immune complexes become trapped in renal glomeruli, as in lupus erythematosus (Chapter 4). Another relatively common type of immune-complex glomerulonephritis is associated with proliferation of mesangial cells and accumulation of immune complexes containing immunoglobulin A (IgA) within the cells.

## Anti-GBM Glomerulonephritis

Glomerulonephritis caused by autoantibodies directed against glomerular basement membranes (*anti-GBM glomerulonephritis*) is a type of autoimmune disease. It is a relatively uncommon cause of acute glomerulonephritis.

It is possible to distinguish immune-complex glomerulonephritis from anti-GBM glomerulonephritis by special studies performed on kidney tissue obtained by renal biopsy.

Case 15-1 illustrates the clinical features of glomerulonephritis that lead to renal failure and demonstrates the use of renal biopsy.

### Case Study 15-1

A 51-year-old man was admitted to the hospital because of cough, chest pain, and weight loss. Physical examination was essentially normal. The urine contained a moderate amount of protein and many red cells. Blood urea nitrogen was 87 mg/dL (normal range 10 to 20 mg/dL). Blood pH was reduced to 7.2 (normal range 7.35 to 7.45). Plasma bicarbonate was reduced to 15 meq/L (normal range 24 to 28 meq/L). A renal biopsy revealed an active glomerulonephritis (Figure 15-5B). By means of special studies, immunoglobulins and complement were identified uniformly attached to the glomerular basement membranes. The lesion was interpreted as glomerulonephritis secondary to antiglomerular basement membrane antibodies. The patient was referred to another center for dialysis and further treatment.

# Nephrotic Syndrome

The term **nephrotic syndrome** refers to a group of abnormalities characterized by an excessive loss of protein in the urine. Urinary excretion of protein is so great that the body is unable to manufacture protein fast enough to keep up with the losses and the concentration of protein in the blood plasma falls. This, in turn, causes significant edema owing to the low plasma osmotic pressure (Chapter 9). Nephrotic syndrome may be caused by a number of different types of renal diseases in which injury to the glomerulus allows proteins to leak through the damaged basement membrane. Because the albumin molecule is much smaller than the globulin molecule, a disproportionately large amount of albumin is lost in the urine. The osmotic pressure of the plasma falls to such an extent that

**nephrotic syndrome**
(nef-rä´tik sin´drōm) A generalized edema resulting from excessive protein loss in the urine, causd by various types of renal disease.

excessive amounts of fluid leak from the capillaries into the interstitial tissues and body cavities. Patients with nephrotic syndrome have marked leg edema, and fluid often collects in the abdominal cavity (called **ascites**); sometimes fluid also accumulates in the pleural cavities (called **hydrothorax**).

Nephrotic syndrome occurs most frequently in children, usually caused by a relatively minimal abnormality in the foot processes of the glomerular epithelial cells. Nephrotic syndrome caused by this type of glomerular abnormality responds to corticosteroid therapy, and most children recover completely, as illustrated by Case 15-2.

In contrast to the favorable outcome in children, nephrotic syndrome in adults is usually a manifestation of progressive, more serious renal disease, in which there are marked structural changes in the glomeruli. Some cases result from chronic progressive glomerulonephritis; others result from glomerular damage resulting from long-standing diabetes, as described later, or from a connective-tissue disease affecting the kidney, such as lupus erythematosus. Some other relatively uncommon types of kidney disease involving the glomeruli may also produce nephrotic syndrome.

**ascites**
(a-si′tēz) Accumulation of fluid in the abdominal cavity.

**hydrothorax** (hī-drō-thor′ax) Accumulation of fluid in the pleural cavity.

**nephrosclerosis** Thickening and narrowing of the afferent glomerular arterioles as a result of disease.

### Case Study 15-2

A 6-year-old boy complained of abdominal discomfort. His mother noted that his face, abdomen, scrotum, and legs were very edematous. His urine contained large amounts of protein and a few casts. His serum protein and serum albumin were both much lower than normal. Additional studies of serum proteins by electrophoresis were also consistent with nephrotic syndrome. The child was hospitalized, placed on a low-sodium diet, and treated with adrenal corticosteroid hormones. The edema gradually subsided, and the corticosteroids were gradually discontinued. He was discharged after a 2-week hospitalization.

## Arteriolar Nephrosclerosis

Arteriolar nephrosclerosis (sometimes simply called **nephrosclerosis**) is a complication of severe hypertension. Because of the extreme elevation of the systemic blood pressure, the small arterioles and arteries

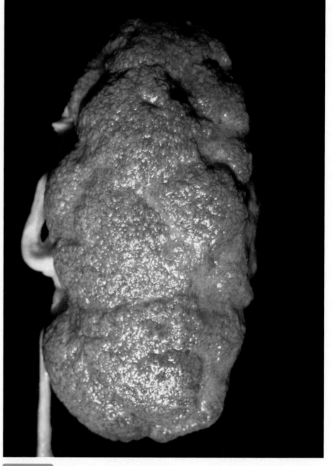

Figure 15-6   Irregular scarring of kidney as a result of nephrosclerosis.

throughout the body are called on to carry blood at a much higher pressure than normal. As a result, the blood vessels undergo severe degenerative changes characterized by thickening and narrowing of the lumens; this reduces blood flow through the narrowed arterioles. The name of the disease, which means literally "sclerosis of the arterioles of the nephrons," refers to these characteristic renal vascular changes. Glomerular filtration is reduced because the arterioles are greatly narrowed. The renal tubules, which are also supplied by the glomerular arterioles, also undergo degenerative changes. Eventually, the kidneys become shrunken and scarred as a result of reduction of their blood supply (Figure 15-6). Severe nephrosclerosis may lead to renal insufficiency, as well as causing cardiovascular system damage resulting from the severe hypertension.

## Diabetic Nephropathy

Persons with long-standing diabetes mellitus often develop progressive renal damage. The glomerular basement membranes exhibit characteristic nodular and diffuse thickening called diabetic glomerulosclerosis

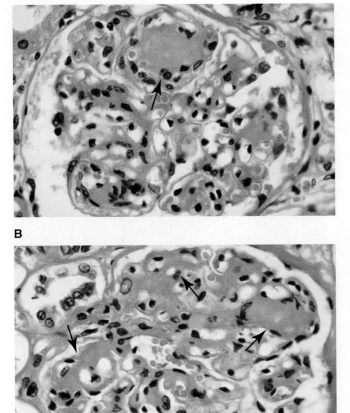

**A,** Nodular glomerulosclerosis. Nodular areas of glomerular basement membrane thickening (*arrow*) are characteristic of diabetes. **B,** Diffuse glomerulosclerosis. Diffuse glomerular basement membrane thickening (*arrows*) also occurs in diabetes, but it may also occur in other types of glomerular disease.

( Figure 15-7 ), which disturbs glomerular function. Usually there is also severe sclerosis of the glomerular arterioles, impairing the flow of blood to the glomeruli and tubules. Sometimes the general term *diabetic nephropathy* (*nephros* = kidney + *path* = disease) is used when referring to both the glomerular and the arteriolar lesions.

Clinically, the condition is characterized by progressive impairment of renal function that may eventually lead to renal failure. Protein leaks through the diseased glomeruli and is lost in the urine. In some patients, so much protein is lost that nephrotic syndrome develops. There is no specific treatment that can arrest the progression of the disease. A renal transplant may be required if the patient develops renal failure. (Diabetes mellitus and its complications are considered with pancreatic disease in Chapter 16.)

## Gout-Associated Nephropathy

Persons with gout, described in Chapter 22, have a higher than normal concentration of relatively insoluble uric acid in their blood and body fluids, which leads to periodic episodes of acute joint inflammation (gouty arthritis) caused by precipitation of uric acid as sodium urate crystals in their joints. Although the skeletal manifestations of gout are well-known, gout also frequently affects the kidneys and urinary tract. Many patients develop kidney stones, described later in this chapter. Sodium urate crystals may also precipitate from the tubular filtrate within the Henle's loop and in the collecting tubules within the renal pyramids where the tubular filtrate is very concentrated. The precipitates obstruct and damage the renal tubules, which is followed by scarring and impaired renal function, a condition called **urate nephropathy** ( Figure 15-8 ).

# Infections of the Urinary Tract

Urinary tract infections are common and may be either acute or chronic. An infection that affects only the bladder is called **cystitis** (*cystis* = bladder). If the upper urinary tract is infected, the term is **pyelonephritis** (*pyelo* = pelvis + *nephros* = kidney + *itis* = inflammation). Most infections are caused by gram-negative intestinal bacteria. These organisms often contaminate the perianal and genital areas and gain access to the urinary tract by ascending the urethra.

Free urine flow, large urine volume, and complete emptying of the bladder protect against urinary tract infections because any bacteria that enter the bladder are soon flushed out during urination instead of being retained to multiply in the bladder urine. An acid urine is an additional defense against infection because most bacteria grow poorly in an acid environment. On the other hand, several conditions predispose to urinary tract infections:

1. Any condition that impairs free drainage of urine increases the likelihood of infection because stagnation of urine favors multiplication of any bacteria that enter the urinary tract.
2. Injury to the mucosa of the urinary tract, as by a kidney stone (calculus) or foreign body, disrupts the protective epithelium, permitting bacteria to invade the deeper tissues and set up an infection.
3. Introduction of a catheter or instrument into the bladder may carry bacteria into the urinary tract when the catheter or instrument is introduced and may also injure the bladder mucosa.

**urate nephropathy** (nĕf-rop´-uh-thē) Kidney damage caused by precipitation of urate crystals within the kidney tubules of a person with gout.

**cystitis** (sis-tī´tis) Inflammation of the bladder.

**pyelonephritis** (pī´el-ō-nef-rī´tis) A bacterial infection of the kidney and renal pelvis.

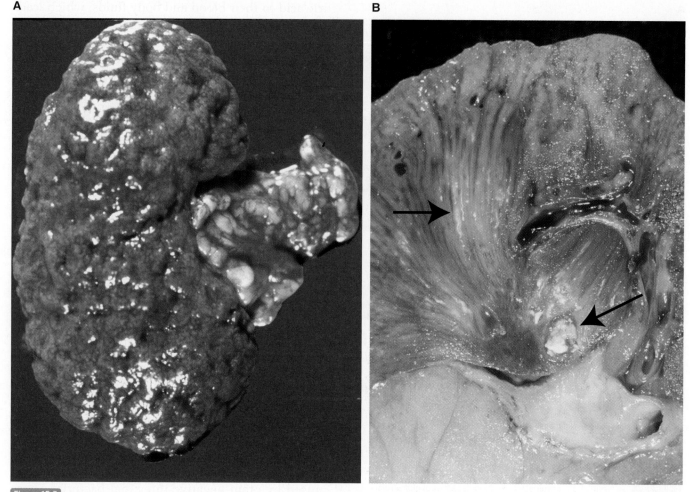

**Figure 15-8** **A,** Urate nephropathy showing multiple depressed scars involving kidney cortex caused by kidney damage resulting from tubular obstruction by urate crystals. **B,** Section of kidney revealing white urate deposits within renal pyramid (*upper arrow*) and large urate deposit near tip of pyramid (*lower arrow*).

## Cystitis

Cystitis is more common in women than in men, because the short female urethra allows infectious organisms to enter the bladder more easily. Young, sexually active women are especially predisposed because sexual intercourse promotes transfer of bacteria from the distal urethra into the bladder and may cause minor injury to the mucosa at the base of the bladder (trigone). Cystitis is also common in older men who cannot empty their bladders completely because of an enlarged prostate gland. The urine remaining in the bladder after voiding favors multiplication of bacteria and may lead to infection.

The manifestations of cystitis result from congestion and inflammation of the bladder (vesical) mucosa. The patient complains of burning pain on urination and a desire to urinate frequently. The urine contains many bacteria and leukocytes. Cystitis is not usually a serious problem and generally responds promptly to antibiotics. Sometimes, however, the infection may spread into the upper urinary tract to affect the renal pelvis and kidney.

## Pyelonephritis

Most cases of pyelonephritis are secondary to spread of infection from the bladder (*ascending pyelonephritis*), but occasionally, the organisms are carried to the kidneys through the bloodstream (*hematogenous pyelonephritis*). The symptoms of pyelonephritis are those of an acute infection, together with localized pain and tenderness over the affected kidney. Histologically, the infected portion of the kidney is infiltrated by masses of leukocytes and bacteria, and many of the renal tubules in the inflamed area are filled with leukocytes (Figure 15-9). Because cystitis and pyelonephritis are frequently associated, the patient also experiences urinary frequency and pain on urination; the urine contains many bacteria and leukocytes. Treatment is with appropriate antibiotics, together with measures directed at correcting any abnormalities in the

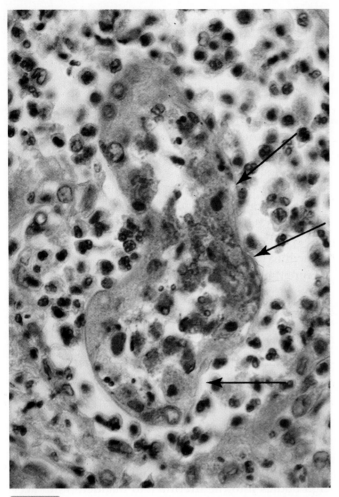

**Figure 15-9** Acute pyelonephritis. The tubule in the center of field contains masses of bacteria that extend through wall of tubule (*middle arrow*). Some tubule cells are necrotic (*upper* and *lower arrows*). Many neutrophils surround the tubules (original magnification × 400).

lower urinary tract that may impede drainage of urine and predispose to infection.

### Vesicoureteral Reflux and Infection

Normally, effective mechanisms prevent urine from flowing upward from the bladder into the ureters during urination. Sometimes, however, these mechanisms are defective, permitting urine to flow retrograde (reflux) into one or both ureters when the bladder contracts during urination. This condition is called **vesicoureteral reflux.** It predisposes to urinary tract infection by preventing complete emptying of the bladder. The urine forced into the ureters during voiding flows back into the bladder at the completion of urination; so residual urine remains in the bladder ( Figure 15-10 ). Bacteria also may be carried into the upper urinary tract by the reflux of urine; this predisposes to pyelonephritis.

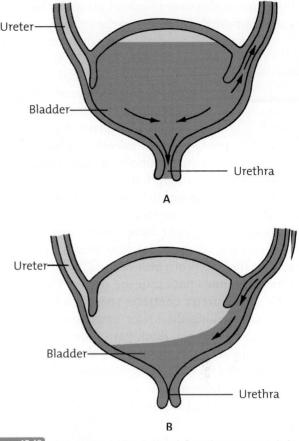

**A**

**B**

**Figure 15-10** Vesicoureteral reflux. **A,** Urine is forced up one ureter during voiding (*right side* of illustration) because of defective function of the vesicoureteral valve. **B,** Urine flows back into bladder after voiding, which prevents complete emptying of bladder and predisposes to infection.

# Calculi

Stones may form anywhere in the urinary tract. They are usually called calculi (singular, **calculus**), which is a Latin word meaning "little stone" or "pebble." Most are composed either of uric acid or of a mixture of calcium salts. Three factors predispose to stone formation: increased concentration of salts in the urine, infection of the urinary tract, and urinary tract obstruction.

A greatly increased excretion of salts in the urine causes the urine to become supersaturated, and the salts may precipitate to form calculi, especially if the urine is concentrated. For example, in the disease called gout (Chapter 22), excretion of uric acid is often greatly increased, which may cause uric acid to precipitate from the urine and form uric acid calculi. In conditions characterized by hyperfunction of the parathyroid glands, which regulate calcium metabolism (Chapter 20), excessive calcium is excreted in the urine, often with the subsequent formation of urinary tract calculi composed of calcium salts.

**vesicoureteral reflux** (ves′i-kō-ūr-ēt′er-al) Retrograde flow of urine from the bladder into the ureter during voiding.

**calculus** A stone formed within the body, as in the kidney or gallbladder.

Infection predisposes to calculi primarily by reducing the solubility of the salts in the urine. Clusters of bacteria also serve as sites where urinary salts may crystallize to form the stone.

Obstruction of the outflow of urine predisposes to stone formation by causing stagnation of urine, and urinary salts tend to precipitate. Stagnation also predisposes to infection, which further increases the likelihood of stone formation.

Most calculi are small, but occasionally they may gradually increase in size to form large branching structures that adopt the contour of the renal pelvis and calyces where they have formed. This kind of structure is called a staghorn calculus because it vaguely resembles the antlers of a male deer ( Figure 15-11 ). Smaller stones sometimes pass into the ureter. The smooth muscle of the ureter contracts spasmodically to propel the stone along the ureter, causing renal colic—paroxysms of intense flank pain radiating into the groin. Frequently, the rough edges of the stone injure the lining of the ureter, causing red blood cells to appear in the urine. Many stones can be passed through the ureter and excreted in the urine, but some become impacted in the ureter and must be removed.

In the past, stones forming in the pelvis or calyces that were too big to pass through the ureter had to be removed surgically. Now methods are available that can break up the stones into small pieces that can be excreted in the urine, avoiding an operation. This type of stone-breaking procedure is called **lithotripsy** (*litho* = stone + *tripsy* = crushing).

The usual way to fragment calculi involves positioning the recumbent patient on a specially designed table. Above the table is x-ray equipment capable of visualizing the location of the stone within the kidney. Below the table is a device to generate electrically produced shock waves capable of fragmenting the stone. When the exact location of the stone has been determined by x-ray examination, the shock-wave–generating equipment is focused very precisely on the kidney stone, and shock waves directed at the stone fragment the stone into fine particles that are excreted in the urine.

Sometimes stones form in the bladder. Usually this stone formation is secondary to the combined effect of infection and stasis of urine, which decrease the solubility of dissolved salts in the urine. Sometimes bladder calculi can be removed through the bladder by means of a cystoscope. The stones are first broken up by an instrument passed through the cystoscope into the bladder and are then flushed out.

# Foreign Bodies

It is not uncommon for people to insert various foreign bodies into the urethra and bladder either accidentally or as a means of sexual stimulation. Such objects must be removed because they may induce infection and may perforate the bladder wall. Frequently, the objects can be removed by means of a cystoscope passed into the bladder through the urethra. Sometimes, however, it is necessary to perform an operation in which the bladder is opened and the object is removed. The following two cases illustrate some of the clinical problems presented by intravesical (*intra* = within + *vesica* = bladder) foreign bodies ( Figure 15-12 ).

### Case Study 15-3

An elderly woman was admitted to the hospital emergency room complaining of lower abdominal pain and burning on urination. An x-ray of the abdomen revealed a rectal thermometer lying horizontally within her bladder. A cystoscope was inserted into the bladder, and the thermometer was manipulated into a vertical position and then extracted through the urethra.

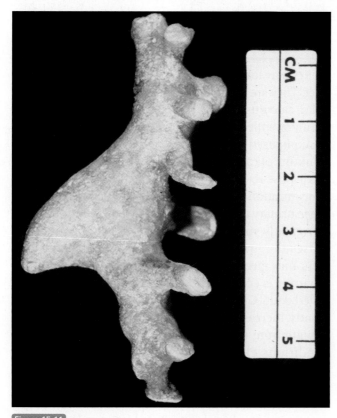

Figure 15-11  Large staghorn calculus of kidney.

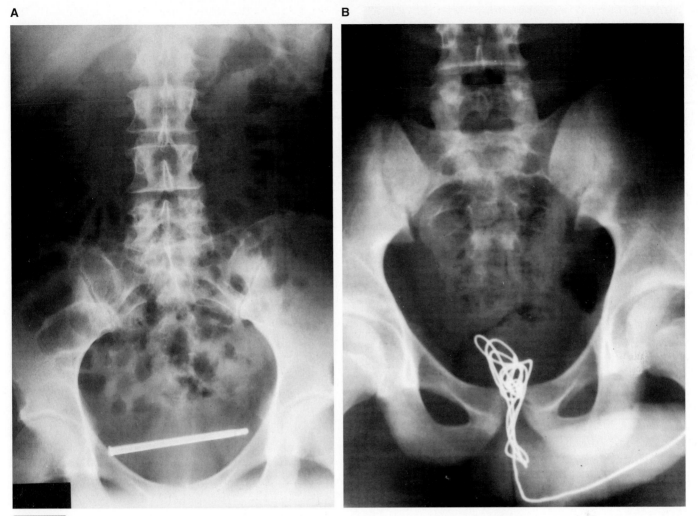

**Figure 15-12** X-ray films illustrating foreign bodies in bladder. **A,** Thermometer (Case 15-3). **B,** Electrical wire (Case 15-4).

### Case Study 15-4

A 15-year-old boy inserted a long piece of stiff electrical wire into his bladder through his penis. The wire coiled within the bladder and could not be extracted. It was necessary to open the bladder and remove the wire through the bladder. Fortunately, neither the urethra nor the bladder were damaged by the wire, and the patient made an uneventful recovery.

# Obstruction

In order for urine to be excreted normally, the urinary drainage system that transports the urine must permit free flow of urine. Obstruction or marked narrowing of the system at any point (*stricture*) causes the system proximal to the blockage to dilate progressively because of the pressure of the retained urine. Dilatation of the ureter is called **hydroureter**. Dilatation of the renal pelvis and calyces is called **hydronephrosis** (*hydro* = water + *nephros* = kidney + *osis* = condition) ( Figure 15-13 ). The distention of the calyces and pelvis in turn causes progressive atrophy of the kidney on the affected side because of the high pressure of the urine within the obstructed drainage system. Eventually, if the obstruction is not relieved, the affected kidney is reduced to a thin shell of atrophic parenchyma covering the overdistended pelvis and calyces.

Which part of the drainage system is affected by the obstruction depends on the location of the block. Obstruction to the outflow of urine from the bladder,

**hydroureter**
A dilatation of the ureter secondary to obstruction of the urinary drainage system, often associated with coexisting dilatation of the renal pelvis and calyces (*hydronephrosis*).

**hydronephrosis** (hydro-nef-rō′sis) A dilatation of the urinary drainage tract proximal to the site of an obstruction.

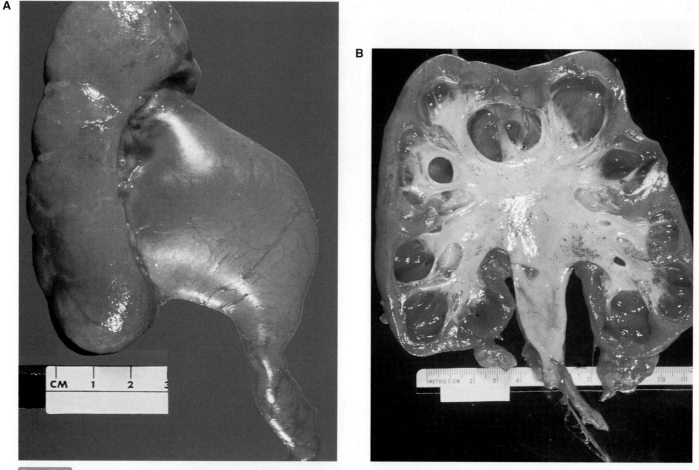

**Figure 15-13** **A,** Marked hydronephrosis and hydroureter. **B,** Bisected hydronephrotic kidney, illustrating enlargement of calyces with atrophy of the renal parenchyma caused by the increased pressure exerted by the urine within the distended renal pelvis and calyces.

as by an enlarged prostate gland or stricture in the urethra, leads to bilateral hydronephrosis and hydroureter, as well as causing overdistention of the bladder ( Figure 15-14A ). Hydronephrosis and hydroureter are unilateral if the obstruction is located low in the ureter,

as might be caused by an obstructing calculus impacted in the ureter or an obstructing tumor of the ureter ( Figure 15-14B ). If the obstruction is located at the junction of the renal pelvis and ureter, as might be caused by scarring of the ureter in this area, a unilateral

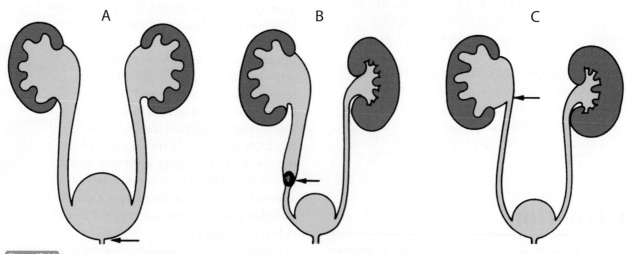

**Figure 15-14** Possible locations and results of urinary tract obstruction. The *arrows* indicate sites of obstruction. **A,** Bilateral hydronephrosis and hydroureter with distention of the bladder caused by urethral obstruction. **B,** Unilateral hydroureter and hydronephrosis caused by obstruction of the distal ureter. **C,** Unilateral hydronephrosis caused by obstruction at the ureteropelvic junction.

hydronephrosis develops, but the ureter on the affected side is of normal caliber ( Figure 15-14C ).

Stagnation of urine secondary to obstruction of the drainage system may lead to further complications. Stagnation predisposes to infection and to stone formation caused by precipitation of urinary salts. A cycle may become established in which hydronephrosis leads to infection and urinary calculi; these in turn may increase the degree of urinary tract obstruction and cause further progression of the hydronephrosis.

- Diagnosis of urinary tract obstruction is usually made by means of a pyelogram or by CT scan (procedures described in Chapter 1). These procedures demonstrate the dilatation of the urinary tract. Treatment is directed toward relieving the obstruction by appropriate means before the kidneys are irreparably damaged.

# Renal Tubular Injury

The blood supply to the renal tubules is derived from the efferent glomerular artery, and minor degrees of tubular injury are seen in many diseases affecting the renal glomeruli. Renal tubular injury in the absence of glomerular disease may be encountered in two situations: tubular necrosis as a result of impaired renal blood flow and tubular necrosis caused by toxic drugs and chemicals. Any condition associated with shock and marked drop in the blood pressure leads to impaired blood flow to the kidneys, which often causes degeneration and necrosis of renal tubules. Many drugs and chemicals that are ingested or absorbed by the body are excreted by the kidneys. Thus, they may cause direct toxic injury to the tubular epithelium.

Acute tubular necrosis causes severe impairment of renal function characterized by a marked decrease in urine output (*oliguria*) or complete suppression of urine formation (*anuria*). This condition is called *acute renal failure*. The reason why urine output is reduced is not well understood. Apparently, marked constriction of renal arterioles reduces blood flow to the kidneys and decreases glomerular filtration. Other factors also may contribute to the reduction of urine output. Many of the tubules are blocked by casts and necrotic debris. The damaged tubular epithelium also has lost its capacity for selective tubular reabsorption. After a period of several weeks, tubular function is slowly restored by regeneration of the damaged epithelium, but several months may be required before renal function returns completely to normal. During the period of acute renal failure, waste products must be removed from the blood by means of dialysis (described in a later section) until tubular function has been restored.

# Renal Cysts

## Solitary Cysts

Solitary cysts of the kidney are relatively common. They vary in diameter from a few millimeters to about 15 centimeters. They are not associated with impairment of renal function and are of no significance to the patient.

## Congenital Polycystic Kidney Disease

Although several different conditions are associated with the formation of kidney cysts, the most common and clinically most important of these conditions is congenital polycystic kidney disease. It is a very common hereditary disease transmitted as a Mendelian dominant trait that affects as many as 1 in 400 persons. Two different genes, designated *PKD1* and *PKD2* (for polycystic kidney disease), located on separate chromosomes are involved. About 85 percent of cases result from mutation of *PKD1*. In most of the others, the mutation involves *PKD2*, which is associated with later onset and slower progression of the disease. A few unfortunate persons have mutations of both *PKD1* and *PKD2*, which causes severe and rapidly progressive disease. The disease is characterized by disturbed proliferation of tubular epithelial cells, leading to the formation of cysts that become detached from the tubules. The epithelium lining the cysts secretes fluid that accumulates within the cysts and causes them to enlarge. As the cysts gradually increase in size, they cause progressive enlargement of both kidneys, where they compress and destroy adjacent renal tissue. Eventually, almost no normal kidney tissue remains, and renal failure supervenes ( Figure 15-15 ). Sometimes small numbers of cysts also form in the liver, but usually they do not disturb liver function. Some affected persons also have small cystlike outpouchings extending from the cerebral arteries at the base of the brain, which are called congenital cerebral aneurysms. Congenital aneurysms and their complications are discussed in Chapter 21.

Because renal tissue is destroyed slowly, renal insufficiency does not usually occur until the patient reaches middle age, and some patients do not experience problems until they are in their 60s. Some experience periodic urinary tract infections or episodes of bloody urine (hematuria) caused by bleeding into one of the enlarging cysts. Some patients also develop hypertension, which often accompanies renal failure.

Polycystic kidney disease can often be suspected by physical examination, which reveals the greatly enlarged kidneys. The diagnosis can be confirmed in several ways. Ultrasound examination or a CT scan of the

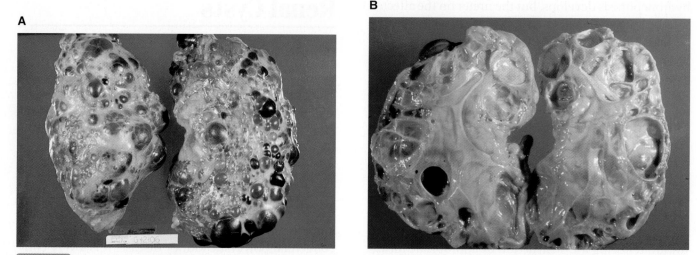

**Figure 15-15** **A,** Greatly enlarged abnormal kidneys characteristic of congenital polycystic kidney disease. **B,** Cut surfaces of diseased kidneys, illustrating multiple large cysts. No normal renal tissue remains.

abdomen reveals the large cystic kidneys. An intravenous pyelogram (IVP) reveals the distortion of the pelves and calyces caused by the cysts. There is no specific treatment. When the kidneys fail, dialysis treatments or a kidney transplant may be required.

The following case illustrates some of the characteristic features of congenital polycystic kidney disease.

### Case Study 15-5

A 67-year-old man was admitted to the hospital after having sustained a severe heart attack. Marked enlargement of both kidneys was detected on physical examination, and there was also clinical and laboratory evidence of severe renal insufficiency. The patient had seven brothers and sisters, four of whom had died between the ages of 40 and 60 of renal failure as a result of congenital polycystic kidneys. The patient eventually died in the hospital of heart failure in conjunction with chronic renal failure. The autopsy revealed greatly enlarged polycystic kidneys. There were also a few cysts within the liver.

# Tumors of the Urinary Tract

Tumors may arise from the epithelium of the renal tubules in the cortex of the kidney, from the transitional epithelium lining the urinary tract, or rarely from remnants of embryonic tissue within the kidney.

## Renal Cortical Tumors

Benign tumors called renal cortical adenomas sometimes arise within the kidney. Usually, they are small and of no clinical significance. Malignant tumors, called renal cortical carcinomas, are more common ( Figure 15-16 ). Often, the first manifestation of a cortical carcinoma is blood in the urine (hematuria) as a result of ulceration of the epithelium of the pelvis or calyces caused by the growing tumor. Often, the tumor eventually invades the renal vein and gives rise to distant metastases. The tumor can be diagnosed by means of a pyelogram (Chapter 1), which reveals the distortion of the pelvis and calyces caused by the tumor, or by means of the CT scan, which demonstrates a mass within the kidney. Treatment is by resection of the kidney (nephrectomy).

## Transitional Cell Tumors

Almost all tumors arising from the transitional epithelium of the urinary tract are malignant and are called *transitional cell carcinomas*. Most arise from bladder epithelium, are of low-grade malignancy, and carry a good prognosis. The tumors are often quite vascular, and they tend to bleed; so hematuria may be the first manifestation of the neoplasm. Bladder tumors can be visualized by means of a cystoscope inserted into the bladder through the urethra and often can be resected by means of a similar type of instrument inserted through the urethra. Sometimes it is necessary to resect part of the bladder in order to remove the tumor completely.

## Nephroblastoma (Wilms Tumor)

An unusual highly malignant tumor composed of primitive cells sometimes arises in the kidney of infants and young children. Histologically, the tumor bears

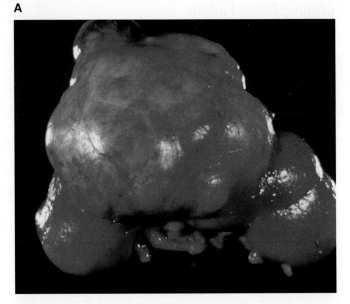

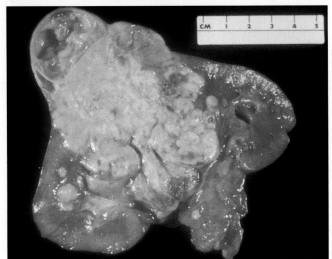

Large renal cortical carcinoma. **A,** External surface. **B,** Longitudinal section of kidney and tumor.

some resemblance to the structure of an embryonic kidney and is called a nephroblastoma or **Wilms tumor**. The neoplasm often metastasizes widely. Treatment is by nephrectomy followed by radiotherapy and anticancer chemotherapy.

# Diagnostic Evaluation of Kidney and Urinary Tract Disease

A variety of methods are used to detect disease of the kidneys and urinary tract, to evaluate the degree to which renal function is disturbed, and to define the type of disease present.

## Urinalysis

The most widely used diagnostic test is an examination of the urine, which is called a **urinalysis**. The examination is useful for detecting whether urinary tract disease is present and for detecting other systemic diseases that alter renal function. The examination includes determinations of urine pH (*acidity*) and specific gravity (a measure of urine concentration) and simple tests for glucose and protein. The urinalysis may also include tests for bile pigment, acetone, and other constituents that may appear in the urine in association with various diseases. A sample of the urine is also centrifuged, and the sediment is examined microscopically. If the urinalysis is normal, renal disease is unlikely. Alternatively, the presence of red cells and protein in the urine may indicate that damage to the glomerular filter has permitted these substances to leak into the glomerular filtrate or that bleeding is occurring somewhere in the urinary tract. Renal casts, which are collections of protein and cells molded into the shape of the kidney tubules, are an indication of glomerular disease. Leukocytes and bacteria in the urinary sediment indicate urinary tract infection.

Additional tests may be performed on the urine, as indicated by the patient's clinical condition. If a urinary tract infection is suspected, for example, the urine is cultured for pathogenic bacteria and sensitivity tests are performed if bacteria are present.

## Clearance Tests

Impairment of renal function can be recognized by measuring the concentration in the blood of various substances, such as urea and creatinine, which are waste products excreted by the kidneys. Elevated levels indicate impaired renal function, and the degree of elevation is a measure of the degree of impairment. Even before elevated levels of waste products are present in the blood, impaired renal function can be detected by means of renal function tests called **clearance tests**. Clearance tests provide a rough estimate of the degree of kidney damage, and periodic clearance tests can be used to follow the progress of renal disease. A gradual fall in the renal clearance of a substance means that renal function is declining.

Clearance tests measure the ability of the kidneys to remove various substances from the blood and excrete them in the urine. The most frequently used clearance test measures the clearance of the waste product

**Wilms tumor** A malignant renal tumor of infants and children.

**urinalysis** (ur-in-al´i-sis) A commonly performed chemical and microscopic analysis of the urine.

**clearance test** (klēr´ans) A test of renal function that measures the ability of kidneys to remove (clear) a substance from the blood and excrete it in the urine.

**creatinine**

(krē-at'in-ēn) A waste product derived from the breakdown of a compound present in muscle (phosphocreatine) that is excreted in the urine.

creatinine, which is a breakdown product of a compound present in muscle. The result, expressed as milliliters of plasma cleared of creatinine per minute, represents the glomerular filtration rate. The clearance is usually determined from a formula using the serum creatinine, along with the person's age, gender, and lean body weight. The clearance is slightly lower in women than in men, and the normal range is 85–105 mL per minute.

## Additional Techniques

Many other specialized procedures can be used to study the kidneys and urinary tract, including various x-ray examinations, ultrasound examinations, and cystoscopy. These examinations are described in Chapter 1. X-ray examination of the abdomen, for example, can identify the size and location of the kidneys and can detect radiopaque calculi in the kidneys or urinary tract. CT scans and pyelograms can detect anatomic abnormalities within the kidneys, such as cysts and tumors, and many abnormalities of the urinary drainage system, such as hydronephrosis. Other specialized procedures using radioisotopes can measure renal blood flow and renal excretory function.

Sometimes the clinician cannot make an exact diagnosis concerning the type of renal disease without resorting to biopsy of the kidney. This can be accomplished by introducing a small biopsy needle through the skin of the flank directly into the substance of the kidney. A small bit of kidney tissue is removed for histologic study. Examination of the biopsy material by the pathologist often permits an exact diagnosis as to the nature and extent of the renal disease, which serves as a guide to proper treatment.

# Renal Failure (Uremia)

Renal failure is an inability of the kidneys to adequately perform their normal regulatory and excretory functions. Function may decline rapidly, which is called *acute renal failure*, or slowly but progressively, which is called *chronic renal failure*.

## Acute Renal Failure

This condition results from necrosis of renal tubules caused by impairment of blood flow to the kidney or by the effects of toxic drugs that damage the kidney tubules, as described previously in the section dealing with renal tubular injury.

## Chronic Renal Failure

In contrast to acute renal failure, this condition is a gradual deterioration of renal function resulting from chronic renal disease. Approximately 50 to 75 percent of all cases of chronic renal failure result from diabetes and hypertension. Chronic pyelonephritis, congenital polycystic renal disease, chronic glomerulonephritis, and autoimmune diseases involving the kidney account for most of the remainder.

A normal kidney contains about one million nephrons. In chronic renal failure, renal function declines as the population of nephrons decreases, although relatively normal renal function can be maintained until the number of functioning nephrons falls below 20 to 30 percent of normal. Unfortunately, many types of chronic renal disease tend to progress because of the way the surviving nephrons respond to the declining renal function ( Figure 15-17 ). The surviving nephrons are forced to "work harder" in order to accomplish the functions previously performed by a full complement of nephrons. Each of the remaining nephrons receives a larger volume of blood to process at a higher than normal pressure. The high blood volumes and pressures damage the arterioles and glomerular capillaries, which leads to thickening of the walls of glomerular arterioles with narrowing of their lumens (arteriolosclerosis) along with glomerular capillary injury followed by scarring (glomerulosclerosis). The tubules are also damaged because the blood vessels that supply the glomeruli also supply the tubules. Consequently, a vicious cycle is created in which the reduced number of functioning nephrons indirectly damages the overworked surviving nephrons, many of which become scarred and cease to function. As more nephrons are lost, an additional burden is placed on those that still survive, which eventually causes many of them to fail. As this process continues, progressively more nephrons are lost at an increasing rate, until eventually renal function deteriorates to the point where the kidneys are no longer able to perform their regulatory and excretory functions. The patient experiences severe derangements of fluid, electrolyte, and acid–base balance. Various acids that would normally be excreted by the kidneys are retained, which disturbs the normal pH of body fluids, leading to a condition called metabolic acidosis described in Chapter 19. The failing kidneys can't produce erythropoietin to stimulate bone marrow function, and the patient becomes anemic.

Renal failure is sometimes called **uremia**. This term refers to the characteristic retention of urea in the blood when the kidneys fail. **Urea** is a normal by-product of

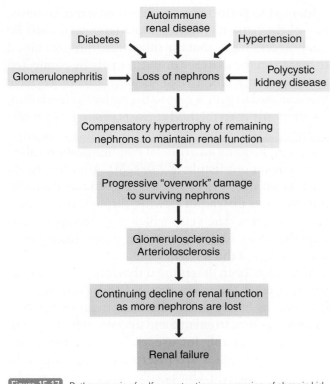

Pathogenesis of self-perpetuating progression of chronic kidney disease.

protein metabolism and is excreted in the urine. It is not a toxic compound and is only one of many substances that accumulate in the blood when the kidneys fail. The amount of urea in the blood, however, correlates with the degree of retention of other waste products and with the clinical manifestations of deteriorating renal function. Therefore, measurement of the concentration of urea in the blood (blood urea nitrogen test, or BUN) provides a rough estimate of the severity of the kidney failure. Another commonly used measure of renal functional impairment is the level of creatinine in the blood.

Symptoms of renal failure are nonspecific. They begin to appear when about 80 percent of renal function has been lost and are quite pronounced by the time renal function has fallen to 5 percent of normal. Symptoms include weakness, loss of appetite, nausea, and vomiting. Production of red cells by the bone marrow decreases, and the patient becomes moderately anemic. Waste products are not eliminated and increase to toxic levels. Excess salt and water are retained by the failing kidneys, resulting in weight gain as a result of retained fluid ("water weight"). The blood volume increases because of fluid retention, and the blood pressure also tends to rise as the intravascular volume increases. Before effective treatment was available the patient in chronic renal failure eventually lapsed into a coma, often had convulsions, and died. Now the

outlook for patients with renal failure has improved dramatically because of two effective methods of treatment:

1. Hemodialysis and peritoneal dialysis, which remove waste products from the patient's blood. Both methods are equally effective, and each has advantages and disadvantages. Every year many new patients with advanced renal disease begin dialysis. Some will continue on dialysis indefinitely. Others will rely on dialysis until a kidney becomes available for transplantation.
2. Renal transplantation, using kidneys from living related donors or recently deceased persons (cadaver donors). Transplantation is the most desirable option; however, kidneys for transplantation are in very short supply, and the average wait for a cadaver donor may be as long as 4 years.

## Hemodialysis

**Hemodialysis** substitutes for the functions of the kidneys. Waste products from the patient's blood diffuse across a semipermeable membrane into a solution (the *dialysate*) on the other side of the membrane. The rate of diffusion is determined by several factors: the concentration of the substances on the two sides of the membrane, the rate of blood flow and flow of the dialysate through the dialyzer, and the characteristics of the dialyzer membrane. Waste products, which are present in high concentrations in the patient's blood, diffuse from the blood into the dialysate because of differences in the concentration on the two sides of the membrane. Usually, the patient's blood is dialyzed by an "artificial kidney" machine. This type of hemodialysis is called extracorporeal hemodialysis (*extra* = outside + *corpus* = body) because the blood is transported outside the patient's body for dialysis in the artificial kidney and then returned by means of a system of tubes connected to the patient's circulatory system.

Hemodialysis is usually performed in an outpatient dialysis center three times per week for 3 or 4 hours during each dialysis session, but it can be performed at home with the assistance of a family member who has been given special training along with the patient. During dialysis, plastic tubes connect the patient's circulation to the dialyzer in the artificial kidney machine. One tube transmits blood to the dialyzer unit where the blood is cleansed and excess fluid is removed, and

**uremia** (ur-ē′mi-yuh) An excess of urea and other waste products in the blood, resulting from renal failure.

**urea** (ū-rē′yuh) The nitrogen waste product derived from protein metabolism and excreted in the urine.

**hemodialysis** (hēm-ō-dī-al′i-sis) A dialysis procedure by which waste products are removed from the blood of patients in chronic renal failure, usually by means of an artificial kidney machine.

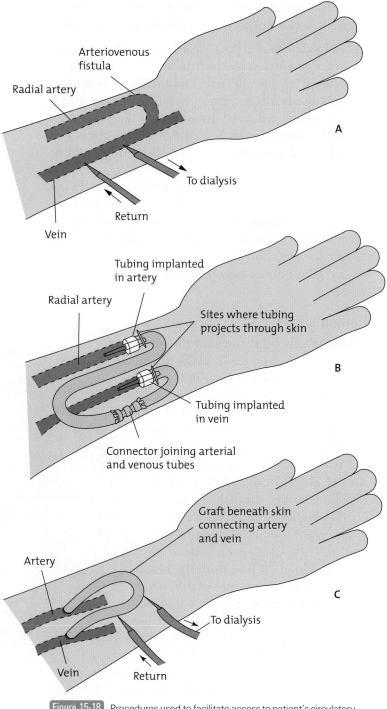

**Figure 15-18** Procedures used to facilitate access to patient's circulatory system for hemodialysis. **A,** Arteriovenous fistula created between radial artery and adjacent vein. **B,** Permanently implanted tubes in radial artery and vein project through skin and are interconnected between dialysis treatments. **C,** Graft of synthetic material or bovine artery connects patient's artery and vein.

In order to perform hemodialysis on a regular basis, one of the patient's arteries and a large vein must be easily accessible so that the tubes that transport blood to and from the dialyzer unit can easily be connected to the patient's blood vessels. Several methods have been devised to gain access to the patient's circulation. A commonly used method consists of surgically interconnecting the radial artery in the wrist and an adjacent vein, forming an artificial communication called an arteriovenous fistula ( Figure 15-18A ). After the fistula has been created, arterial blood is short-circuited directly into the vein instead of flowing through the peripheral capillaries. The vein, which now receives blood directly under high pressure, becomes much larger and develops a thick wall.

After it has been determined that long-term dialysis will be needed, the arteriovenous fistula is created several months before the first dialysis treatment so that the vein has time to enlarge and thicken. When the vein has become suitable for use, dialysis treatments are begun. Two needles are inserted through the skin directly into the vein. One needle is attached to the tube that delivers blood to the dialyzer, and the second needle is attached to the tube that returns the blood to the patient.

Less commonly, other procedures are used to gain access to the patient's circulation for dialysis. Various types of arteriovenous shunts can be created. In one procedure, two plastic tubes are permanently implanted, one in the radial artery and another in an adjacent vein. Both tubes protrude through the skin and are joined by a short connecting piece ( Figure 15-18B ). During dialysis, the connector is removed and the implanted arterial and venous tubes are attached to the tubes that convey blood to and from the dialyzer. At the completion of dialysis, the arteriovenous communication is reestablished until the next treatment. In another method, an arteriovenous fistula is created by connecting a large artery and vein in the forearm by a graft made either from synthetic material or from a specially treated segment of a cow artery (called a bovine graft). The graft is placed beneath the skin, and needles are inserted through the skin directly into the graft to connect the patient's circulation to the dialyzer ( Figure 15-18C ).

There are many types of artificial kidney machines. Many are quite compact, and portable units are available. Improvements in the design and operation of the machines are being made continually. The essential component of the artificial kidney machine is the dialyzer. Attached to it are the tubes that carry blood to and from the patient and the tubes that carry dialysate to and from the unit. There are three basic types of

the other tube conveys the blood from the dialyzer back to the patient's circulation. Before dialysis begins, the clotting time of the patient's blood is prolonged by administration of heparin to prevent the blood from clotting as it flows through the dialyzer.

dialyzers: coil dialyzers, parallel plate dialyzers, and hollow fiber dialyzers (Figure 15-19). The hollow fiber dialyzer illustrated in Figure 15-19C is quite compact and efficient, and is the most commonly used type. The dialyzer consists of a bundle of hollow synthetic fibers through which the blood passes. The dialysate circulates around the outside of the fibers in the opposite direction.

## Peritoneal Dialysis

Peritoneal dialysis uses the patient's own peritoneum as the dialyzing membrane (Figure 15-20). In order to perform peritoneal dialysis, a large plastic tube must first be inserted into the patient's abdominal (peritoneal) cavity and fixed in position by suturing it to the skin. The dialysis procedure consists of instilling several liters of dialysis fluid through the tube into the peritoneal cavity and allowing the fluid to remain within the peritoneal cavity for a variable period of time. During this time, waste products diffuse across the peritoneum from the underlying blood vessels into the dialysis fluid that fills the peritoneal cavity. Dialysis fluid is then withdrawn and fresh fluid is instilled. Peritoneal dialysis can be performed by means of an automated system in which the machine automatically fills and drains the peritoneal cavity at night while the patient is asleep. Another similar method is called *continuous ambulatory peritoneal dialysis*. In this procedure, 2 liters of fluid remain within the peritoneal cavity all the time. The patient replaces the fluid with fresh dialysis fluid four or five times a day. Patients carry out their usual activities when they are not draining and refilling their peritoneal cavities.

## Renal Transplantation

When the kidneys fail, a normal kidney sometimes can be transplanted from either a close relative or a recently deceased person (cadaver donor).

Unless the transplanted kidney comes from an identical twin whose tissues contain identical HLA antigens, the transplant will invariably contain foreign HLA antigens that the patient lacks. (The HLA system is considered in Chapter 2.) Consequently, the patient's immunologic defenses will respond to the foreign antigens and attempt to destroy (reject) the foreign kidney unless the patient's immune system is suppressed by drugs or other agents (Chapter 4).

The likelihood that a transplanted kidney will survive depends on how closely the HLA antigens match those of the patient. The more closely they resemble one another, the better the chances of survival. More than 90 percent of transplanted kidneys survive for 5 years when the transplanted kidney is obtained

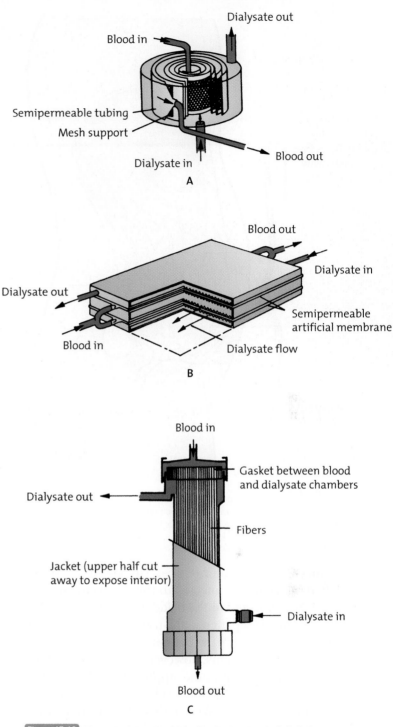

Figure 15-19 Types of dialyzers, as described in the text. **A**, Coil dialyzer. **B**, Plate dialyzer. **C**, Hollow fiber dialyzer.

from a close relative whose HLA antigens very closely resemble those of the patient. The survival rate of cadaver transplants has improved greatly in recent years and now is almost as good as transplants from living related donors.

In the transplant operation, the transplanted kidney is usually placed in the iliac area outside the peritoneal cavity. The renal artery of the transplanted kidney is

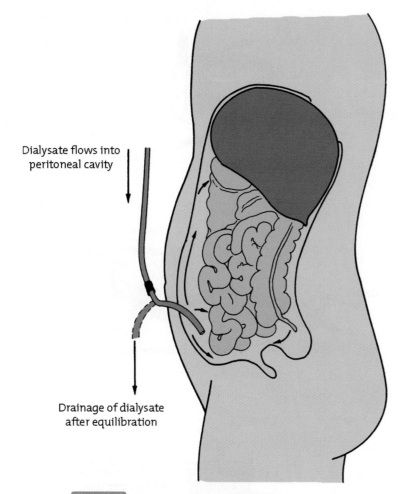

Dialysate flows into
peritoneal cavity

Drainage of dialysate
after equilibration

**Figure 15-20** Principle of peritoneal dialysis. Dialysate fills peritoneal cavity. Waste products diffuse (*arrows*) from blood vessels beneath peritoneum into dialysate. Fluid is drained after equilibration.

Based on new studies on a selected group of transplant patients, in the future it may not always be necessary to continuously suppress the immune system in order to prevent rejection of the transplant. These studies indicate that the immune system can be "taught" to recognize the foreign HLA antigens as part of the patient's own antigens. The key to success involves suppressing the patient's own immune system first before the kidney is transplanted, and then administering bone marrow from the kidney donor into the circulation of the patient. The donor blood cells become established in the patient's bone marrow because the weakened immune system is unable to reject the foreign cells. Eventually the patient ends up with two different cell populations, the patient's own cells and the transplanted cells, and the immune system "learns" that both must be the body's own cells. Consequently, continuous suppression of the immune system may no longer be required in all dialysis patients. In at least some instances the transplanted kidney cells can be manipulated so that they may no longer be recognized as foreign by the patient's immune system. In these initial studies, several patients have been followed for up to 5 years without requiring drugs to suppress the immune system,

connected to the internal iliac (hypogastric) artery. The renal vein is connected to the iliac vein, and the ureter is connected to the bladder ( **Figure 15-21** ). In the great majority of patients, the transplant is successful and "takes over" for the patient's own nonfunctional kidneys. Some patients, however, reject the transplant despite intensive immunosuppressive therapy. Most rejections occur within the first few months after transplantation. Should this occur, the patient resumes dialysis treatments until another kidney suitable for transplantation becomes available.

Although a well-functioning transplanted kidney permits the patient to lead a relatively normal life, the patient with a renal transplant may have other problems. Immunosuppressive drugs must be continued indefinitely to prevent rejection of the foreign kidney, and adverse side effects sometimes result from these drugs. The immunosuppressed patient is also more susceptible to infection because the body's immune defenses have been weakened so that the transplant can survive.

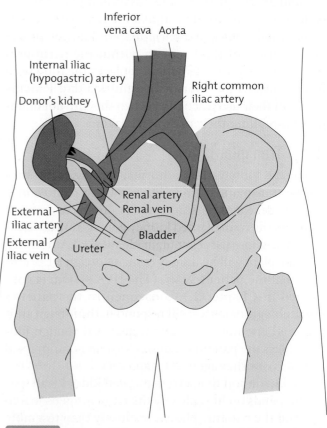

Inferior
vena cava  Aorta

Internal iliac
(hypogastric) artery

Donor's kidney

Right common
iliac artery

External
iliac artery

Renal artery
Renal vein

External
iliac vein

Ureter

Bladder

**Figure 15-21** Method of kidney transplantation in an adult. A transplanted kidney is placed in the iliac region. Artery and vein of transplant are connected to patient's iliac artery and vein, and the ureter of the transplant is connected to the bladder.

which is a remarkable accomplishment. Hopefully, continued progress at inducing the transplant cells and those of the recipient to live together in harmony will do much to simplify the life of the transplant recipient.

# Structure and Function of the Male Reproductive System

The male reproductive system is very closely associated with the urinary system that began during prenatal development when the duct system of the developing kidneys (the mesonephric ducts) was used to form the male reproductive duct system. The close association continued as the components of the male reproductive system and their physiologic functions merged with those of the urinary duct system. The prostate gland surrounds the urethra at the base of the bladder and the secretions of the prostate, seminal vesicles, and ejaculatory ducts that make up seminal fluid enter and are discharged through the urethra. Because of the close relationship, an infection or other disease affecting one system often can involve the other system as well.

The components of the male reproductive system are the *penis*, the *prostate* and certain accessory glands, the *testes*, and a duct system for transporting sperm from the testes to the urethra. The transport duct system begins as the *epididymides* (singular, *epididymis*), which are closely applied to the testes, and continues as the two *vasa deferentia* (singular, *vas deferens*). The two vasa extend upward in the spermatic cords, are joined by the seminal vesicles, and enter the prostatic urethra as the ejaculatory ducts. The urethra is divided into a long *penile urethra* and a short segment transversing the prostate gland, called the *prostatic urethra*. It is conventional to speak of the distal penile urethra as the *anterior urethra* and the prostatic urethra and adjacent proximal part of the penile urethra as the *posterior urethra*. Figure 15-22 illustrates the anatomy of the male reproductive system. A working knowledge of how these structures are interrelated is necessary in order to understand the spread of inflammatory disease in the male reproductive tract and the various complications that may result.

The prostate is a spherical gland about 5 centimeters in diameter that surrounds the urethra just below the base of the bladder ( Figure 15-23A ). It is composed of numerous branched glands arranged in two major groups intermixed with masses of smooth muscle and fibrous tissue ( Figure 15-23B ). *The inner group of glands* surrounds the urethra as it passes through the prostate,

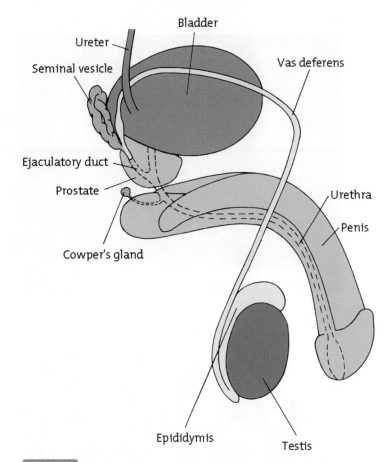

**Figure 15-22** A side view of the male reproductive system. Seminal fluid consists of sperm mixed with secretions of seminal vesicles, prostate gland, and Cowper's (bulbourethral) glands. The testes, excretory ducts, seminal vesicles, and Cowper's glands are paired structures.

and the *outer*, or *main group of glands*, makes up the bulk of prostatic glandular tissue ( Figure 15-23C ). The prostate secretes a thin alkaline fluid containing a high concentration of an enzyme secreted by prostatic epithelial cells. The prostatic secretions are discharged into the urethra during ejaculation through very fine ducts that open near the orifices of the ejaculatory ducts. Secretions mix with sperm and the secretions of the seminal vesicles to form the *seminal fluid*.

The two testes (also called testicles), which originally developed within the abdomen, occupy separate compartments within the scrotum. In the fetus, the testes descend through the inguinal canals into the scrotum, bringing their blood vessels, nerves, and excretory ducts with them as the spermatic cords and usually have completed their descent about 1 month before birth. To guide descent of the testes, a band of fibrous tissue called a **gubernaculum** (a Latin word meaning "rudder" or "guide") extends from the inferior surface of each testis through the inguinal canal into the scrotum

**gubernaculum**
(goo′-ber-nak′-ū-lum)
A band of fibrous tissue extending from the fetal testis into the scrotum that promotes descent of the testis.

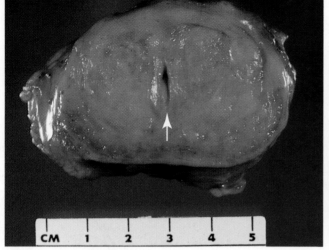

A

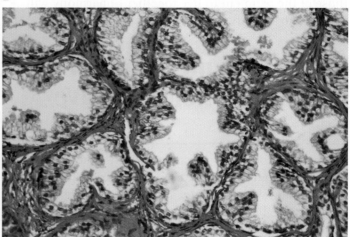

B

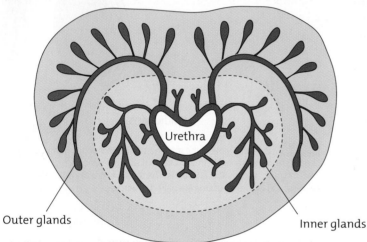

C

Outer glands

Urethra

Inner glands

**Figure 15-23** Normal prostate. **A,** Cross-section of prostate that surrounds urethra (*arrow*). **B,** Histologic appearance of glandular and fibromuscular tissue (original magnification × 100). **C,** Diagrammatic cross-section indicating arrangement of inner and outer groups of glands.

where it attaches. As the gubernaculum shortens, it guides each testis into the scrotum, where a fibrous remnant of the gubernaculum remains to anchor each testis within its scrotal compartment. Normally a broad band of connective tissue attaches each testis within the scrotum, which allows the testis some mobility, but the broad attachment prevents rotation of the testis on its axis, which would also twist the spermatic cord and obstruct the blood vessels supplying the testis.

As the testes descend, fingerlike projections of peritoneum called *vaginal processes* project from the peritoneal cavity into the scrotal compartments, and the testes descend into the scrotum posterior to the vaginal processes. After the testes have completed their descent, the proximal parts of the vaginal processes fuse, which obliterates the communications between the peritoneal cavity and the scrotum, but the distal part of each vaginal process persists as a small peritoneum-lined sac called the *tunica vaginalis*, which surrounds

the anterior half of each testis ( Figure 15-24 ). If the proximal part of a vaginal process does not fuse normally, the vaginal process remains as a communication between the peritoneal cavity and the scrotum, which may allow a loop of intestine to extend into the scrotum. This condition is called a *congenital inguinal hernia*. (Hernias are considered in Chapter 17.)

The testes, which are activated by gonadotropic hormones at puberty, have two major functions: production of sperm by sperm-producing cells called *germ cells*, which occurs within the testicular tubules, and production of the male hormone testosterone, which occurs in clusters of cells located between the tubules called *interstitial cells* or *Leydig cells*. The two types of cells have different temperature requirements. The testosterone-producing cells function at normal body temperature, as do most other cells. The sperm-producing germ cells require a temperature that is several degrees lower than body temperature, and the

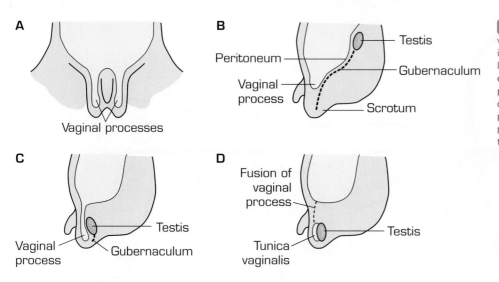

A

Vaginal processes

B

Peritoneum
Vaginal process
Testis
Gubernaculum
Scrotum

C

Vaginal process
Testis
Gubernaculum

D

Fusion of vaginal process
Tunica vaginalis
Testis

**Figure 15-24** Descent of testes. **A**, Anterior view illustrating vaginal processes extending into scrotum. **B**, Lateral view prior to testicular descent, illustrating the gubernaculum extending from the testis into the scrotum posterior to the vaginal process. **C**, Testis descends into scrotum posterior to vaginal process. **D**, Proximal part of the vaginal process obliterated; distal part persists as tunica vaginalis.

scrotum contains muscles that automatically raise or lower the testes, bringing the testes closer to the body if the scrotal temperature is too low, or relaxing to move the testes away from the body if the scrotal temperature is too high. Maintaining a lower than normal scrotal temperature is very important because an elevated scrotal temperature impairs sperm production (spermatogenesis). Moreover, sperm-producing cells are damaged and eventually destroyed if the testes do not descend normally into the scrotum and are continually subjected to the higher intra-abdominal temperature.

# Gonorrhea and Nongonococcal Urethritis

*Gonorrhea* is a relatively common disease. The gonococcus, spread by sexual contact, initially causes an acute inflammation of the anterior urethra. However, the inflammation may spread into the posterior urethra, prostate, seminal vesicles, and epididymides. The gonococcus may also cause an acute inflammation of the rectal mucosa. Occasionally, healing of the gonorrheal inflammation in the posterior urethra may be associated with considerable scarring, leading to narrowing of the urethra and thus to urinary tract obstruction. Inflammatory obstruction of the vasa deferentia may block sperm transport and lead to sterility. *Nongonococcal urethritis*, caused by chlamydia, causes an acute urethritis and clinically is very similar to gonorrhea. (Sexually transmitted diseases are considered in Chapter 6.)

# Prostatitis

*Acute prostatitis* develops when an acute inflammation of the bladder or urethra spreads into the prostate. It may follow a gonococcal infection of the posterior

urethra. *Chronic prostatitis* is a mild chronic inflammation of the prostate that is quite common and causes few symptoms.

# Benign Prostatic Hyperplasia

Moderate enlargement of the prostate gland is relatively common in older men and usually involves the inner group of glands surrounding the urethra (Figure 15-25). The hyperplasia results from stimulation of the gland by a potent male sex hormone called *dihydrotestosterone*, which is formed in the prostate from testosterone by a prostatic enzyme. Prostatic enlargement is significant only if it obstructs the bladder neck, leading to incomplete emptying of the bladder, or causes complete urinary tract obstruction. An enlarged obstructing prostate causes difficulty in urinating and

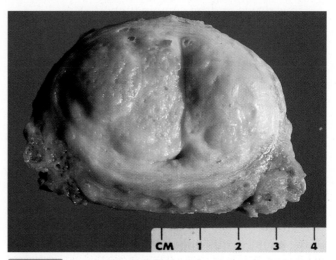

CM    1    2    3    4

**Figure 15-25** Cross-section of prostate showing nodules of hyperplastic tissue compressing urethra.

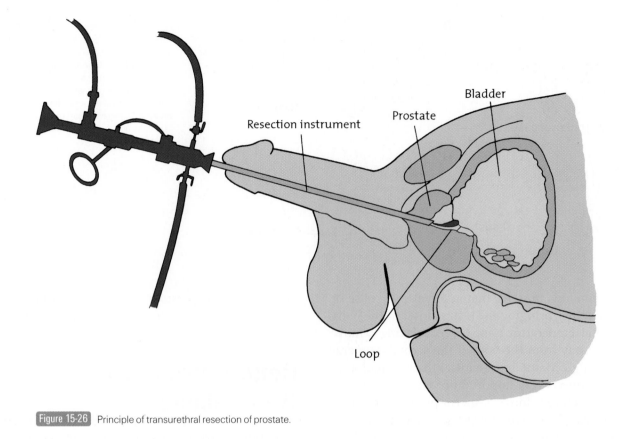

**Figure 15-26** Principle of transurethral resection of prostate.

may lead to various other complications caused by urinary retention and stagnation of urine in the bladder, such as cystitis, pyelonephritis, hydronephrosis, and stone formation.

There are many ways to treat benign prostatic hyperplasia. These depend on various factors, such as the size of the gland, the severity of the urinary symptoms, the patient's age and health, and of course the patient's preference. Treatment options include

1. Oral medications to shrink the prostate using various drugs or drug combinations.
2. Various outpatient procedures that destroy excess prostate tissue and reduce the size of the gland by using laser, microwave, or radio wave treatment, or by means of heat coagulation or freezing.
3. Surgical resection of obstructing prostatic tissue.

An obstructing prostate that prevents complete emptying of the bladder can be treated surgically. It is a very effective treatment and remains the "gold standard" against which all other treatments are compared, but it is an invasive procedure and is used less frequently than in previous years. The procedure relieves the urinary obstruction by "reaming out" the enlarged part of the gland that is encroaching on the urethra and blocking outflow of urine. This is usually accomplished by a procedure called a transurethral resection of the prostate (usually simply called TUR or TURP). A hollow tubular instrument is inserted through the penis into the urethra, and the site of the obstruction is visualized. Then, by means of a snarelike cutting instrument, pieces of the enlarged prostate are shaved off and removed ( Figure 15-26 ). This procedure enlarges the urethral opening so that the patient can void normally. The resected tissue is examined histologically by the pathologist to establish the diagnosis of benign prostatic hyperplasia and exclude prostatic carcinoma as a cause of the obstruction ( Figure 15-27 ). The lining of the urethra covering the enlarged prostate is removed along with the obstructing part of the gland, but the epithelial lining soon regenerates and the continuity of the urethral lining is restored.

Two different types of oral medications are used to treat benign prostatic hyperplasia. One type blocks transmission of the nerve impulses that cause contraction of the prostate and bladder neck smooth muscle cells, which relaxes the muscle cells so that they do not compress the urethra, which makes it easier to urinate. The second type inhibits the prostatic enzyme that converts testosterone to dihydrotestosterone. As a result, the prostate is no longer stimulated by dihydrotestosterone, and it decreases in size. The use of both drugs given together is more effective than either drug given separately. Whichever method of treatment is

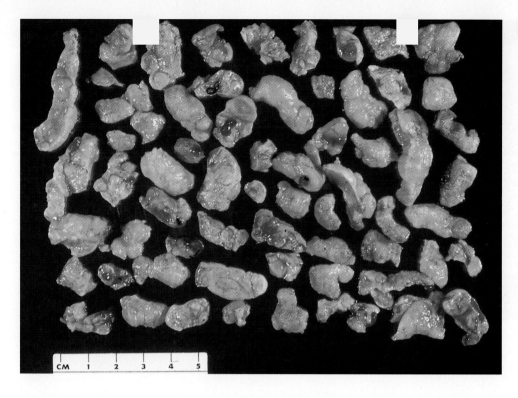

Figure 15-27 Appearance of tissue removed by transurethral resection.

used, however, the patient must continue taking the oral medications in order to maintain their beneficial effects.

# Carcinoma of the Prostate

*Carcinoma of the prostate* is the most common carcinoma in men, affecting primarily older men whose average age at the time of diagnosis is 68 years. The tumor usually originates in the outer group of prostatic glands, in contrast to benign prostatic hyperplasia, which involves the inner group of glands surrounding the urethra. The diagnosis of prostatic carcinoma is being made about 10 years earlier than in previous years, which is related to the use of prostate-specific antigen (PSA) as a screening test to detect prostate carcinoma. PSA is secreted by prostatic epithelial cells, and elevated levels appear in the blood of many patients with prostate cancer. The test is not specific for prostate carcinoma, however, because some patients with benign prostatic hyperplasia and other types of benign prostatic disease also may have higher than normal PSA levels. The diagnosis of prostatic carcinoma is established by needle biopsy of the prostate in which a needle is inserted into a suspected abnormal area in the prostate through the rectum or perineum. Often ultrasound examination is used to locate dense areas in the prostate, which assists in selecting the site for biopsy.

Patients in the early stages of prostate carcinoma may be completely free of symptoms, and the tumors are identified only by routine rectal examination as an area of irregularity or nodularity on the posterior surface of the prostate when palpated through the rectum by the examiner's finger. In other patients, the first manifestations may appear when the growing tumor partially obstructs the bladder neck, causing the same type of symptoms as in patients with benign prostatic hyperplasia. The tumor may eventually infiltrate the tissues surrounding the prostate and metastasize to the bones of the spine and pelvis.

Treatment depends on the degree of differentiation of the tumor, the age of the patient, and how far the tumor has spread at the time of diagnosis. A well-differentiated localized tumor in an elderly man may progress slowly and may not produce symptoms for as long as 10 years. Many patients in whom prostatic carcinoma is diagnosed fall into this group, and may elect to be followed by their physician without any treatment unless the tumor appears to be progressing as determined by a progressive rise of PSA and other indications that the tumor is enlarging. However, it may be many years before this occurs and the need for treatment may not even arise during the patient's lifetime. Depending on the patient's age and expected longevity, an elderly man may be more likely to die of some other disease before a well-differentiated tumor has progressed to the stage where more active treatment of the tumor would be required.

A small, localized prostatic carcinoma can be treated by removing the entire prostate and surrounding tissues.

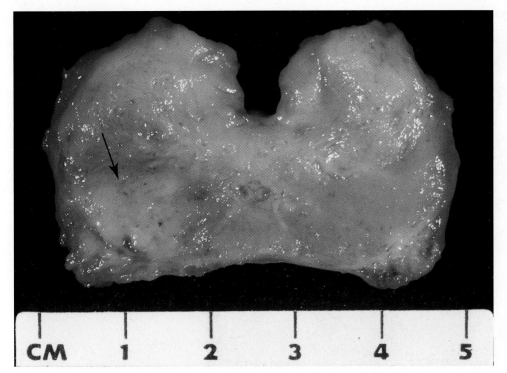

Figure 15-28 A cross-section of resected prostate illustrating a small carcinoma arising from outer prostate glands (*arrow*).

This procedure is called a radical prostatectomy ( Figure 15-28 ). Although this operation may eradicate the tumor, it usually also disrupts the nerve supply to the penis, which leads to permanent inability to achieve an erection of the penis (**impotence**). In other cases, the tumor is treated by irradiation rather than surgery. Radical prostatectomy alone or combined with radiation therapy appears to improve survival in many patients. There is considerable controversy, however, about the effectiveness of radical surgery or radiation therapy in older men with localized well-differentiated carcinoma of the prostate. Many physicians believe that treatment does not improve survival in this group of patients, that the treatment causes more disability and complications than the tumor, and that a slowly growing prostatic carcinoma in an older man is best left alone. In contrast, a less well-differentiated tumor in a younger man requires more aggressive treatment.

**impotence**
Inability of the male to achieve an erection.

When a prostatic carcinoma has advanced to the stage when it has spread beyond the prostate and has metastasized, it is often possible to induce regression of the tumor by altering the level of male sex hormones in the body. Most prostatic carcinomas are dependent on the male sex hormone for their continued growth. Therefore, many advanced prostatic tumors can be treated effectively either by surgical removal of the testes, eliminating the source of the male sex hormone, or by drugs that suppress output of pituitary gonadotropic hormone, thereby inhibiting testicular testosterone secretion. Either method of treatment usually causes regression of the tumor.

# Cryptorchidism

Sometimes the testis does not descend normally into the scrotum, a condition called either *cryptorchidism* (*crypto* = hidden + *orchis* = testis) or *cryptorchism*. Usually an undescended testis is located within the abdominal cavity, but it sometimes may be within the inguinal canal. In some newborn infants one or both testes may not have descended into the scrotum, but testicular descent often will occur normally within about 6 months after birth. If the testes are not in the scrotum by the time the infant is 1 year old, the cryptorchid testis should be surgically brought into the scrotum because progressive damage to sperm-producing germ cells begins as early as 6 months after birth, and the longer the testis is retained within the abdomen, the more marked the germ cell damage. In contrast, the testosterone-producing interstitial cells are unaffected and will function normally at puberty when stimulated by gonadotropic hormones even though sperm production is no longer possible because the germ cells have been destroyed ( Figure 15-29 ). An undescended testis also increases the long-term risk of testicular carcinoma, which is about 20 times more frequent in persons with an undescended testis than in the general population.

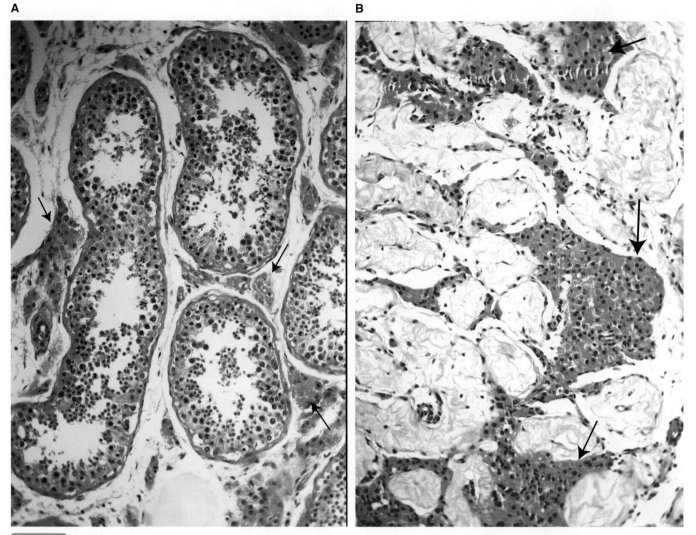

**Figure 15-29** Photographs comparing normal scrotal testis with intra-abdominal testis. **A,** Normal testis showing active spermatogenesis within testicular tubules. The clusters of cells between the tubules are interstitial cells (*arrows*). **B,** Intra-abdominal testis showing marked atrophy and fibrosis of testicular tubules. The large cluster of cells between the tubules are interstitial cells that function normally at body temperature. They appear quite prominent because of the marked tubular atrophy (original magnification × 160).

# Testicular Torsion

If the fibrous tissue derived from the gubernaculum that attaches the testis to the scrotum is a relatively long and narrow band rather than a short broad attachment, the testis may undergo a rotary twist on its axis, which also twists the spermatic cord and interrupts the blood supply to the testis ( Figure 15-30A ). The thin-walled veins in the cord are compressed first, which impedes return of venous blood from the testis, but flow through the arteries continues for a time, leading to marked engorgement of the testis with blood, which is soon followed by complete hemorrhagic necrosis of the testis, called a hemorrhagic infarction ( Figure 15-30B ). This condition is more likely to occur in young persons between ages 10 to 25 years, but may occur at any age and may even occur in the fetus during prenatal descent of the testis, as illustrated in Case 15-6.

A testicular torsion is characterized by an acute onset of severe testicular pain associated with swelling of the involved testis and is an acute surgical emergency. If the torsion can be untwisted and the testis is properly anchored in the scrotum within a few hours after onset of the torsion, the testis probably can be salvaged, but the longer the delay, the less likely the possibility that the testis will survive. Because the abnormal mobility of the testis within the scrotum that caused the torsion is likely to be present in the other testis as well, usually the other testis is surgically anchored in the scrotum so that it cannot undergo torsion.

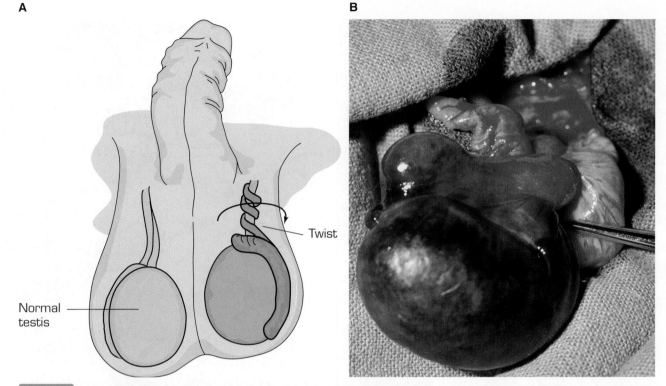

**Figure 15-30** Causes and effect of testicular torsion. **A,** Rotary twist also twists spermatic cord, interrupting blood supply to testis. Normally the epididymis is located along the posterior surface of the testis, but the torsion has rotated the testis and also rotated the epididymis anteriorly. **B,** Hemorrhagic infarction of testis caused by torsion.

In the figure, the labels read: "Normal testis" and "Twist".

## Case Study 15-6

A 6-pound 10-ounce male infant was delivered at term to a 27-year-old mother after an uneventful labor and delivery. The infant appeared normal at birth except for a markedly enlarged and discolored right half of the scrotum. The scrotum was incised revealing a necrotic testis adherent to the scrotal skin. Histologic examination revealed complete infarction of the testicle with associated inflammation and fibrous tissue proliferation in response to the testicular necrosis.

# Scrotal Abnormalities

## Hydrocele

**hydrocele**
(hī′-drō-cēl) An accumulation of excess fluid within the tunica vaginalis of the testis.

Normally the sac-like tunica vaginalis contains only a very small amount of fluid ( Figure 15-31A ), but sometimes a much larger amount of fluid accumulates in the sac, which is called a **hydrocele** (*hydro* = water + *cele* = swelling). This is not a serious condition, and no treatment is required unless the hydrocele causes marked scrotal swelling and is uncomfortable ( Figure 15-31B ). The fluid can be aspirated as a temporary solution, but the fluid usually accumulates again. The long-term solution is surgical excision of the sac. When the physician examines a patient with a hydrocele, he or she usually also performs a careful examination of the testis and scrotum, which may be supplemented by an ultrasound examination in order to exclude the possibility of a testicular tumor or some other condition associated with the hydrocele.

## Varicocele

The term *varicocele* (*varix* = dilated vein + *cele* = swelling) refers to varicose veins that develop within the spermatic cord veins that drain blood from the testis, caused by failure of the vein valves to function properly ( Figure 15-31C ). This is the same reason that varicose veins form in other locations, as described in Chapter 10. Normally functioning valves in the spermatic cord veins promote venous blood flow away from the testes and prevent backflow, but poorly functioning valves allow blood to pool in the veins, which become markedly dilated. Generally, a varicocele does not cause symptoms. Occasionally, however, a varicocele may reduce fertility by impairing spermatogenesis,

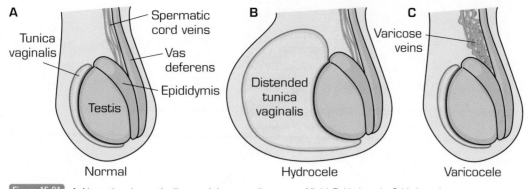

**Figure 15-31** **A,** Normal tunica vaginalis containing a small amount of fluid. **B,** Hydrocele. **C,** Varicocele.

a result of the higher scrotal temperature caused by warm venous blood pooling in the varicose scrotal veins. A varicocele can be treated surgically if it causes scrotal discomfort or impairs fertility. Otherwise no treatment is required.

# Erectile Dysfunction

## Physiology of Penile Erection

The penis consists primarily of three cavernous bodies, which are cylinders of extremely vascular erectile tissue. The two laterally placed corpora cavernosa are surrounded by dense fibrous tissue capsules; the midline corpus spongiosum surrounds the penile urethra. Each cylinder is composed of a spongy meshwork of endothelium-lined blood sinuses supported by trabeculae (partitions) composed of connective tissue and smooth muscle. The blood sinuses of the erectile tissue are supplied by arteries and drained by veins. Normally the arteries are constricted so that very little blood flows into the cavernous bodies and the vascular sinuses are collapsed. During sexual excitement, however, parasympathetic nerve impulses arising from the sacral part of the spinal cord release the neurotransmitter nitric oxide, which causes relaxation of the smooth muscle in the walls of the penile arteries and in the trabeculae between the sinuses. As a result, the penile arteries dilate, and the sinuses in the cavernous bodies expand. Blood pours under high pressure into the blood sinuses within the cavernous bodies. The greatly increased arterial blood flow and rising pressure within the blood sinuses compress the draining veins, which retards outflow of blood from the penis and contributes to the engorgement of the blood sinuses. The penis rapidly becomes rigid and erect ( Figure 15-32 ).

Erectile dysfunction is an inability to achieve and maintain a penile erection of sufficient rigidity to penetrate the vagina and maintain the erection during sexual intercourse. This is a relatively common problem that increases in frequency with advancing age. Penile erection is a complex process. First, sexual desire is required to initiate the physiologic events that increase blood flow to the penis. Second, the arteries supplying the cavernous bodies must dilate enough to deliver a large volume of blood to the penis. Third, the pressure of the blood within the cavernous bodies must be sufficiently high to compress the draining veins. Blood must flow into the penis faster than it drains out, or an erection cannot be maintained.

# Causes of Erectile Dysfunction

To achieve and sustain a penile erection, the sensory, motor, and autonomic nerve supply to the penis must be normal, and the blood vessels supplying the penis must be able to deliver an adequate volume of blood to the penis. Various factors may disturb these physiologic processes. These include

1. A low testosterone level, which inhibits sexual desire and arousal.
2. Damage to the nerves supplying the penis resulting from radical prostate surgery or neurologic diseases.
3. Impaired blood supply to the penis, resulting from arteriosclerosis of the blood vessels that deliver blood to the penis, as may occur in persons with systemic arteriosclerosis or long-standing, poorly controlled diabetes.
4. Some drugs used to treat hypertension that target the autonomic nervous system, which also affect the autonomic nerves supplying the penis.
5. Stress, emotional factors, and many chronic illnesses, which may impair the person's quality of life and also adversely affect sexual performance.

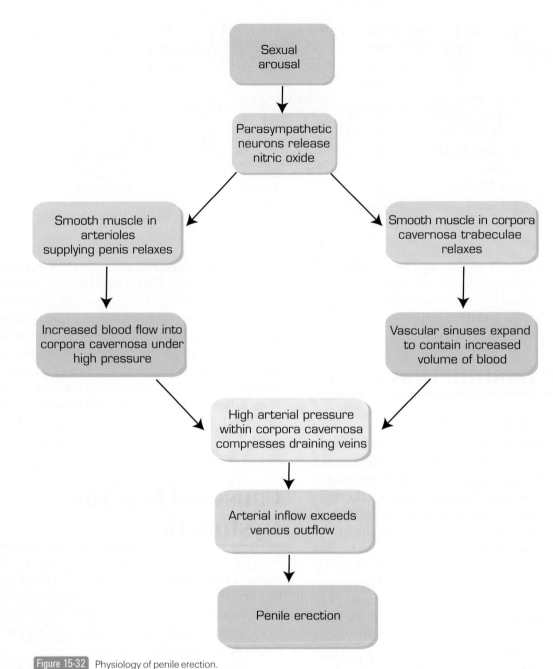

Figure 15-32  Physiology of penile erection.

**phosphodiesterase**
(fahs-foh-di-ester'-ase)
An enzyme that breaks down cyclic guanosine monophosphate (cGMP). A drug that inhibits phosphodiesterase inhibits cGMP breakdown, which prolongs its action, thereby facilitating penile erection in men with erectile dysfunction.

## Treatment

Many different medical and surgical procedures can be used to treat erectile dysfunction, depending on the cause of the dysfunction and the individual's preference. One well-known treatment involves the use of drugs that inhibit an enzyme called **phosphodiesterase** in order to promote increased blood flow to the penis. The best known of these drugs is sildenafil, better known by its trade name Viagra. The sequence of events involved in penile erection and the role of phosphodiesterase inhibitor drugs are as follows:

1. Sexual arousal stimulates parasympathetic neurons supplying the penis to release the neurotransmitter nitric oxide.

2. Nitric oxide diffuses into smooth muscle cells where it promotes the formation of a compound called cyclic guanosine monophosphate (cGMP), which in turn causes relaxation of the smooth muscle cells in the penile arteries and in the trabeculae within the corpora cavernosa. Blood under pressure fills the cavernous bodies, causing the penis to become rigid and erect.

3. Although cGMP is formed continuously as long as parasympathetic nerve impulses continue to release nitric oxide, the duration of action of the cGMP molecules is relatively brief because cGMP is broken down by a phosphodiesterase enzyme.

4. Phosphodiesterase inhibitor drugs such as sildenafil inhibit the enzyme, thereby prolonging the vasodilator effect of cGMP, which helps sustain the erection.

# Carcinoma of the Testis

Testicular tumors are uncommon and usually develop in young men. Most arise from the germinal epithelium of the testicular tubules and are malignant. There are several different types. The type with the most favorable prognosis is called a **seminoma**. (This term is another exception to standard terminology. It means literally a tumor of semen-producing epithelium. In this case, the term refers to a malignant neoplasm, not a benign tumor.) Another type of testicular tumor is a malignant teratoma, which is composed of many different types of malignant tissues, as described in Chapter 8. Some other testicular tumors resemble placental trophoblastic tissue. One tumor of this type is called an **embryonal carcinoma**. Another is called a choriocarcinoma, which is the same kind of tumor that arises from trophoblastic tissue in the uterus, as described in Chapter 14. Testicular cancers are treated by extensive surgical resection of the testicle, the spermatic cord, and sometimes the regional lymph nodes as well. In some cases, radiation and anticancer chemotherapy also are used.

# Carcinoma of the Penis

Carcinoma of the penis is uncommon; it is almost never encountered in a circumcised male (Figure 15-33). It was considered that the secretions that accumulate

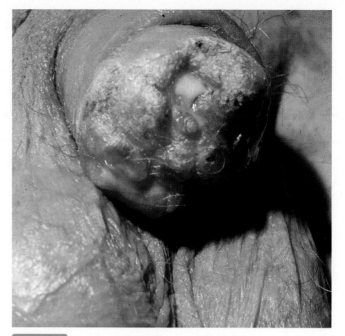

**Figure 15-33** Large carcinoma of penis involving foreskin.

under the foreskin of the penis are carcinogenic, and this accumulation is prevented by circumcision. However, carcinogenic strains of the papillomavirus, the same virus that causes cervical dysplasia and carcinoma in women, can be transmitted by sexual intercourse, and probably is responsible for penile carcinoma in uncircumcised men. Probably the papillomavirus grows well beneath an intact foreskin but does not thrive if the foreskin has been removed. Treatment usually consists of partial or complete resection of the penis.

**seminoma**
(sem-in-ō′ma)
One type of malignant tumor of testis.

**embryonal carcinoma**
A malignant testicular tumor in which the malignant cells have features resembling rapidly growing trophoblastic tissue.

# CHAPTER REVIEW

## Summary

Our kidneys perform many important functions for us. The glomeruli filter our blood and the tubules process the filtrate, reclaiming the desirable components and excreting the waste products. The kidneys help regulate our blood pressure and blood volume (via the renin–angiotensin–aldosterone system) and maintain a normal hemoglobin concentration in our bloodstream

(by producing erythropoietin as needed to stimulate red blood cell production in the bone marrow).

An inflammation of the glomeruli is called glomerulonephritis. Immune-complex glomerulonephritis usually follows a beta-streptococcal infection, in which circulating streptococcal antigens combine with anti-streptococcal antibodies in the bloodstream to form immune complexes that are trapped in the glomeruli and incite an inflammation. Antiglomerular basement membrane (anti-GBM) glomerulonephritis is an autoimmune disease in which the inflammation is caused by autoantibodies combining with glomerular antigens.

Nephrotic syndrome results from glomerular injury in which leakage of blood proteins (primarily albumin) from the glomerular filtrate exceeds the body's capacity to replenish the protein. The blood osmotic pressure falls, allowing escape of excess fluid from the circulation that is responsible for the edema and ascites characteristic of the condition. In children the condition results from a temporary minimal change in the glomeruli with return of renal function to normal, but in adults it is a manifestation of more severe permanent glomerular damage that has a less favorable prognosis.

Hypertension damages the glomerular arterioles (arteriolar nephrosclerosis), which is followed by secondary degenerative changes in the glomeruli and tubules. Long-duration poorly controlled diabetes causes characteristic diffuse and nodular glomerulosclerosis called diabetic nephropathy, which may lead to renal failure. Gout, which is a metabolic disease often associated with arthritis and characterized by a high blood uric acid, can also damage the kidney as well as the joints. Uric acid (as sodium urate) is not very soluble in body fluids and may precipitate in Henle's loop and collecting tubules, causing progressive renal damage. The condition is called gout nephropathy.

Urinary tract infections are common especially in young sexually active women, and are usually caused by gram-negative bacteria. Infection localized to the bladder is called cystitis, and causes pain and burning on urination. Impaired drainage of urine, as may occur in an older man with an enlarged prostate who cannot empty his bladder completely, predisposes to bladder infection; as does injury to the bladder mucosa, or insertion of catheters or other instruments into the bladder. Usually bladder infections respond promptly to antibiotics.

Extension of a bladder infection into the kidney is called pyelonephritis and is a more serious condition which may damage the kidneys. Vesicourethral reflux refers to bladder urine entering the ureter during voiding, which predisposes to bladder infection because the urine forced into the ureter during voiding flows back into the bladder after voiding, which prevents complete emptying of the bladder.

Kidney stones (calculi) may form in the urinary tract. Three factors predispose: infection, stasis of urine, or an excessively high concentration of calcium salts or sodium urate (uric acid) in the urine. A calculus blocking the urinary drainage system may cause pain (renal colic) and may lead to distention of the urinary tract proximal to the obstruction (hydronephrosis–hydroureter). Several methods are available to deal with urinary tract calculi. Foreign bodies inserted into the urinary tract may injure the bladder and predispose to infection.

The renal tubules may be damaged either by toxic chemicals that damage the tubules as the toxin-containing tubular filtrate flows through the renal tubules, or as a result of impaired blood supply to the kidney caused by a fall in systemic blood pressure. Urine output falls precipitously, but usually tubular function returns slowly to normal. Renal dialysis may be required until renal function returns.

Occasionally a single fluid-filled cyst forms in the kidney that does not disturb renal function. However, polycystic kidney disease, a Mendelian dominant genetic disease, is a serious problem characterized by formation of multiple progressively enlarging cysts that gradually destroy the function of the kidneys as the cysts enlarge; manifestations of renal failure usually do not arise until middle age.

Several different types of tumors arise in the urinary tract in both children and adults, each having different manifestations and prognosis. Many different diagnostic tests are available to evaluate renal function. End-stage renal disease is treated by dialysis and by renal transplantation. Recent advances in transplantation methods appear promising and may reduce the need for immunosuppressive therapy to prevent rejection of the transplant.

The normal structure and function of the male reproductive system are described. The testes along with the kidneys develop posterior to the peritoneal cavity and the gubernacula direct the testes into the scrotum. Descent is not completed until relatively late in prenatal development. The germ cells will form the sperm and the interstitial cells will form testosterone after puberty. Germ cells require lower scrotal temperature and are damaged if a lower temperature is not maintained, but interstitial cells can function normally at body temperature.

Urethral infections may be caused by the gonococcus or by *Chlamydia* and respond to appropriate treatment. Acute prostatitis results from spread of an infection from the bladder or urethra. Chronic prostatitis is a mild inflammation that causes few symptoms. Benign prostatic hyperplasia is a common problem in older men and may impair complete emptying of the bladder, which predisposes to bladder infection, calculi, and hydronephrosis. Transurethral resection of the obstructing prostate tissue (TUR) is effective but other more conservative methods of treatment are becoming popular.

Carcinoma of the prostate is the most common malignant tumor in men, which is usually a slowly growing well-differentiated tumor in elderly men that can be treated conservatively, but may be less well differentiated and more aggressive in younger men. The prostatic specific antigen test (PSA) can be used to screen for asymptomatic carcinoma, followed by transrectal biopsy to confirm the diagnosis. Treatment recommendations are based on the age of the patient and the differentiation of the tumor, which can vary from limited treatment to radical prostatectomy or radiation therapy. Radical prostatectomy is an extensive procedure with significant complications, and may not be appropriate for elderly men with well-differentiated slowly growing tumors. PSA is often used to monitor response to treatment.

Cryptorchidism refers to a testis that has not descended into the scrotum and leads to loss of germ cells that require a lower temperature for spermatogenesis, but interstitial cells can function normally at body temperature. An undescended testis is sterile, and carries a relatively high risk of malignancy. Testicular torsion shuts off blood flow to the testis, which causes hemorrhagic infarction of the involved testis. Early recognition and prompt treatment may salvage the testis. A hydrocele is an accumulation of excess fluid in the Tunica vaginalis. Varicose veins in the spermatic cord draining the testis are called varicoceles and usually do not require treatment. Malignant tumors of the testis are relatively uncommon, occur in younger men, and respond to aggressive treatment. Many of the tumors produce products (alpha fetoprotein and human chorionic gonadotropin) that can be used to aid diagnosis and monitor response to treatment. Carcinoma of the penis, which rarely occurs in circumcised men, is caused by a carcinogenic papillomavirus and requires surgical treatment.

Erectile dysfunction refers to inability to maintain a penile erection of sufficient rigidity to engage in sexual intercourse. The problem is usually related to vascular disease that impairs blood flow to the penis, and may respond to drugs that promote improved blood flow.

## Questions for Review

1. What is the difference between glomerulonephritis and pyelonephritis? What is the relationship between glomerulonephritis and beta-streptococcal infection? What factors predispose to urinary tract infection?

2. What is the difference between nephrotic syndrome and nephrosclerosis? Why does edema develop in a patient with nephrosis?

3. What are the common causes of urinary tract obstruction? What are its effects on the kidneys and the lower urinary tract?

4. What conditions lead to renal tubular necrosis? What are its clinical manifestations?

5. What is uremia? What are its manifestations? How is it treated? What is the role of urea in producing the clinical manifestations of uremia?

6. What methods does the clinician use to establish a diagnosis of renal disease?

7. What is congenital polycystic kidney disease? What are its clinical manifestations? What is its pattern of inheritance? How is it treated?

8. What is the difference between acute and chronic renal failure?

9. What is the difference between hemodialysis and peritoneal dialysis?

10. Why does a kidney transplant from a donor who is a close relative usually have a greater likelihood of survival than does a cadaver transplant?

11. How does diabetes affect the kidneys? What are the clinical manifestations? How does gout affect the kidneys?

12. What are the components of the male reproductive system?

13. What is benign prostatic hyperplasia? What are its clinical manifestations? How is it treated?

14. What is the effect of castration on prostatic carcinoma?

15. What factors predispose to the development of carcinoma of the penis? How may the disease be prevented?

16. What is cryptorchidism? What are the clinical manifestations? How is the condition treated? Why should it be treated?

17. What is a testicular torsion? What are its manifestations and complications? How is the condition treated?

18. A young man has an undescended testis within the abdomen. How does this affect testicular function? What complications may result from this condition?

## Supplementary Reading

Chertow, G. M. 2004. A 43-year-old woman with chronic renal insufficiency. *Journal of the American Medical Association* 291:1252–59.

A case discussion dealing with the problems and solutions in a patient with chronic renal disease based on the pathophysiology of chronic renal failure.

Feldman, D. R., Bosl, G. J., Sheinfeld, J., and Motzer, R. J. 2008. Medical treatment of advanced testicular cancer. *Journal of the American Medical Association* 299:672–84.

Testicular carcinoma is a young man's disease and is the most common type of cancer diagnosed between the ages of 15 to 35 years. Classification and treatment of advanced testicular tumors are described in which tumors were classified based on histologic features, sites of metastases, and degree of elevation of serum tumor markers. New more aggressive treatment has improved the cure rate from 25 percent in the 1970s to nearly 80 percent now, but was associated with significant toxic effects. Impaired fertility also occurred in patients who had a retroperitoneal lymph node dissection to supplement resection of the testis and chemotherapy. Disruption of the sympathetic retroperitoneal nerves concerned with emission and ejaculation was responsible for the infertility.

Johansson, J. E., Andren, O., Andersson S. O., et al. 2004. Natural history of early, localized prostate cancer. *Journal of the American Medical Association* 291:2713–19.

Two hundred ninety-one older men with early prostate carcinoma (diagnosed before the use of PSA testing) were followed without initial treatment for 21 years. During the first 15 years the cancers progressed slowly but behaved more aggressively in the patients followed beyond 15 years, possibly related to dedifferentiation of the original tumor. Radical prostatectomy reduced cancer-related mortality by 50 percent, but many of the patients died of other conditions; so there was no change in overall mortality.

McVay, K. T. 2007. Erectile dysfunction. *New England Journal of Medicine* 357:2472–81.

A discussion of the pathophysiology of erectile dysfunction. Treatments are described.

Meyer, T. W., and Hostetter, T. H. 2007. Uremia. *New England Journal of Medicine* 357:1316–25.

Current concepts and discussion of the pathophysiology of chronic renal failure.

Mulley, A. G. 1986. Shock-wave lithotripsy: Assessing a slam-bang technology. *New England Journal of Medicine* 314:845–47.

Lithotripsy is a well-engineered, highly selective application of brute force. Applications in fracturing gallstones are also described.

Morgentaler, A. 2004. A 66-year-old man with sexual dysfunction. *Journal of the American Medical Association* 291:2994–3003.

An excellent summary of the pathophysiology of erectile dysfunction together with the applications and limitations of various methods of treatment.

Pettersson, A., Richiardi, L., Nordenskjold, A., et al. 2007. Age at surgery for undescended testis and risk of testicular cancer. *New England Journal of Medicine* 356:1835–41.

Cryptorchidism is associated with impaired fertility and is a risk factor for testicular cancer. From 5 to 10 percent of all men with testicular carcinoma have a history of cryptorchidism. Testes undescended at birth may descend spontaneously within the first few months after birth but are unlikely to descend spontaneously thereafter. Germ cell development rapidly deteriorates in an undescended testis. Surgical correction (orchiopexy) positions and fixes the testis in the scrotum, and is performed on infants as young as 6 months, both to preserve germ cell function and to reduce the risk of later development of testicular cancer. This study of 17,000 men surgically treated for cryptorchidism considered the age at which the procedures were performed. Treatment for undescended testis prior to puberty decreases the risk of testicular carcinoma but is less effective when performed after puberty.

Rhoden, E. L., and Morgentaler, A. 2004. Risks of testosterone-replacement therapy and recommendations for monitoring. *New England Journal of Medicine* 350:482–92.

Testosterone replacement therapy is used to treat men with low testosterone levels and it improves libido, bone density, muscle mass, and red cell production but also has some undesirable effects. Testosterone stimulates prostate growth and enlargement. Because many older men harbor small asymptomatic prostate carcinomas, the testosterone may also stimulate tumor growth as well. The administered testosterone also exerts a negative feedback effect on pituitary gonadotropin output (Chapter 20), which inhibits sperm production and impairs fertility. Some men also may experience breast tenderness and breast enlargement, possibly because some of the testosterone is converted to estrogen within the body. Men over 40 years of age should be evaluated to exclude occult prostate carcinoma before beginning treatment, and the level of prostate specific antigen (PSA) should be monitored periodically to ensure that an undetected occult prostate carcinoma is not being activated by the testosterone treatment.

Rubin, H. R., Fink, N. E., Plantinga, L. C., et al. 2004. Patient ratings of dialysis care with peritoneal dialysis vs hemodialysis. *Journal of the American Medical Association* 291:697–703.

New patients beginning dialysis must choose between hemodialysis and peritoneal dialysis. Although not all patients requiring dialysis are suitable candidates for peritoneal dialysis, those who chose peritoneal dialysis were more likely to be working full time or part time and were more satisfied with their care than were hemodialysis patients.

Stanford, J. L., Feng, Z., and Hamilton, A. S., et al. 2000. Urinary and sexual function after radical prostatectomy for clinically localized prostate cancer: The prostate cancer outcomes study. *Journal of the American Medical Association* 283:354–60.

In a large group of patients 8.4 percent were incontinent, and 59.9 percent were impotent at 18 or more months after surgery. Despite the level of incontinence and sexual dysfunction, 75.5 percent of the men were satisfied with their treatment.

Starzl, T. E. 2008. Immunosuppressive therapy and tolerance of organ allografts (Editorial). *New England Journal of Medicine* 358:407–10.

The author reviews three landmark articles in the same issue of the January 24, 2008, journal in which combined kidney and bone marrow stem cells induced formation of two cell populations that "tricked" the immune system into recognizing the antigens of both cell populations as normal antigens for the patients. The immune system did not respond and immunosuppression was not required to maintain the transplants. Details of the other cases reported are also provided.

Stevens, L. A., Coresh, J., Greene, T, and Levey, A. S. 2006. Assessing kidney function—measured and estimated glomerular filtration rate. *New England Journal of Medicine* 354:2743–83.

Clearance calculated from serum and urine creatinine values overestimate the glomerular filtration rate because of tubular secretion of creatinine. The Cockcroft–Gault formula provides a reasonably good estimate. A reduction of GFR to less that 60 ml per minute (related to body surface area) defines chronic kidney disease.

Walsh, P., DeWeese, T. L., and Eisenberger, M. A. 2007. Localized prostate carcinoma. *New England Journal of Medicine* 357:2696–2705.

Patients with small well-differentiated tumors can be managed by observation without immediate treatment. Available evidence suggests that with careful monitoring every 6 months and biopsies at regular intervals, deferring treatment until there are signs of progression is unlikely to affect the likelihood of cure. The alternative options of surgery and radiation therapy along with its potential benefits and side effects should also be presented, and the patient can choose how he wants to proceed.

Wilson, P. D. 2004. Polycystic kidney disease. *New England Journal of Medicine* 350:151–64.

A review of pathogenesis, genes involved, and clinical manifestations. Affected patients may have other problems, including an increased risk of aortic aneurysms and heart valve defects, cysts in the liver, pancreas, and intestines, and congenital cerebral aneurysms.

## Interactive Activities

### Matching 1

Match the items in the left column with the characteristic or property in the right column

**Disease**

1. Polycystic kidney disease
2. Gout
3. Pyelonephritis
4. Post-streptococcal glomerulonephritis
5. Diabetes

**Characteristics or Manifestations**

A. Kidney infection
B. Mendelian dominant trait
C. Nodular and diffuse glomerular basement membrane thickening
D. Urate crystals plug tubules
E. Antigen–antibody immune complexes trapped in glomeruli

### Matching 2

Match the disease or condition in the left column with its characteristic features in the right column.

1. Cryptorchidism
2. Hydrocele
3. Varicocele
4. Testicular torsion
5. Prostate hyperplasia

A. Dilated spermatic cord veins
B. Twisted spermatic cord
C. Overgrowth of prostatic tissue
D. Undescended testis
E. Excess fluid in tunica vaginalis

## Fill in the Blanks

1. The infectious agents that are the two main causes of acute urethritis acquired by sexual contact are _____ and _____. These infections are treated by _____.

2. Varicose veins of the spermatic cord are called a _____ and excess fluid in the processus vaginalis is called a _____.

3. Prostatic epithelial cells secrete a protein called _____, which also can be detected in the bloodstream. Higher than normal levels are detected in the bloodstream of men with a disease called _____.

4. Testicular carcinomas are uncommon tumors. Many of these tumors produce a hormone called _____ and a protein antigen called _____.

5. A testicular malignant tumor that is composed of many different types of immature tissues is called a/an _____.

6. Carcinoma of the penis is an uncommon tumor that almost never occurs in circumcised men. The agent responsible for the carcinoma is a/an _____.

7. The fibrous cord that guides the testis into the scrotum is called the _____.

8. Failure of the proximal end of the tunica vaginalis to close after the testis has entered the scrotum may be complicated by a condition called a/an _____.

## True or False

Indicate whether the following statements are true or false by writing T or F at the end of the statement.

1. Most prostate carcinomas arise from the inner group of prostatic glands surrounding the prostatic urethra.____

2. Prostate-specific antigen is secreted by prostatic epithelial cells.____

3. Most prostate carcinomas are very poorly differentiated, grow rapidly, and have a very poor prognosis.____

## Critical Thinking

1. Mary Smith's 7-year-old son was seen by a physician because of swelling of his legs and abdomen, and his urinalysis contained a large amount of protein. His condition has been diagnosed as nephrotic syndrome. Mary wants to know why the kidney disease caused her child's legs and abdomen to swell, and what the expected outcome of the disease will be (prognosis). What would you tell her?

2. Peter Jones is a middle-aged man with gout who has periodic episodes of gouty arthritis. He has heard that gout may damage his kidneys and he wants to know whether this is true. If it is, he wants to know why, and whether he can reduce his risk of kidney damage. What would you tell him?

3. Sally Smith experienced an episode of burning on urination and urinary frequency. A health-care practitioner performed a urinalysis and told her that she had many bacteria and white blood cells in her urine and told her that she had a urinary tract infection. She recovered promptly after receiving an antibiotic. Sally wants to know why she developed the infection, and what factors predispose to developing a urinary tract infection. What would you tell her?

4. John Smith's grandfather is 78 years old. During a routine medical exam a prostatic specific antigen (PSA) test was performed and reported as elevated. A needle biopsy of the prostate was reported as a well-differentiated carcinoma of the prostate. He asks you for your opinion on treatment methods and what he should do. What would you tell him?

5. Your classmate Martin Jones has an undescended left testis that has never caused any problems, but he has heard that the testis should be removed. He questions whether this is really necessary and what he should do. What would you tell him?

6. Arnold Anderson has heard that carcinoma of the penis is caused by a virus and wonders whether this is true. If so, he wants to know how the virus is transmitted and how he can protect himself. What would you tell him?

# The Liver, Biliary System, and Pancreas

## LEARNING OBJECTIVES

1. Describe the normal structure of the liver, and explain the functions of the liver as they relate to the major diseases of the liver.

2. List the major causes of liver injury, and describe their effects on hepatic function.

3. Compare the three major types of viral hepatitis in terms of their pathogenesis, incubation period, incidence of complications, and frequency of carriers. Explain the diagnostic tests used to identify each type of viral infection, and describe methods of prevention.

4. Explain the adverse effects of excess alcohol intake on liver structure and function.

5. Explain how gallstones are formed, and describe their causes and effects.

6. Compare the three major causes of jaundice.

7. Describe the pathogenesis and treatment of acute pancreatitis.

8. Describe the pathogenesis, manifestations, complications, and prognosis of pancreatic cystic fibrosis.

9. Differentiate between the two principal types of diabetes mellitus with respect to pathogenesis, incidence, manifestations, complications, and treatment.

10. Understand pregnancy-associated diabetes and its pathogenesis and prognosis. How is it treated?

# Structure and Function of the Liver

The liver is the largest organ in the body. It has a roughly triangular shape and is located beneath the diaphragm in the upper abdomen ( Figure 16-1 ). It is a complex organ with many functions. These are concerned mainly with the following:

1. Metabolism of ingested carbohydrates, protein, and fat delivered through the portal circulation
2. Synthesis of various substances, including plasma proteins and proteins taking part in blood clotting
3. Storage of vitamin B$_{12}$ and other materials
4. Detoxification and excretion of various substances

The liver has a double blood supply. About three-quarters of the blood flow is provided by the *portal vein*, which drains the spleen and gastrointestinal tract. Portal blood is rich in nutrients absorbed from the intestines but low in oxygen content. The rest of the blood, which comes from the *hepatic artery*, has a high oxygen content but is low in nutrients. Blood flowing from the hepatic artery and the portal vein mixes as the blood flows through the liver and is eventually collected into the right and left hepatic veins, which drain into the inferior vena cava.

The liver cells are arranged in the form of long, wide plates interconnected at various angles to form a lattice. The hepatic sinusoids occupy the spaces between the plates ( Figure 16-2A ).

Branches of the hepatic artery, portal vein, bile ducts, and lymphatic vessels travel together within the liver and are called the **portal tracts** ( Figure 16-2B ). The terminal branches of both the hepatic artery and the portal vein discharge their blood into the hepatic sinusoids ( Figure 16-2C ). In histologic sections, the liver plates appear as cords surrounded on each side by sinusoids that converge toward the central veins. The portal tracts appear at the periphery. This anatomic configuration, which is called a **liver lobule**, is illustrated diagrammatically in Figure 16-3A .

Blood flow in the liver is from portal tracts through the sinusoids into central veins ( Figure 16-3B ). Consequently, the liver cells nearest the portal tracts receive the most oxygen and nutrients, and those nearest the central veins are much less well supplied. Because of their relatively poor nutritional state, the liver cells nearest the central veins are more vulnerable to injury from toxic agents or circulatory disturbances, as occurs in shock and heart failure, than are the cells nearer the portal tracts.

The small terminal bile channels, called **bile canaliculi**, collect the bile made by the liver cells, which drains into the bile ducts traveling in the portal tracts. The direction of the bile flow is opposite that of the blood flow in the sinusoids (Figure 16-3B). The bile ducts gradually converge to form larger ducts, which finally unite as the large right and left hepatic ducts. The two hepatic ducts join to form the common hepatic duct. The gallbladder joins the common hepatic duct by means of the cystic duct to form the common bile duct that enters the duodenum.

**portal tract** Branch of hepatic artery, portal vein, and bile duct located at periphery of liver lobule.

**liver lobule** A histologic subdivision of the liver in which columns of liver cells converge toward a central vein and portal tracts are located at the periphery.

**bile canaliculus** (kan-alik'u-lus) Small terminal bile channel located between liver cords.

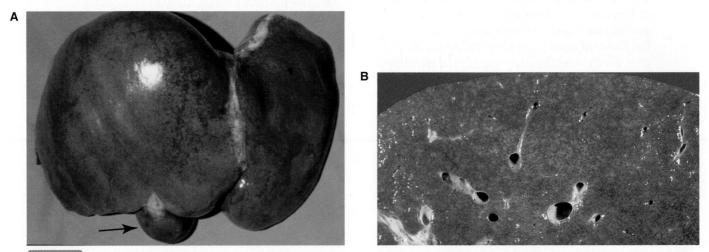

**A**

**B**

Figure 16-1 **A,** A normal liver viewed from above to show its superior and anterior surfaces. The gallbladder is located on the undersurface of the liver, and the fundus of the gallbladder projects slightly beyond the anterior edge of the liver (*arrow*). **B,** Section of liver illustrating the uniform appearance of the hepatic parenchyma and the large blood vessels (branches of the portal vein) transporting blood into the liver from the gastrointestinal tract.

**A**

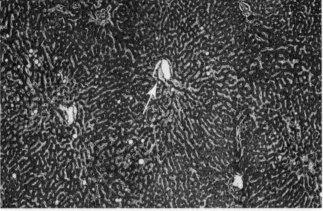

**B**

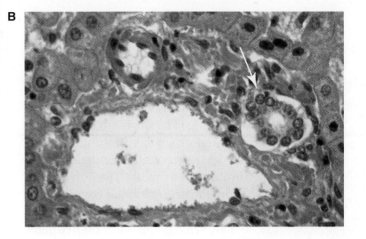

**C**

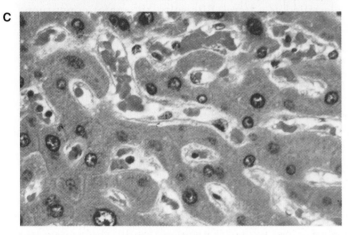

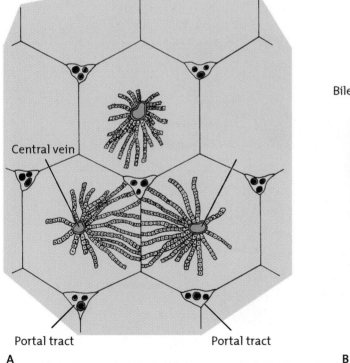

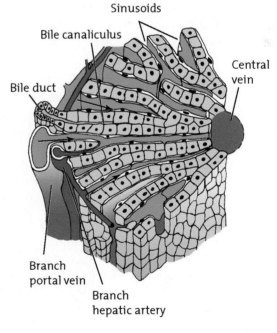

**Figure 16-2** Photomicrographs showing the cellular structure of a normal liver. **A,** Low-magnification photomicrograph illustrating plates of liver cells, which appear as cords in histologic sections, and sinusoids between cords, which drain into central veins. *Arrow* indicates central vein (original magnification × 25). **B,** Higher magnification illustrating portal tract. *Arrow* indicates bile duct. Branch of hepatic artery is *above* and *left* of bile duct and branch of portal vein is *left* and *below* bile duct (original magnification × 400). **C,** High magnification of liver cell cords and hepatic sinusoids (original magnification × 400).

Central vein

Central vein

Portal tract        Portal tract

**A**

Sinusoids

Bile canaliculus

Bile duct

Central vein

Branch portal vein

Branch hepatic artery

**B**

**Figure 16-3** **A,** Concept of liver lobule, consisting of cords of cells radiating toward central vein with portal tracts at periphery. Lobules are outlined in diagram. **B,** Blood flow in sinusoids toward central vein; flow of bile toward portal tract.

# Bile

## Formation and Excretion

Bile pigment is a product of the breakdown of red blood cells. Red cells normally survive for about 4 months. The worn-out erythrocytes are broken down by the mononuclear phagocytes (reticuloendothelial cells) throughout the body. The iron derived from the hemoglobin is conserved by the body and reused to synthesize new hemoglobin. The iron-free heme pigment forms bilirubin. Because the breakdown of red cells proceeds in mononuclear phagocytes throughout the body, small quantities of bile pigment are continually present in the blood. When the blood passes through the liver, the bilirubin is removed by the liver cells. Excretion is accomplished by combining the bilirubin with other substances, a process called *conjugation*, which requires certain specific enzymes. Most of the bilirubin is conjugated with glucuronic acid and excreted as *bilirubin glucuronide*. The **conjugated bilirubin** is much more soluble and less toxic than the unconjugated material. The bile pigment is excreted into the small bile channels between the liver cell cords; it is collected into large ducts at the periphery of the lobules that eventually unite to form the major bile ducts. Figure 16-4 summarizes the basic anatomy of the biliary duct system.

## Composition and Properties

**Bile** is an aqueous solution containing various dissolved substances excreted by the liver. In addition to conjugated bilirubin, it contains bile salts, lecithin, cholesterol, water, minerals, and other materials that have been detoxified by liver cells and excreted. **Cholesterol** is a lipid with a complex ring structure that is classified as a *sterol*. **Bile salts**, the major constituent of bile, are derivatives of cholesterol and certain amino acids. They function as detergents because of their molecular structure, which contains both a lipid-soluble (*hydrophobic*) and a water-soluble (*hydrophilic*) part. **Lecithin** is a phosphorous-containing lipid (phospholipid) that has detergent properties similar to bile salts. Bile is secreted continually and is concentrated and stored in the gallbladder. During digestion the gallbladder contracts, which squirts bile into the duodenum. Bile does not contain digestive enzymes but functions as a biologic detergent. Bile salts emulsify fat into small globules, increasing the surface area so that the fat can be acted on more readily by pancreatic enzymes. Digestion of fat is much less efficient in the absence of bile.

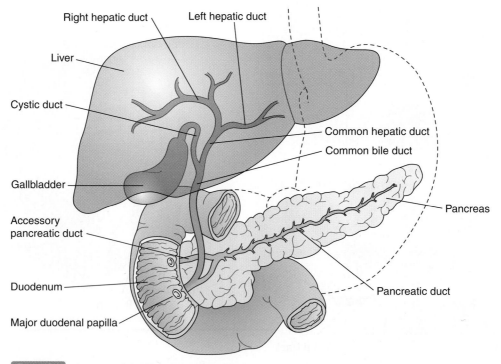

Right hepatic duct — Left hepatic duct

Liver

Cystic duct

Common hepatic duct

Common bile duct

Gallbladder

Pancreas

Accessory pancreatic duct

Duodenum

Pancreatic duct

Major duodenal papilla

**Figure 16-4** Anatomy of the biliary duct system. Right and left hepatic ducts form the common hepatic duct, which is joined by the cystic duct to form the common bile duct that opens into the duodenum along with the pancreatic duct through a common channel.

# Causes and Effects of Liver Injury

The liver is vulnerable to injury by many agents. Histologically, liver injury may be manifested by necrosis of liver cells, by accumulation of fat within the liver cell cytoplasm, or by a combination of the two. Some injurious agents primarily cause cell necrosis, whereas others chiefly induce fatty change in liver cells.

The effect of hepatic injury depends on the extent of damage induced by the injurious agent. If liver injury is mild, the liver cells will completely recover, restoring liver function to normal. Fortunately, this is the usual outcome. If the injury is extremely severe, large amounts of liver tissue are completely destroyed, and not enough liver may remain to sustain life. If the patient does survive, healing of the severe injury may be associated with severe scarring, and liver function may never return to normal. Multiple episodes of relatively mild liver injury may have a cumulative effect, leading to scarring and permanent impairment of liver function. Similarly, any chronic or progressive injury may cause scarring and impairment of function.

Liver cell injury caused by drugs, chemicals, alcohol, or toxins can produce fatty change in liver cells rather than necrosis. Figure 16-5 diagrams the general causes and possible effects of various degrees of liver injury.

Clinically, the most common types of liver disease characterized by injury to liver cells are *viral hepatitis*, and liver cell injury associated with consuming excessive amounts of alcoholic beverages, which is called *alcoholic liver disease*. Chronic liver cell injury from any cause may in turn be followed by diffuse scarring throughout the liver, which is called *cirrhosis*.

# Viral Hepatitis

The term *viral hepatitis* applies to several clinically similar infections. Two of these diseases, hepatitis A and hepatitis B, have been recognized as separate diseases since the early 1940s. Subsequently, a third type of viral hepatitis was recognized as a separate entity called hepatitis C. These three types account for most cases of viral hepatitis. Two additional types of viral hepatitis occur less frequently. One type, called hepatitis D or

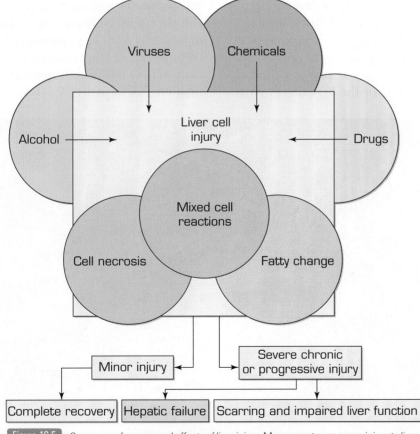

Figure 16-5    Summary of causes and effects of liver injury. Many agents can cause injury to liver cells, manifested either as fatty change, necrosis, or a combination of both. Mild injury is followed by complete recovery. Severe, chronic, or progressive injury may lead to hepatic failure or diffuse scarring with impaired hepatic function.

delta hepatitis, occurs in persons already infected with the hepatitis B virus. Another type, called hepatitis E, is found primarily in third world countries and is infrequently encountered in North America.

## Clinical Manifestations and Course

Viral hepatitis is a type of liver injury, and the comments regarding the course and outcome of any liver injury also apply to viral hepatitis. All of the hepatitis viruses produce similar histologic changes in the liver that are characterized by diffuse inflammation throughout the liver lobules associated with liver cell swelling and necrosis of individual liver cells, as illustrated in Figure 16-6 . The clinical manifestations of viral hepatitis are quite variable and correlate with the degree of liver cell injury and associated inflammation. Manifestations vary from a severe illness with jaundice and markedly abnormal liver function tests, to asymptomatic or very mild disease without jaundice but with abnormal liver function tests. Persons with few symptoms of infection could easily escape detection, which is sometimes called *subclinical hepatitis*. Despite the absence of symptoms, these subjects can transmit the infection to others.

The outcome of viral hepatitis depends primarily on which virus caused the infection. Most cases of hepatitis caused by the hepatitis A virus (HAV) are quite mild, and patients recover completely without complications. An unfavorable outcome occurs in only a very small percentage of cases. In contrast, persons infected with hepatitis B virus (HBV) or the hepatitis C virus (HCV) may become chronic carriers of the virus and develop chronic progressive hepatitis that eventually leads to cirrhosis and liver failure. Table 16-1 summarizes the salient features of the three major types of viral hepatitis.

## Hepatitis A

*Hepatitis A virus* (HAV) is an RNA virus that has a relatively short 2–6 weeks incubation period. The virus is excreted in oropharyngeal (nose and throat) secretions and in the stools during the late-incubation period and for about 2 weeks after the onset of symptoms. Transmission is by direct person-to-person contact or by fecal contamination of food or water. Food- or waterborne infections frequently occur in epidemics. The infection is self-limited, and there are no chronic carriers of the virus. Antibody to HAV, which appears in the blood after recovery, provides immunity against HAV but not against other hepatitis viruses. If a susceptible person is exposed to hepatitis A, gamma globulin provides protection if administered within 14 days of exposure. An inactivated hepatitis A vaccine is available. It is recommended for immunizing persons who are at relatively high risk of becoming infected, such as health-care workers who have frequent contact with infected persons and persons traveling in foreign countries where there is a high incidence of hepatitis A in the population. Many physicians also recommend routine immunization of children, especially if they live in communities where there is a high incidence of hepatitis A.

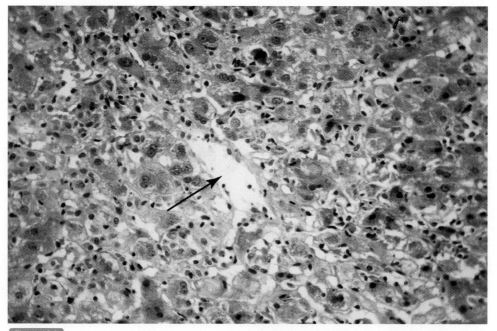

Figure 16-6 Acute viral hepatitis. Cords of liver cells extending from central vein (*arrow*) have lost their orderly arrangement and appear disrupted by swelling of liver cells, necrosis of individual cells, and scattered aggregates of inflammatory cells throughout the liver lobules (original magnification × 100).

## Table 16-1  Comparison of Three Major Types of Viral Hepatitis

|  | Hepatitis A | Hepatitis B | Hepatitis C |
|---|---|---|---|
| Type of virus | RNA | DNA | RNA |
| Incubation period | 2–6 weeks | 6 weeks–4 months | 3–12 weeks |
| Method of transmission | Fecal–oral contaminated food or water | Blood or body fluids | Blood or body fluids |
| Antigen–antibody test results | Anti-HAV (confers immunity) | Infected persons are HbsAg positive and lack anti-HBs<br><br>Immune persons lack HbsAg and have anti-HBs | HCV RNA in blood indicates virus in blood and active infection<br><br>Anti-HCV denotes infection (does not confer immunity) |
| Complications | No carriers or chronic liver disease | 10 percent become chronic carriers and may develop chronic liver disease | 75 percent become carriers and many develop chronic liver disease |
| Prevention of disease after exposure | Gamma globulin | Hepatitis B immune globulin | None available |
| Immunization available | Yes | Yes | No |

## Hepatitis B

*Hepatitis B virus* (HBV) is a DNA virus composed of an inner core and an outer coat. The core consists of a double strand of DNA and an enzyme (*DNA polymerase*) enclosed within a protein shell. The DNA strand and its inner protein shell together are called the **hepatitis B core antigen** (abbreviated HBcAg). The outer coat composed of lipid and protein is called **hepatitis B surface antigen** (abbreviated HBsAg). The core antigen and surface antigen together form the complete virus particle.

In contrast to hepatitis A, hepatitis B has a much longer incubation period, which varies from 6 weeks to 4 months. When an individual becomes infected, the virus invades the liver and multiplies within the hepatic cells. The core of the virus is produced in the nucleus, and the surface antigen is produced in the cytoplasm. For some unexplained reason, much more surface antigen is produced within the infected cells than is necessary to coat the virus particles, and the large excess is released into the bloodstream, where it can be detected by special laboratory tests. Such blood is called *surface-antigen (HBsAg) positive.* Although the laboratory tests detect only the surface antigen, HBsAg-positive blood is infectious because it also contains complete virus particles ( Figure 16-7 ).

In the course of an infection, the surface antigen first appears during the incubation period and can be detected during the first few weeks of the infection. Normally, it does not persist in the blood for more than 2 or 3 weeks. Then antibodies begin to appear, both to the core of the virus (anti-HBc) and to the surface antigen (anti-HBs) ( Figure 16-8 ).

Most infected individuals eliminate the virus from the bloodstream in a few weeks and recover completely, but about 10 percent become chronic carriers of the virus. Some of the carriers develop chronic hepatitis, which causes progressive liver damage. About 1 percent of the United States population are asymptomatic chronic carriers of the virus, and their blood is infectious. The carrier rate is much higher among drug abusers and men who have sexual relations with other men. In some

**hepatitis B core antigen** The antigen contained in the core of the hepatitis B virus.

**hepatitis B surface antigen** The coating of the hepatitis B virus that is also found in great excess in the blood of infected patients.

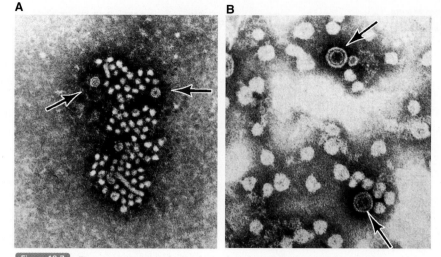

**Figure 16-7** Electron photomicrographs of complete virus particles (*arrows*) and excess surface antigen in blood of patient with hepatitis B. **A,** Original magnification × 130,000. **B,** Original magnification × 290,000 (from Dane, D. S., Cameron, C. H., and Briggs, M. 1970. Viruslike particles in serum of patients with Australia-antigen-associated hepatitis. *Lancet* 1:695–98. Used by permission).

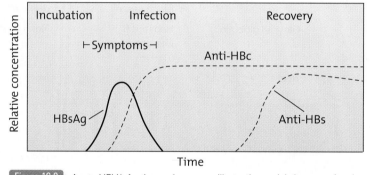

**Figure 16-8** Acute HBV infection and recovery, illustrating serial changes of major antigens and antibodies used to aid in the diagnosis of HBV infection and monitor its course.

population groups, the carrier rate may approach 20 percent.

Worldwide, more than 350 million people are infected with the hepatitis B virus, and about one million people each year die of the complications of the disease. Some antiviral drugs are available that can suppress viral multiplication and slow disease progression in persons who have active hepatitis and circulating virus in their bloodstream.

HBV is not excreted in the stool. Consequently, transmission does not occur by means of contaminated food or water. Most HBV infections result from contact with the blood or secretions of HBsAg-positive individuals. Drug abusers may transmit the virus by sharing needles and syringes. Physicians, dentists, nurses, laboratory personnel, and other health professionals may become infected from contact with blood of HBsAg-positive patients. Improperly sterilized dental instruments or instruments used for ear piercing also may

transmit HBV. Because HBV is present in saliva, vaginal secretions, and seminal fluid, infection may be spread by close family contacts or sexual contacts. An HBsAg-positive mother may transmit the virus to her newborn infant, who usually acquires the infection from maternal blood and vaginal secretions at the time of delivery. Formerly, many cases followed blood transfusions; however, this is no longer true because all blood collected for transfusion is now tested routinely for HBsAg, and antigen-positive blood is not used for transfusion.

A vaccine is available to immunize against HBV. Universal vaccination is recommended, and HBV vaccination is included in vaccination schedules recommended for infants and children. Hepatitis B-immune globulin provides some protection to nonimmunized persons if administered promptly after exposure to the virus, and is given routinely to newborn infants born to HBsAg-positive mothers.

## Hepatitis C

The *hepatitis C virus* (HCV) is an RNA virus that is transmitted by infected blood and body fluids as is HBV, but HCV infection is an even more serious problem than HBV infection for several reasons:

1. HCV is a frequent cause of chronic hepatitis in the United States, accounting for almost half of the reported cases.
2. Most HCV-infected persons are unable to eliminate the virus and become chronic carriers. About 1 to 2 percent of the population are chronic carriers of the virus, and their blood and body fluids are infectious. Many of the chronic carriers will develop chronic hepatitis, which in turn is followed by cirrhosis in many of the infected persons.
3. There are no agents like gamma globulin that can protect an uninfected person who has been exposed to the virus, as by an accidental needle stick when drawing blood from an infected person.
4. There is no available immunizing agent that can be used to establish an active immunity against the virus, and none is likely to be developed in the foreseeable future.

HCV-infected persons may experience symptoms of hepatitis, but many infected persons have few symptoms of infections, and some may not even know that they have become infected. Infected persons develop antibodies against HCV, but antibodies may not appear for several months after the infection. Viral RNA, a measure of virus particles in the circulation, is an indication of active infection, and the amount of viral RNA can be measured in the blood of infected persons to monitor the course of the infection.

In the past, HCV infections sometimes followed blood transfusion of HCV-infected blood or use of blood products such as antihemophilic globulin prepared from infected blood. However, in 1992 a screening test to identify anti-HCV antibody became available as a diagnostic test for HCV infection. As soon as the test became available, it was used routinely by blood banks as a screening test. HCV-antibody–positive blood could be identified and not be used for transfusion. As a result, infections acquired by blood transfusion or use of blood products are no longer a problem.

Currently, most HCV infections are acquired from infected blood or body fluids in much the same ways that HBV and HIV infections are acquired. The Centers for Disease Control and Prevention, which monitors HBV infections, estimates that about 60 percent of HCV infections occur in injection drug users who share virus-contaminated needles. In 20 percent of cases, the infection was acquired by sexual contact, although HCV is not as easily transmitted by sexual practices as is HBV. About 10 percent of cases result from other types of blood and body fluid exposures, such as household contacts, occupational exposures of health-care workers, and virus transmission from mother to infant during childbirth. In another 10 percent of cases the source of infection could not be determined.

Many people may have become infected by virus-contaminated blood or blood products before routine HCV blood testing procedures were available, but have no symptoms. Nevertheless, they are at risk of developing chronic hepatitis and its associated complications. Other persons in the past may have engaged in practices that put them at risk of becoming infected, such as injecting drugs, but they were unaware of the risks at the time. Most infected individuals can't rid themselves of the virus and the HCV infection becomes chronic, although they may not have symptoms of active infection. Although an unfavorable outcome occurs in only a small percentage of infected persons, this is still a large number of people at risk of serious liver disease because HCV infection is so prevalent.

Because of the serious late complications that can occur in some infected persons, the Centers for Disease Control and Prevention recommends that the following groups of high-risk individuals be tested for possible asymptomatic HCV infection:

1. Persons who have ever injected illegal drugs, even persons who injected drugs only once or a few times and do not consider themselves drug users.
2. Persons who received antihemophilic globulin or other clotting factor concentrates before 1987, when the manufacturing processes used were not adequate to eliminate the virus from the concentrates.
3. Persons who received blood transfusions before 1992, when screening blood for HCV was not available, or who had other contacts with blood before 1992, such as hemodialysis or organ transplants.
4. Health-care personnel who had been exposed to blood or body fluids, as might have occurred following an accidental needle stick while drawing blood.
5. Children born to HCV-infected mothers because about 5 percent of infants born to infected mothers become infected.

Because of the potential late complications of HCV infection, all HCV-positive persons should be referred for further medical evaluation. Those who have chronic hepatitis, as demonstrated by abnormal liver function tests, viral RNA in their blood, and a liver biopsy demonstrating chronic inflammation in the liver, should be treated by drugs that inhibit viral multiplication. Hopefully, treatment will minimize or prevent the late complications resulting from the infection.

## Hepatitis D (Delta Hepatitis)

This type of hepatitis is caused by a small defective RNA virus that can only infect persons who are already infected with HBV because the virus is unable to produce its own outer viral coat and can reproduce itself only by coating itself with HBsAg produced by HBV, thereby forming complete but hybrid virus particles composed of a delta virus core and an HBsAg outer layer. Delta hepatitis is less common than other types of viral hepatitis, and most cases in the United States are found among intravenous drug abusers who became infected by sharing contaminated needles.

## Hepatitis E

Hepatitis E is caused by an RNA virus that is transmitted by the fecal–oral route, like the hepatitis A virus; most of the cases are in third world countries, where outbreaks have been traced to contaminated water supplies. Only a few cases have been reported in North America, and usually the infected persons acquired the disease while traveling outside the United States.

## Other Hepatitis Viruses

Other viruses may at times cause a mild hepatitis. These include the Epstein-Barr (EB) virus, which causes infectious mononucleosis (Chapter 11), and another somewhat similar virus called cytomegalovirus, which may also cause an infection resembling infectious mononucleosis.

## Sexually Transmitted Hepatitis

All types of viral hepatitis can be transmitted by sexual practices among persons of the same sex or between heterosexual couples. The hepatitis A virus is excreted in the stool of infected subjects and may also contaminate the anal–genital skin. Consequently, the virus is readily transmitted by anal–oral and oral–genital sexual activity. Hepatitis B virus, which is present in the blood and secretions of infected individuals, is transmitted primarily by anal intercourse, and hepatitis C also may be transmitted in this way. Minor abrasions of the anal, rectal, and genital mucosa of sexual partners permits transfer of virus-infected blood and body fluids between partners.

The following case illustrates the usual clinical and laboratory features of viral hepatitis as a result of HBV infection.

### Case Study 16-1

A 22-year-old man was seen by a physician because of upper abdominal discomfort, nausea, loss of appetite, and jaundice. The patient noted that his urine had become darker in color. He was homosexual and stated that a sexual partner had suffered a similar illness recently. Physical examination revealed a jaundiced young man with a slightly enlarged, tender liver. There were no findings to suggest chronic liver disease. Laboratory studies revealed a slight elevation of bilirubin and abnormalities of several liver-function tests. Tests for hepatitis B surface antigen were positive. The patient was considered to have hepatitis B, probably contracted through sexual activities with a partner who either had active hepatitis or was a chronic carrier of the virus. The patient made an uneventful recovery. Hepatitis B surface antigen was no longer detected in the blood 3 weeks later, and antibody to hepatitis B surface antigen appeared during convalescence.

# Fatty Liver

Fatty liver is a special type of liver injury in which fat accumulates in liver cells ( Figure 16-9 ). A number of injurious agents are capable of disrupting the metabolic processes within the liver cells, leading to an accumulation of fat globules within the liver cell cytoplasm ( Figure 16-10 ). In the United States, the most common cause of fatty liver is excessive alcohol ingestion, but a number of volatile solvents, drugs, chemicals, and some poisons can cause fat accumulation in liver cells. Obese persons and many persons with diabetes also accumulate excess fat in the liver. Fatty liver is also a characteristic feature of a condition called *Reye's syndrome*, which is described later in the chapter. Heavy fat infiltration impairs liver function, but the effect is reversible, and the liver cells return to normal when the injurious agent is no longer present.

## Alcoholic Liver Disease

The term *alcoholic liver disease* refers to a group of structural and functional changes in the liver resulting from excessive alcohol consumption. The severity

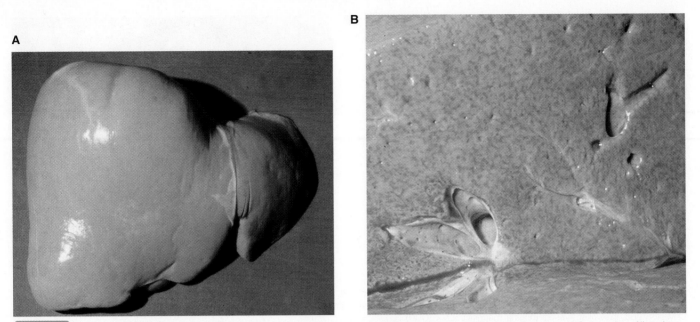

**Figure 16-9** Fatty liver. **A,** The liver appears yellow because of a large amount of fat within liver cells, but otherwise appears normal. **B,** A section of liver that appears normal except for the yellow color caused by the fat.

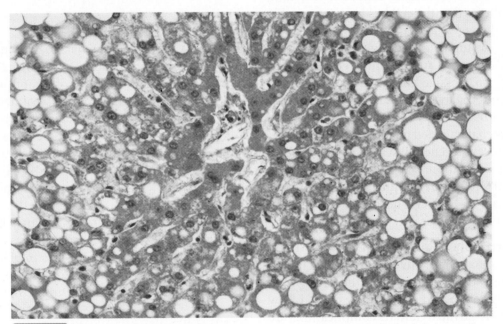

**Figure 16-10** Photomicrograph of fatty liver. Liver cord cells in center of photograph appear relatively normal. Other cells contain large fat globules that appear as clear spherical vacuoles within liver cells in photograph (original magnification × 100).

of the liver injury and its rate of progression are determined not only by how much alcohol is consumed, but also how long the person has been drinking excessively.

It is convenient to subdivide alcoholic liver disease into three stages of progressively increasing severity: (1) alcoholic fatty liver, (2) alcoholic hepatitis, and (3) alcoholic cirrhosis.

**Alcoholic Fatty Liver** This is the mildest form of alcoholic liver disease. If the subject stops drinking, the liver function gradually returns to normal, and the fat globules in the liver cells disappear as the liver cells process the accumulated fat.

**Alcoholic Hepatitis** This is the next stage in the progressive liver injury caused by alcohol. Heavy alcohol intake not only promotes fatty change in liver cells, but causes other degenerative changes as well and may actually induce liver cell necrosis. A rather characteristic feature of severe alcoholic liver injury is the accumulation of irregularly shaped, pink deposits within the cytoplasm of the liver cells. These structures, which

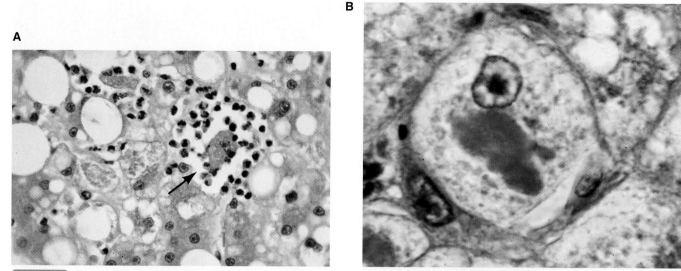

**A**

**B**

> **Mallory body** An irregular red-staining structure in the cytoplasm of injured liver cells, usually resulting from alcohol-induced liver injury.

are called **Mallory bodies** or alcoholic hyalin, indicate that the cell has been irreparably damaged. Neutrophilic leukocytes also accumulate in response to the liver cell necrosis, and the injury is followed by progressive fibrous scarring throughout the liver. The term *alcoholic hepatitis* is used to refer to this type of liver injury, which is characterized not only by fatty change, but also by liver cell degeneration with Mallory bodies and leukocyte infiltration ( Figure 16-11 ). In this case, the term *hepatitis* refers to the inflammatory cell infiltration secondary to liver cell necrosis and does not imply an infection, as in viral hepatitis.

**Alcoholic Cirrhosis** This is the third and most advanced stage of alcoholic liver injury. It is characterized by diffuse scarring throughout the liver, which disturbs liver function and also impedes blood flow through the liver. Cirrhosis and its complications are described in the following section. In the United States, a large number of cases of cirrhosis are related to heavy alcohol ingestion and follow repeated episodes of alcoholic hepatitis. It is generally considered that a person must drink more than 1 pint of whiskey daily, or its equivalent in other alcoholic beverages, for 10 to 15 years in order to develop alcoholic cirrhosis. However, there is considerable individual variation in susceptibility to alcoholic liver injury. Occasionally, the disease develops more rapidly, and it has been seen in teenagers and young adults.

The following clinical summary illustrates the clinical features seen in a young man who died of severe alcoholic liver disease.

**Case Study 16-2**

A 33-year-old man had been drinking heavily for many years and was in the habit of consuming about 1 quart of liquor per day. Recently, he had noticed weakness and loss of appetite. The physical examination revealed that he was slightly jaundiced. His liver was enlarged, and there was moderate ascites. Laboratory studies revealed a reduced serum albumin and a moderate elevation of serum bilirubin.

Other tests of liver function were abnormal. The clinical impression was severe alcoholic liver disease. Despite intensive therapy, the patient's condition did not improve, and he eventually died of chronic liver failure. The autopsy revealed fatty change in liver cells and active alcoholic hepatitis with many Mallory bodies in the cytoplasm of the liver cells, and the early stages of cirrhosis.

# Cirrhosis

The term **cirrhosis** refers to diffuse scarring of the liver from any cause ( Figure 16-12 ). Any substance capable of injuring the liver may cause cirrhosis under certain conditions. The two most common causes of cirrhosis are

1. Alcoholic liver disease, resulting from repeated episodes of alcoholic hepatitis followed by scarring.

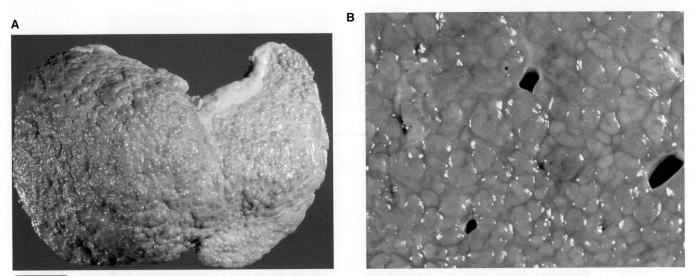

**A**

**B**

**Figure 16-12** Advanced hepatic cirrhosis illustrating elevated nodules of liver tissue surrounded by depressed areas of scar tissue. **A,** Exterior of liver. **B,** A closer view of the liver in cross section.

## A Closer Look

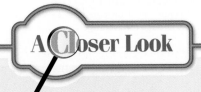

*The term* cirrhosis *refers to advanced liver cell damage, often caused by long-term heavy drinking of alcoholic beverages. The unusual origin of the term is interesting, as is the physician who coined the term.* René Laennec, the same physician who discovered the stethoscope, named the disease. The condition is characterized by accumulation of fat in the liver associated with progressive scarring that interferes with blood flow through the liver. The condition is usually caused by heavy alcohol

consumption, a disease as common in the 1800s as it is today. At autopsy, the liver is often enlarged, nodular, and has a yellow–tan color caused by the fat within the damaged liver cells. Laennec was impressed by the yellow–tan (tawny) color of the liver and coined the term *cirrhosis*, from the Greek word *kirros*, which means yellow–tan. Even today alcohol-related cirrhosis is often called Laennec cirrhosis.

2. Chronic hepatitis caused by HBV or HCV infections, which eventually leads to diffuse liver scarring. In many parts of Asia and Africa, where a large proportion of the population are chronic carriers of HBV, chronic HBV infection is the major cause of cirrhosis.

Less common causes of cirrhosis include

1. An episode of severe liver necrosis, such as after an attack of severe viral hepatitis.
2. Various other drugs and chemicals that damage liver cells.
3. Some genetic diseases that directly or indirectly lead to liver damage such as hemochromatosis (Chapter 11).

4. Long-standing bile duct obstruction, which causes a special type of cirrhosis called **biliary cirrhosis**.

## Derangements of Liver Structure and Function

In cirrhosis, the liver is converted into a mass of scar tissue containing nodules of degenerating and regenerating liver cells, proliferating bile ducts, and inflammatory cells ( Figure 16-13 ). The normal architectural pattern of the liver is completely disorganized, and the intrahepatic branches of

**cirrhosis of the liver** (si-rō′sis) A disease characterized by diffuse intrahepatic scarring and liver cell degeneration.

**biliary cirrhosis** Diffuse liver cell damage and scarring with distortion of liver cell structure and function (cirrhosis) caused by obstruction of bile ducts.

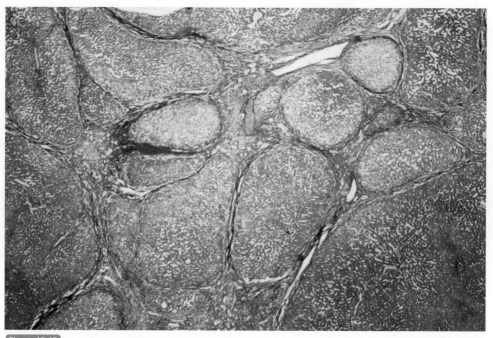

Figure 16-13 A low-magnification photomicrograph of cirrhotic liver illustrating nodules of liver cells circumscribed by dense scar tissue (blue–green stain). The normal architectural pattern is lost. The number of functioning liver cells is reduced and replaced by scar tissue, and the scar tissue disrupts blood flow through the liver. Compare with Figure 21-2 (original magnification × 25).

the hepatic artery and portal vein are constricted by scar tissue.

The two major functional disturbances in cirrhosis are impaired liver function and portal hypertension.

**Impaired Liver Function** As a result of liver cell damage, scarring, and impairment of blood supply to the liver caused by scarring, the number of functioning liver cells is greatly reduced. Eventually, a patient with cirrhosis may die of liver failure.

**Portal Hypertension** Normally, the portal vein blood passes through sinusoids into the hepatic veins and then into the inferior vena cava. In cirrhosis, venous return through the portal system is impaired, and the pressure in the portal vein rises because the blood flow is obstructed by scar tissue. The high pressure affects the portal capillaries, and this contributes to excessive leakage of fluid from the capillaries. Eventually, the abdomen becomes distended by fluid that accumulates within the abdominal cavity (*ascites*) ( Figure 16-14 ).

A reduced concentration of albumin in the blood also contributes to ascites because albumin is crucial to maintaining the normal colloid osmotic pressure of the blood, which is the force that tends to hold fluid in the capillaries (Chapter 9). Albumin, which is produced by the liver, is reduced in cirrhosis because the cirrhotic liver is unable to manufacture this protein in sufficient quantities; consequently, the colloid osmotic pressure of the blood is lower than normal, and fluid leaks from the portal capillary bed.

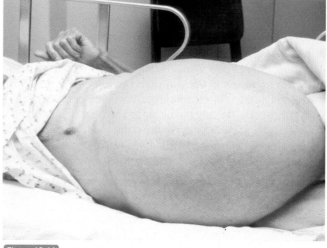

Figure 16-14   Marked ascites in patient with advanced cirrhosis.

Because of the obstruction of portal venous return, a collateral circulation develops in an attempt to bypass the intrahepatic obstruction and deliver portal blood directly into the systemic circulation. Anastomoses develop where tributaries of portal and systemic veins are closely associated, and they shunt blood from the portal system of veins where the pressure is high into the veins of the systemic circulation where the pressure is much lower ( Figure 16-15 ). The communications that are most important clinically are the anastomoses developing between veins around the stomach and spleen, which drain into the portal vein, and the esophageal veins that eventually drain into the superior

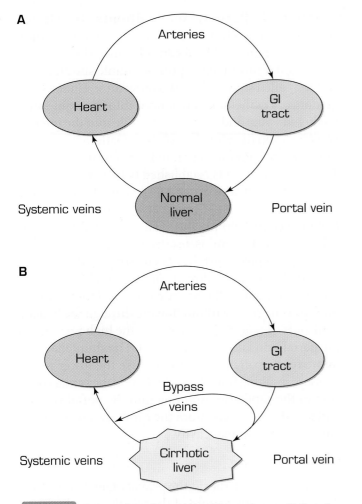

**A**

Arteries

Heart → GI tract

Systemic veins          Portal vein

Normal liver

**B**

Arteries

Heart      GI tract

Bypass veins

Systemic veins          Portal vein

Cirrhotic liver

**Figure 16-15** A comparison of normal blood flow pathways with those in cirrhosis. **A,** Normal flow pattern. The heart pumps blood through the aorta to the gastrointestinal tract from which blood collects in portal vein and flows through hepatic sinusoids into hepatic veins, then into vena cava, and finally, back to heart to be repumped. **B,** The flow pattern in cirrhosis. Blood pumped to gastrointestinal tract is collected in portal vein; however, flow through hepatic sinusoids is interrupted by intrahepatic scarring, and portal vein pressure rises. Bypass channels shunt blood into superior or inferior vena cava in order to return blood to the heart. Bypass veins cannot handle increased blood flow under increased pressure and become dilated.

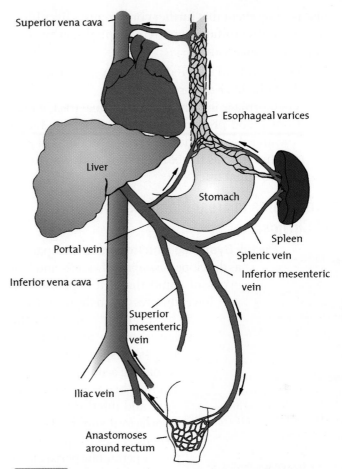

**Figure 16-16** Formation of collateral venous channels (described in the text) that return blood to the systemic circulation when portal blood flow is impeded by cirrhosis. The *arrows* indicate direction of blood flow.

vena cava by way of the intercostal veins and azygos veins. The esophageal veins are not equipped to handle the increased blood flow and high pressure and therefore become dilated and form *varicose veins*, which are called *esophageal varices* (plural of *varix*). **Esophageal varices** are thin-walled vessels covered by a thin layer of esophageal epithelium and frequently rupture, leading to profuse and sometimes fatal hemorrhage.

Other anastomoses develop between branches of the portal vein and the veins draining the abdominal wall that eventually flow into either the superior or the inferior vena cava. Still other anastomoses develop around the rectum between branches of the inferior mesenteric veins and the iliac veins, permitting blood to flow through the iliac veins into the inferior vena cava.

**Figure 16-16** demonstrates the collateral circulation that delivers blood into the systemic circulation when blood flow through the liver is obstructed by scar tissue. The collateral channel blood flow reduces the engorgement of the abdominal organs, but the elevated portal pressure does not return to normal.

**Hepatic Encephalopathy** Hepatic encephalopathy (*encephalon* = brain + *pathy* = disease) is a deterioration of brain function characterized by impaired consciousness, confusion, disorientation, and eventually coma. The condition results from toxic substances that accumulate in the bloodstream and are normally detoxified and excreted by the liver, a task that the cirrhotic liver is unable to accomplish efficiently. Not all of the toxic products have been identified, but many of them are products of protein digestion, especially ammonia, which comes from deamination of amino acids, and other products derived from bacterial decomposition of material in the colon. In a person with advanced liver

**esophageal varices** (var′i-sēz) Dilated (varicose) veins of the esophagus, which are often present in patients with cirrhosis of the liver.

disease, any event that further compromises liver function may precipitate hepatic encephalopathy. Two important causes are

1. An episode of binge drinking in a subject with alcoholic liver disease.
2. A hemorrhage into the gastrointestinal tract, which drops blood pressure and reduces hepatic blood flow, and also provides more toxic products of protein digestion as the blood is broken down within the intestinal tract.

## Procedures to Treat Manifestations of Cirrhosis

**splenorenal shunt**
(splē′no-rē′nul) Surgically created anastomosis between splenic vein and renal vein, performed to lower portal pressure in the treatment of esophageal varices.

**portacaval shunt** (por′tuh-kay′vul) Surgically created anastomosis between the portal vein and the vena cava, performed to lower portal pressure in the treatment of esophageal varices.

**transjugular intrahepatic portosystemic shunt** A nonsurgical method used to lower portal vein pressure in a person with cirrhosis by connecting an intrahepatic branch of the portal vein to a hepatic vein branch.

**Portal–Systemic Anastomoses** If a patient has developed esophageal varices and is at risk of hemorrhage, it is possible to lower the pressure in the portal system by surgically connecting the splenic vein to the renal vein side-to-side (**splenorenal shunt**) or making a side-to-side connection between the portal vein and inferior vena cava (**portacaval shunt**). A shunt decompresses the portal system by permitting portal blood to flow directly into the inferior vena cava ( Figure 16-17 ). Blood no longer is forced to circumvent the scarred liver by collateral channels. The dilated esophageal veins decrease in size, and the risk of hemorrhage from varices is greatly reduced.

**Intrahepatic Portosystemic Shunts** In selected patients a nonsurgical portal–systemic communication can be accomplished by means of a procedure called a **transjugular intrahepatic portosystemic shunt**, which is often called simply the TIPS procedure. Under x-ray guidance, a catheter is introduced into the right internal jugular vein and passed retrograde into the inferior vena cava and then into one of the hepatic veins (which drain blood from the liver into the inferior vena cava). Then a connection is established between a branch of the hepatic vein and a large intrahepatic branch of the portal vein to create a tract between portal vein and hepatic vein within the liver. The tract is dilated, and a device (called a stent) is inserted to keep the tract open.

When the procedure has been completed, much of the portal blood flows directly from a portal vein branch directly into one of the hepatic veins and then into the inferior vena cava, without flowing through the hepatic sinusoids ( Figure 16-18 ). As a result, the high pressure in the portal vein falls toward normal. The shunt may also improve the patient's ascites because the lower portal pressure resulting from the shunt lowers the venous pressure in the capillaries draining into the portal system, and less fluid is forced from the capillaries to accumulate in the abdominal cavity.

## Biliary Cirrhosis

In some types of cirrhosis, the primary target of the liver damage is the epithelium of the bile ducts rather than the functional cells (hepatocytes) of the liver lobules. This type of cirrhosis is called biliary cirrhosis to

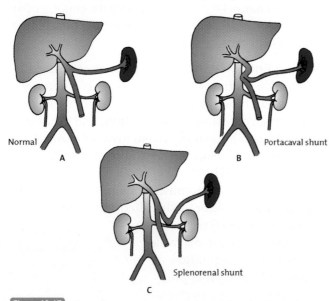

Figure 16-17 Operative procedures to create portal–systemic anastomoses for treatment of esophageal varices. **A,** Normal anatomic relation. **B,** Portacaval shunt. **C,** Splenorenal shunt.

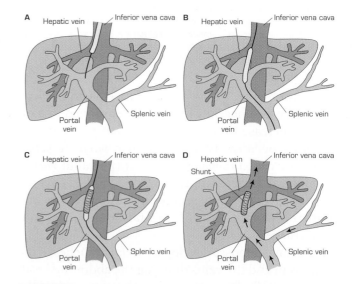

Figure 16-18 The TIPS procedure. **A,** Intrahepatic communication (tract) established between the hepatic and portal vein. **B,** Angioplasty balloon dilates tract. **C,** Expandable metal stent inserted into tract and dilated by angioplasty balloon. **D,** Completed shunt between hepatic artery and portal vein lowers portal vein pressure. Esophageal varices become smaller as portal vein pressure falls.

distinguish it from the more common type of cirrhosis in which liver cell injury involves primarily the hepatocytes. There are two main types of biliary cirrhosis. The first, which is called *primary biliary cirrhosis*, is an autoimmune disease that targets the small intrahepatic bile ducts. The second, called *secondary biliary cirrhosis* or *obstructive biliary cirrhosis*, results from long-standing obstruction of the large extrahepatic bile ducts.

### Primary Biliary Cirrhosis

This is a slowly progressive chronic disease characterized by inflammation and destruction of the small intrahepatic bile ducts. Bile excretion is disrupted and is followed by scarring, which begins in the portal tracts and eventually spreads into the liver lobules. The disease appears to be caused by autoantibodies that are directed against bile duct epithelial cells, which can be demonstrated by appropriate laboratory tests.

Because excretion of bile is impeded, products accumulate in the blood that are normally excreted in the bile, including bile pigment (bilirubin), bile salts, and cholesterol. Accumulation of bile pigment in the blood causes the skin to become yellow, which is called jaundice, and the bile salts that accumulate irritate the skin, which becomes very itchy. Unfortunately, there is no effective treatment for this condition, which progresses slowly over many years and eventually leads to liver failure. Ultimately, a liver transplant may be required.

### Secondary (Obstructive) Biliary Cirrhosis

This condition is caused by long-standing blockage of the large extrahepatic bile ducts. Common causes of bile duct obstruction are

1. A gallstone blocking the common bile duct.
2. Carcinoma arising in the head of the pancreas that blocks the common channel transporting both bile and pancreatic secretions into the duodenum.
3. Carcinoma arising from the common bile duct that blocks the duct, as illustrated in Figure 16-19.

The bile duct obstruction leads to stasis of bile within the ducts. The pressure within the ducts rises, and the larger ducts become dilated. The elevated intraductal pressure is transmitted back into the smaller intrahepatic bile ducts and from there into the small bile channels (bile canaliculi) that carry bile from the liver lobules into the bile ducts within the portal tracts at the periphery of the lobules. The elevated intraductal pressure and bile stasis damage the intrahepatic bile ducts, which is followed by portal tract inflammation and scarring.

The clinical manifestations of the extrahepatic bile duct obstruction are much the same as those caused by primary biliary cirrhosis. Treatment consists of various surgical procedures to unblock the obstructed bile duct. If this is not possible, some type of surgical procedure is used to bypass the obstruction and reestablish bile flow into the duodenum.

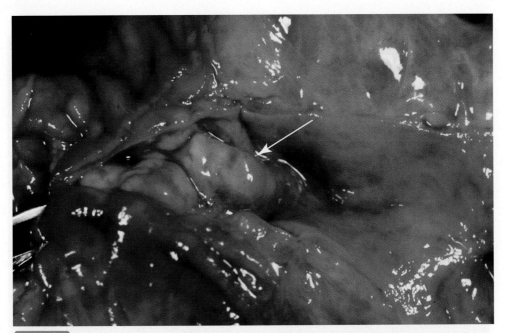

**Figure 16-19** Carcinoma arising from common bile duct (*arrow*) blocking outflow of bile into duodenum. Common bile duct has been opened and is distended, a result of the increased pressure of the bile within the common duct caused by the duct obstruction.

# Reye's Syndrome

**Reye's syndrome** (rhymes with "eye") is a relatively uncommon acute illness that develops in infants and children after a mild viral infection and is characterized by both marked swelling of the brain with neurologic dysfunction and accumulation of fat within the cytoplasm of liver cells associated with impaired liver function. Clinically, the illness manifests as a sudden onset of vomiting and impaired consciousness, which may progress to delirium and coma. Laboratory tests reveal the disturbed liver function that is related to the accumulation of fat in the liver cells, and some patients become jaundiced. In severely affected patients, the mortality rate is about 25 percent, and some of the survivors may be left with neurologic abnormalities or psychiatric disturbances. There is no specific treatment.

Current evidence indicates that Reye's syndrome is related in some way to acetylsalicylic acid (aspirin) given to treat the fever and discomfort associated with the viral infection. The aspirin may increase the injurious effects of the virus or interact with the virus to cause the liver and brain injury. Therefore, acetaminophen (for example, Tylenol) is recommended instead of aspirin to treat symptoms of viral infections in infants and children.

**Reye's syndrome**
(Rīz) A disease characterized by a fatty liver and neurologic disturbances, probably related to aspirin administration in association with a viral infection.

**cholelithiasis** (kō´lē-lith-ī´uh-sis) Formation of gallstones.

**micelle** (mi-sell´) An aggregate of bile salt and lecithin molecules by which cholesterol is brought into solution in bile.

# Cholelithiasis

The formation of stones within the gallbladder is called **cholelithiasis** (*chole* = bile + *lith* = stone). Gallstones are very common and are estimated to develop in about 20 percent of the population. Most gallstones are composed entirely or predominantly of cholesterol, and they form because the bile contains more cholesterol than can be held in solution by the available bile salts and lecithin ( Figure 16-20 ).

## Factors Affecting the Solubility of Cholesterol in Bile

Because cholesterol is a lipid, it is not soluble in an aqueous solution such as bile but is brought into solution by bile salts and lecithin, which aggregate in clusters called **micelles**. In a micelle, the lipid-soluble (*hydrophobic*) parts of the bile salt molecules are oriented toward the center of the cluster, and the opposite water-soluble (*hydrophilic*) ends face outward. Cholesterol becomes soluble by dissolving in the hydrophobic center of the micelles, and the cholesterol-containing micelles dissolve in the bile because the peripheral hydrophilic parts of the bile salt molecules are water soluble. Lecithin participates in the formation of the micelles by fitting between the molecules of the bile salts ( Figure 16-21 ).

The solubility of cholesterol in bile depends not only on its cholesterol content, but also on its content of bile salts and lecithin, because these substances are needed to hold the cholesterol in solution. Cholesterol

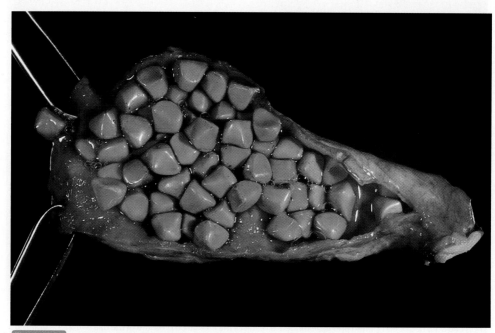

Figure 16-20    Opened gallbladder filled with gallstones composed of cholesterol.

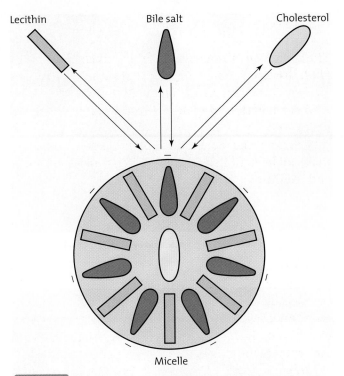

Lecithin    Bile salt    Cholesterol

Micelle

Figure 16-21    The manner in which cholesterol dissolves in micelles composed of bile salts and lecithin. If the bile salt concentration is insufficient relative to that of cholesterol, cholesterol will precipitate and form gallstones.

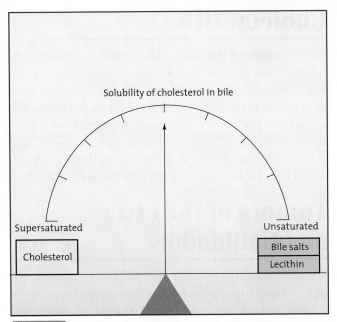

Solubility of cholesterol in bile

Supersaturated    Unsaturated

Cholesterol    Bile salts
                Lecithin

Figure 16-22    "Board-and-fulcrum" concept illustrating factors that affect solubility of cholesterol in bile.

remains soluble provided its concentration is not excessive in relationship to the amounts of available bile salts and lecithin. If there is an excess of cholesterol relative to bile salts and lecithin, the bile becomes supersaturated with cholesterol and cholesterol crystals may precipitate. On the other hand, if there is an excess of bile salts and lecithin relative to cholesterol, more cholesterol can dissolve in the bile. These relationships can be conceptualized by a board on a fulcrum, one end of the board being weighted by cholesterol and the other end by bile salts and lecithin. Variations in the "weight" on either end of the board cause corresponding changes in the solubility of the cholesterol in the bile ( Figure 16-22 ).

Whenever bile contains a relative excess of cholesterol, it becomes supersaturated with cholesterol, and under proper conditions, the cholesterol may precipitate to form the beginnings of gallstones. This situation may arise because of an increased excretion of cholesterol in the bile, a reduced excretion of bile salts and lecithin, or a combination of both factors. As long as the bile remains supersaturated, cholesterol crystals continue to accumulate around those that have already precipitated, and the gallstones slowly increase in size. Eventually, the gallbladder may become filled with gallstones, the end stage of a process that began several years earlier.

## Complications of Gallstones

Gallstones that remain in the gallbladder do not cause symptoms. Unfortunately, gallstones are sometimes extruded into the cystic duct or common bile duct when the gallbladder contracts after a fatty meal, and they may become impacted within the biliary ducts. This event causes severe abdominal pain called **biliary colic**. The pain results from spasm of the smooth muscle in the ducts combined with forceful contractions of the gallbladder that attempt to propel the stone through the ducts. Sometimes a stone can be passed through the ducts into the duodenum, but often it becomes impacted. If the stone lodges in the cystic duct, bile can neither enter nor leave the gallbladder, but flow of bile from the liver into the duodenum is not disturbed even though storage of bile in the gallbladder is no longer possible. If the stone blocks the common duct, bile can no longer be excreted into the duodenum, and it accumulates in the bloodstream. This condition is called *obstructive jaundice*.

## Treatment of Gallstones

The standard treatment of gallstones producing symptoms is surgical removal of the diseased gallbladder. In the past, it was necessary to perform a major surgical operation to remove the gallbladder. Now, most cholecystectomies can be performed by means of a laparoscopic procedure through very small incisions in the abdomen.

**biliary colic**  Abdominal pain that results when a gallstone enters the biliary duct system.

# Cholecystitis

Inflammation of the gallbladder is called cholecystitis (*chole* = bile + *cyst* = bladder + *itis* = inflammation). It is a relatively common disease. Chronic cholecystitis appears to predispose an individual to develop gallstones. As previously described, impaction of a gallstone in the neck of the gallbladder or the cystic duct may precipitate an acute cholecystitis if the gallbladder is the site of a preexisting chronic inflammation.

# Tumors of the Liver and Gallbladder

Primary tumors of the liver and gallbladder are uncommon. Primary carcinoma of the liver is quite rare in the United States and Canada but is a common malignant tumor in Asian and African countries. The current evidence indicates that chronic carriers of the hepatitis B virus (HBV) not only have a relatively high incidence of chronic liver disease, but also carry an increased risk of developing a primary liver carcinoma, suggesting that chronic HBV infection predisposes both to liver injury and to liver cancer. The frequency of primary liver cancer in Asia and Africa is probably related to the high incidence of chronic HBV carriers in these populations. Failure of the body's immune defenses to destroy the infected liver cells and eliminate the virus leads to a smoldering chronic infection that may eventually lead to cirrhosis and predisposes to liver cancer. Patients with chronic HCV infections also are at risk of cirrhosis and liver cancer ( Figure 16-23 and Figure 16-24 ).

In contrast to the infrequency of primary liver cancer in developed countries, the liver is a common site

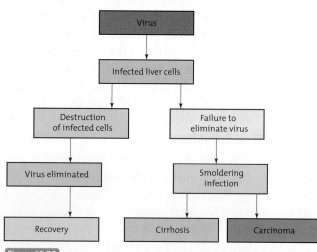

Figure 16-23 Possible outcomes of hepatitis B and hepatitis C infections. Failure to eliminate virus leads to chronic infection, which may be complicated by cirrhosis and liver cancer.

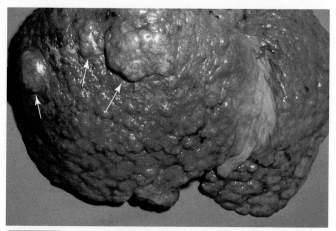

Figure 16-24 Cirrhosis of liver complicated by primary liver cell carcinoma (*arrows*).

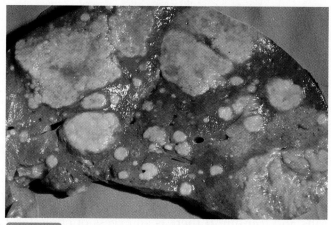

Figure 16-25 A cross-section of liver containing multiple nodules of metastatic carcinoma.

of metastatic carcinoma ( Figure 16-25 ). Carcinoma arising in the gastrointestinal tract may spread to the liver when tumor cells are carried to the liver in the portal venous blood. Tumors from the breast, lung, and other sites also often spread to the liver. The tumor cells are carried in the blood delivered to the liver by the hepatic artery. Sometimes enlargement of the liver as the result of metastatic carcinoma may be the first sign of a malignant tumor that originated in some other part of the body. Various diagnostic procedures can be used to identify tumors in the liver. The computed tomographic (CT) scan described in Chapter 1 is a very effective means of detecting cysts and tumors in the liver.

# Jaundice

**Jaundice** is a yellow discoloration of the skin and the sclerae (whites of the eyes) that results from accumulation of bile pigment (bilirubin) in the tissues and body fluids. This accumulation can have several causes. Bile pigment is derived from the breakdown of red cells, as described elsewhere in this text. The pigment is

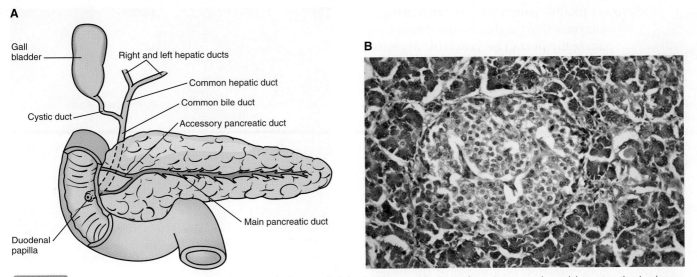

**Figure 16-26** **A,** Duct system of pancreas. The main pancreatic duct usually joins the common bile duct to form a common channel that enters the duodenum by a single opening at the apex of a nipplelike projection called the duodenal papilla (ampulla of Vater). A much smaller accessory pancreatic duct, illustrated in the diagram, is frequently present and opens into the duodenum by a separate opening proximal to the duodenal papilla. **B,** A photomicrograph of pancreatic islet surrounded by exocrine pancreatic tissue.

extracted from the blood by the liver cells, conjugated, and excreted into the biliary ducts. It is convenient to classify jaundice on the basis of the disturbance responsible for the retention of bile pigment. On this basis, jaundice is classified as *hemolytic*, *hepatocellular*, or *obstructive*. The cause of the jaundice usually can be classified correctly, based on laboratory tests (liver function tests) in conjunction with the clinical features.

## Hemolytic Jaundice

In conditions associated with accelerated breakdown of red cells, excessive bile pigment is delivered to the liver, beyond the liver's ability to conjugate and excrete the pigment. Therefore, unconjugated bile pigment accumulates in the blood. Hemolytic jaundice is sometimes seen in adults with hemolytic anemia, but it is encountered most frequently in newborn infants with hemolytic disease as a result of blood group incompatibility between mother and infant (Chapter 14).

## Hepatocellular Jaundice

If the liver is severely damaged, as in hepatitis or cirrhosis, conjugation of bilirubin is impaired. Moreover, the excretion of conjugated bilirubin is hampered because of injury to liver cells and disruption of small bile channels that lie between liver cell cords. As a result, conjugated bilirubin leaks back into the blood through the ruptured intrahepatic bile channels.

## Obstructive Jaundice

In obstructive jaundice, the extraction and conjugation of bilirubin by liver cells are not impaired, but jaundice develops because the bile duct is obstructed, preventing delivery of bile into the duodenum. Often the obstruction is caused by an impacted stone in the common duct. Carcinoma of the head of the pancreas is another common cause of common bile duct obstruction. As indicated in Figure 16-26, the common duct passes very close to the head of the pancreas as it enters the duodenum. Therefore, a pancreatic tumor frequently compresses and invades the common duct. As previously described, long-standing common bile duct obstruction leads to obstructive biliary cirrhosis.

**jaundice** (jawn´dis) Yellow color of the skin that results from accumulation of bile pigment within the blood.

# Biopsy of the Liver

Many times, the exact cause and extent of liver disease in a given patient are difficult to determine. In such cases, a biopsy of the liver can be performed by inserting a needle through the skin directly into the liver and extracting a small bit of liver tissue. This can be examined microscopically by the pathologist, and generally, an exact diagnosis of the nature and severity of the liver disease can be made. This information can provide a basis for proper treatment.

# The Pancreas: Structure and Function

The pancreas is actually two glands in one: a digestive gland and an endocrine gland. The *exocrine tissue* of the pancreas, which is concerned solely with digestion, secretes an alkaline pancreatic juice rich in digestive enzymes into the duodenum through the *pancreatic duct*. The powerful digestive enzymes break down proteins, carbohydrates, and fats. The *endocrine tissue* of the pancreas consists of multiple small clusters of cells scattered throughout the gland called the pancreatic islets or **islets of Langerhans**, which discharge their secretions directly into the bloodstream. The islets indirectly supplement the digestive (exocrine) functions of the pancreas by secreting hormones that regulate carbohydrate metabolism by controlling the concentration of glucose in the bloodstream, and also have effects on protein and fat metabolism as well. Each islet is composed of several different types of cells. The three main types are **alpha cells**, **beta cells**, and **delta cells**. *Alpha cells* secrete a hormone called *glucagon*, which raises blood glucose; the more numerous *beta cells* secrete *insulin*, which lowers blood glucose in response to a rise in blood glucose after eating, restoring blood glucose to normal. *Delta cells* produce a hormone called *somatostatin*, which inhibits secretion of both glucagon and insulin. Three other relatively rare cell types also have been described, and they produce hormones concerned primarily with regulating gastrointestinal functions. Figure 16-26 illustrates the anatomy and cellular structure of the pancreas. Diseases of the exocrine pancreas are considered first, followed by diseases of the endocrine pancreas.

# Pancreatitis

## Acute Pancreatitis

Acute pancreatitis is caused by escape of pancreatic juice from the ducts into the substance of the pancreas, which leads to destruction of pancreatic acinar and islet tissue by activated pancreatic enzymes, accompanied by acute inflammation of the affected pancreatic tissue. Some of the enzymes leak from the damaged tissue into the bloodstream, where elevated levels of amylase and lipase can be detected by appropriate laboratory tests. The clinical manifestations of acute pancreatitis depend on how much pancreatic tissue has been damaged. Mild episodes are accompanied by abdominal pain together with elevated pancreatic enzymes detected by blood tests; however, the pain subsides, and the patient recovers. Patients with severe acute pancreatitis have marked abdominal pain and

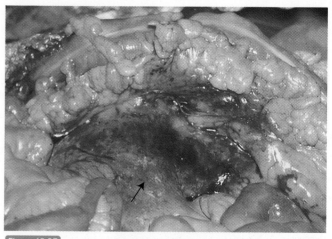

**Figure 16-27** Acute pancreatitis. Transverse colon (*upper part of photograph*) has been elevated to reveal pancreas (*arrow*), which is inflamed and contains large areas of hemorrhage.

tenderness, and they are seriously ill. The activated pancreatic enzymes not only destroy much of the pancreas but also damage pancreatic blood vessels, which lead to marked hemorrhage in the damaged tissues. This condition is often called *acute hemorrhagic pancreatitis* ( Figure 16-27 ).

The pathogenesis of acute pancreatitis usually involves active secretion of pancreatic juice while the pancreatic duct is obstructed at its entrance into the duodenum. The build-up of obstructed secretions greatly increases the pressure within the duct system, causing the ducts to rupture and the pancreatic juice to escape. Two factors predispose to acute pancreatitis: disease of the gallbladder and excessive alcohol consumption.

Pancreatitis often develops in patients with gallstones because in most individuals the common bile duct and common pancreatic duct usually enter the duodenum through a common channel (the *ampulla of Vater*). If a stone becomes impacted in the ampulla, it can obstruct the pancreatic duct and precipitate pancreatitis.

Patients who drink excessive amounts of alcohol also are prone to pancreatitis. Alcohol is a potent stimulus of pancreatic secretions, and it may also induce edema and spasm of the pancreatic sphincter in the ampulla of Vater. Pancreatitis develops because alcohol-induced hypersecretion combined with sphincter spasm leads to high intraductal pressure, followed by duct necrosis and escape of pancreatic juice.

## Chronic Pancreatitis

Chronic pancreatitis results from repeated episodes of mild acute pancreatitis. Each bout of pancreatitis destroys some pancreatic tissue but the inflammation subsides, and the damaged pancreatic tissue is replaced by scar tissue. Eventually, as progressively more pancreatic tissue is destroyed, the affected person has difficulty digesting and absorbing nutrients because there is not enough surviving pancreatic tissue to produce adequate digestive enzymes. The associated destruction of pancreatic islets may also lead to diabetes.

# Cystic Fibrosis of the Pancreas

Cystic fibrosis is a relatively common, serious hereditary disease that is transmitted as an autosomal recessive trait and first becomes manifest in infancy and childhood. The disease has an incidence of about 1 per 3000 in whites but is quite rare in blacks and other races. The abnormal gene involved in the disease results from a mutation of a normal gene called the *CFTR* gene, which stands for *cystic fibrosis transmembrane conductance regulator*, meaning that the gene regulates the movement of salt and water in and out of epithelial cells by means of ion channels located on the cell membranes. A very large number of *CFTR* gene mutations have been identified. Tests have been developed to identify carriers of the more common gene mutations. In some individuals, the disease is relatively mild and compatible with survival into adolescence or adult life. Others, with more severe disease, die in childhood. Modern therapy has improved survival, but nevertheless, the average (median) life expectancy is only about 35 years.

As a result of the gene mutation, there is defective transport across cell membranes of chloride, sodium, and the water molecules in which they are dissolved. Electrolyte and water secretion is deficient in the mucus secreted by the epithelial cells of the pancreas, bile ducts, mucosa of respiratory tract, and other mucus-secreting cells throughout the body. As a result, the mucus becomes abnormally thick and tends to coagulate, forming dense plugs that obstruct the pancreatic ducts, bronchi and bronchioles, and bile ducts.

The most characteristic structural abnormalities are usually in the pancreas. Mucus plugs in the small pancreatic ducts block the secretion of pancreatic juice, which accumulates under increased pressure within the obstructed ducts. Eventually, the ducts become cystically dilated. The pancreatic secretory cells, unable to discharge their secretions into the duodenum, undergo atrophy and are replaced by fibrous tissue. Eventually, the pancreas becomes converted into a mass of cystically dilated ducts surrounded by dense fibrous tissue ( Figure 16-28 ). The name of the disease derives from these characteristic structural abnormalities.

In the lungs, the small bronchi and bronchioles become obstructed by the thick mucous secretions of the epithelial cells lining the respiratory tract. Bronchial obstruction predisposes to pulmonary infection, leading to bronchitis, bronchiectasis, and repeated bouts of pneumonia in the lung distal to the blocked bronchi. Eventually, the lungs are severely damaged by the repeated infections.

The function of sweat glands is also abnormal in cystic fibrosis. The sweat glands are unable to conserve sodium and chloride, and the sweat of affected individuals contains an excessively high salt concentration. This biochemical abnormality has served as the basis of a diagnostic test for cystic fibrosis called a *sweat test*. A small quantity of sweat is collected, and the sodium and chloride concentrations are determined. The salt concentration of the sweat is low in normal persons and high in persons with cystic fibrosis.

Many cystic fibrosis patients need to take capsules containing pancreatic enzymes in order to digest and absorb food properly because their own pancreas has been destroyed by the disease. Various types of treatment are also used to preserve as much pulmonary function as possible. Pulmonary infections caused by antibiotic-resistant bacteria are a serious problem and are difficult to deal with. Lungs so severely damaged by repeated infections that they can no longer function effectively can be treated by lung transplants.

# Diabetes Mellitus

The most important disease of the endocrine pancreas is **diabetes mellitus**, which results either because the pancreatic islets are incapable of secreting sufficient insulin or because the insulin is not being utilized efficiently. One of its major manifestations is an elevated level of glucose in the blood, which is called **hyperglycemia** (*hyper* = excess – *glyc* = sweet – *heme* = blood).

Diabetes is divided into two major groups, depending on whether the diabetes results primarily from insulin deficiency, which is called *type 1 diabetes*, or from an inadequate response to insulin, which is called *type 2 diabetes*. Previously, type 1 diabetes was called insulin-dependent diabetes or juvenile-onset diabetes because it resulted from insulin deficiency and often occurred in children and teenagers. Type 2 diabetes was called non-insulin–dependent diabetes or adult-onset diabetes because the islets produced insulin and the diabetes typically occurred in older adults. The two types of

**diabetes mellitus** (dī-u-bē′tēz mel′lit-is) A metabolic disease characterized by hyperglycemia and caused by insufficient insulin secretion or inefficient utilization of insulin.

**hyperglycemia** (hī-per-glī-sē′mi-uh) Excessively high blood glucose concentration.

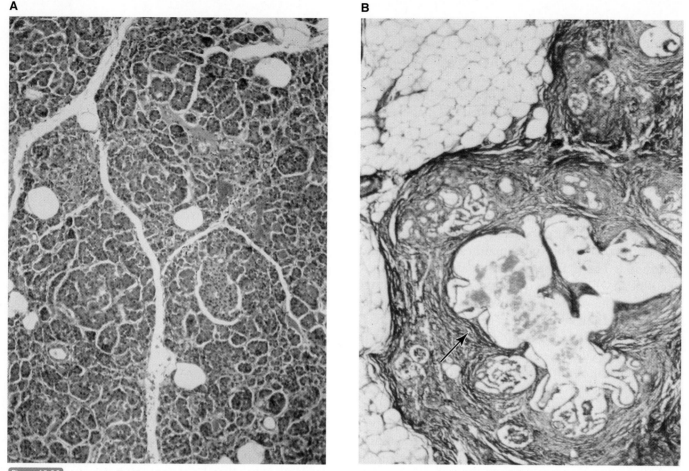

**Figure 16-28** Low-magnification photomicrographs comparing normal pancreas (**A**) with pancreas of patient with cystic fibrosis (**B**). Duct in center of field (*arrow*) exhibits cystic dilatation. Most of pancreatic glandular tissue has undergone atrophy and has been replaced by fibrous tissue (original magnification × 25).

diabetes are not restricted to the age groups implied by this terminology, however, and these terms are used less frequently now. **Table 16-2** compares the major features of the two types.

## Type 1 Diabetes Mellitus

Type 1 diabetes is an autoimmune disease in which cytotoxic and delayed hypersensitivity T lymphocytes attack and destroy the pancreatic islets, assisted by autoantibodies directed against islet cells. The rate at which islets are destroyed by the immune system and the rate at which insulin secretion declines vary among affected subjects. In some, islet cell destruction proceeds rapidly, and in others, the destruction occurs more slowly. In some cases, onset of diabetes follows a viral infection, suggesting that the virus may have induced the disease by injuring or destroying the islets. Type 1 diabetes occurs primarily in children and young

| **Table 16-2** | **Comparison of the Two Major Types of Diabetes Mellitus** | |
|---|---|---|
| | Type 1 | Type 2 |
| Usual age of onset | Childhood<br>Young adulthood | Middle age or later |
| Body build | Normal | Overweight |
| Plasma insulin | Absent or low | Normal or high |
| Complications | Ketoacidosis | Hyperosmolar coma |
| Response to insulin | Normal | Reduced |
| Response to oral antidiabetic drugs | Unresponsive | Responsive |

adults, and affected subjects are prone to develop a condition called **diabetic ketosis** caused by a lack of insulin. There is a hereditary predisposition to type 1 diabetes. Persons who inherit certain HLA-D types are at increased risk of acquiring this type of diabetes. (HLA types and predisposition to disease were considered in Chapter 2.)

## Type 2 Diabetes Mellitus

Type 2 diabetes is by far the more common type and is a more complex metabolic defect. The pancreatic islets secrete normal or increased amounts of insulin, but the tissues are relatively insensitive to the action of insulin and are unable to respond appropriately. (Inadequate response to insulin is called *insulin resistance*.) The condition develops most frequently in older overweight and obese adults. The reason for the impaired response to insulin is not completely understood, but it seems to be related in some way to obesity because weight reduction restores insulin responsiveness and frequently controls the diabetes. Ketosis does not usually occur as a complication of type 2 diabetes, but affected persons may develop another complication called **hyperosmolar coma**, which results from the marked hyperglycemia.

Although insulin resistance plays an important role in the pathogenesis of type 2 diabetes, islet cell function is not completely normal either, because the pancreas is unable to increase insulin output sufficiently to compensate for the insulin resistance.

Type 2 diabetes is a hereditary disease in which genetic factors play an even greater role than in type 1

diabetes, although in most cases we do not know the exact mode of inheritance or the genes that predispose to this type of diabetes. Children of parents who have type 2 diabetes are at significant risk of also eventually becoming diabetic. In some population groups, such as the Pima Indians of Arizona, as many as 40 percent of adults are diabetic.

## Pregnancy-Associated Diabetes

As described in Chapter 14, the high levels of placental hormones in pregnancy cause the pregnant woman to become less responsive to insulin (develop insulin resistance) but most women can compensate by secreting more insulin and the blood glucose does not rise excessively. However, some women are unable to secrete enough additional insulin, and they develop pregnancy-related diabetes caused by their insulin resistance. The condition is called **gestational diabetes**, and is treated by diet along with supplementary insulin if necessary because hyperglycemia is harmful to the developing fetus. Although blood glucose returns to normal after delivery, a woman who has demonstrated significant insulin resistance during pregnancy is at risk of developing permanent diabetes in later years. Pregnancy-related diabetes serves as a "wake-up call"

**diabetic ketosis**
A disturbance of the body's acid–base balance (acidosis) caused by an inability to utilize glucose, which requires the body to use fat as an energy source. Fat metabolism generates excessive amounts of acid ketone bodies, which disrupts the normal alkalinity of body fluids.

**hyperosmolar coma** (hī-per-oz-mō´lär) Coma resulting from neurologic dysfunction caused by hyperosmolarity of body fluids as a consequence of severe hyperglycemia.

**gestational diabetes**
Elevated blood glucose caused by insulin resistance resulting from elevated hormones related to the pregnancy. Blood glucose returns to normal postpartum, but woman has increased risk of diabetes later in life.

to begin taking steps that may avoid later permanent hyperglycemia: by eating a healthy diet, controlling weight, being active, and exercising moderately. A program of this type helps maintain normal blood glucose without promoting excessive insulin secretion, which helps preserve pancreatic beta cell function.

## Diabetes and the Metabolic Syndrome

The term **metabolic syndrome**, also called the *insulin resistance syndrome*, is a group of conditions that often are identified in persons with impaired glucose tolerance or type 2 diabetes, and which can progress to diabetes-associated complications as well as cardiovascular disease and its complications. The metabolic syndrome components include:

1. Obesity, especially when much of the excess fat accumulates in the abdomen
2. Insulin resistance, characterized by high-normal or elevated blood glucose
3. Blood lipid abnormalities that predispose to cardiovascular disease (described in Chapter 10), which is called dyslipidemia
4. Hypertension

Overweight people with excess abdominal fat, as indicated by their waist circumference, should be screened for the other conditions associated with the syndrome by measuring blood pressure, blood glucose, and blood lipids. If other metabolic syndrome-associated abnormalities are detected, treatment to correct or improve the associated conditions can be undertaken.

# Actions of Insulin on Metabolic Processes

Insulin has multiple effects that influence not only carbohydrate metabolism, but protein and fat metabolism as well. The chief sites of insulin action are on liver cells, muscle, and adipose tissue (fat). Insulin promotes entry of glucose into cells and favors utilization of glucose as a source of energy. In muscle and liver cells, it promotes storage of glucose as glycogen. In adipose tissue, insulin favors the conversion of glucose into fat (triglyceride) and storage of the newly formed triglyceride within the fat cells. Insulin also promotes entry of amino acids into the cells and stimulates protein synthesis. The main stimulus for insulin release is elevation of the level of glucose in the blood, as occurs after a meal.

## Fat Metabolism and Formation of Ketone Bodies

When fat is metabolized as a source of energy, it is split first into fatty acids and glycerol. The fatty acids are broken down into two carbon fragments, which are combined with a large carrier molecule called *coenzyme A (CoA)*. The combination is called **acetyl coenzyme A** or *acetyl-CoA*. Some of the acetyl-CoA molecules are normally converted by the liver into compounds called ketone bodies: acetoacetic acid, beta-hydroxybutyric acid, and acetone, as illustrated in Figure 16-29.

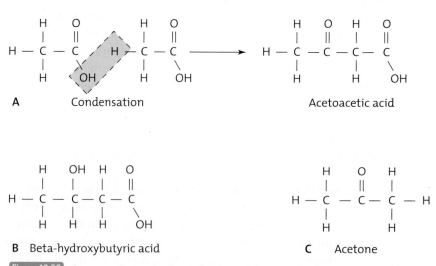

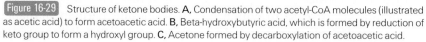

**Figure 16-29** Structure of ketone bodies. **A,** Condensation of two acetyl-CoA molecules (illustrated as acetic acid) to form acetoacetic acid. **B,** Beta-hydroxybutyric acid, which is formed by reduction of keto group to form a hydroxyl group. **C,** Acetone formed by decarboxylation of acetoacetic acid.

# Biochemical Disturbances in Diabetes

In diabetes mellitus, glucose is absorbed normally. However, because of lack of insulin or insulin insensitivity, it is not used normally for energy and is not stored normally as glycogen. Consequently, it accumulates in the bloodstream, resulting in a high level of blood glucose (hyperglycemia). The excessive glucose "spills over" in the urine and is excreted. Because glucose must be excreted in the urine in solution, the body loses excessive amounts of water and electrolytes along with the glucose. This may lead to disturbance in water balance and acid–base balance. (Water and electrolyte balance are discussed in Chapter 19.)

**Diabetic Ketoacidosis**  The person with type 1 diabetes, lacking insulin, is unable to use carbohydrates because insulin is required to promote entry of glucose into the cells where the glucose can be metabolized to yield energy. So the body turns to fat as an energy source. Body fat is split into long-chain fatty acid molecules and glycerol. The fatty acids are broken down by enzymes into two carbon (*acetyl*) fragments, which are joined to coenzyme A to form *acetyl coenzyme A* (acetyl-CoA), but the acetyl-CoA molecules are produced in such large quantities that they cannot be oxidized efficiently to yield energy. Many of the acetyl-CoA molecules condense to form *ketone bodies*, which can

be used as an energy source, but so many ketone bodies are produced that the body can't deal effectively with the excess. This condition is called **ketosis**. The ketone bodies accumulate in the blood and are excreted in the urine, carrying with them more water and electrolytes. The acid ketone bodies can be buffered to some extent by the bicarbonate buffer systems in the bloodstream. If the diabetes is extremely severe, however, so many ketone bodies may be produced that the buffer systems cannot maintain a normal blood pH, and *diabetic acidosis* develops. The term *ketoacidosis* is often used for this type of acidosis because of its relationship to overproduction of ketone bodies. Severe acidosis may lead to coma because acidosis has an adverse effect on cerebral function.

All these effects can be reversed by supplying insulin, which promotes normal utilization of glucose and storage of glycogen. The disturbances of fat and protein metabolism also are reversed by the action of insulin. Figure 16-30 summarizes the major metabolic disturbances in type 1 diabetes.

The following case illustrates the clinical and biochemical disturbances in severe diabetic ketoacidosis.

**acetyl coenzyme A** (acetyl-CoA) A combination of a two-carbon acetate fragment with a complex organic compound called coenzyme A.

**ketosis** (kē-tō′sis) An excess of ketone bodies (acetoacetic acid, beta-hydroxybutyric acid, and acetone) in the blood resulting from utilization of fat as the primary source of energy.

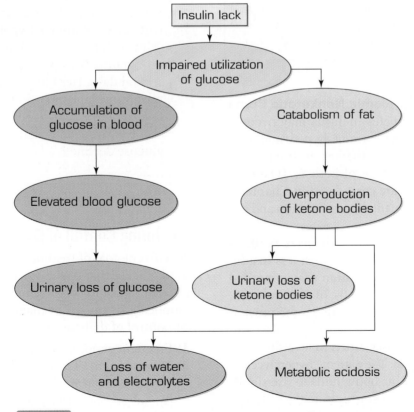

**Figure 16-30**  Major metabolic derangements in type 1 diabetes mellitus.

## Case Study 16-3

A middle-aged woman with diabetes became unconscious while babysitting and was brought to the hospital by ambulance. Her temperature was moderately elevated. Respirations were rapid and deep. Blood pressure was normal. The patient was comatose but responded to painful stimuli. The skin was warm and dry. The remainder of the physical signs was normal. The patient's urine contained large amounts of glucose and a small amount of albumin. There was a strongly positive reaction for acetone and other ketone bodies. Blood glucose was 865 mg/dL (normal range 70–110 mg/dL). Other laboratory studies revealed a low blood pH and reduced plasma bicarbonate of 8 mEq/L (normal range 24–28 mEq/L). The patient was considered to have severe diabetic acidosis probably precipitated by a respiratory infection. She received intensive treatment with intravenous fluids, insulin, and antibiotics. Her condition gradually improved. The following day she was conscious and oriented and was able to take fluids orally. She continued to improve and was eventually discharged from the hospital on a diabetic diet and supplementary insulin therapy.

**Hyperosmolar Hyperglycemic Nonketotic Coma**
Persons with type 2 diabetes mellitus may become comatose as a result of the extreme hyperosmolarity (concentration) of body fluids that results from severe hyperglycemia in the absence of ketosis. (Osmotic pressure and osmolarity are considered in Chapter 2 in connection with movement of materials into and out of cells.)

Although individuals with type 2 diabetes exhibit a reduced responsiveness to insulin, much less insulin is required to inhibit fat mobilization than is needed to promote entry of glucose into cells. In these subjects, the response to insulin is usually sufficient to prevent ketosis but inadequate to prevent hyperglycemia. Consequently, blood glucose rises, often to levels that are from 10 to 20 times normal. The extreme hyperglycemia causes the osmolarity of the body fluids to rise significantly, and water moves by osmosis from the cells into the more concentrated extracellular fluids. The cells become dehydrated, which disturbs the function of neurons and causes coma. Treatment consists of supplying insulin to reduce the hyperglycemia and administering hypotonic fluids to help reduce the hyperosmolarity of the body fluids, as illustrated by the following case.

## Case Study 16-4

A 52-year-old woman who was not previously known to be diabetic had experienced increased urinary output and thirst for the previous 2 weeks and had consumed large quantities of sugar-containing soft drinks. She became progressively more confused and eventually lapsed into coma. She was found by a neighbor and was brought to the hospital by ambulance. On admission she was comatose and dehydrated. Her respiratory rate was not increased. Blood pressure was normal. The urine contained a large amount of glucose but no ketone bodies. Blood pH and bicarbonate were normal. Blood glucose was 1750 mg/dL (normal range 70–110 mg/dL), and the osmolarity of the plasma was 396 mOsm/L (normal range 280–295 mOsm/L). A diagnosis of hyperosmolar nonketotic coma was made, and she was treated with large volumes of hypotonic (0.45 percent) saline solution and with insulin. Her condition gradually improved over the succeeding several days. Her blood glucose gradually fell toward normal and eventually reached 150 mg/dL on the fourth day. Plasma osmolarity also returned to normal as the elevated blood glucose declined.

## Monitoring Control of Diabetes

The current goal of treatment is to achieve control of blood glucose that is as close as possible to normal, as close control of hyperglycemia reduces the long-term complications caused by diabetes. Tests used to monitor control of diabetes include:

1. Frequent periodic measurements of blood glucose.
2. Measurement of a compound in the blood called *glycosylated hemoglobin*, also called hemoglobin $A_{1C}$ (abbreviated $HbA_{1C}$), which is used as an index of long-term control of hyperglycemia.

3. Urine tests for glucose previously were performed frequently to monitor blood glucose indirectly by detecting glucose spilling into the urine when blood glucose was too high, but are not used very often now because they have been replaced by frequent blood glucose tests. However, urine tests are still used in special situations, such as to check for ketone bodies as an indication of diabetic ketosis in persons with type 1 diabetes.

Blood tests can be performed by the diabetic at home or at work. Blood testing products permit diabetics to monitor their own blood glucose at frequent intervals. A drop of blood is drawn by a sterile disposable lancet, collected on a specially treated strip of paper, and inserted into an instrument that displays the glucose concentration.

The glycosylated hemoglobin test is a more complex test that must be done by a medical laboratory but is only necessary every 3 to 6 months. The test monitors how well the blood glucose is being controlled by treatment. Normally a small amount of blood glucose becomes permanently attached to hemoglobin. This glucose–hemoglobin complex is called **glycosylated hemoglobin**, and its concentration is directly proportional to the average blood glucose concentration over the preceding 6 to 12 weeks, unlike the blood glucose test, which only indicates the concentration of blood glucose at the time the sample was collected. In normal persons up to 6 percent of hemoglobin is glycosylated. In persons with very poorly controlled diabetes, the concentration is higher. Diabetics in whom blood glucose levels have been closely controlled can achieve glycosylated hemoglobin levels that are close to normal. Higher levels indicate less satisfactory control of blood glucose and indicate a need for more intensive treatment. In general, the better the long-term control of blood glucose, as indicated by a close to normal glycosylated hemoglobin value, the less likely the development of long-term late diabetic complications.

## Treatment of Diabetes

Treatment of diabetes consists of a diet in which carbohydrate intake is controlled. Type 1 diabetics also require insulin, and the dose should be adjusted in order to control the level of blood glucose as closely as possible. Most type 1 diabetics require several insulin injections spaced throughout the day in order to maintain blood glucose within reasonably normal limits.

Insulin pumps are sometimes useful for type 1 diabetics who are difficult to treat because of their need for frequent insulin injections. An insulin pump is a small battery-operated device that can be attached to the patient's belt. A short length of tubing extends from the pump to a fine (27-gauge) needle that is inserted into the subcutaneous tissue of the abdominal wall and secured with tape. The pump is programmed to deliver a small constant infusion of insulin, supplemented by larger doses just before meals, simulating the release of insulin by the pancreas.

Type 2 diabetic patients can often be managed by diet and weight reduction alone. If they do not respond adequately, oral hypoglycemic drugs are added. Many of these drugs act by promoting the release of insulin from pancreatic islets, and they are only useful for treating type 2 diabetes. If diet, weight reduction, and hypoglycemic drugs don't control the hyperglycemia, insulin is used to regulate blood glucose in the same way that it is used in type 1 diabetes.

**glycosylated hemoglobin** (gli-ko´-sil-ay-ted) Hemoglobin to which glucose molecules have become permanently attached. Concentration is related to concentration of glucose in the blood.

## Complications of Diabetes

Diabetics are liable to develop a number of complications that can be reduced to some extent by proper adherence to diet and other prescribed treatments. They have an *increased susceptibility to infection*, apparently related to the high levels of blood glucose. Pathogenic bacteria seem to grow more readily in the presence of elevated blood glucose levels. They may develop *diabetic coma*, as a result either of *ketoacidosis* or of *the greatly increased osmolarity of body fluids* resulting from hyperglycemia. They have a greater incidence of *arteriosclerosis* and its associated vascular complications such as strokes, heart attacks, and gangrene of the legs and feet as a result of poor circulation. The vascular problems probably result both from abnormalities in fat metabolism associated with diabetes and from the elevated blood lipids frequently found in diabetics. They are also subject to other late complications, which increase in frequency with the duration of the disease. The small blood vessels supplying the retina of the eye often undergo degenerative changes, which may eventually lead to *blindness* in some subjects. The glomerular arterioles and capillaries within the kidneys also undergo degenerative changes, which impair renal function and may result in *renal failure* (Chapter 15). The peripheral nerves may undergo degenerative changes, called *peripheral neuritis*, which cause pain and disturbed sensation in the extremities.

## Other Causes of Hyperglycemia

Other conditions at times may lead to impaired glucose utilization and hyperglycemia, but they are much less common than true diabetes mellitus. These conditions include the following:

1. Chronic pancreatic disease, in which the hyperglycemia results from damage or destruction of pancreatic islets
2. Endocrine diseases associated with overproduction of pituitary or adrenal hormones because these hormones act in various ways to raise blood glucose
3. Ingestion of many different drugs, such as diuretics or antihypertensive drugs, in which glucose utilization is impaired as a side effect of the drug

# Hypoglycemia

The normal pancreas continually monitors the blood glucose and automatically adjusts its output of insulin to maintain the blood glucose level within the normal range. The type 1 diabetic patient, however, must adjust the dose of insulin to match the amount of carbohydrate to be metabolized. If there is insufficient insulin, the blood glucose is too high. If there is too much insulin, the blood glucose is too low, a condition called *hypoglycemia* (*hypo* = under). Two conditions predispose to hypoglycemia in a diabetic patient taking insulin. The first is a reduced intake of food, such as skipping a meal; blood glucose falls because carbohydrate intake is insufficient in relation to the amount of insulin injected. The second condition is increased activity, such as vigorous exercise, which lowers blood glucose by increasing glucose utilization. As a result,

there is a relative excess of insulin. Too much insulin causes a precipitous drop in the level of glucose in the blood and initiates a chain of events called an *insulin reaction*. The adrenal medulla responds to the hypoglycemia by discharging epinephrine (adrenaline), which tends to raise blood glucose by converting liver glycogen into glucose. Epinephrine exerts widespread systemic effects as well: rapid heart rate, rise in blood pressure, constriction of cutaneous blood vessels causing the skin to appear pale, stimulation of sweat glands causing a cold sweat, and stimulation of the nervous system leading to increased excitability, anxiousness, hyperactive reflexes, and tremors.

Neurologic manifestations appear if the blood glucose continues to fall because the nervous system requires glucose to carry out its metabolic processes and begins to malfunction when deprived of its energy source. The subject becomes confused, loses consciousness, may have convulsions, and soon lapses into a deep coma. Prolonged severe hypoglycemia may cause permanent brain damage.

If the patient is still conscious and able to swallow, the insulin reaction can be stopped by ingesting a quick-acting carbohydrate, such as a piece of candy or a glucose tablet.

**Table 16-3** compares the clinical manifestations of insulin shock with those of diabetic ketoacidosis and hyperosmolar nonketotic coma, two other conditions to which the diabetic patient is predisposed.

**Table 16-3**    **Differentiation of Insulin Shock from Ketoacidosis and Hyperosmolar Coma**

| Diagnostic Feature | Insulin Shock | Ketoacidosis | Hyperosmolar Coma |
| --- | --- | --- | --- |
| Food intake | May be insufficient | Normal or excessive | Normal or excessive |
| Insulin | Excessive | Insufficient | Normal or increased |
| Onset of symptoms | Rapid | Gradual (several days) | Gradual (several days) |
| Skin | Cold sweat, pale | Dry and flushed | Dry and flushed |
| Respirations | Normal or shallow | Slow and deep | Usually normal |
| Reflexes | Hyperactive | Depressed | Normal |
| Heart rate | Rapid | Rapid | Usually normal |
| Blood pressure | Normal or slightly elevated | Low | Usually normal |
| Glucose in urine | Absent | Large amount | Large amount |
| Blood glucose | Very low | High | Extremely high |
| Blood bicarbonate and pH | Normal | Low | Normal |
| Acetone in blood and urine | Absent | Present | Absent |

# Tumors of the Pancreas

Carcinoma of the pancreas is relatively common and develops most often in the head of the pancreas. In this location, the neoplasm blocks the common bile duct, resulting in obstructive jaundice. Carcinoma elsewhere in the pancreas is usually far advanced when first detected and produces no specific symptoms.

Sometimes benign tumors arise from the islet cells and produce symptoms as a result of overproduction of hormones. Beta cells give rise to insulin-secreting tumors that cause episodes of severe hypoglycemia similar to those experienced by a diabetic who receives too much insulin.

# CHAPTER REVIEW

## Summary

The liver is the largest organ in the body and performs many important functions. The liver lobule is the basic structural and functional unit. Branches of the hepatic artery, portal vein, and bile duct travel in the portal tracts at the periphery of the lobules. Hepatic artery and portal branches deliver blood into the channels (sinusoids) between the plates of liver cells. From the sinusoids the blood flows into the central veins in the center of the lobules, and from there into the hepatic veins and eventually into the inferior vena. Bile is secreted into small bile channels within the plates of liver cells, flows into larger bile ducts, and is stored in the gallbladder where it is expelled during digestion to mix with pancreatic secretions. Bile consists of bile pigment (bilirubin), a product of red cell breakdown, together with bile salts, lecithin, cholesterol, and other components. Bile functions as a biologic detergent to facilitate fat digestion.

Many conditions can damage liver cells. Common causes include viral hepatitis, alcohol excess, various drugs and toxins, autoimmune diseases that target liver cells, and diseases that obstruct or impede bile flow into the duodenum. Manifestations of liver injury include fatty change in liver cells, liver cell necrosis, or a combination of both conditions. Severe or repeated episodes of liver cell damage may eventually lead to scarring throughout the liver, which is called cirrhosis. The two most common causes of cirrhosis are chronic hepatitis resulting from hepatitis B (HBV) or hepatitis C (HCV) infection, and alcoholic liver disease. Other conditions include biliary cirrhosis caused by an autoimmune disease affecting small bile ducts (primary biliary cirrhosis) or obstruction of larger bile ducts (secondary biliary cirrhosis).

Cirrhosis impairs liver cell function and also disrupts blood flow through the liver. The pressure within the portal system rises, which is followed by accumulation of fluid within the abdominal cavity (ascites) caused by the low serum albumin resulting from the liver disease, and the high portal pressure, which forces more fluid out of the capillaries. The body forms collateral channels to divert blood from the portal system into systemic veins in an attempt lower the pressure in the portal system by diverting some of the portal blood into the systemic venous circulation. One of the venous return pathways are the esophageal veins that become dilated and may rupture, leading to serious life-threatening bleeding. Various surgical methods have been devised to deal with these problems, with variable success.

Gall stones (biliary calculi) may form within the gall bladder, and may be extruded from the gall bladder into the ducts, where they may cause pain (biliary colic) and can also obstruct bile flow through the ducts. Blockage of the common bile duct interrupts bile flow into the duodenum and leads to jaundice. Obstruction of the cystic duct prevents bile storage in the gall bladder but does not impede discharge of bile into the duodenum. Most stones are composed of cholesterol and form when the bile contains more cholesterol than can be held in solution by bile salts and lecithin. The usual treatment for gall stones is to remove the gall bladder, which can be performed by a laparoscopy procedure, and does not require a large surgical incision.

Malignant tumors, either primary or metastatic, may involve the liver. Persons with cirrhosis may develop primary liver cell carcinoma. Deposits of metastatic carcinoma may spread to the liver from carcinoma in other organs, such as colon, lung, or breast.

Jaundice is a common manifestation of liver disease and is classified by its pathogenesis as hemolytic, hepatocellular, or obstructive jaundice. A liver biopsy may help identify the cause of the liver disease when the diagnosis is uncertain.

The pancreas is both an exocrine and endocrine gland. The exocrine cells secrete potent digestive enzymes. The two important hormones secreted by the pancreatic islets are insulin, which lowers blood glucose (beta cells), and glucagon, which raises blood glucose (alpha cells).

The two important diseases of the exocrine pancreas are pancreatitis, and cystic fibrosis of the pancreas. Acute hemorrhagic pancreatitis is a very serious disease. It results from escape of activated enzymes from ruptured ducts caused by duct obstruction, resulting in extensive destruction of the pancreas and associated hemorrhage from damaged pancreatic blood vessels. Chronic pancreatitis results from repeated bouts of less severe pancreatic damage that over time leads to progressive loss of pancreatic digestive enzymes. The other serious pancreatic disease is cystic fibrosis of the pancreas, an autosomal recessive disease caused by a gene mutation affecting transport of salt and water across cell membranes. The result is thick mucus secretion by pancreatic duct epithelium that blocks pancreatic ducts, leading to cystic distention of blocked ducts along with atrophy and fibrosis of pancreatic secretory tissue. Sometimes the fibrosis surrounding the pancreatic islets also disturbs islet cell function to such an extent that diabetes develops. Mucus plugs block bronchioles and predispose to repeated bouts of pulmonary infection, which slowly damages the lungs. Similar mucus plugs blocking bile ducts lead to scarring in liver tissue as well. Sweat gland function is also disturbed. The salt concentration in sweat is much higher than normal, which serves as a diagnostic test for the disease. The severity of the disease varies among affected persons, but long-term prognosis is relatively poor despite intensive treatment.

Diabetes is the other pancreatic disease that targets the pancreatic islets and causes hyperglycemia. Type 1 diabetes is an autoimmune-mediated destruction of islets with loss of insulin secretion. Affected subjects require insulin and are subject to ketoacidosis caused by failure to take enough insulin to metabolize carbohydrates efficiently. Type 2 diabetes results because the tissues don't respond appropriately to insulin, which is called insulin resistance. The pancreas secretes a large amount of insulin, but this may not be enough to overcome the insulin resistance, and eventually the pancreatic islet function begins to fail. Obesity contributes to the insulin resistance, and weight loss may restore blood glucose to normal. Both types of diabetes are associated with both immediate and long-term complications, and both can be reduced by good control of the diabetes. However, excessively tight control of blood glucose may lead to hypoglycemia, which leads to a different set of problems.

The hormones secreted by the placenta in pregnancy lead to insulin resistance, and some pregnant women may not be able to increase their insulin output enough to overcome the insulin resistance, and blood glucose rises. The condition is called pregnancy-associated diabetes and requires treatment because hyperglycemia is harmful to the fetus. Glucose returns to normal after delivery, but the affected woman has an increased risk of developing diabetes later in life.

The metabolic syndrome is a group of manifestations related to insulin resistance, which includes obesity, and other associated abnormalities that contribute to cardiovascular disease and require treatment.

Pancreatic carcinoma is a serious disease with a relatively poor prognosis because the disease is often far advanced before it produces symptoms. The islet cells also give rise to insulin-secreting tumors that may cause hypoglycemia.

## Questions for Review

1. What are some of the principal functions of the liver? How does the blood supply to the liver differ from that to the other organs? Why does severe liver disease cause disturbances in blood clotting?

2. What is the difference between hemoglobin and bilirubin? How does conjugated bilirubin differ from unconjugated bilirubin? What is the difference between bilirubin and bile? What role does bile play in digestion?

3. What are the possible causes and effects of liver injury? What is the usual outcome of a liver injury?

4. What is viral hepatitis? What are its major symptoms? How is hepatitis transmitted?

5. What is the difference between hepatitis A and hepatitis B?

6. What effect does alcohol have on the liver? What types of liver disease are associated with excessive alcohol ingestion?

7. What is cirrhosis? What liver diseases may lead to cirrhosis? Why does portal hypertension develop in patients with cirrhosis? Why do ascites develop in patients with cirrhosis? Why do esophageal varices develop?

8. What is jaundice? How is jaundice classified? Under what circumstances do gallstones cause jaundice?

9. What factors predispose to the development of gallstones?

10. What is the difference between viral hepatitis and alcoholic "hepatitis"?

11. What is the difference between acute and chronic pancreatitis?

12. What are the major metabolic disturbances in type 1 diabetes? How does insulin correct these disturbances?

13. What are the major complications of diabetes?

14. Which type of diabetes can be treated by diet alone?

15. What is meant by the following terms: *sweat test*, *hyperosmolar nonketotic hyperglycemic coma*, *ketoacidosis*, and *ketone bodies*?

16. What is cystic fibrosis of the pancreas? What are its clinical manifestations? What is its pattern of inheritance?

17. What is hypoglycemia? What are its clinical manifestations? How is it treated?

18. What are the major differences between diabetic ketoacidosis and insulin shock?

## Supplementary Reading

Abrahamson, M. J. 2007. A 74-year-old woman with diabetes. *Journal of the American Medical Association* 297:197–204.

A case-based discussion emphasizing that the metabolic disorder affects over 20 million people in the United States, of which 90 percent have type 2 diabetes. The basic disturbance is insulin resistance associated with impaired beta cell insulin production. In most persons who develop diabetes the insulin resistance progresses for many years before type 2 diabetes finally results. Treatment with oral medications that stimulate insulin secretion by beta cells is effective but supplementary insulin is needed by many patients to control the hyperglycemia. Oral drugs that act by promoting insulin secretion may hasten the failure of beta cell function.

American Diabetes Association. 2000. Type 2 diabetes in children and adolescents. *Pediatrics* 105:671–80.

A review of current concepts. Type 2 diabetes is becoming more frequent in this age group, related primarily to obesity. Children with type 2 diabetes usually have a family history of diabetes, and those of non-European ancestry are disproportionately represented.

Beckman, J. A., Creager, M. A., and Libby, P. 2002. Diabetes and atherosclerosis: Epidemiology, pathophysiology, and management. *Journal of the American Medical Association* 287:2570–81.

The prevalence of type 2 diabetes in children and in the developing nations is rising substantially. Most patients with diabetes die of the complications of atherosclerosis.

Boyle, M. P. 2007. Adult cystic fibrosis. *Journal of the American Medical Association* 298:1787–93.

New methods of treatment and emphasis on nutritional support have greatly increased the survival of patients with cystic fibrosis, and have also documented a number of mild cases that survive into middle age. The article describes principles of diagnosis and treatment, and describes the various complications resulting from the disease. The author suggests that the disease should be considered in adult patients presenting with any one of three conditions: bronchiectasis, chronic sinusitis with nasal polyps, or infertility in males. The value of the sweat test for screening is emphasized. The effectiveness of current treatment is illustrated by a 52-year-old man with cystic fibrosis who had few health or activity-limiting problems until his 40s.

Callery, M. P., and Freedman, S. D. 2008. A 21-year-old man with chronic pancreatitis. *Journal of the American Medical Association* 299:2589–94.

Evaluation and treatment of chronic pancreatitis is considered based on the case history of a young man with pancreatitis having its onset at age 11 and recurring periodically. Causes and methods of treatment are discussed, including a rather limited role of surgical treatment. Some uncommon cases are caused by gene mutations, one of which is a different mutation of the same gene responsible for cystic fibrosis. Pancreatitis may also be a manifestation of an autoimmune disease targeting pancreatic tissue.

Centers for Disease Control and Prevention. 1993. Hepatitis E among U.S. travelers. *Morbidity and Mortality Weekly Report* 42:1–4.

Hepatitis E outbreaks in third world countries are related to contaminated water supplies. Although the infection is not established in the United States, a few cases have been reported, and cases of hepatitis E may become more frequent among residents of states at the U.S.–Mexico border. Gamma globulin does not contain anti-HEV antibodies; thus gamma globulin does not provide protection against infection.

Hoofnagel, J. H., and Seeff, L. B. 2006. Peginterferon and ribavirin for chronic hepatitis C. *New England Journal of Medicine* 355:2444–51.

Hepatitis C is often silent and most infected patients have few symptoms of infection. Persisting infection leads to cirrhosis in 20 to 30 percent of infected patients, and from 1 to 4 percent of patients with cirrhosis also develop hepatocellular carcinoma each year. Liver cell injury in infected patients results from activation of the immune system in which natural killer cells and cytotoxic T cells attempt to eliminate the virus-infected liver cells. Hepatitis C progresses more rapidly in HIV infected persons. Treatment is recommended for all subjects with detectable hepatitis C viral RNA in their bloodstream, elevation of serum enzyme levels indicating liver damage, and a positive liver biopsy indicating the characteristics and the severity of the liver cell injury. A 48-week course of treatment consists of weekly subcutaneous injection of pegylated interferon (a long-acting interferon produced by attaching polyethylene glycol to the interferon molecule) and twice daily oral doses of ribavirin. Unfortunately, the course of therapy has a high rate of side effects.

Isselbacher, K. J. 1977. Metabolic and hepatic effects of alcohol. *New England Journal of Medicine* 296:612–16.

Describes the metabolism of alcohol by the liver and effects of alcohol on carbohydrate, protein, and fat metabolism. Describes alcohol-related disorders.

Kaplan, M. M, and Gershwin, M. E. 2005. Primary biliary cirrhosis. *New England Journal of Medicine* 353:1261–73.

Long-term outcome of this autoimmune disease has improved in recent years. Autoimmune damage to the liver appears to be related to antibodies directed against a bacterial or viral antigen that cross-reacts with similar antigens within liver cell mitochondria, and such antibodies are considered diagnostic of the disease. Treatment with a bile acid (ursodeoxycholic acid) appears promising.

Krawitt, E. L. 2006. Autoimmune hepatitis. *New England Journal of Medicine* 354:54–66.

Another autoimmune disease that appears to be caused by antibodies formed as a result of a viral infection in which antiviral antibodies cross-react with similar antigens in liver cells. Has many features similar to primary biliary cirrhosis and the two conditions may be related.

Lauer, G. M., and Walker, B. 2001. Hepatitis C virus infection. *New England Journal of Medicine* 345:41–52.

A review of the current status of the disease and methods of treatment. In the United States, 1.8 percent of the population is positive for HCV antibodies, and 75 percent of seropositive persons have circulating virus in their bloodstream, indicating active HCV infection.

Ludwig, D. S., and Ebbeling, C. B. 2001. Type 2 diabetes mellitus in children. *Journal of the American Medical Association* 286:1427–30.

In prior years, type 2 diabetes occurred primarily in older overweight adults, and type 1 diabetes occurred in children and young adults. Now, as many as half the new cases of diabetes in children are classified as type 2, which is related to the increasing prevalence of overweight children. Insulin resistance related to overweight causes the pancreas to secrete more insulin, eventually leading to failure of beta-cell function. Many factors have contributed to childhood obesity and its most serious complication, which is type 2 diabetes.

Mokdad, A. H., Bowman, B. A., and Ford, E. S. 2001. The continuing epidemic of obesity and diabetes in the United States. *Journal of the American Medical Association* 286:1195–200.

As body mass index rises, so does the prevalence of type 2 diabetes.

Navarro, V. J., and Senior, J. R. 2006. Drug-related hepatotoxicity. *New England Journal of Medicine* 354:731–39.

Describes and classifies hepatotoxic drugs based on their clinical presentation and approaches to treatment. Acetaminophen is a commonly encountered hepatotoxin.

Seef, L. B., et al. 2000. Forty-five-year follow-up of hepatitis C virus infection in healthy young adults. *Annals of Internal Medicine* 132:105–11.

The rate of HCV infection was determined from reexamination of frozen serum specimens collected from military recruits between 1948 and 1954 and revealed a 0.1 percent infection rate in whites and a 1.8 percent infection rate in African Americans. A 45-year follow-up revealed that liver disease occurred in 11.8 percent of HCV-positive persons and 2.4 percent of HCV-negative persons. One HCV-positive person died of liver disease. Healthy HCV-positive persons are at low risk of progressing to end-stage chronic liver disease.

Steffen, R., Kane, M. A., Shapiro, C. N., et al. 1994. Epidemiology and prevention of hepatitis A in travelers. *Journal of the American Medical Association* 272:885–89.

Hepatitis A vaccine (or gamma globulin if vaccine not available) is recommended for all nonimmune travelers visiting developing countries.

# Interactive Activities: Liver and Biliary System

## Matching 1

Match the disease or condition in the left column with its most likely result of the condition or the condition with which it is associated in the right column.

| Disease or Condition | Result or Response to the Condition |
|---|---|
| 1. Reye's syndrome | A. Occurs frequently in persons with cirrhosis |
| 2. Excess alcohol consumption | B. Primary biliary cirrhosis |
| 3. Autoimmune disease involving the liver | C. Carcinoma of colon |
| 4. Primary carcinoma of liver | D. Bile contains excess cholesterol |
| 5. Metastatic carcinoma within liver | E. Virus infection treated with aspirin |
| 6. Cholelithiasis | F. Calculus passing through bile duct |
| 7. Biliary colic | G. Fatty liver with inflammation and Mallory bodies |
| 8. Pancreatic carcinoma blocks common bile duct | H. Obstructive (secondary) biliary cirrhosis |

## Matching 2

Match the disease or condition in the left column with its manifestations or characteristic features in the right column.

| Disease or Condition | Manifestations or Characteristic Features |
|---|---|
| 1. Type 1 diabetes | A. Hyperglycemia despite increased insulin secretion, often related to obesity |
| 2. Type 2 diabetes | B. Ketosis |
| 3. Pregnancy-associated diabetes | C. Increased long-term risk of diabetes |
| 4. Complication of type 1 diabetes | D. High blood pressure (hypertension) |
| 5. Complication of type 2 diabetes | E. Autoimmunity-related islet cell destruction |
| 6. Long-term effect of pregnancy-associated diabetes | F. Insulin resistance caused by placental hormones |
| 7. Carcinoma of pancreas blocking common bile duct | G. Jaundice |
| 8. Feature associated with the metabolic syndrome | H. Coma caused by increased osmolarity of body fluids |

## True or False

Indicate whether the following statements are true or false by writing T or F at the end of the statement.

1. The infectious particle in the blood of persons with HBV infection is HBV surface antigen.____

2. Most HCV-infected persons are unable to eradicate the virus and become chronic carriers of the virus.____

3. Many HCV-infected persons do not show manifestations of their infection. They are asymptomatic.____

4. Primary biliary cirrhosis is an autoimmune disease in which the autoantibody is directed against bile duct epithelial cells.____

5. Secondary biliary cirrhosis is caused by long-standing obstruction of the common bile duct.____

6. Cholesterol causes cirrhosis.____

7. A gallstone blocking the cystic duct causes jaundice.____

8. Bile contains fat-digesting enzymes that facilitate fat absorption.____

9. The high pressure in the portal venous system in persons with cirrhosis leads to formation of connections between the portal and systemic circulation in an attempt to lower the pressure.____

10. In most cases of HCV infection, the virus was transmitted to the infected person by virus-contaminated food or water.____

11. Cystic fibrosis of the pancreas is transmitted as a Mendelian dominant trait.____

12. Type 2 diabetes is associated with increased insulin secretion by the pancreas.____

13. The metabolic syndrome is characterized by obesity, high-normal or elevated blood glucose, blood lipid abnormalities that predispose to cardiovascular disease, and hypertension.____

14. With proper treatment most persons with cystic fibrosis of the pancreas have a normal life expectancy.____

15. Thick mucus obstructing bronchioles predisposes to pulmonary infections and progressive lung damage in persons with cystic fibrosis.____

16. An insulin-secreting benign tumor of islet cells raises blood glucose._____
17. Ketone bodies are toxic compounds that damage the pancreas._____
18. Hyperglycemia in pregnancy is harmful to the fetus._____

## Critical Thinking

1. John Jones and his male partner frequently engage in sexual activities. John knows that hepatitis B and C, as well as HIV, are transmitted by blood and body fluids, but another partner told him that hepatitis A can also be transmitted by sex acts between partners. He asks for your opinion. If this is true, how can John reduce his risk? What would you tell him?

2. Peter Smith has had a problem for many years with excess alcohol consumption and now has cirrhosis with ascites and dilated esophageal veins. His physician has recommended that he have a procedure performed to connect a branch of the portal vein to a systemic vein in order to lower the portal pressure and reduce his risk of bleeding from a ruptured esophageal vein. He asks you why the dilated esophageal veins (varices) developed and how a procedure could improve the situation. Peter also wants to know if the procedure will cause the scarred liver to return to normal if he stops drinking. What would you tell him?

3. Naomi Foster had a routine medical examination and was essentially normal, but her blood pressure was slightly elevated (140/92). She was moderately overweight but not obese. A group of laboratory tests performed during her examination was normal except for a blood glucose that was slightly elevated (135 mg/dL). Does she have a problem? If so, what is it? What should she do about it?

4. Arnold Foster has a drinking problem, although he does not consider himself to be an alcoholic. He has experienced several episodes of upper abdominal pain, and his doctor told him he has pancreatitis. He is concerned about this diagnosis and wonders whether this is a serious problem and what he should do about it. What would you tell him?

# The Gastrointestinal Tract

## 17

1. Identify the major types of cleft lip and cleft palate deformity.

2. Explain the pathogenesis of dental caries and periodontal disease, and describe prevention and treatment.

3. Name and describe the three most common lesions of the esophagus that lead to esophageal obstruction.

4. Explain the pathogenesis and treatment of peptic ulcer. Describe the major complications of peptic ulcer.

5. Describe the common types of chronic and acute enteritis and their clinical manifestations.

6. Differentiate between appendicitis and Meckel diverticulitis in terms of pathogenesis, clinical manifestations, and treatment.

7. Understand the major disturbances of bowel functioning and the harmful effects of eating disorders on health.

8. Describe the pathogenesis of diverticulitis, and explain the role of diet in development of the lesion.

9. Name the causes, clinical manifestations, and complications of intestinal obstruction, carcinoma of the colon, and diverticulosis of the colon. Explain their treatment.

# Structure and Functions

The gastrointestinal tract, which is concerned with the digestion and absorption of food, comprises the oral cavity and related parts of the face, the esophagus, the stomach, the small and large intestines, and the anus.

# Cleft Lip and Cleft Palate

Embryologically, the face and palate are formed by coalescence of proliferating masses of cells that merge to form the facial structures and to separate the nasal cavity from the mouth. In the upper part of the face, the areas of coalescence are located on either side of the midline in a line that passes through the upper lip and jaw and extends into each nostril. The palate is formed by two shelflike masses of tissue that grow medially and fuse in the midline to close the communication between nose and mouth. If these developmental processes are disturbed, defects may result in the upper lip and jaw (**cleft lip**) or in the palate (**cleft palate**).

Cleft lip and palate are common abnormalities that frequently occur in combination. The incidence of these abnormalities is about 1 per 1000 births. Both cleft lip and cleft palate follow a multifactorial pattern of inheritance (Chapter 7). The incidence is significantly higher among the children of parents who have previously given birth to an infant with a cleft lip or palate and among the children of parents who themselves have a cleft lip or palate. The various types of cleft lip and palate that are encountered clinically are illustrated in Figure 17-1 .

Cleft lip may be unilateral or bilateral and may range in severity from a relatively minor defect in the mucosa of the lip to a large cleft extending deeply into the upper jaw. In the most severe deformity, the cleft extends completely through the upper jaw into the floor of the nose (complete cleft) and may also extend posteriorly into the palate ( Figure 17-2 ).

# Abnormalities of Tooth Development

The teeth are specialized structures developed in the tissues of the jaws. Each tooth consists of a solid portion called **dentine**, which forms the bulk of the tooth; an **enamel** crown covering the exposed surface of the tooth; and a central pulp cavity containing nerve fibers,

**cleft lip** Defect in the upper lip of variable degree, as a result of a developmental disturbance.

**cleft palate** Defect in hard palate allowing communication between oral cavity and nasal cavity, as a result by a developmental disturbance.

**dentine** (den´tēn) Bony structure of the tooth.

**enamel** Dense outer covering of the exposed surface of the tooth.

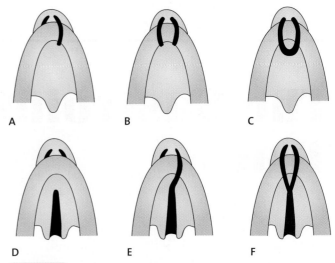

**Figure 17-1** Types of cleft lip and palate abnormalities viewed from below. **A,** A unilateral cleft lip extending into the nose but not extending posteriorly into the palate. **B,** A bilateral cleft lip extending into the nose but not extending into the palate. **C,** A bilateral cleft lip extending into the nose and palate. **D,** A midline cleft palate. **E,** A cleft palate with unilateral cleft lip extending into the nose. **F,** A cleft palate with bilateral cleft lip extending into the nose.

lymphatics, and blood vessels. The root of the tooth, which is embedded in the jaw, is covered by a thin layer of bonelike tissue called cementum, and the tooth is anchored in the jaw by dense connective-tissue fibers.

There are two sets of teeth. The first set, called the *temporary* or *deciduous teeth*, consists of a total of 20 teeth (10 in each jaw) that erupt in childhood. Eventually, these temporary teeth are replaced by a second, permanent set of 32 teeth. When the permanent teeth begin to grow, they press against the roots of the temporary teeth. This causes resorption of the roots and loosening of the temporary teeth, which eventually fall out and are replaced by the permanent teeth.

Each deciduous and permanent tooth develops from a separate tooth bud. The deciduous teeth are formed before birth and erupt during childhood. The permanent teeth do not begin to develop until after birth and erupt at various times in late childhood and adolescence. Calcium is deposited in the dentine and enamel of the tooth as it is being formed.

## Missing Teeth and Extra Teeth

The absence of one or more teeth is relatively common and is often a familial trait that follows a multifactorial pattern of inheritance ( Figure 17-3 ). It results from failure of one or more tooth buds to develop. Sometimes an extra tooth bud forms, resulting in an extra tooth.

## Abnormalities of Tooth Enamel Caused by Tetracycline

Enamel forms within the developing teeth at specific times. If the antibiotic tetracycline is administered while enamel is being formed in the teeth, the antibiotic

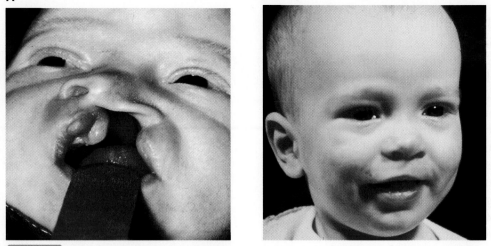

Figure 17-2  **A,** Cleft lip and palate in a 2-week-old infant. **B,** The same child at 14 months of age after surgical correction of the defect.

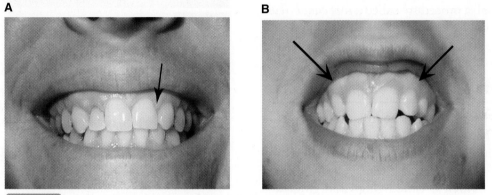

Figure 17-3  Congenital absence of teeth. **A,** Mother lacks the left lateral incisor (*arrow*). Left canine (cuspid) tooth is located lateral to left central incisor. Compare the appearance of the left side with the opposite side in which all teeth are present. **B,** Daughter lacks both lateral incisors. The canine teeth (*arrows*) are adjacent to the central incisors.

is deposited with calcium in the enamel and causes permanent yellow–gray to brown discoloration in the crowns. The antibiotic may also disturb the formation of the enamel. If a tetracycline antibiotic is taken by a pregnant woman, the drug crosses the placenta and enters the fetal circulation, where it becomes incorporated in the enamel of the developing teeth. If administered to infants and children, tetracycline is deposited in the crowns of the permanent teeth that are undergoing enamel formation at the time the antibiotic is ingested. Tetracycline antibiotics should not be given to pregnant women or to infants and children during the time when enamel is forming in the developing permanent teeth. This period extends through infancy and childhood to about the age of 8 years.

# Dental Caries and Its Complications

The oral cavity contains a diverse collection of both aerobic and anaerobic bacteria. Masses of these bacteria intermixed with bacterial products and proteins from saliva form aggregates called **dental plaque** that adhere to the teeth and predispose to tooth decay.

**Caries,** the term for tooth decay, is caused by mouth bacteria acting on bits of retained food material, such as sugar and highly refined, starchy foods. Bacterial fermentation liberates organic acids that erode the covering enamel, exposing the underlying dentine, which is attacked by the acids and invaded by mouth bacteria, which forms a dental cavity. The affected area appears discolored and is quite soft when probed with a dental instrument. Dental x-rays reveal the cavity as an area of decreased density in the affected tooth.

If the cavity is not treated and continues to enlarge, the decay eventually reaches the dental pulp. The bacteria invade the pulp and incite an inflammation that causes the throbbing pain characteristic of a toothache. Unchecked, the infection may spread to the apex of the tooth root, which is embedded in the jawbone, and from there spread to the bone surrounding the dental root. The result may be an abscess surrounding the apex of the tooth.

**dental plaque**
Masses of bacteria, bacterial products, and salivary proteins adherent to teeth, which predisposes to tooth decay.

**caries** (ka´rēz) Tooth decay.

## Prevention and Treatment

The incidence of tooth decay can be reduced by proper mouth hygiene, including frequent brushing of the teeth and use of dental floss to remove food particles that promote bacterial growth. Fluoride added to water supplies and toothpaste helps to prevent cavities by promoting formation of a more acid-resistant tooth structure that resists decay. Dental caries is treated by removing the decayed area and packing the defect with some type of dental filling material. After infection of the pulp and dental root has occurred, more extensive treatment is required. Antibiotics may be needed if there is an acute infection or abscess at the apex of the tooth. After the infection is under control, the entire pulp cavity must be cleaned out and packed with dental filling material, a procedure called a *root canal treatment*. Sometimes the tooth cannot be salvaged and must be extracted.

# Periodontal Disease

Masses of bacteria and debris accumulating around the base of the teeth may incite an inflammation. Initially, the inflammation affects only the gums surrounding the roots of the teeth, which is called *gingivitis* (*gingiva* = gum). Later, the inflammation extends between the teeth and the adjacent gums, leading to the formation of small pockets of infection between the teeth and gums. This condition is called **periodontal disease** (*peri* = around + *dens* = tooth). If pus is discharged from the margins of the infected gums, the descriptive term *pyorrhea* (*pyo* = pus + *rhea* = flow) is often used. The infection may spread into the tooth sockets that anchor the teeth in the jawbone, causing the teeth to loosen and eventually fall out. Various methods of treatment to the gums and teeth may control or arrest the condition, which is an important cause of loss of teeth.

**periodontal disease** (per-i-ō-don´tal) An inflammation of the gums around the roots of the teeth.

# Inflammation of the Oral Cavity

An inflammation of the oral cavity is called *stomatitis* (*stoma* = mouth). It may be caused by a number of irritants and infectious agents. Common irritants are alcohol, tobacco, and hot or spicy foods. Infectious agents include the herpesvirus and some other viruses, the fungus *Candida albicans* (which also causes vaginal infections), and various bacteria.

Canker sores are another relatively common inflammatory disease involving the oral cavity. A canker sore

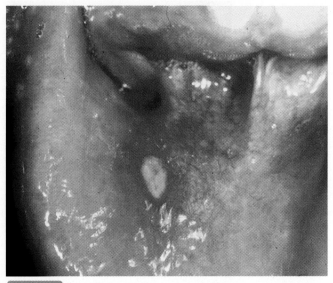

**Figure 17-4** Superficial shallow ulcer of oral mucosa caused by canker sore.

appears as a small painful superficial ulcer of the oral mucosa surrounded by a narrow zone of inflammation that appears as a red border surrounding the ulcer ( Figure 17-4 ). We do not know what causes canker sores, and there is no specific treatment for this condition, although various measures can reduce the discomfort caused by the ulcers.

# Tumors of the Oral Cavity

Carcinoma of the oral cavity, which may arise from the squamous epithelium of the lips, cheek, tongue, palate, or back of the throat, is relatively common ( Figure 17-5 ). It is treated by surgical resection or by radiation therapy.

# Diseases of the Esophagus

The esophagus is a muscular tube extending from the pharynx to the stomach with sphincters at both upper and lower ends. The upper sphincter relaxes to allow passage of swallowed food, which is propelled down the esophagus by rhythmic peristaltic contractions. The lower esophageal sphincter (called the gastroesophageal or cardiac sphincter) relaxes when the food reaches the lower end of the esophagus and allows the food to pass into the stomach. Some of the more important conditions affecting the esophagus include the following:

1. Failure of the lower (cardiac) sphincter to function properly
2. Tears in the lining of the esophagus from retching and vomiting
3. Esophageal obstruction as a result of carcinoma, food impaction, or stricture

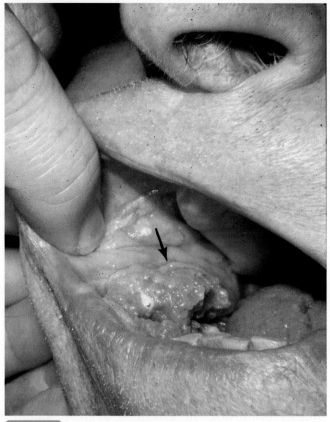

**Figure 17-5** Squamous cell carcinoma of oral mucosa (*arrow*), which appears as an irregular overgrowth of tissue arising from the mucosa of the cheek.

injecting botulinum toxin into the sphincter through an esophagoscope. The toxin blocks the transmission of nerve impulses from the nerve plexuses to the muscle fibers for several months, which relaxes the sphincter and relieves the patient's symptoms.

**Incompetent Cardiac Sphincter and Its Complications** In this relatively common condition, acid gastric juice leaks back into the esophagus through the improperly closed incompetent lower esophageal sphincter. The squamous epithelial lining of the esophagus, which was not "designed" to tolerate high-acid secretions, becomes irritated and inflamed, which is called **reflux esophagitis**. In some patients the squamous mucosal lining may actually become ulcerated and scarred. Sometimes the squamous lining responds to the acidity by undergoing a change (metaplasia) into a more acid-resistant columnar gastric-type mucosa. This condition, which is called **Barrett esophagus** after the person who first described it, may lead to additional problems. Unfortunately, the metaplastic columnar epithelium is frequently abnormal and poses an increased risk of developing adenocarcinoma arising in the abnormal columnar epithelium. Treatment of reflux esophagitis consists of avoiding lying down soon after eating because the recumbent position promotes reflux, sleeping with the head of the bed elevated to minimize reflux, and avoiding alcoholic beverages because alcohol not only stimulates gastric acid secretion but also tends to relax the lower esophageal sphincter, which facilitates reflux. Drugs that reduce secretion of gastric acid and antacids that neutralize gastric acid are helpful.

Symptoms of esophageal disease include difficulty in swallowing together with variable degrees of substernal discomfort or pain. Complete obstruction of the esophagus leads to inability to swallow, which is often associated with regurgitation of food into the trachea, causing episodes of choking and coughing.

## Cardiac Sphincter Dysfunction

The two major disturbances of cardiac sphincter function are failure of the cardiac sphincter to open properly, which is called **cardiospasm**, and inability of the sphincter to remain closed properly, which is called an *incompetent cardiac sphincter*, and leads to a condition called *reflux esophagitis*.

**Cardiospasm** Sometimes the cardiac sphincter fails to open properly, caused by a malfunction of the nerve plexuses in the esophagus that control its functions. As a result, food cannot pass normally into the stomach, and the smooth muscle in the wall of the esophagus must contract more vigorously to force the food past the constricted sphincter. Treatment consists of periodic stretching of the sphincter by means of an instrument introduced into the esophagus or by surgically cutting the muscle fibers in the constricted area. An alternative treatment in selected cases consists of

## Gastric Mucosal Tears

Retching and vomiting may cause tears in the mucosa of the gastroesophageal junction where the esophagus passes through the diaphragm or in the lining of the distal esophagus, and these tears can bleed profusely ( Figure 17-6 ). The repetitive, intermittent, vigorous contractions of the abdominal muscles associated with vomiting raise intra-abdominal pressure and forcefully jam the upper part (cardia) of the stomach against the opening in the diaphragm through which the esophagus passes, causing tears in the mucosa. This vomiting-related complication most often follows the retching and vomiting related to excess alcohol intake but may follow vomiting from any cause, including self-induced vomiting to control weight.

**cardiospasm**
(kar-dē-o-spazm)
Spasm of the lower gastroesophageal (cardiac) sphincter.

**reflux esophagitis**
Inflammation of the lining of the esophagus caused by reflux of acidic gastric secretions through an incompetent lower gastroesophageal sphincter.

**Barrett esophagus**
A condition in which the epithelial lining of the esophagus changes from squamous to columnar type, usually as a result of reflux esophagitis.

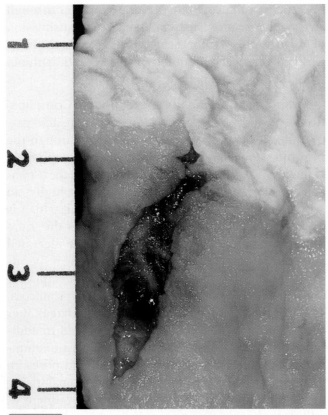

**Figure 17-6** Gastric mucosal tear caused by retching and vomiting. The opaque mucosa in the *upper part* of the photograph is the normal stratified squamous mucosa of the esophagus. The 2-centimeter-long tear extends distally from the gastroesophageal junction and caused a fatal gastric hemorrhage.

## Esophageal Obstruction

**Carcinoma of the Esophagus** Carcinoma may arise anywhere in the esophagus, either from the squamous epithelium or from the columnar epithelium associated with Barrett esophagus. The tumor gradually narrows the lumen of the esophagus, frequently infiltrates the surrounding tissues, and may invade the trachea.

**Stricture** A stricture is a narrowing caused by scar tissue. Reflux esophagitis with ulceration and scarring may lead to a stricture. Esophageal scarring may also result from accidentally or deliberately swallowing a corrosive chemical that causes necrosis and inflammation. Severe scarring eventually follows. A common cause of esophageal stricture in children is accidental swallowing of commercial lye solutions (used for cleaning clogged drains).

# Gastritis

Inflammation of the stomach is called *gastritis*, and the inflammation may be either acute or chronic. Many patients with gastritis have few symptoms, but some experience abdominal discomfort and nausea.

## Acute Gastritis

In most cases, acute gastritis is a self-limited inflammation of short duration. However, at times, the acute inflammation may be quite severe and may be complicated by ulceration of the mucosa with bleeding from the ulcerated areas. Patients in whom the acute gastritis is associated with mucosal ulceration often have more pronounced symptoms, and the ulcerated areas may bleed profusely.

There are many causes of acute gastritis, but most are caused by nonsteroidal anti-inflammatory drugs such as aspirin, ibuprofen, and naproxen. These drugs are widely used to treat symptoms of arthritis and related musculoskeletal pain problems. The drugs act by inhibiting an enzyme called *cyclooxygenase* that is required for the synthesis of prostaglandins, which are potent mediators of inflammation (Chapter 3). Prostaglandins, however, are produced by many different cells and have many different functions. Those produced by gastric epithelial cells help protect the stomach from the damaging effects of gastric acid by promoting the secretion of mucin to coat and protect the stomach lining. Nonsteroidal anti-inflammatory drugs reduce inflammation by inhibiting the synthesis of prostaglandin mediators of inflammation, but they also inhibit the synthesis of the prostaglandins that help protect the gastric mucosa. Consequently, the mucosa becomes more vulnerable to injury from acid gastric juice.

Excess ingestion of alcoholic beverages is another common cause of acute gastritis because the alcohol is a gastric irritant and also stimulates gastric acid secretion.

## Chronic Gastritis and Its Complications: The Role of *Helicobacter pylori*

Many cases of chronic gastritis are related to growth (colonization) of a small, curved, gram-negative organism called *Helicobacter pylori* on the surface of the gastric mucosa. This unique organism grows in the layer of mucus covering the epithelial cells lining the stomach, where it can be identified by special bacterial stains, by culture, or by other specialized tests. The organism produces an enzyme called *urease* that decomposes urea, a normal by-product of protein metabolism that is present in small amounts in blood and body fluids. Decomposition of urea yields ammonia, a substance that neutralizes the gastric acid and allows the organism to flourish in an acid environment that would destroy other bacteria. *Helicobacter* also produces enzymes that can break down the layer of protective mucus that covers the epithelial surface. Presumably, the chronic gastritis is caused by the ammonia and other products produced by the organism that damage the gastric mucosa of susceptible persons.

Colonization of the gastric mucosa by *Helicobacter pylori* is very common, and not all persons who harbor the organism have chronic gastritis. The organism is spread from person-to-person in households by close contacts. The spread of the organisms appears to be by mouth-to-mouth contact and also by the fecal–oral route because the organism has been cultured from both dental plaque material and from fecal material.

There are also some uncommon but important long-term harmful effects of *Helicobacter* infection. Chronic gastritis caused by this organism slightly increases the risk of two different gastric tumors: gastric carcinoma and malignant lymphoma arising from lymphocytes in the gastric mucosa (called mucosa-associated lymphoid tissue). The gastric carcinoma risk occurs because the gastritis often leads to atrophy of the gastric mucosa and causes the gastric epithelium to change into an abnormal intestinal-type epithelium (a process called intestinal metaplasia). It is these cellular changes in the gastric mucosa that predispose to gastric carcinoma. The lymphoma risk probably results because the gastritis overstimulates the mucosa-associated lymphoid tissue, which may lead to unregulated growth of lymphocytes that eventually progresses to gastric lymphoma.

# Peptic Ulcer

Peptic ulcer is a chronic ulcer that usually involves the distal stomach or proximal duodenum ( Figure 17-7 ). The ulcer results from digestion of the mucosa by acid gastric juice. Persons who secrete large volumes of acid gastric juice are prone to ulcers.

The initial event is probably a small, superficial erosion of the gastric or duodenal mucosa. Gastric acid and pepsin begin to digest the deeper tissues, which have been denuded of covering epithelium. Attempts at healing in the presence of continuing digestion eventually lead to considerable scarring at the base of the ulcer. Clinically, ulcers produce pain that is usually relieved by ingestion of food or antacids that neutralize the gastric acid.

*Helicobacter pylori*, the same organism that is associated with chronic gastritis, also plays an important role in the pathogenesis of both gastric and duodenal ulcers. Presumably the organism injures the mucosa and initiates the mucosal erosion that eventually develops into a chronic ulcer. The mucosal damage caused by the gastritis disturbs various functions of gastric mucosal cells that regulate gastric acid secretion and causes the mucosa to secrete excess acid. Peptic ulcer has complications: hemorrhage (bleeding), perforation, and obstruction. An ulcer that erodes into a large blood vessel may cause severe hemorrhage. An ulcer may also erode completely through the wall of the stomach or duodenum, causing a perforation of the wall. Sometimes the scarring that follows healing of a gastric ulcer may be so severe as to cause obstruction of the outlet of the stomach, called the pylorus, preventing the stomach from emptying properly.

Peptic ulcer is generally treated by antacids, which neutralize the excess gastric acid and promote healing of the ulcer, or by drugs that block the secretion of

**A**

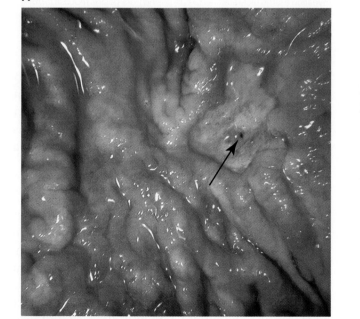

**B**

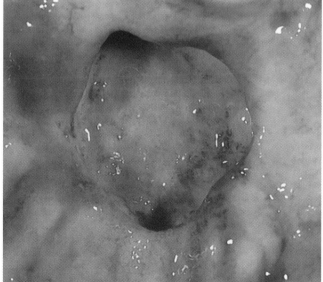

Figure 17-7    Peptic ulcers. **A,** Gastric ulcer, which eroded a blood vessel in the base of the ulcer (*arrow*) and bled profusely. **B,** Large chronic duodenal ulcer.

acid by the gastric epithelial cells. Because of the strong correlation between *Helicobacter pylori* and peptic ulcers, patients with ulcers who are colonized by this organism are often treated not only with drugs to neutralize gastric acid or suppress its secretion, but also with antibiotics and other medications to eradicate *Helicobacter pylori*.

# Carcinoma of the Stomach

At one time, carcinoma of the stomach was the most common malignant tumor in men, but the incidence has been decreasing. The initial symptom may be only vague upper abdominal discomfort. Sometimes the first manifestation is an iron deficiency anemia, the result of chronic blood loss from the ulcerated surface of the tumor. Gastric carcinoma is treated by resection of a large part of the stomach together with the surrounding tissues and draining lymph nodes ( Figure 17-8 ). Unfortunately, a gastric carcinoma is often far advanced by the time it causes symptoms; consequently, long-term survival of patients with stomach carcinoma is relatively poor. Sometimes gastric carcinoma may produce symptoms similar to those of a benign peptic ulcer. At times it may be difficult for the physician to determine whether a patient has a benign peptic ulcer of the stomach or an ulcerated gastric carcinoma. The distinction can usually be made by gastroscopy, an examination in which a flexible gastroscope is passed into the stomach so that the physician can visualize the lesion and take biopsy specimens from various areas.

**colitis** (kō-lī′tis) Inflammation of the colon, such as chronic ulcerative colitis.

**gastroenteritis** Inflammation of the stomach and intestine.

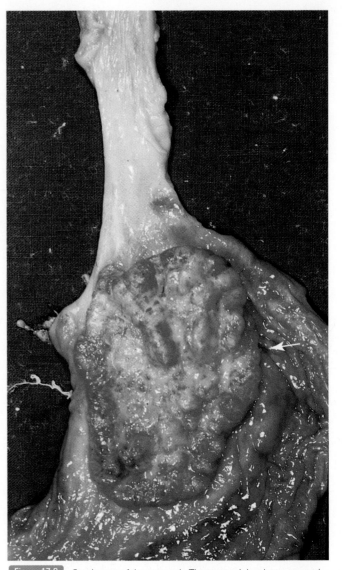

Figure 17-8 Carcinoma of the stomach. The stomach has been opened revealing a large ulcerated neoplasm arising from gastric mucosa (*arrow*) and extending upward to gastroesophageal junction. Esophagus is seen in *upper part* of photograph.

# Inflammatory Disease of the Intestine

The intestine may be the site of both acute and chronic inflammation. The term **enteritis** (*enteron* = bowel) is a general term, but usually refers to an inflammation of the small intestine, and the term **colitis** denotes inflammation restricted to the colon. **Gastroenteritis** indicates an inflammation of both the stomach and intestine. The general term bowel can refer to any part of the intestinal tract, either small intestine, colon, or both.

## Acute Enteritis

Acute intestinal infections are usually caused by known pathogens or their toxins, as described in Chapter 5. They are generally of short duration and may subside

without specific treatment, or may respond to appropriate antibiotics or other agents. Clinical manifestations include nausea, vomiting, abdominal discomfort, and passage of many loose stools. In severe infections, the bowel mucosa may be ulcerated, and the diarrheal stools may be bloody.

## Chronic Enteritis

Chronic enteritis is less common and more difficult to treat. The two important types of chronic enteritis are *Crohn disease* and *chronic ulcerative colitis*. Often the two diseases are grouped together under the general term *chronic inflammatory bowel disease*. Both diseases tend to be chronic, with periodic flare-ups manifested by cramplike abdominal pain and diarrhea, followed by periods when the disease is inactive. During periods

*Crohn disease was not the original name of the disease described by Dr. Crohn and his associates, and its pathogenesis was different from what they had postulated.*

In 1932, Burrill Bernard Crohn and two colleagues, Leon Ginzburg and Gordon Oppenheimer, published a description of 14 patients with a previously unknown chronic inflammatory disease of the distal ileum, which they called *regional ileitis*. Crohn thought that it was caused by a pathogenic mycobacterium because some of the histologic features of the inflammation suggested a mycobacterial infection. However, no organism was ever isolated that could account for the disease, which currently is considered to be an autoimmune disease. Later it was found that the disease could affect other parts of the small intestine, and even the colon. Consequently, the term *regional ileitis* was dropped and the disease was named Crohn disease after the first author of the article describing the disease. Crohn practiced in New York and usually admitted his patients to Mount Sinai Hospital. After his publication, patients were referred to him from all over the United States, as well as some foreign countries, and his practice flourished. He eventually became head of the gastroenterology department at Mount Sinai Hospital. He moved to Connecticut when he retired, where he died in 1983. No organism was ever identified as the cause of the disease.

of activity, the affected persons may also have systemic manifestations, including joint inflammation, eye inflammation, and various types of skin nodules and skin infections. These two diseases appear to be autoimmune diseases as described in Chapter 4. Although the diseases have many similarities, there are also significant differences between them.

## Crohn Disease

**Crohn disease** is a chronic inflammation and ulceration of the bowel mucosa with marked thickening and scarring of the bowel wall ( Figure 17-9 ). The distal ileum is a frequently involved site. The inflammation often affects scattered areas of the small bowel, leaving normal intervening segments of bowel (called "skip areas") between the areas of severe disease. Occasionally affected persons have such severe thickening and scarring of an involved segment of bowel that the lumen becomes greatly narrowed or even completely blocked, which impedes passage of bowel contents. Crohn disease was originally called regional ileitis because the inflammatory process is often localized to the distal ileum, but now we know that the disease is not restricted to the ileum. Other parts of the small intestine may also be involved, and the disease may involve the colon as well.

> **Crohn disease**
> (krō′-n) A chronic autoimmune disease characterized by segmental areas of inflammation and scarring within the intestine, often involving primarily the distal ileum. Also called *regional ileitis*.

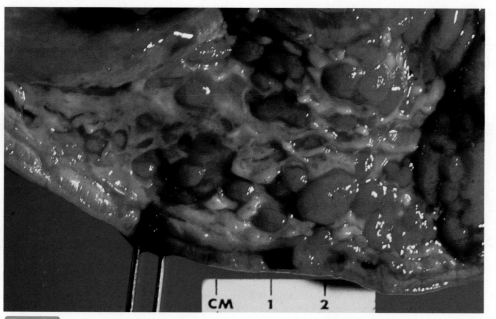

Figure 17-9    Crohn disease. Mucosa is ulcerated and covered by inflammatory exudate.

**Chronic Ulcerative Colitis** In contrast to Crohn disease, chronic ulcerative colitis targets the colon, not the small intestine. The inflammation is limited to the mucosa, and the bowel wall is not thickened as in Crohn disease. Frequently, the disease begins in the rectal mucosa but may spread progressively until eventually the entire colon is involved. In severe cases, the ulcerated mucosa may bleed profusely, leading to bloody diarrhea, and at times the inflammatory process becomes so extensive that it leads to a perforation of the colon with escape of bowel contents into the peritoneal cavity. Affected persons with long-standing disease also may develop carcinoma arising in the diseased regions of the colon or rectum.

**Treatment of Chronic Enteritis** Treatment of inflammatory bowel disease involves symptomatic and supportive measures, including antibiotics and corticosteroid hormones to control disease symptoms during flare-ups, and immunosuppressive drugs. Eventually surgical resection of severely diseased bowel segments may be required in many patients. Persons with severe and extensive chronic ulcerative colitis may require total removal of the entire colon and rectum, both to control the disease and also to eliminate the risk of colon carcinoma, which is prone to occur in patients with long-standing chronic disease.

## Antibiotic-Associated Colitis

Some persons taking broad-spectrum antibiotics develop mild diarrhea. Others, unfortunately, develop severe bloody diarrhea with abdominal pain, fever, and other systemic manifestations, which may be life-threatening. In the mild cases, the intestinal mucosa is slightly inflamed. In the more severely affected persons, there are multiple ulcerations of the colonic mucosa, and the ulcerated areas are covered by masses of fibrin and inflammatory cells.

The broad-spectrum antibiotics cause the colitis by changing the intestinal bacterial flora. Most of the normal flora is destroyed by the broad-spectrum antibiotic. This allows overgrowth of an anaerobic spore-forming intestinal bacterium called *Clostridium difficile* (pronounced dif-fís-sill) that is not inhibited by the antibiotic. The organism produces two toxins that cause the intestinal inflammation and necrosis.

The diagnosis of antibiotic-associated colitis is established by detection of the bacterial toxin in the stool and by identification of the organism in stool cultures. Treatment consists of stopping the antibiotic, and in severe cases, giving a drug that inhibits anaerobic bacteria (metronidazole), or an antibiotic (vancomycin), which inhibits growth of the organism.

## Appendicitis

*Appendicitis* is the most common inflammatory lesion of the bowel, caused primarily to the narrow caliber of the appendix, the base of which often becomes plugged by firm bits of fecal material. Because of the obstruction, the secretions normally produced by the epithelial cells lining the appendix drain poorly from the area distal to the blockage. The accumulated secretions create pressure within the appendiceal lumen. This compresses the blood vessels in the mucosa, impairing its viability ( Figure 17-10 ). Bacteria normally present in the appendix and colon invade the devitalized wall, causing an acute inflammation.

Clinically, appendicitis is characterized by generalized abdominal pain that soon becomes localized to the right lower part (quadrant) of the abdomen. Examination of the abdomen reveals localized tenderness over the appendix when pressure is applied to the abdomen by the fingers of the examiner. Often the patient also experiences pain when the pressure is released suddenly (rebound tenderness). In addition, there is usually reflex contraction of the abdominal

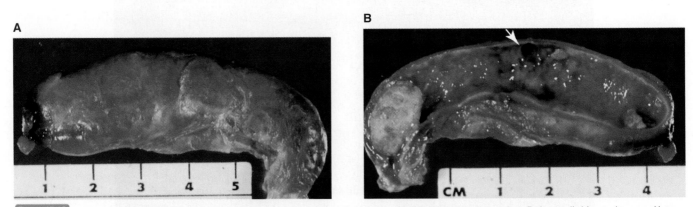

**Figure 17-10** Acute appendicitis. **A,** Exterior of appendix is swollen, congested, and covered with inflammatory exudate. **B,** Appendix bisected to reveal interior. Pus within lumen has been removed. Mucosa is congested and ulcerated (*arrow*). The base of the appendix (*left side* of photograph) is plugged by a firm mass of fecal material.

muscles (abdominal rigidity) in response to the underlying inflammation. Laboratory tests reveal that the number of polymorphonuclear leukocytes in the blood also is increased as a result of the infection.

Sometimes it may be difficult to distinguish appendicitis from other conditions with similar manifestations, such as acute gastroenteritis or a gynecologic problem in a young woman such as a fallopian tube infection (salpingitis) or ruptured ovarian cyst. When the diagnosis is uncertain, other diagnostic studies such as ultrasound or CT examination, or even a laparoscopy may help establish the correct diagnosis and lead to appropriate treatment.

Mild cases of appendicitis may heal spontaneously. More severe inflammation may lead to rupture of the appendix and peritonitis. For this reason, it is essential to identify appendicitis and remove the appendix in any patient in whom appendicitis is suspected.

## Meckel Diverticulum

During embryonic development, the small intestine is connected for a time to the yolk sac of the embryo by means of a narrow tubular channel called the *vitelline duct* (*vitellus* = yolk). Normally, the duct disappears along with the yolk sac, and no trace persists in the adult. In about 2 percent of persons, however, a remnant of the vitelline duct persists as a small tubular outpouching from the distal ileum about 12 to 18 inches proximal to the cecum. This structure is called a **Meckel diverticulum** ( Figure 17-11 ). Normally, a Meckel diverticulum has the same type of epithelial lining as that lining the small intestine, but sometimes part of the epithelial lining consists of acid-secreting gastric

mucosa. Most Meckel diverticula are asymptomatic, but sometimes the diverticulum becomes infected, causing the same symptoms and complications as an acute appendicitis. If a Meckel diverticulum contains misplaced (ectopic) gastric mucosa, the acidic "gastric juice" secreted by the diverticulum may cause a peptic ulcer of the diverticulum, which may be complicated by bleeding or perforation, as may occur with peptic ulcers in the stomach or duodenum. Whenever an operation is performed for a suspected appendicitis or other gastrointestinal problem, the surgeon always checks to see whether the patient's symptoms are caused by an inflammation or other problem in an unsuspected Meckel diverticulum.

**Meckel diverticulum** (dī-vur-tik′kū-lum) A tubular outpouching from the distal ileum; remnant of the vitelline duct.

# Disturbances of Bowel Function

## Food Intolerance

Some patients manifest crampy abdominal pain, abdominal distention, flatulence (excessive gas in the intestinal tract), and frequent loose stools as a result of food intolerance. The two most common types are

1. Lactose intolerance
2. Intolerance to the wheat protein gluten

**Lactose Intolerance**  Lactose is a disaccharide found in milk and dairy products. During digestion, lactose must be split into its two component monosaccharides,

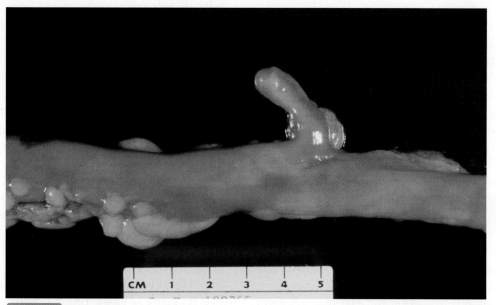

Figure 17-11  Meckel diverticulum of ileum.

glucose and galactose, before it can be absorbed. This process is accomplished by an enzyme called *lactase*, which is present on the mucosal surface of the epithelial cells in the small intestine. The enzyme is abundant in infants and young children. In many populations, however, the concentration of lactase gradually declines to very low levels during adolescence and early adult life. The enzyme is deficient in about 20 percent of adult whites, 70 percent of American blacks, 90 percent of American Indians, and almost all Asians.

Persons in whom lactase is deficient are unable to digest lactose. Consequently, lactose cannot be absorbed and remains within the intestinal lumen, instead of being absorbed normally, leading to abdominal discomfort, cramps, and diarrhea. Some of the unabsorbed lactose is fermented by bacteria in the colon, yielding lactic acid and other organic acids that further raise the intraluminal osmotic pressure and contribute to the person's discomfort. The symptoms are related to ingestion of dairy products and abate promptly when intake of dairy products is reduced or discontinued. Lactose-free milk and other low lactose-free dairy products are also available.

**Gluten Intolerance** *Gluten*, a protein found in wheat and other grains, imparts the elasticity to bread dough. Some persons become hypersensitive to this protein and develop a chronic diarrhea associated with impaired absorption of fat and other nutrients. Clinically, the condition is characterized by passage of frequent large, bulky stools containing much unabsorbed fat, associated with weight loss and vitamin deficiencies as a result of the impaired intestinal absorption. The hypersensitivity also leads to atrophy of the villi in the small intestine. This condition is called gluten enteropathy (*enteron* = bowel + *pathy* = disease) or nontropical sprue.

Diagnosis is made on the basis of the clinical features and is confirmed if biopsy of the small intestinal mucosa reveals atrophy of the intestinal villi. The specimen for biopsy is obtained by a flexible biopsy device with a small capsule on the end that is swallowed by the patient. The device is positioned in the upper jejunum and is manipulated so that a small bit of intestinal mucosa enters the capsule. Then the capsule is closed, cutting off and retaining a piece of mucosa.

Treatment by a gluten-free diet promptly cures the condition, and the intestinal villi return to normal.

## Irritable Bowel Syndrome

Some patients exhibit episodes of crampy abdominal discomfort, loud gurgling bowel sounds, and disturbed bowel function. Frequent loose stools sometimes alternate with periods of constipation and excessive amounts of mucus are secreted by the colonic mucosal glands. These manifestations are frequently quite distressing to the affected individual, but no structural or biochemical abnormalities can be identified to account for the functional disturbances. This condition is often called the irritable bowel syndrome.

The diagnosis of irritable bowel syndrome is one of exclusion. The physician must rule out infections as a result of pathogenic bacteria and intestinal parasites, food intolerance, and various types of chronic enteritis such as Crohn disease and chronic ulcerative colitis. Treatment consists of measures that improve intestinal motility. Sometimes substances that increase the bulk of the stool provide relief of symptoms. Other medications also are available that can provide relief from some of the distressing symptoms of this condition.

# Eating Disorders

Eating disorders are conditions in which food intake is inappropriate and harmful because it leads to serious health consequences. Excessive food intake leading to obesity, which has many harmful effects on health, is the most prevalent disorder. However, abnormal eating habits associated with anorexia nervosa and bulimia nervosa also pose serious health problems for the affected persons.

# Obesity

## Causes of Obesity

Fat is the storage form of energy. Any caloric intake that exceeds requirements is stored as adipose tissue and weight is gained. Each excess pound of body weight represents the storage of approximately 3500 calories. Weight is lost if caloric intake is reduced below the amount required for normal metabolic processes. Many genetic, environmental, and hormonal factors play a role in regulating body weight by affecting appetite and food intake, and by influencing the metabolic pathways that convert food into energy or into adipose tissue. It is sometimes said that obesity is caused by an endocrine gland malfunction. In rare instances, hypothyroidism contributes to obesity by reducing the body's metabolic rate. Adrenal cortical hyperfunction may be associated with increased deposition of fat and an abnormal distribution of body fat. These are uncommon situations. Most obese individuals have no detectable endocrine or metabolic disturbances. In the vast majority of cases, obesity is the result of overeating, and can be "cured" by reducing food intake.

Current data indicate that 60 percent of Americans are overweight. Half of the persons in this overweight group are classified as obese, which is defined as 20 percent or more over ideal body weight, or a body mass index of 30 or more. (Body mass index is a calculated value based on weight in kilograms divided by the square of height in meters.) Moreover, the prevalence of obesity has increased about 8 percent in the last decade. About 6 percent of women and 3 percent of men are more than 100 percent over their ideal body weight, which is called morbid obesity.

## Health Consequences of Obesity

Overweight persons have a higher incidence of diabetes, hypertension, cardiovascular disease, and several other diseases than do persons of normal weight. Therefore, being significantly overweight is undesirable, and extreme obesity is a major health hazard. Obese persons have a mortality rate almost twice that of normal individuals. The excess fat is harmful to the cardiovascular system in three ways:

1. Blood volume and cardiac output must increase to nourish the excess adipose tissue, which overworks the heart.
2. Obese persons are prone to develop high blood pressure, which places a further strain on the heart and blood vessels.
3. Blood lipids are often elevated, which predisposes to arteriosclerosis of the coronary arteries.

Other systems also are adversely affected. Large masses of adipose tissue may impair normal pulmonary ventilation, producing various types of respiratory difficulty and increased susceptibility to pulmonary infection.

The high incidence of diabetes in obese persons is the result of an impaired ability to utilize insulin efficiently (Chapter 16). Musculoskeletal disabilities are frequent because the excess weight places undue stress on the bones, joints, and ligaments.

## Treatment of Obesity

Most overweight persons are too heavy because they are eating too much and are not active enough. Obesity virtually always results from overeating and can be abolished by reducing food intake and becoming more active. However, the results of treatment of obesity by dieting have been surprisingly poor because obese individuals are either unable or unwilling to reduce their caloric intake.

Because of the limited success of treating obesity by diet various other measures have been proposed. Drugs that suppress appetite have been used. As a last resort, massive obesity is sometimes treated by surgical

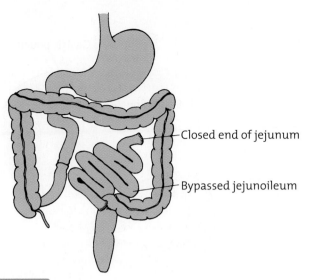

Figure 17-12 Ileal bypass procedure.

procedures. One of the first weight-reduction operations was called an ileal bypass, which produced weight loss primarily by preventing absorption of food from the small intestine. The stomach was connected to a very short segment of small intestine but most of the small intestine was bypassed, which greatly restricted food absorption ( Figure 17-12 ). Unfortunately this drastic procedure led to so many late complications caused by inadequate absorption of nutrients that it had to be abandoned.

Intestinal bypass was replaced by other operations that controlled food intake primarily by reducing the capacity of the stomach. The surgical procedures are often grouped together under the general term of *stomach stapling operations* and are usually performed as laparoscopic procedures (described in Chapter 1). The best known and most widely used of the weight-loss procedures is called the *Roux-en-Y gastric bypass*, named after the man who devised it (Roux) and the Y-shaped connection made between the small bowel loops in the procedure.

In a gastric bypass, a line of staples is placed across the upper part of the stomach. This divides the stomach into two compartments, a very small upper compartment having a volume of only about 15 milliliters, and a much larger lower compartment that is continuous with the duodenum. Then the jejunum is divided. The distal cut end is anastomosed (connected) to the gastric pouch, and the proximal cut end is connected by means of a second anastomosis to the jejunum distal to the anastomosis between the jejunum and gastric pouch ( Figure 17-13 ). When the procedure is completed, food from the gastric pouch empties directly into the jejunum. The main part of the stomach no longer receives food. Gastric secretions can drain into the duodenum normally, but the secretions enter the

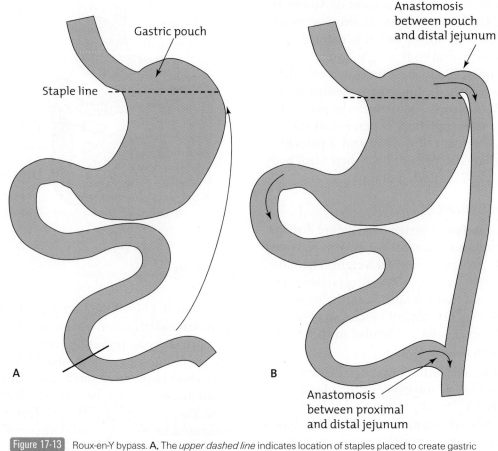

**Figure 17-13** Roux-en-Y bypass. **A,** The *upper dashed line* indicates location of staples placed to create gastric pouch. The *lower solid line* indicates the site where the jejunum is divided. The *arrow* indicates how the distal segment of jejunum is moved for anastomosis with gastric pouch. **B,** Completed bypass illustrating proximal and distal anastomoses. The *arrows* indicate direction of movement of gastric contents, as described in text.

jejunum distal ("downstream") to the segment of jejunum receiving the contents from the gastric pouch.

Gastric bypass induces weight loss because the upper compartment of the stomach is so small that it soon becomes overdistended with food when the individual starts to eat. The subject feels "stuffed" and has to stop eating. Weight is lost by enforced reduction of food intake, but absorption of nutrients is also impaired to some extent because gastric contents are shunted into the distal jejunum, bypassing absorption from the proximal part of the small intestine.

Adjustable gastric banding is another laparoscopic procedure to control food intake, which uses an inflatable saline-filled adjustable gastric band that is applied to the upper part of the stomach. The band compresses the stomach to form a small upper gastric pouch that is almost completely separated from the rest of the stomach except for a very small channel that allows the upper gastric pouch to empty slowly into the lower part of the stomach. The amount of compression applied to the inflatable band, which controls the rate of gastric emptying, can be adjusted by adding or removing

saline through a port placed under the skin of the abdomen. The procedure has the advantage of not requiring a major redesign of the gastrointestinal tract, but banding does not lead to as much weight loss as the gastric bypass (Figure 17-14).

# Anorexia Nervosa and Bulimia Nervosa

These two conditions are characterized by profound eating disturbances. Although they are characterized as separate disorders, there is considerable overlap between the two conditions. A more recently recognized condition called *binge eating disorder*, which occurs in older overweight and obese persons, is probably best considered as a variation of bulimia.

## Anorexia Nervosa

In this condition the affected persons have a false perception of being too fat when they are actually much

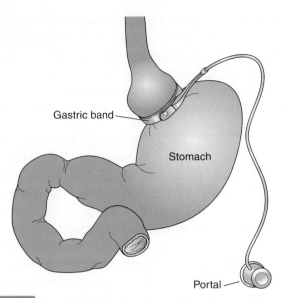

**Figure 17-14** Principle of the adjustable gastric-banding procedure. Adjustable band filled with saline limits capacity of stomach by constricting outflow from stomach above the band. Rate of gastric emptying can be regulated by adding or removing saline from the band.

too thin, and they continue to lose weight by restricting food intake and exercising excessively. The condition occurs much more frequently in women than in men, and is more prevalent in Western countries where a slim body is considered ideal and excessive weight is thought to be undesirable. Fashion models, ballet dancers, and other groups in which a slender body is required, are disproportionately represented.

Often **anorexia nervosa** begins in adolescent girls during puberty as their bodies change along with the distribution of their body fat, which is perceived as getting fat from overeating, and is followed by dieting and exercise to deal with the perceived overweight. As their weight loss accelerates, other measures may be taken to reduce weight, such as self-induced vomiting or taking laxatives. The excessive weight loss disrupts many of the body's physiologic processes. Menstrual periods cease, thyroid function declines, fluid and electrolyte disturbances develop, and bones become fragile from loss of calcium (osteoporosis). Extreme emaciation is a life-threatening condition that may lead to death if the condition is not treated.

Severe anorexia nervosa is difficult to treat; both the medical and psychological problems associated with the condition must be dealt with. Medical treatment requires correcting the physiologic disturbances caused by the fasting, which may require intravenous fluids and whatever other methods are needed to restore health. Psychologic treatment requires the assistance of a psychiatrist or clinical psychologist experienced in dealing with eating disabilities. The affected person needs to acquire a more realistic perception of her or his own body, needs to understand what may have led to the eating problem, and needs to learn how to adjust eating habits to prevent a recurrence of the condition.

## Bulimia Nervosa

This condition is another method of weight control that is characterized by repeated episodes of binge eating (rapidly eating an excessively large amount of food) followed by purging (self-induced vomiting) to counteract the effects of the bingeing, and is followed by guilt and remorse at the inability to control the binge–purge behavior. The purging may be supplemented by taking laxatives to decrease food absorption by promoting rapid passage of digested food through the small intestine. The condition occurs most often in young women. Their body weight may fluctuate in relation to their binge–purge behavior but they don't become emaciated. Their friends and relatives often are not aware of their problem because they look normal and they are not aware of their binge–purge behavior, which is carefully concealed.

**Bulimia nervosa** carries with it some serious health problems. Repeated self-induced vomiting leads to dental problems caused by the corrosive effect of the gastric acid on the tooth enamel. The repeated loss of excess gastric juice may lead to metabolic alkalosis and electrolyte disturbances (Chapter 19). One of the most serious effects of self-induced vomiting is a tear in the mucosa of the stomach near the gastroesophageal junction, which can bleed profusely and may be fatal, as illustrated in Figure 17-6. Treatment of bulimia nervosa involves the same medical and psychological approaches used to deal with anorexia nervosa.

## Binge Eating Disorder

The condition called a *binge eating disorder* is characterized by binge eating without compensatory purging to restrict the excess calories contributed by the binge eating, and leads to weight gain. The condition occurs in overweight and obese older adults, with both genders represented in roughly equal proportions. The binge eating complicates the problems of the obese person who is trying to lose weight, and it is estimated that up to 20 percent of persons in weight-loss programs may have a binge eating problem. The same approach used to motivate a person to lose weight also applies when dealing with the additional problem posed by the binge eating.

**anorexia nervosa** Excessive self-induced weight loss because of a false perception of being fat.

**bulimia nervosa** Weight control by compulsive overeating followed by self-induced vomiting and other methods in order to prevent weight gain.

# Diverticulosis and Diverticulitis of the Colon

Outpouchings of the mucosa of the colon often project through weak areas in the muscular wall of the large intestine. These outpouchings are called diverticula (singular, **diverticulum**), and the condition is called **diverticulosis** ( Figure 17-15 and Figure 17-16 ). This is an acquired condition, in contrast to a Meckel diverticulum, which is a congenital abnormality. Diverticula, which usually occur in the distal colon, are encountered with increasing frequency in older patients where they can be demonstrated easily by x-ray examination of the colon ( Figure 17-17 ). Highly refined, low-residue diets predispose to diverticula because stools are small and hard, and high intraluminal pressure must be generated by peristalsis to propel the stool through the colon. This high intracolonic pressure forces the mucosa through weak areas in the muscular wall. In contrast, people who subsist on high-residue diets have large, bulky stools that can be propelled through the colon easily at low intraluminal pressures, and diverticula occur infrequently among them.

Most diverticula are asymptomatic, but occasionally problems arise. Bits of fecal material may become trapped within these pouches and incite an inflammatory reaction called **diverticulitis**. The inflammation may be followed by considerable scarring. Occasionally, perforation of a diverticulum may occur, leading to an abscess in the pelvis. Sometimes blood vessels in the mucosa of the diverticulum may become ulcerated by abrasion from the fecal material, resulting in bleeding. Diverticula attended by such complications as infections, perforation, or bleeding are often treated by surgical resection of the affected segment of bowel.

**diverticulum**
(dī-vur-tik′u-lum) An outpouching from an organ, as from the mucosa of the colon, which projects through the muscular wall.

**diverticulitis**
(dī-vur-tik-u-lī′tis) An inflammation of a diverticulum.

**diverticulosis**
(dī-vur-tik-u-lō′sis) A condition characterized by an outpouching of the colonic mucosa through weak areas in the muscular wall.

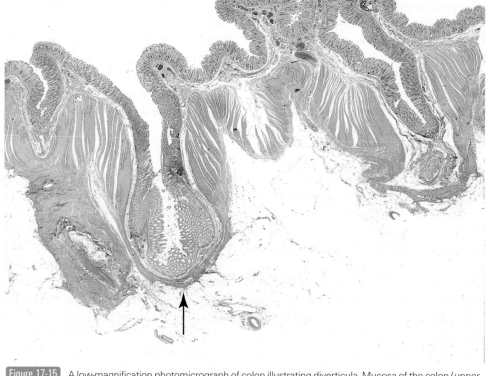

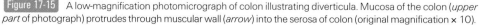
**Figure 17-15** A low-magnification photomicrograph of colon illustrating diverticula. Mucosa of the colon (*upper part* of photograph) protrudes through muscular wall (*arrow*) into the serosa of colon (original magnification × 10).

**A**

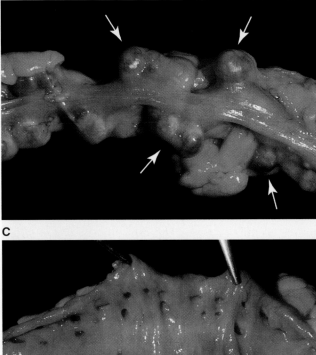

**C**

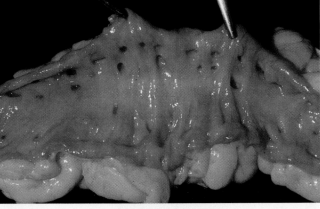

**B**

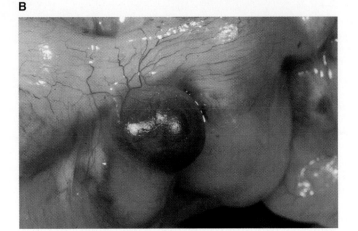

**Figure 17-16** Diverticulosis of colon. **A,** Exterior of colon illustrating several diverticula projecting through wall of colon (*arrows*). **B,** A closer view of diverticulum. **C,** Interior of colon, illustrating openings of multiple diverticula. Several of the openings are well demonstrated in the mucosa just below the clamps.

# Intestinal Obstruction

If the normal passage of intestinal contents through the bowel is blocked, the patient is said to have an *intestinal obstruction*. The site of the blockage may be either the small intestine (*high intestinal obstruction*) or the colon (*low intestinal obstruction*). Bowel obstruction is always serious. The severity of the symptoms depends on the location of the obstruction, its completeness, and whether there is interference with the blood supply to the blocked segment of bowel.

Obstruction of the *small intestine* causes severe, crampy pain as a result of vigorous peristalsis, reflecting the attempt of the intestine to force bowel contents past the site of obstruction. This is associated with vomiting of copious amounts of gastric and upper-intestinal secretions, resulting in loss of large quantities of water and electrolytes. As a consequence, the patient becomes dehydrated and develops pronounced fluid and electrolyte disturbances. Symptoms are much less acute when the distal colon is obstructed. There may be mild, crampy abdominal pain and moderate distention of the abdomen. However, vomiting with associated loss of fluid and electrolytes is not as serious a

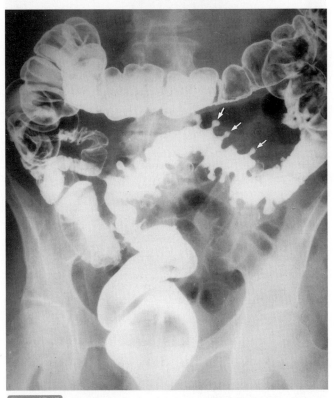

**Figure 17-17** Diverticula of colon demonstrated by injection of barium contrast material into colon (barium enema). Diverticula filled with contrast material appear as projections from the mucosa (*arrows*).

problem as in high intestinal obstruction. Disturbances of fluid and electrolytes do not develop as rapidly.

The common causes of intestinal obstruction are as follows:

1. Intestinal adhesions
2. Hernia
3. Volvulus
4. Intussusception
5. An obstructing tumor

## Adhesions

Adhesive bands of connective tissue (adhesions) may form within the abdominal cavity after surgery ( Figure 17-18 ). Sometimes a loop of bowel becomes kinked, compressed, or twisted by an adhesive band, causing obstruction proximal to the site of the adhesion.

## Hernia

A **hernia** is a protrusion of a loop of bowel through a small opening, usually in the abdominal wall. The herniated loop pushes the peritoneum ahead of it, forming the hernia sac. Inguinal hernia is quite common in men ( Figure 17-19 ). A loop of small bowel protrudes through a weak area in the inguinal ring and may descend downward into the scrotum. Umbilical and femoral hernias occur in both sexes. In an umbilical hernia a loop of bowel protrudes through a weak area in the abdominal wall where the umbilical blood vessels from the placenta entered the abdomen in the fetus ( Figure 17-20 ). In a femoral hernia, a loop of intestine extends under the inguinal ligament along the course of the femoral vessels into the groin.

**hernia** (her′nē-yuh) A protrusion of a loop of bowel through a narrow opening, usually in the abdominal wall.

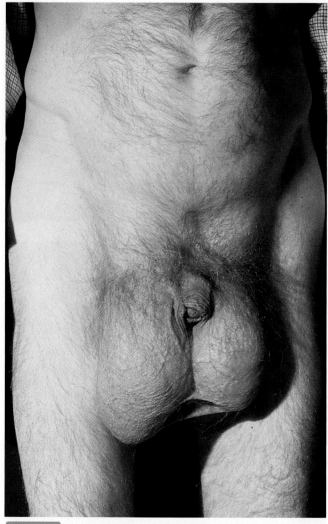

**Figure 17-19**   Large bilateral inguinal hernias extending into the scrotum.

If a herniated loop of bowel can be pushed back into the abdominal cavity, the hernia is said to be *reducible*. Occasionally, a herniated loop becomes stuck and cannot be reduced. This is called an *incarcerated hernia*. Sometimes the loop of bowel is so tightly constricted by the margins of the defect that allowed the herniation

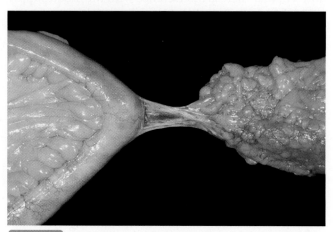

**Figure 17-18**   Fibrous adhesion between loop of small intestine (*left side* of photograph) and omentum.

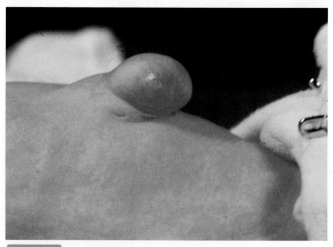

**Figure 17-20**   A large umbilical hernia in an infant.

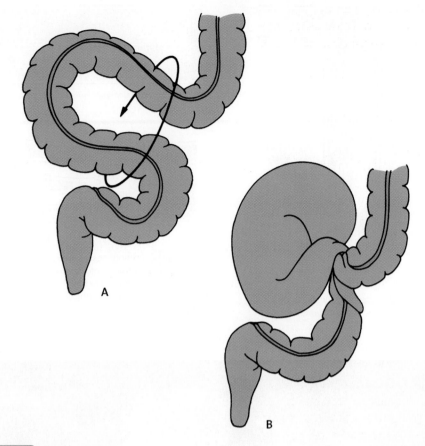

**Figure 17-21** Pathogenesis of volvulus. **A,** Rotary twist of sigmoid colon on its mesentery. **B,** Obstruction of colon and interruption of its blood supply caused by volvulus.

that the blood supply to the herniated bowel is obstructed, causing necrosis of the protruding segment of bowel. This is called a *strangulated hernia* and requires prompt surgical intervention.

## Volvulus and Intussusception

A **volvulus** is a rotary twisting of the sigmoid colon on the fold of peritoneum that suspends the bowel from the posterior wall of the abdomen, which is called the sigmoid mesocolon ( **Figure 17-21** ). The blood supply to the twisted segment also is impaired because the blood vessels supplying the bowel travel in the mesentery, and they are compressed when the bowel and mesentery become twisted.

An **intussusception** is a telescoping of one segment of bowel into an adjacent segment. This is a common cause of intestinal obstruction in children and usually results from vigorous peristalsis that telescopes the terminal ileum into the proximal colon through the ileocecal valve ( **Figure 17-22** ). In adults, the condition is usually secondary to a benign tumor of the bowel that is supported by a narrow stalk. A tumor of this type is often called a pedunculated tumor, the name being derived from the stalk (pedicle) that supports it (*pediculus* = little foot). As the tumor is propelled by a

peristaltic wave, the base of the tumor exerts traction on the bowel wall at its site of attachment, causing the proximal segment of bowel to be pulled into the distal segment ( **Figure 17-23** and **Figure 17-24** ).

# Tumors of the Bowel

Carcinoma of the colon may obstruct the distal colon and is a common cause of low intestinal obstruction. Tumors of the small intestine are uncommon, whereas benign pedunculated polyps of the colon occur quite frequently. Usually they do not cause symptoms, but occasionally the tip of the polyp may become eroded and cause bleeding. Often a polyp can be removed by inserting a flexible instrument called a colonoscope into the bowel through the rectum and cutting the narrow stalk.

In contrast, *carcinoma of the colon* is a common tumor that may arise anywhere in the large intestine or rectum. Carcinoma arising in the cecum and right half of the colon generally does not cause obstruction of the bowel because

**volvulus**
(vol′vū-lus) A rotary twisting of the intestine on its mesentery, with obstruction of the blood supply to the twisted segment.

**intussusception** (in′tus-us-cep′shun) A telescoping of one segment of bowel into an adjacent segment.

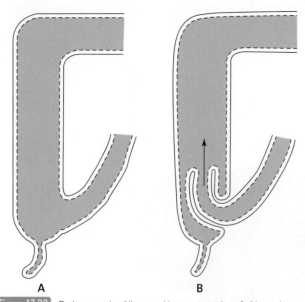

Figure 17-22 Pathogenesis of ileocecal intussusception. **A,** Normal anatomic relationships. **B,** Vigorous peristalsis carries distal ileum into cecum. *Dashed line* indicates mucosa.

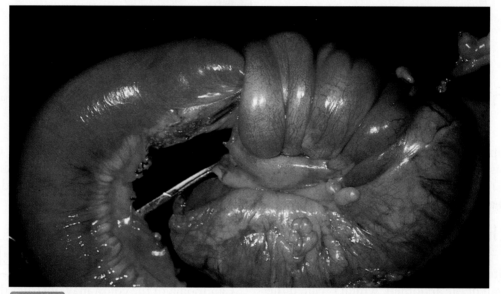

Figure 17-23 Pathogenesis of intussusception caused by tumor. **A,** Pedunculated tumor protrudes into lumen of bowel. **B,** Peristalsis propels tumor and produces traction on its base causing proximal segment of bowel to be telescoped into distal segment. *Dashed line* indicates mucosa.

Figure 17-24 Intussusception of colon as a result of colon tumor. Midportion of colon is swollen because of telescoping of the proximal segment (*left side* of photograph) into distal segment (*right side* of photograph).

the caliber of this portion of the colon is large and the bowel contents are relatively soft. However, the tumor often becomes ulcerated and slow chronic blood loss from the ulcerated surface of the tumor often leads to chronic iron deficiency anemia, as described in Chapter 11. The patient with a carcinoma of the right half of the colon may consult a physician because of weakness and fatigue caused by the anemia, without experiencing any symptoms referable to the intestinal tract.

Carcinoma of the distal part of the colon, which has a much smaller caliber than the proximal colon, often causes partial obstruction of the bowel and leads to symptoms of lower intestinal obstruction.

Figure 17-25 illustrates the progressive growth of a colon carcinoma, which gradually encircles the bowel wall and greatly narrows or completely obstructs the lumen. Figure 17-26 illustrates almost complete obstruction of the descending colon by a colon carcinoma, as demonstrated by a barium enema.

# Mesenteric Thrombosis

The blood supply to the gastrointestinal tract is derived from several large arteries arising from the aorta. The blood supply to most of the bowel is provided by the superior mesenteric artery. This vessel supplies blood

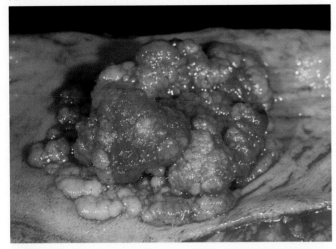

**A**

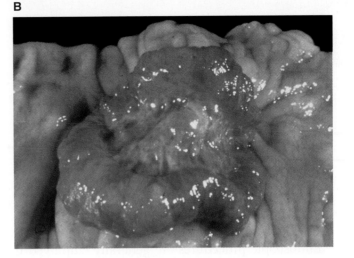

**B**

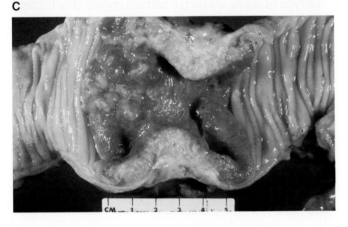

**C**

**Figure 17-25** Stages in the progressive growth of a colon carcinoma. **A,** Broad-based overgrowth of neoplastic epithelium. No ulceration or invasion of bowel wall. **B,** Central necrosis within more advanced carcinoma. Tumor invades bowel wall. **C,** Ulcerated far-advanced colon carcinoma, which completely encircles the bowel wall, reducing the caliber of the lumen, and extends completely through the bowel wall.

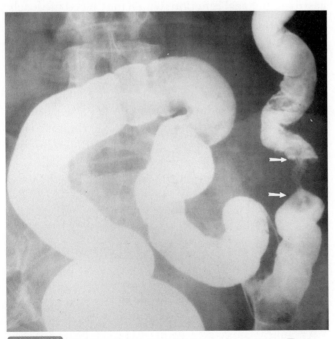

**Figure 17-26** Colon carcinoma demonstrated by barium enema. The tumor narrows the lumen of the colon, which appears as a filling defect in the column of barium (*arrows*).

to the entire small intestine and the proximal half of the colon. The arteries supplying the gastrointestinal tract may develop arteriosclerotic changes and become occluded by thrombosis in the same way as may other arteries. Thrombosis of the superior mesenteric artery leads to an extensive infarction of most of the bowel.

# Hemorrhoids

**Hemorrhoids** are varicosities of the venous plexus that drains the rectum and anus. Constipation and increased straining during bowel movements predispose to their development. Symptoms of hemorrhoids can often be relieved by a high-fiber diet rich in fruits and vegetables, which promotes large, bulky stools that can be passed without excessive straining. Stool softeners and local application of rectal ointments may also provide temporary relief. Hemorrhoids can be removed surgically if they do not respond to more conservative therapy.

**hemorrhoids** (hem'or-oyds) Varicosities of anal and rectal veins.

# Diagnostic Evaluation of Gastrointestinal Disease

Unfortunately, the gastrointestinal tract cannot be examined as easily as many other parts of the body. However, it is possible to visualize the interior of the esophagus, the stomach, the duodenum, and the entire colon by endoscopic procedures using specially designed instruments that are inserted into the gastrointestinal tract either through the oral cavity or the anus. Endoscopy is described in Chapter 1 in the section on diagnostic procedures.

Endoscopic procedures are generally employed if the patient experiences symptoms suggesting disease of the esophagus, stomach, or colon. Abnormal areas in the mucosa can be visualized, biopsied, and examined histologically.

Areas that cannot be visualized directly can be studied by radiologic examination. Examination of the upper gastrointestinal tract is accomplished by having the patient ingest a radiopaque material (contrast medium), allowing the clinician to visualize the transport of the material through the intestinal tract by x-ray studies. Any areas where the motility of the bowel appears abnormal, indicating disease, can be seen on the film. This technique also allows the clinician to visualize the contours of the gastrointestinal mucosa and thereby to identify the location and extent of disease affecting the bowel mucosa, such as ulcer, stricture, tumor, or an area of chronic inflammation. The colon can be studied in a similar manner by instilling radiopaque material into the bowel through the anus in order to outline the contours of the large intestine. This type of study is called a barium enema (see Figures 17-17 and 17-26). Other diagnostic methods are also used for specific indication (CT and MRI described in Chapter 1).

# CHAPTER REVIEW

## Summary

Failure of normal prenatal development of facial structures leads to various types of cleft lip and palate, which can be corrected surgically. Dental abnormalities are relatively frequent. Missing or extra teeth occur in about 2 percent of our population and often run in families but usually do not cause any problems. The complications of tooth decay and periodontal disease together can be minimized or even prevented by proper dental care. Oral inflammation is common, especially canker sores and oral herpes as well as other conditions that irritate the oral mucosa. Squamous cell carcinoma also occurs in the mouth and throat, and is difficult to cure.

The esophageal sphincter doesn't always function properly. It may not open normally (cardiospasm), which impedes transit of food into the stomach, or may not close properly, which allows acid gastric juice to reflux into the esophagus. The acid gastric juice irritates the esophageal mucosa and may also lead to long-term complications (Barrett's esophagus). Retching and vomiting may tear the lining of the stomach close to the gastroesophageal junction, which may bleed profusely. Gastric and duodenal ulcers are caused by acid gastric juice, and are often associated with *Helicobacter pylori* infection. Treatment of ulcers requires antacid therapy supplemented by antibacterial therapy to eradicate *Helicobacter* if the organism is demonstrated to be associated with the ulceration. Carcinoma of the stomach also may be ulcerated and difficult to distinguish from a benign ulcer without an examination by gastroscopy and biopsy of the ulcer.

Inflammation of the intestine may be acute or chronic. The two common types of chronic enteritis are Crohn disease and chronic ulcerative colitis, which are both autoimmune diseases; and tend to be difficult to treat. Antibiotic-associated colitis, as the name implies, is caused by an antibiotic that suppresses the normal bacterial flora of the colon, allowing overgrowth of the toxin-producing spore-forming anaerobic bacterium *Clostridium difficile*.

Appendicitis is very common and can be a very serious problem if the disease is not recognized and treated.

The inflammation is caused by an obstruction at the base of the appendix that is usually caused by fecal material, which blocks escape of intestinal gland secretions. Mucosal ulceration is followed by invasion of the appendix wall by intestinal bacteria living within the lumen of the appendix.

Several disturbances of intestinal function result from food intolerance to lactose or wheat protein (gluten), and sometimes the cause of the dysfunction can't be determined (irritable bowel syndrome). Eating disturbances result when normal eating patterns are abnormal or deranged. Obesity is the biggest eating problem in our society and leads to many complications, especially diabetes and cardiovascular disease. Various surgical treatment methods are used to reduce the capacity of the stomach and reduce absorption of nutrients from the small intestine when medical therapy is unsuccessful. Other eating problems include anorexia and bulimia nervosa, and binge eating disorders.

Low-residue diets and chronic constipation predispose to colon diverticula, which are common and often asymptomatic, but occasionally may become inflamed or may bleed, which require surgical treatment. Passage of bowel contents may be impeded by many different conditions (intestinal obstruction), and its manifestations depend on what part of the bowel is blocked by the obstruction. Treatment is to restore the normal transit of bowel contents, which may require a surgical procedure, such as resecting an obstructing bowel carcinoma.

Hemorrhoids, which are varicose veins of the anorectal mucosa, are very common problems that are more of an annoyance than a health hazard. They usually respond to conservative measures but can be treated surgically if they cause problems.

## Questions for Review

1. What is a cleft palate? What is its usual mode of inheritance? How is it treated?
2. What factors effect the development of dental caries? What complications may result from dental caries? What are the causes and possible effects of periodontal disease?
3. What are some of the major causes of esophageal obstruction? What symptoms are produced by esophageal obstruction?
4. What is peptic ulcer? In what part(s) of the gastrointestinal tract are peptic ulcers encountered? What factors contribute to the development of peptic ulcers? What are the complications of a peptic ulcer?
5. What is the difference between Crohn disease and chronic ulcerative colitis? Diverticulosis and diverticulitis?
6. What is a Meckel diverticulum? Where is it located? What clinical manifestations can it produce?
7. What are eating disorders? How are they treated?
8. What is intestinal obstruction? What symptoms does it produce? What are some of the common causes of intestinal obstruction?
9. What is the pathogenesis of acute appendicitis?
10. What symptoms and physical findings are likely to be encountered in a patient with a carcinoma of the colon? Why?
11. What is an intussusception? How is it caused? What is the difference between volvulus and intussusception?

## Supplementary Reading

Cummings, D. E., and Flum, D. R. 2008. Gastrointestinal surgery as a treatment for diabetes (Editorial). *Journal of the American Medical Association* 299:341–43.
    Obese patients with diabetes who had laparoscopic adjustable gastric-banding procedures to treat their diabetes lost weight and 73 percent had remission of their diabetes. Patients who had a Roux-en-Y gastric bypass procedure sustained a greater response than gastric-banding patients. It appears likely that the gastric bypass increases insulin sensitivity but also improves beta-cell function.

DeMaria, E. J. 2007. Bariatric surgery for morbid obesity. *New England Journal of Medicine* 356:2176–83.
    A discussion of the applications and limitations of the various types of surgical procedures available to reduce food intake by reducing the size of the stomach and/or impairing absorption of nutrients from

the small intestine. Some of the newer laparoscopic procedures are described.

Eckel, R. 2008. Nonsurgical management of obesity in adults. *New England Journal of Medicine* 358:1941–50.

Nonsurgical treatment is described for obese patients whose body mass index is not high enough to be considered for bariatric surgery. Patients should be encouraged to set realistic goals, record food intake, and record their weight at least weekly. Applications and limitations of weight-loss drugs are considered.

Hossain, P., Kawar, B., and Nahas, M. E. 2007. Obesity and diabetes in the developing world—A growing challenge. *New England Journal of Medicine* 356:213–15.

The rates of obesity have tripled in developing countries that have adopted a Western lifestyle characterized by decreased physical activity and overconsumption of cheap high-calorie foods, and affects children as well as adults. Type 2 diabetes, cardiovascular disease, and some cancers have followed the obesity epidemic. These problems are severe in middle-income countries of Eastern Europe, Latin America, and Asia, but are rare in developing countries that continue to observe their traditional lifestyle. The obesity–diabetes–hypertension triad also targets the kidneys, leading to development of diabetic nephropathy in one-third of persons with diabetes, and its incidence has increased greatly in Asia, where diabetic nephropathy is the most common cause of end-stage renal disease in 9 of 10 Asian countries.

Nishioka, N. S., and Lauwers, G. 2006. Case 10-2006: A 66-year-old woman with Barrett's esophagus with high-grade dysplasia. *New England Journal of Medicine* 354:1403–09.

Partial resection of the esophagus has many complications and less aggressive treatment is preferred. Various methods can be used to replace areas of dysplasia with normal squamous epithelium, which are described and discussed.

Paulson, E. K., Kalady, M. F., and Pappas, T. N. 2003. Suspected appendicitis. *New England Journal of Medicine* 348:236–42.

The three signs most predictive of appendicitis are right lower quadrant pain, abdominal rigidity, and migration of pain from the epigastrium to the right lower quadrant. Diagnosis in women is more difficult because of other conditions related to ovarian or tubal disease. Abdominal CT or ultrasound study is helpful for evaluating confusing cases.

Service, G. J., Thompson, G. B., Service, J., et al. 2005. Hyperinsulinemic hypoglycemia with nesidioblastosis after gastric-bypass surgery. *New England Journal of Medicine* 353:249–54.

Gastric bypass ameliorates obesity-related complications, and diabetes improves rapidly even before there has been significant weight loss, apparently because the bypass of nutrients into the distal jejunum induces the release of intestinal hormones that stimulate pancreatic islets to increase insulin secretion. In some bypass patients, the prolonged islet stimulation causes hyperplasia of islets, which is called nesidioblastosis (*nesidion* = islet). The islet hyperplasia leads to excess insulin secretion, which leads to hypoglycemia (see also editorial by Cummings in the same issue pages 300–301).

Suerbaum, S., and Michetti, P. 2002. Helicobacter pylori infection. *New England Journal of Medicine* 347:1175–86.

A current review article with an extensive bibliography. Reviews the evolution of the infection, diagnostic methods for detecting the infection, and methods of treatment. Proposes explanation for the high frequency of infection.

Uemura, N., Okamota, S., Yamamoto, S., et al. 2001. Helicobacter pylori infection and the development of gastric cancer. *New England Journal of Medicine* 345:784–89.

Gastric cancer develops in persons with *Helicobacter pylori* infection but not in uninfected persons. Persons with gastritis associated with marked gastric atrophy and intestinal metaplasia are at risk.

# Interactive Activities

## Matching

Match the abnormalities in the right column with the disease in the left column.

**Disease or Condition**

1. Crohn disease (regional ileitis)

2. Meckel diverticulitis

3. Mesenteric artery thrombosis

4. Chronic ulcerative colitis

5. Antibiotic-associated colitis

6. Nontropical sprue

7. Lactose intolerance

8. Irritable bowel syndrome

9. Colon diverticulosis

10. Colon diverticulitis

11. Intussusception

12. Colon volvulus

**Abnormality**

A. Protrusion of colon mucosa through weak area in bowel wall

B. Hypersensitivity to wheat protein (gluten)

C. Inflammation of colon diverticula

D. Inflammation and ulceration of colon mucosa

E. Chronic inflammation and ulceration of distal ileum

F. Deficiency of lactase enzyme

G. Overgrowth of *Clostridium difficile* in colon

H. Inflammation of congenital small-bowel diverticulum

I. Disturbed bowel function without structural changes

J. Rotary twist of sigmoid colon on its mesentery

K. Telescoping of proximal colon into distal colon

L. Extensive necrosis of entire small bowel and proximal half of colon

## True or False

Indicate whether the following statements are true or false by writing T or F at the end of the statement.

1. Cardiospasm results from failure of the *upper* esophageal sphincter to open normally._____

2. Canker sores are caused by herpes simplex virus type 1._____

3. Barrett esophagus increases the risk of esophageal carcinoma._____

4. Most persons with bulimia nervosa are underweight and frequently emaciated._____

5. *Helicobacter pylori* may cause chronic gastritis._____

6. Crohn disease only occurs in the colon._____

7. Meckel diverticulum results from chronic constipation._____

8. A sigmoid colon volvulus is a rotary twisting of the sigmoid colon on its mesentery, which obstructs blood flow to the twisted segment, and blocks passage of bowel contents through the colon._____

9. Of the procedures used to promote weight loss, gastric banding leads to greater weight loss than a Roux-en-Y gastric bypass._____

10. Self-induced vomiting can cause a tear of the gastric mucosa that may bleed profusely._____

## Critical Thinking

1. Susan Martin is a middle-aged obese woman with diabetes and hypertension. She says that she has tried various weight-reduction diets that lead to temporary weight loss but she soon gains back the lost weight. She is concerned about her diabetes, and is considering a surgical procedure. She asks your opinion about her problem. What would you tell her?

2. Steven Smith is a 35-year-old man who experiences episodes of upper abdominal discomfort, and his physician tells him that the discomfort is caused by reflux of acid gastric contents into his distal esophagus. He wants to know what he should do to relieve his discomfort, and whether there are any long-term complications caused by the gastric reflux. What would you tell him?

# 18 Nutrition and Disease

1. What are the major nutrients needed by the body? What are their functions?

2. What are the essential components of a well-balanced diet?

3. Understand the main causes of malnutrition and the persons at risk.

4. Understand the difference between kwashiorkor and marasmus. Why do children with kwashiorkor become edematous?

5. What are the causes and effects of the following vitamin deficiencies: vitamin D, vitamin K, vitamin $B_{12}$, folic acid, and citric acid?

6. Name five minerals required by the body. What are their functions?

# Nutrient Requirements and Their Functions

Our body is a well-designed "machine" that is constructed to perform the many activities of daily living. Like any machine, it requires:

1. Fuel to power the machine
2. A system to convert the power source to useable energy
3. Periodic maintenance to replace worn-out components

In our body, the fuel is the food we eat, along with the water we drink. Vitamins and minerals are the components that function along with cell enzymes to convert the fuel to energy, and the periodic maintenance is accomplished by replacing worn-out cell components and cells when they no longer function properly.

## Food and Water

Our food is composed of the various combinations of carbohydrates, proteins, and fats along with vitamins, minerals, and water. All of these are provided in a well-balanced diet. The carbohydrates, proteins, and fats needed to produce energy are large complex molecules. They must first be broken down by enzymes in our gastrointestinal tract into simple compounds that can be absorbed and processed to yield energy, which is measured in calories (kilocalories).

Carbohydrates and proteins each provide 4 calories per gram, but fat has a much higher energy content of 9 calories per gram. The number of calories needed to supply the body's needs depends of the person's body size, gender, age, and amount of physical activity. Body size determined from height and weight is converted to *body mass index* (BMI), a number calculated by dividing body weight in kilograms by the square of the height in meters. BMI can be obtained most conveniently from tables that convert height and weight data directly to BMI, which is considered to be a more accurate assessment of body weight than height–weight measurements. Ranges have been established for underweight, normal weight, overweight, and obesity (Table 18-1). Adult body weight is stable when calorie intake matches the number of calories required to supply the body's needs. Each 3500 calories consumed in excess of requirements adds 1 pound of body weight; conversely, losing weight requires cutting 3500 calories over requirements for each pound lost.

**Carbohydrates** Carbohydrates provide a quick source of energy. Monosaccharides, which are simple 6-carbon molecules such as glucose and fructose, and disaccharides, which consist of two monosaccharide molecules joined together, such as sucrose and lactose, can be converted quickly into energy. Complex carbohydrates, found in wheat and other grains, cereals, corn, beans, and root vegetables such as potatoes, are much larger molecules composed of long chains of glucose molecules joined together. They can be converted to energy, as are

| Table 18-1 | **Adult Body Mass Index Chart** |

| BMI | 19 | 20 | 21 | 22 | 23 | 24 | 25 | 26 | 27 | 28 | 29 | 30 | 31 | 32 | 33 | 34 | 35 |
|---|---|---|---|---|---|---|---|---|---|---|---|---|---|---|---|---|---|
| **Height** | | | | | | | | Weight in Pounds | | | | | | | | | |
| 4'10" | 91 | 96 | 100 | 105 | 110 | 115 | 119 | 124 | 129 | 134 | 138 | 143 | 148 | 153 | 158 | 162 | 167 |
| 4'11" | 94 | 99 | 104 | 109 | 114 | 119 | 124 | 128 | 133 | 138 | 143 | 148 | 153 | 158 | 163 | 168 | 173 |
| 5' | 97 | 102 | 107 | 112 | 118 | 123 | 128 | 133 | 138 | 143 | 148 | 153 | 158 | 163 | 158 | 174 | 179 |
| 5'1" | 100 | 106 | 111 | 116 | 122 | 127 | 132 | 137 | 143 | 148 | 153 | 158 | 164 | 169 | 174 | 180 | 185 |
| 5'2" | 104 | 109 | 115 | 120 | 126 | 131 | 136 | 142 | 147 | 153 | 158 | 164 | 169 | 175 | 180 | 186 | 191 |
| 5'3" | 107 | 113 | 118 | 124 | 130 | 135 | 141 | 146 | 152 | 158 | 163 | 169 | 175 | 180 | 186 | 191 | 197 |
| 5'4" | 110 | 116 | 122 | 128 | 134 | 140 | 145 | 151 | 157 | 163 | 169 | 174 | 180 | 186 | 192 | 197 | 204 |
| 5'5" | 114 | 120 | 126 | 132 | 138 | 144 | 150 | 156 | 162 | 168 | 174 | 180 | 186 | 192 | 198 | 204 | 210 |
| 5'6" | 118 | 124 | 130 | 136 | 142 | 148 | 155 | 161 | 167 | 173 | 179 | 186 | 192 | 198 | 204 | 210 | 216 |
| 5'7" | 121 | 127 | 134 | 140 | 146 | 153 | 159 | 166 | 172 | 178 | 185 | 191 | 198 | 204 | 211 | 217 | 223 |
| 5'8" | 125 | 131 | 138 | 144 | 151 | 158 | 164 | 171 | 177 | 184 | 190 | 197 | 203 | 210 | 216 | 223 | 230 |
| 5'9" | 128 | 135 | 142 | 149 | 155 | 162 | 169 | 176 | 182 | 189 | 196 | 203 | 209 | 216 | 223 | 230 | 236 |
| 5'10" | 132 | 139 | 146 | 153 | 160 | 167 | 174 | 181 | 188 | 195 | 202 | 209 | 216 | 222 | 229 | 236 | 243 |
| 5'11" | 136 | 143 | 150 | 157 | 165 | 172 | 179 | 186 | 193 | 200 | 208 | 215 | 222 | 229 | 236 | 243 | 250 |
| 6' | 140 | 147 | 154 | 162 | 169 | 177 | 184 | 191 | 199 | 206 | 213 | 221 | 228 | 235 | 242 | 250 | 258 |
| 6'1" | 144 | 151 | 159 | 166 | 174 | 182 | 189 | 197 | 204 | 212 | 219 | 227 | 235 | 242 | 250 | 257 | 265 |
| 6'2" | 148 | 155 | 163 | 171 | 179 | 186 | 194 | 202 | 210 | 218 | 225 | 233 | 241 | 249 | 256 | 264 | 272 |
| 6'3" | 152 | 160 | 168 | 176 | 184 | 192 | 200 | 208 | 216 | 224 | 232 | 240 | 248 | 256 | 264 | 272 | 279 |
| | Healthy Weight | | | | | | Overweight | | | | | Obese | | | | | |

Locate the height of interest in the leftmost column and read across the row for the height to the weight of interest. Then follow the column to the top of the row that lists the body mass index (BMI). BMI of 19 to 24 is healthy weight range. BMI of 25 to 29 is the overweight range, and BMI of 30 and above is the obese range.

*Source:* US Departments of Agriculture and Health and Human Services: *Dietary Guidelines for Americans*, 6th ed. Washington, DC: US Government Printing Office, 2005. Chart from Insel, P., Turner, R. E., and Ross, D. 2007. *Nutrition*, 3rd ed. Sudbury, MA: Jones and Bartlett Publishers.

monosaccharides, but at a much slower rate because the chains first must be broken by enzymes into individual glucose molecules before they can be processed to yield energy. Carbohydrates in excess of the body's energy requirements can be stored as glycogen in muscle and in the liver, and as fat in adipose tissue.

**Proteins**  Proteins are long chains of amino acids bonded together that must first be broken down into individual amino acids before they can be used to make new proteins needed to replace worn-out cells and tissues. There are 20 different amino acids. Most can be synthesized within the body from other components, but nine amino acids (called *essential amino acids*) can't be synthesized and must be obtained from the proteins in the food we eat. Minimal protein requirements are about 0.8 grams per kilogram of body weight in adults, although a normal balanced diet has a much higher protein content. If the diet contains more protein than the body needs, the excess is converted to fat and stored in adipose tissue.

**Fats**  Fats (triglycerides) are composed of three long-chain fatty acid molecules joined to a glycerol molecule. When fat is broken down to yield energy, the long fatty acid molecules are broken into 2-carbon fragments which, along with glycerol, are used to yield the energy stored within the triglyceride. The body can synthesize glycerol and most fatty acids from other components, but two fatty acids (called *essential fatty acids*) can't be synthesized and must be obtained from our diet. Fat intake should be less than 30 percent of total calories in the diet, and much lower in persons with high blood cholesterol, especially if they have coronary heart disease (Chapter 10).

## Vitamins and Minerals

Vitamins are organic compounds that function along with cell enzymes to convert food into energy. There are two major groups: *water soluble vitamins* (citric acid, the B vitamins, and folic acid) that are relatively easy to absorb, and *fat soluble vitamins* (vitamins A, D, E, and K) that must be absorbed along with dietary fat. Conditions that impair fat digestion or absorption, such as bile duct, liver, or pancreatic disease, also reduce absorption of fat-soluble vitamins.

Minerals are necessary for proper functioning of body cells. Some are needed in relatively large amounts, such as sodium, chloride, calcium, magnesium, and phosphate. Others are required in only trace amounts, such as copper, iodine, selenium, and zinc. Minerals play an important role in many body functions, such as bone formation, hemoglobin synthesis, metabolic processes regulated by thyroid hormones, and regulation of fluid and electrolyte balance.

# Achieving a Balanced Diet: Food Groups and Food Guides

A well-balanced diet can supply us with all the nutrients we need in appropriate amounts to achieve and maintain good health, and deficient diets lead to disease. The acceptable percentages of nutrients in a balanced diet are carbohydrates 45–65 percent, proteins 10–15 percent, and fats 20–35 percent. Nutrition guides to healthy eating are provided by the United States and Canadian government agencies, and various food guide pyramids are provided and updated periodically. Diets high in fruits, vegetables, whole-grain foods, and protein from meats, poultry, and low-fat dairy products are emphasized, with reduced consumption of saturated fats, trans fats, and cholesterol.

# Malnutrition

## Causes of Malnutrition

Malnutrition means that the intake of nutrients is inadequate, either because there is insufficient food, or the food is not being utilized efficiently. The usual causes fall into four categories:

1. *There is not enough food available.* In developing countries there may not be enough food to supply the population as a result of crop failure, natural disaster, poor food distribution, an unstable government, or other causes that impact food production or delivery. Often, infants and children are disproportionately affected because they have a greater need for nutrients to sustain their rapid growth rate during infancy and childhood.

   In modern industrialized countries, sometimes the food and other nutrients that are adequate for a normal healthy person may become insufficient when requirements increase greatly, as after major surgical procedures, severe burns, or other conditions that increase the body's need for nutrients. Consequently, food intake becomes inadequate to provide for the increased demand.

2. *Diseases or other disorders interfere with intake, absorption, or metabolism of nutrients.* Chronic pancreatic disease disrupts digestive functions by impairing adequate flow of digestive enzymes into the bowel; chronic liver, biliary tract, and pancreatic disease (Chapter 16) interfere with absorption and processing of nutrients in the liver. Many of the diseases characterized by damage to the

lining of the gastrointestinal tract, such as chronic inflammatory bowel disease (Chapter 17), interfere with food digestion and absorption.

3. *Drugs given to treat cancer and various other diseases may reduce food intake by decreasing appetite, by causing nausea or vomiting, or by interfering with the digestion and absorption of nutrients.*

4. *Age-related conditions may interfere with nutrition.* Elderly persons often eat less and their digestive processes may function less efficiently. Those living alone may not bother to prepare meals regularly. Some may have problems chewing and swallowing food, or may have had a stroke or other neurologic problem that makes eating difficult. Emotional problems such as loneliness and depression may also decrease interest in food.

## Malnutrition in Children

All foods provide calories to supply energy. Deficiency of carbohydrates and fats reduces the supply of available energy, but a protein deficiency presents a special problem because it deprives the body of amino acids to make the proteins required for normal body functions. Malnutrition that deprives the body of both energy and protein is called *protein-energy malnutrition* (PEM) or *protein-calorie malnutrition*. This condition is most prevalent in developing countries where food supplies are limited. All organs systems are involved. Heart, liver, kidneys, and other organs become smaller and function less efficiently. Impaired immune system function causes increased susceptibility to infection. As the malnutrition progresses, so does the progressive decline of organ functions. Severe untreated malnutrition is potentially fatal.

The two characteristic manifestations of malnutrition in children are called *kwashiorkor* and *marasmus* ( Table 18-2 ), although there are intermediate forms with features of both. Kwashiorkor results from a diet that is more deficient in protein than in other nutrients, and usually occurs in children between 18–24 months of age. In many cultures breastfeeding of the first child is continued until the next child is born. When the first child is weaned, the supply of protein-rich milk is no longer available. Kwashiorkor develops in the displaced child in whom protein-deficient foods provide most of the calories that replace the protein-rich breast milk. A characteristic feature of this condition is edema of the tissues as demonstrated by swollen legs, and by a swollen abdomen that is caused by accumulation of fluid in the peritoneal cavity. The edema is caused by protein deficiency. Protein is required to make the blood protein *albumin* that is made by the liver. One of its major functions is to maintain the normal osmotic

| Table 18-2 | Marasmus and Kwashiorkor Compared | | |
|---|---|---|---|
| Condition | Usual Cause | Result | Manifestations |
| Marasmus | Protein and nonprotein nutrients both deficient | Starvation caused by inadequate food | Retarded growth. Marked emaciation. Loss of subcutaneous fat and muscle. |
| Kwashiorkor | Protein deficiency greater than deficiency of other nutrients | Child displaced from breastfeeding by birth of second child | Low blood albumin leads to edema of limbs and accumulation of fluid in abdomen. Changes in hair color. Weight loss but not emaciated. |

pressure of the blood, which regulates the flow of fluid between the blood and the fluid surrounding the tissue cells (extracellular fluid), as described in Chapter 9. Albumin concentration falls when protein is deficient in the diet, which causes excess fluid to leak from the bloodstream and accumulate in the tissues. The protein deficiency may also cause the color of the hair to change, which may acquire a reddish cast, or may cause the hair to acquire alternating dark and light bands.

In contrast, marasmus is severe malnutrition caused by starvation in a young child. Growth stops and muscle and body fat are depleted. Organs atrophy. The child is frail and apathetic, but the edema characteristic of kwashiorkor does not occur.

Treatment consists of supplying adequate nutrients together with vitamins and minerals before the malnutrition-induced organ damage has progressed to such a degree that response to treatment is unlikely to be successful.

## Malnutrition in Adults

In Western countries and other industrialized countries most cases of malnutrition are caused primarily by diseases that impair food intake, digestion, or absorption, or by conditions that increase nutrient and protein requirements. Other groups at risk are persons living in poverty, the elderly, persons who consume alcohol in excess, drug abusers, persons with AIDS or advanced cancer, and persons with eating disorders such as anorexia and bulimia nervosa (Chapter 17).

**Identifying Persons at Risk of Malnutrition** Malnutrition should be suspected in adults who have lost weight and whose intake or absorption of nutrients has decreased for any reason, or whose nutrient requirements have increased significantly as a result of disease. Prevention and early detection of malnutrition in high-risk patients facilitate early treatment. More advanced malnutrition takes longer to correct.

**Evaluation and Treatment** Nutritional deficiencies often involve not only inadequate food nutrients, but also multiple vitamin and mineral deficiencies. Weight loss of 5 to 10 percent of normal body weight can usually be tolerated but as weight loss increases, so do the manifestations of the protein-energy deficiency. Extreme emaciation is a life-threatening condition, and loss of over 30 percent of body weight may be fatal.

The initial clinical evaluation of patients in whom malnutrition is suspected is supplemented by laboratory tests to assess the extent of organ and tissue damage, including determination of serum albumin as an index of protein deficiency. Medical treatment requires correcting any fluid and electrolyte disturbances and other physiologic disturbances caused by the deficiencies, followed by slowly increasing calorie and protein intake, preferably by oral feeding. Appropriate vitamin and mineral supplements are also provided, along with whatever additional measures are necessary to restore health.

## Alcohol: Its Role in Malnutrition

Drinking modest amounts of alcoholic beverages is considered acceptable in many cultures and even provides some health benefits by favorably influencing blood lipids and other physiologic processes that may help protect us from heart disease (described in Chapter 10). Although not classified as a nutrient, alcohol provides 7 calories per gram, which is almost as many calories as in fat. So alcohol can be categorized as a "high-calorie non-nutrient."

Excess alcohol intake can cause serious problems. Rapidly drinking large amounts of alcohol in a short period of time can be lethal, as documented by many reports of fatal alcohol intoxication resulting from binge drinking among college students. Chronic alcohol use may lead to dependence on alcohol, which can progress to alcohol addiction in susceptible individuals, and the unfortunate person becomes "an alcoholic." Alcoholism is a common cause of malnutrition because the alcoholic is substituting non-nutritive "empty calories" from alcohol for calories from food, which supply the nutrients, vitamins, and minerals that the body needs. Many of the harmful results of alcoholism are related

not only to the organ damage caused by excess alcohol, such as alcoholic liver disease described in Chapter 16, but also from the associated vitamin deficiencies that accompany an inadequate diet.

# Vitamins: Their Sources and Functions

Vitamins function as catalysts for many biochemical reactions. Fat-soluble vitamins A, D, E, and K are absorbed along with fat from the gastrointestinal tract, transported in the circulation along with fat and stored in the liver, and also in adipose tissue. Excessive amounts of fat-soluble vitamins (megadoses) that exceed the liver's storage capacity may cause toxic effects. With the exception of vitamin $B_{12}$, water-soluble vitamins, such as the other B vitamins and vitamin C, are not stored in the body, and any excess in the body is excreted in the urine.

## Fat-Soluble Vitamins

**Vitamin A** Vitamin A is present in dairy products, fruits and vegetables, and foods that are fortified with vitamin A. Some vitamin A is absorbed as a precursor compound and converted in the body to the active vitamin. There are three different forms of this vitamin. One form is part of the photoreceptor pigments in the retina that are concerned with vision, and a deficiency impairs the ability of the retina to respond to dim light, which is an early symptom of the deficiency called *night blindness*. Other forms of vitamin A regulate the maturation of epithelial cells, and play a role in bone growth and reproductive function. Rarely, disturbed epithelial cell growth and differentiation may lead to increased keratinization of the skin, and changes in the epithelium of the eye can lead to severe eye damage.

**Vitamin D** Many dairy products are fortified with vitamin D. Vitamin D is sometimes called "the sunshine vitamin" because vitamin D is synthesized by the action of sunlight on a cholesterol precursor in the skin to form an intermediate compound that is carried in the circulation to the liver where further processing occurs, and finally to the kidney where the synthesis is completed to form the active compound (calcitriol). A person exposed to sunlight in the summer can store enough vitamin D in the liver to have adequate supplies for the rest of the year.

Vitamin D functions along with parathyroid hormone (Chapter 20) to regulate the level of calcium in the blood and the deposition of calcium salts in bone matrix to form sturdy, rigid bone. In children vitamin D deficiency leads to impaired calcium deposition (ossification) of growing bone, which leads to bending and bowing of the poorly calcified bone. This condition, which is called **rickets**, rarely occurs now because milk and dairy products are fortified with vitamin D, and vitamin supplements are given routinely to children. In adults the comparable condition is called **osteomalacia**, which literally means "softening of bones."

Although rickets and osteomalacia are rare, current studies suggest that vitamin D deficiency occurs more frequently than suspected. Two factors are responsible: age, and use of sunscreens. Age is a factor because adults over 65 are less able to form vitamin D from cholesterol precursors in response to sunlight than are younger persons. Use of sunscreens to protect the skin from sun damage prevents the penetration of sunlight into the skin to start the synthesis of vitamin D. Penetration of sunlight into the skin also is less efficient in African Americans and other persons with dark skin because the melanin pigment in the skin impedes the penetration of sunlight to activate vitamin D synthesis. Persons living in northern parts of the country who have less sunlight exposure also don't make as much vitamin D.

Large doses of vitamin D are toxic. Blood calcium rises and the excess calcium is deposited in body tissues. Calcium is withdrawn from bone to raise blood calcium, which leads to loss of bone density.

**Vitamin E**  Vitamin E is a group of four compounds found in vegetable oils that was shown to be necessary for reproduction in rats, and is called *tocopherol*, which means "promoting childbirth." The important compound is called alpha tocopherol. Its main function is as an *antioxidant*, which is a compound that inactivates potentially cell-damaging toxic molecules (those having unpaired electrons) that form when compounds are oxidized during metabolic processes. Vitamin E is found in many foods, especially those made with vegetable oils. Its antioxidant properties may possibly help protect against some chronic diseases such as coronary artery disease, although clinical studies have not provided any strong evidence to support these claims.

**Vitamin K**  Vitamin K was named for Koagulation (spelled with a *K*). Its major function is to activate four proteins made by the liver that play an essential role in the coagulation of the blood (Chapter 9). The vitamin K compounds are called quinones. There are two different types. Vitamin $K_1$ (phylloquinones) is found in food: green leafy vegetables, vegetable oils, meat, liver, and some fish products. Vitamin $K_2$ (menaquinones) is made by our own intestinal bacteria and absorbed from the colon. Because vitamin K is a fat-soluble vitamin, its absorption from food is compromised by diseases that impair fat digestion or absorption. Absorption of vitamin K made by intestinal bacteria is abolished if broad-spectrum antibiotic treatment destroys the bacteria that make the vitamin.

Newborn infants are vulnerable to vitamin K deficiency because they lack the intestinal bacteria required to make vitamin K and are not yet consuming foods that contain the vitamin. Consequently, they are prone to episodes of bleeding, which is called *hemorrhagic*

**rickets**
Impaired calcification of bone in a growing child, caused by vitamin D deficiency, which leads to bowing of leg bones when weight bearing is attempted.

**osteomalacia** (ostēō-măh-lāy'see-yăh) Impaired calcification of bone in an adult caused by vitamin D deficiency, which also contributes to bone loss caused by osteoporosis.

## A Closer Look

*Vitamin D is different from other vitamins. Its major role is to regulate many important physiologic functions in our bodies, where it functions more like a hormone than a vitamin.*

In addition to its important role in promoting calcium absorption and calcification of bone, vitamin D inhibits proliferation of actively dividing cells, including cancer cells, and promotes maturation of normal cells. It promotes the functions of the immune system, which helps us fight infections and protects us against diseases. We can make vitamin D from sunlight exposure, which converts a cholesterol precursor in our skin to the first stages of vitamin D production, which is transported to the liver for further processing and then to the kidney to make the finished product. If we have dark skin, are using sunscreen, stay indoors, or wear clothing that almost completely covers our body, the sun may not have an opportunity to start the synthesis in the skin. Liver or kidney disease may impede later stages of vitamin D synthesis. Most physicians say that we are not getting enough vitamin D and should consider vitamin D supplements. Drinking milk, which is fortified with vitamin D, provides a high-grade nutrient as well as the vitamin D.

*disease of the newborn.* In order to prevent this condition, all newborn infants receive an injection of vitamin K to prevent bleeding caused by lack of the vitamin.

## Water-Soluble Vitamins

The B vitamins and vitamin C comprise the water-soluble vitamin group. There are several members of the B-vitamin group that were designated originally by number, such as vitamin $B_1$, $B_2$, $B_3$, and so on, but now they are usually designated by specific names, except for vitamin $B_6$ and $B_{12}$, which retain their number designations. The B vitamins participate along with enzymes in many energy-generating chemical reactions, and only the major B vitamins will be described. Because of their importance, thiamin ($B_1$), riboflavin ($B_2$), and niacin ($B_3$) are routinely added to fortify grain products, and recently folic acid also was added.

**Thiamin**  Thiamin (Vitamin $B_1$) is derived primarily from enriched grain products, although pork, some nuts and seeds, and a few other foods contain significant amounts of thiamin. In industrialized countries thiamin deficiency usually results from heavy alcohol consumption, which supplies calories but at the expense of required nutrients. Deficiency leads to peripheral nerve degeneration (peripheral neuritis) and a more serious degeneration of brain tissue characterized by confusion, loss of memory, difficulty in walking, and other features of brain degeneration. This condition, which is prone to occur in alcoholics, is called the Wernicke–Korsakoff syndrome.

Another manifestation of thiamin deficiency called *beriberi* is not often encountered in industrialized countries. The condition is characterized by peripheral nerve degeneration causing pain and weakness, which is associated with atrophy of leg muscle innervated by the damaged nerves. Sometimes cardiac function is also impaired, which leads to heart failure and heart failure-related accumulation of edema fluid in the legs and lungs.

**Riboflavin**  Riboflavin (vitamin $B_2$) is present in most plant and animal foods: milk, yogurt, grain products, and cereals have been enriched with riboflavin. Riboflavin deficiency is uncommon, and is characterized by mouth problems (stomatitis). The tongue becomes smooth and sore. Fissures and cracks appear in the skin at the angles of the mouth, the skin of the lips becomes sore and swollen; sometimes skin on other parts of the body becomes inflamed (dermatitis).

**Niacin**  Niacin (vitamin $B_3$) is present in meat, poultry, whole-grain and enriched grain products, and can also be made in the body from the amino acid tryptophan.

A deficiency leads to a disease called *pellagra*, and its manifestations can be remembered by the "3 Ds": dermatitis, diarrhea, and dementia. Untreated, the disease may be fatal.

**Vitamin $B_6$**  Vitamin $B_6$ is required for many metabolic reactions and the major dietary sources are from fortified ready-to-eat cereals, potatoes and other starchy vegetables, and foods containing meat, fish, or poultry. Vitamin $B_6$ deficiencies are rare but may occur occasionally in persons addicted to alcohol. Manifestations are anemia, dermatitis, and neurologic symptoms such as depression and confusion.

**Vitamin $B_{12}$ and Folic Acid**  Vitamin $B_{12}$ and folic acid (folate) are both required for normal DNA synthesis, and for normal maturation of both red and white blood cells. Vegetarians are at risk of vitamin $B_{12}$ deficiency unless they take vitamin supplements or eat vitamin $B_{12}$-fortified cereals. Folic acid is present in green leafy vegetables and grain products fortified with folic acid. A deficiency of either vitamin $B_{12}$ or folic acid or both may lead to an anemia in which the red cells are larger than normal (macrocytic anemia) as described in Chapter 11. Folic acid helps prevent congenital malformations called neural tube defects, described in Chapter 21, which was one of the reasons advanced in favor of folic acid fortification of grain and cereal products. Absorption of vitamin $B_{12}$, described in Chapter 11, is a more complex process than absorption of folic acid. Diseases or other conditions that impair vitamin $B_{12}$ absorption may lead to permanent neurologic damage as well as anemia.

**Vitamin C**  Vitamin C is present in many fruits and vegetables. Good sources are potatoes and tomatoes, citrus fruits of all types, vegetables, and vitamin-enriched juice drinks. One of its important functions is its role in the formation of collagen, a protein forming the dense connective tissue that supports and stabilizes individual body components. Vitamin C deficiency causes *scurvy*, which results from formation of poorly constructed collagen that lacks tensile strength and does not provide proper support for body tissues. Bleeding usually results because the defective collagen in the connective tissue surrounding bones and joints and supporting blood vessels is of such poor quality that blood vessels break, which leads to skin and mucous membrane hemorrhages, bleeding gums, and bone pain caused by areas of hemorrhage under the periosteum surrounding the bones.

Table 18-3 summarizes the spectrum of diseases caused by vitamin deficiencies.

## Table 18-3 Diseases and Conditions Caused by Vitamin Deficiencies

| Vitamin | Disease or Condition |
|---|---|
| Vitamin A | Night blindness; advanced deficiency may lead to severe eye damage |
| Vitamin D | Rickets in children; osteomalacia in adults |
| Vitamin E | An antioxidant; may help protect against various chronic diseases |
| Vitamin K | Impaired blood coagulation predisposes to bleeding in adults and hemorrhagic disease of newborn infants (preventable by prophylactic injection of vitamin K) |
| Thiamin | Peripheral neuritis, Wernicke–Korsakoff syndrome, beriberi |
| Riboflavin | Stomatitis, glossitis, dermatitis |
| Niacin | Pellagra (dermatitis, diarrhea, dementia) |
| Vitamin $B_6$ | Anemia, dermatitis, neurologic disease |
| Vitamin $B_{12}$ | Macrocytic anemia |
| Folic acid | Macrocytic anemia; neural tube defects in newborn infants |
| Vitamin C | Scurvy |

## A Closer Look

***Scurvy still occurs and may be hard to recognize.***
Scurvy is one of the earliest recorded diseases, and its successful treatment with oranges and lemons was recorded in an article published in 1753. But cases of scurvy are still encountered, and may not be as easy to recognize as you might think, as documented in a recently published article in a prominent medical journal (Duggan, C. P., Westra, S. J., and Rosenberg, A. E. 2007. Case 23-2007: A 9-year-old boy with bone pain, rash, and gingival hypertrophy. *New England Journal of Medicine* 357:392–400.)

A 9-year-old boy with a mental disorder (autism) was seen by a physician because of hip and knee pain that made it difficult for him to walk, and a skin rash, followed by swollen gums, and bleeding in the skin. Several diagnostic possibilities were considered, and extensive studies were performed, which led to the diagnosis of scurvy. The bone pain was caused by bleeding in the connective tissue (periosteum) covering the bone. Treatment consisted of vitamin C and pediatric multivitamins.

# Minerals

Many minerals are necessary for proper functioning of body cells. The major minerals, which are required in relatively large quantities are sodium, chloride, calcium, magnesium, and phosphate. Their functions in the regulation of fluid and electrolyte balance are considered in Chapter 19. The body also requires very small amounts of other minerals. These include: (1) iodine for thyroid hormone synthesis, (2) iron for hemoglobin synthesis, (3) fluoride for strong bones and teeth and to help prevent tooth decay, (4) copper, which is present in many compounds that function as antioxidants to prevent cell damage from free radicals generated during oxidation reactions related to cell metabolism, and (5) zinc and selenium, which are required for proper functioning of many enzyme systems.

# CHAPTER REVIEW

## Summary

Food provides calories, and vitamins help convert food into energy. Food groups and food guides promote proper food selection to achieve a balanced diet by helping select appropriate quantities of food from each food group. Failure to attain a balanced diet leads to malnutrition, which may result from (1) not enough available food, (2) a disease that interferes with food intake, absorption, or utilization, or increases the requirement for nutrients that exceeds the quantity available, (3) drugs given to treat disease that have side effects that interfere with food uptake or utilization, or (4) age-related conditions that may hamper food uptake or utilization. Alcoholism leads to malnutrition by replacing non-nutritive alcohol calories for nutrients. Protein-energy malnutrition in children leads to marasmus and kwashiorkor caused by inadequate nutrients. In adults most cases result from diseases that cause poor digestion, absorption, or utilization of nutrients rather than inadequate availability of nutrients, and improvement of the nutritional status requires treatment of the underlying disease. In general, evaluation and treatment of malnutrition involves: (1) assessing the extent of the malnutrition-related organ damage,

(2) gradually increasing nutrient intake, and (3) simultaneously treating any associated organ damage.

Vitamin deficiencies often coexist with malnutrition, and many are relatively common. Vitamin A deficiency causes night blindness; vitamin D deficiency adversely affects bone growth and calcification, but also has many effects on cell proliferation and immune system function. Vitamin K is required for normal blood coagulation, and deficiency leads to bleeding problems, especially in newborn infants, which can be prevented by giving vitamin K to all newborn infants. The B vitamins are involved in energy-generating chemical reactions, and deficiencies can have widespread effects on the nervous system as well as other tissues. Vitamin C deficiency impairs formation of the collagen fibers that make up the body's connective-tissue framework. The deficiency leads to widespread effects as seen in persons with scurvy, a disease that is still encountered. Minerals play many roles in our cells and tissues. Some are present in large amounts, such as sodium and chloride, and others are needed in only minimal quantities (trace minerals) but nevertheless have important functions.

## Questions for Review

1. What is body mass index (BMI) and how is it used?
2. How does the body break down food to be processed to yield energy?
3. What conditions cause malnutrition?
4. Compare the causes of malnutrition in children living in undeveloped countries with malnutrition in adults living in the United States and Canada.
5. What is the difference between marasmus and kwashiorkor? Why do children with kwashiorkor become edematous?
6. How is alcoholism responsible for malnutrition? What diseases or conditions may result from alcohol-related malnutrition?
7. What are the fat soluble vitamins? What conditions predispose to deficiency of these vitamins?
8. What are the effects of deficiencies of the following vitamins: vitamin K, vitamin D, niacin, folic acid, vitamin $B_{12}$?

## Supplementary Reading

Beers, M. D., ed. *Merck Manual of Diagnosis and Therapy*, 18th ed. 2006 West Point, PA: Merck Manuals Department.
    Comprehensive source of health-related topics.

Brender, E. 2005. Vitamin D. *Journal of the American Medical Association* 394:2386.
    A short one-page article designed for patient education describing the amount of sunlight exposure

required to ensure adequate vitamin D (10–15 minutes twice per week) absorption; the diseases resulting from the deficiency (rickets and osteomalacia); persons at risk of deficiency (breastfed infants receiving less than 2 cups a day of vitamin D-fortified formula or milk; persons with dark pigmented skin; very limited sun exposure; fat malabsorption diseases; liver or kidney disease, who are unable to perform the later stages of vitamin D activation; and those in the northern hemisphere where sunlight is limited during winter.

Holick, M. F. 2007. Vitamin D deficiency. *New England Journal of Medicine* 357:266–81.

Most cells and tissues in the body have vitamin D receptors, and the vitamin has many effects unrelated to the skeletal system. Vitamin D inhibits cell proliferation of both normal cells and cancer cells, and promotes normal differentiation of cells. Vitamin D is required for normal immune system function, which may explain why black Americans, who are often vitamin D deficient, are more prone to tuberculosis than are whites, and tend to have more aggressive disease. People living farther from the equator (where sunlight is most intense and prolonged) have a greater risk of a number of diseases than are persons living closer to the equator.

Current recommendations for vitamin D supplements are too low, and many persons are vitamin D deficient.

Insel, P., Turner, R. E., and Ross, D. 2007. *Nutrition*, 3rd ed. Sudbury, MA: Jones and Bartlett.

A valuable resource on nutrition.

## Interactive Activities

### Matching

Match the disease or condition in the left column with the vitamin deficiency in the right column.

| | |
|---|---|
| 1. Pellagra | A. Vitamin A deficiency |
| 2. Macrocytic anemia | B. Vitamin C deficiency |
| 3. Night blindness | C. Thiamin deficiency |
| 4. Osteomalacia | D. Niacin deficiency |
| 5. Scurvy | E. Vitamin $B_{12}$ deficiency |
| 6. Wernicke–Korsakoff syndrome | F. Vitamin D deficiency |

### Critical Thinking

1. A middle-aged-man with AIDS has been living alone and caring for himself. He has lost about 10 pounds in the last few months. He has had moderate diarrhea and has no appetite. Do you think he has a nutritional deficiency? Why or why not? If he does, why did it develop? How should he be treated?

2. Mary Smith just delivered a healthy baby girl and was told that the baby received an injection of vitamin K. She wants to know why this was done. What would you tell her?

3. John Jones is a middle-aged-man who has had a serious drinking problem for several years. After a recent bout of prolonged heavy drinking he began to notice tingling pain in his legs and weakness of his leg muscles, and he has also had difficulty remembering recent events. How would you evaluate his recent problems?

# 19

# Fluids and Electrolytes

1. Explain the basic concepts relating to the regulation of the concentration of electrolytes in the body. List the major ions in the intracellular and extracellular water, and define units of concentration.

2. Describe the common disturbances of water balance and their pathogenesis.

3. Explain the physiologic mechanisms concerned with the control of pH.

4. Describe the pathogenesis of the four common disturbances of acid–base balance and the body's compensatory mechanisms.

5. Define the role of the kidneys and the lungs in the regulation of acid–base balance.

## Body Water and Electrolytes

About 70 percent of the body consists of water. Most is within cells as *intracellular water*. The remainder, called *extracellular water*, is within the interstitial tissues surrounding the cells and in the blood plasma. The body water contains dissolved mineral salts (**electrolytes**) that dissociate in solution, yielding positively charged ions (**cations**) and negatively charged ions (**anions**). The body fluids are electrically neutral, and the sum of the positively charged ions in solution is always balanced by the sum of the negatively charged ions. In disease, the concentrations of the individual ions may vary, but electrical neutrality is always maintained.

To help remember the distribution of water and contained electrolytes within the body, it may be convenient to use the "rule of thirds." Approximately two-thirds of the body weight is water, and two-thirds of the water is within the cells. The remaining one-third is extracellular, and most of the extracellular fluid is in the tissues surrounding the cells (interstitial fluid). The rest is in the blood and lymph within vessels in the interstitial tissues. The water content of a woman's body is about 10 percent lower than a man's body of comparable size because a woman has more body fat, which contains very little water.

For purposes of description, it is convenient to give separate consideration to disturbances of body water and abnormalities in the concentrations of electrolytes. This separation is artificial, however, because all body fluids contain dissolved mineral salts. If the electrolyte concentration of the body changes, there is usually a corresponding change in body water. Conversely, changes in body water are usually associated with changes in electrolyte concentrations.

# Interrelations of Intracellular and Extracellular Fluid

Fluid and electrolytes diffuse freely between the intravascular and interstitial fluids. However, the capillaries are impermeable to protein so the interstitial fluid contains very little protein.

The fluid within the cells is separated from the interstitial fluid by the cell membrane, which is freely permeable to water but relatively impermeable to sodium and potassium ions. The principal extracellular ions are sodium ($Na^+$) and chloride ($Cl^-$), whereas the principal intracellular ions are potassium ($K^+$) and phosphate ($PO_4^{3-}$). The differences in the concentration of the ions on different sides of the cell membrane are a result of the metabolic activity of the cell.

In general, the amount of sodium in the body determines the volume of the extracellular fluid because this is the chief extracellular cation, and the amount of potassium in the body determines the volume of the intracellular fluid because this is the chief intracellular cation.

# Units and Concentration of Electrolytes

In dealing with disturbances of electrolytes, the clinician is concerned primarily with concentrations of the various ions and with the interrelation of positively and negatively charged ions with one another, rather than with the actual number of milligrams or grams of the various salts dissolved in the plasma. Therefore, the concentrations of electrolytes are expressed in units that define their ability to combine with other ions.

The quantity that expresses "combining weight" is termed the *equivalent weight*. An equivalent weight is the molecular weight of a substance in grams divided by its valence. When one equivalent weight of a substance is dissolved in a solution to make one liter (1 L), the concentration is *one equivalent per liter*. For a mono-

valent substance, this is the same as a one molar solution, expressed as *one mole per liter*.

As an example, the equivalent weight of sodium chloride is determined by adding 23 g (atomic weight of sodium) to 35.5 g (atomic weight of chloride) and dividing by the valence (which is one), to equal 58.5 g of sodium chloride, the equivalent weight.

In body fluids, the concentrations of electrolytes are low and are usually expressed in *milliequivalents per liter* (abbreviated mEq/L) rather than in equivalents, although some physicians prefer to express concentrations of monovalent ions in millimoles per liter (abbreviated mmol/L), which is the same as mEq/L, when dealing with monovalent ions. A milliequivalent is 1/1000 of an equivalent. Concentrations of ions expressed in milliequivalents have equal combining properties, even though their equivalent weights are not equal. For example, a milliequivalent of bicarbonate ion is equal in electrical and ionic characteristics to a milliequivalent of chloride ion, even though the molecular weight of bicarbonate is greater than that of chloride.

**electrolyte** (ē-lek′trō-līt) A compound that in solution dissociates into positive and negative ions.

**cation** (kat′ī-on) An ion that carries a positive charge.

**anion** (an′ī-on) An ion carrying a negative charge.

# Regulation of Body Fluid and Electrolyte Concentration

The amount of water and electrolytes in the body represents a balance between the amounts ingested in food and fluids and the amounts excreted in the urine, through the gastrointestinal tract, in perspiration, and as water vapor excreted by the lungs. The kidneys are important in controlling the concentration of body water and electrolytes. Under the influence of adrenal cortical and posterior pituitary hormones, the kidneys regulate the internal environment of the body by selectively excreting or retaining water and electrolytes as required to maintain a uniform composition of the body fluids.

# Disturbances of Water Balance

## Dehydration

The most common disturbance of water balance is dehydration, which may be caused by inadequate water intake or excess water loss. Most cases of dehydration seen in medical practice result from excessive loss of fluid from the gastrointestinal tract as a consequence of vomiting or diarrhea. Fluid intake is usually decreased, contributing to the dehydration. Occasionally, comatose or debilitated patients become dehydrated because of inadequate intake of fluid.

## Overhydration

Overhydration is less common than dehydration. Sometimes overhydration results from administering too much fluid intravenously, but may also occur when a person with impaired renal function drinks a large amount of fluid, which the kidneys are unable to excrete efficiently. Drinking a large amount of water may also change the concentration of the electrolytes in the extracellular fluid, even in a person with normal renal function. As the ingested water is absorbed into the circulation, the water increases the volume of the extracellular fluid, which lowers its sodium ion concentration (hyponatremia) as the fluid becomes more dilute. Marked hyponatremia may have serious and sometimes life-threatening consequences. This condition may occur in an infant who is given water to supplement formula feedings or when the infant's formula is prepared with too much water and is too dilute. Infants under 6 months of age are at greatest risk, as their kidneys are relatively immature and they are less able to excrete the excess water. Another group at risk includes athletes engaging in strenuous sports, such as marathon runners, who consume excessive amounts of water while exercising in order to prevent dehydration. Their renal function also may be compromised during vigorous exercise because renal blood flow falls and urine output declines as blood is diverted from the kidneys to actively exercising muscles.

# Disturbances of Electrolyte Balance

In general, the same conditions that produce disturbances of water balance also disturb the electrolyte composition of the body fluids. Most electrolyte disturbances result from depletion of body electrolytes. Depletions of sodium and potassium generally occur together, often because of loss of electrolytes along with water from the gastrointestinal tract as a result of vomiting or diarrhea. Large amounts of sodium and potassium may also be lost in the urine as a result of prolonged use of diuretics. Diuretics are substances that promote excretion of salts and water by the kidneys by impairing reabsorption of

**buffer**
A substance that minimizes change in pH of a solution when an acid or base is added.

these substances from the glomerular filtrate; they are often administered to patients with heart failure, cirrhosis of the liver, and some types of kidney diseases. Loss of large amounts of electrolytes may also accompany excessive excretion of water in the urine in uncontrolled diabetes, as a result of the diuretic effect of the excreted glucose (Chapter 16), or in renal tubular disease, in which the regenerating renal tubules are unable to conserve electrolytes and water (Chapter 15).

# Acid–Base Balance

The body may be considered an acid-producing machine that generates large amounts of organic and inorganic acids in consequence of normal metabolic processes. It produces various nonvolatile acids such as sulfuric, phosphoric, and uric acid from the breakdown of proteins. It forms ketone bodies in the oxidation of fat (Chapter 16) and produces lactic acid from breakdown of glucose when oxygen supplies are insufficient. Large amounts of carbon dioxide also are formed as by-products of intracellular metabolic processes, and some of the carbon dioxide dissolves in body fluids to form *carbonic acid*.

Despite the large amounts of acid produced, the body fluids remain slightly alkaline, and their pH is maintained within the narrow range of 7.38 to 7.42. The body is able to maintain the alkalinity of body fluids because it has three regulatory mechanisms that neutralize and eliminate the acids as rapidly as they are formed:

1. The buffer systems of the blood
2. The lungs, which regulate the carbonic acid concentration
3. The kidneys, which control bicarbonate concentration

## Buffers

*The buffer systems of the blood* are the first line of defense against change in pH. In a general sense, a buffer is anything that cushions a blow or absorbs an impact. Chemically, a **buffer** may be defined as a weak acid and a salt of the acid or as a weak base and its salt. Buffers minimize change in hydrogen ion concentration by converting strong (completely ionized) acids and bases into weaker (less completely dissociated) acids and bases.

The major buffer system of the blood is the *sodium bicarbonate–carbonic acid system*. This system is of major importance because both components of the buffer system are present in large amounts, and the concentration of each component can be regulated by the body. The concentration of carbonic acid (dissolved carbon dioxide) is controlled by the lungs, and the concentration of bicarbonate is controlled by the kidneys. Although the bicarbonate–carbonic acid buffer system is not the only buffer system of the body, the system is in equilibrium with the other buffer systems. Therefore, measurement of the components of this system provides an overall evaluation of the acid–base status of the patient.

## Control of Carbonic Acid by the Lungs

The lungs excrete carbon dioxide and regulate the carbonic acid content of the blood. Carbonic acid is derived from the carbon dioxide produced along with water as a by-product of the metabolic activity of the cells. Carbon dioxide is quite soluble in blood plasma; some of the dissolved gas reacts with water to form the weak carbonic acid, which partially dissociates to form hydrogen ions and bicarbonate ions. The three forms are in equilibrium with one another as follows:

$$\text{Dissolved } CO_2 \text{ in plasma} \leftrightarrow H_2CO_3 \leftrightarrow H^+ + HCO_3^-$$

The carbon dioxide gas dissolved in plasma is in equilibrium with the carbon dioxide gas in the pulmonary alveoli. The alveolar carbon dioxide concentration is usually expressed in terms of the pressure exerted by the gas, which is called its partial pressure (designated $PCO_2$), as described in Chapter 15. Consequently, an equilibrium exists between alveolar $PCO_2$ and the various forms of $CO_2$ in the plasma, as follows:

$$\text{Alveolar } PCO_2 \leftrightarrow \text{plasma } PCO_2 \leftrightarrow H_2CO_3 \leftrightarrow H^+ + HCO_3^-$$

The carbon dioxide content of alveolar air and the alveolar $PCO_2$ vary with the rate and depth of respiration. If alveolar $PCO_2$ changes, there is a corresponding change in the amount of carbon dioxide dissolved in the plasma and in the amount of carbonic acid formed by the dissolved carbon dioxide. An increase in the rate and depth of respiration (hyperventilation) always lowers alveolar $PCO_2$ by exchanging inspired air containing almost no $CO_2$ for an equivalent amount of alveolar air containing a relatively large amount of $CO_2$. The fall in alveolar $PCO_2$ in turn leads to a corresponding decrease in the concentration of carbonic acid and carbon dioxide in the plasma. Conversely, alveolar $PCO_2$ rises if the rate and depth of pulmonary ventilation decrease; the concentration of carbon dioxide and carbonic acid in the plasma increase correspondingly.

## Control of Bicarbonate Concentration by the Kidneys

The kidneys regulate bicarbonate concentration in the plasma by selectively reabsorbing filtered bicarbo-

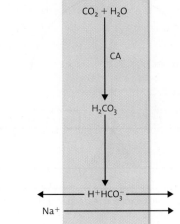

Tubular filtrate    Tubule cell    Blood plasma

**Figure 19-1** Formation and excretion of hydrogen ions by renal tubular epithelial cells in exchange for sodium. CA indicates carbonic anhydrase.

nate as necessary to meet the body's requirements. In addition, the kidneys can manufacture bicarbonate to replace the amounts lost in buffering acids produced as a consequence of normal metabolic processes. These two bicarbonate-regulating functions depend on the secretion of hydrogen ions by the renal tubules in exchange for sodium ions, which are simultaneously reabsorbed from the tubular filtrate into the circulation as illustrated in **Figure 19-1**. Under the influence of the enzyme carbonic anhydrase, carbonic acid ($H_2CO_3$) is formed from carbon dioxide ($CO_2$) and water ($H_2O$) within the tubular epithelial cells and dissociates into hydrogen ($H^+$) and bicarbonate ($HCO_3^-$) ions. The hydrogen ions enter the tubular filtrate in exchange for sodium ions ($Na^+$). The bicarbonate ions enter the bloodstream along with the sodium ions that have been absorbed from the filtrate.

## Relationship Between pH and Ratio of Buffer Components

In any buffer system, the pH depends on the ratio of the two components and not on the absolute quantities of the components. For the bicarbonate–carbonic acid buffer system at normal body pH of 7.4, the normal ratio consists of 20 parts of sodium bicarbonate and one part of carbonic acid.

Another way of visualizing the bicarbonate–carbonic acid relationship is to think of a board on a fulcrum. One side of the board is weighted by 20 parts of sodium bicarbonate, and the other side is weighted by one part of carbonic acid. The fulcrum is placed so that the board is exactly in balance, corresponding to a body pH of 7.4. Variations in the "weight" of either the sodium bicarbonate or the carbonic acid can be

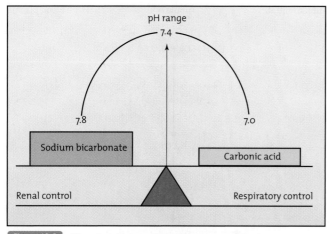

**Figure 19-2** "Board-and-fulcrum" concept of normal bicarbonate–carbonic acid relationships.

visualized as unbalancing the board, resulting in a shift of pH to a new level, either higher or lower than the normal value ( Figure 19-2 ).

# Disturbances of Acid–Base Balance

A disturbance in which blood pH is shifted to the acid side of the physiologic range is called **acidosis**. It may be caused by an excess of carbonic acid or by a reduced amount of bicarbonate. **Alkalosis** is a shift in the opposite direction, which may result from a decrease in carbonic acid or an excess of bicarbonate. These possibilities allow classification of acid–base disturbances into four large categories:

1. Metabolic acidosis (decrease in bicarbonate)
2. Respiratory acidosis (increase in carbonic acid)
3. Metabolic alkalosis (increase in bicarbonate)
4. Respiratory alkalosis (decrease in carbonic acid)

The term *metabolic* is applied when the disturbance lies primarily in the bicarbonate member of the buffer pair. The term *respiratory* indicates that the primary disturbance lies in the carbonic acid component of the buffer.

The various forms of acid–base disturbance are compared in Table 19-1 .

## Compensatory Mechanisms Responding to Disturbances in pH

If the acid–base disturbance shifts the pH outside of the physiologic range, various control measures are activated to resist the change in pH. Compensatory mechanisms attempt to preserve the normal 20:1 ratio of bicarbonate to carbonic acid and thereby return the

**Table 19-1** **Comparison of Common Acid–Base Disturbances**

| Disturbance | Primary Abnormality | Compensation | Usual Causes |
|---|---|---|---|
| Metabolic acidosis | Excess endogenous acid depletes bicarbonate | Hyperventilation lowers $PCO_2$; kidney excretes more hydrogen ions and forms more bicarbonate | Renal failure; ketosis; overproduction of lactic acid |
| Respiratory acidosis | Inefficient excretion of carbon dioxide by lungs | Formation of additional bicarbonate by kidneys | Chronic pulmonary disease |
| Metabolic alkalosis | Excess plasma bicarbonate | None | Loss of gastric juice; chloride depletion; excess corticosteroid hormones; ingestion of excessive bicarbonate or other antacids |
| Respiratory alkalosis | Hyperventilation lowers $PCO_2$ | Increased excretion of bicarbonate by kidneys | Severe anxiety with hyperventilation; stimulation of respiratory center by drugs; central nervous system disease |

pH to physiologic range. For example, if the concentration of carbonic acid rises as a result of pulmonary disease, there is a compensatory increase in bicarbonate that tends to restore the ratio of the two constituents and maintain pH in the physiologic range. Conversely, if there is a decrease in bicarbonate, compensation involves a decrease in the concentration of carbonic acid to maintain a relatively normal ratio. If one member of the buffer pair is disturbed by disease, the compensation is achieved by the other member of the buffer pair. The compensations are the body's attempt to minimize the extent of the pH change resulting from a disease-related change affecting one member of the buffer pair by changing the other member. This provides a short-term solution to the acid–base disturbance. The long-term correction of the acid–base balance derangement involves treating successfully the underlying disease or condition that caused the pH disturbance, which may not always be possible.

For the student attempting to grasp the fundamentals of the major disturbances in acid–base balance, the "board-and-fulcrum" concept shown in Figure 19-2 is frequently helpful. The "weight" of carbonic acid is controlled by respiration, and the "weight" of bicarbonate is controlled by renal excretion or conservation of bicarbonate. The student should consider two things: (1) the nature of the primary disturbance and how it will "unbalance" the board, and (2) the steps that the body should take to bring the board back into balance. These are the compensatory mechanisms, and they generally consist of "adding weight" or "subtracting weight" from the other member of the board. Admittedly, this is a mechanical oversimplification of a complex process, but it is a helpful learning device.

The two most common clinical disturbances of acid–base balance are metabolic acidosis and respiratory acidosis.

## Metabolic Acidosis

*Metabolic acidosis*, a common problem in medical practice, occurs when the amount of acid generated exceeds the body's buffering capacity. The concentration of bicarbonate in the plasma falls because it is consumed in neutralizing the excess acid ( Figure 19-3A ). Three of the more common conditions leading to metabolic acidosis are

1. Renal failure (uremia)
2. Ketosis (overproduction of ketone bodies)
3. Lactic acidosis (excessive production of lactic acid)

Renal failure is the end stage of many different types of kidney disease, as described in Chapter 15. Metabolic acidosis occurs because the failing kidneys are unable to excrete efficiently the various acid waste products that are produced by the body's normal metabolic processes. Ketosis results from overproduction of the acid ketone bodies' acetoacetic acid and beta-hydroxybutyric acid, which are derived from the metabolism of fat.

**acidosis** A disturbance in the acid–base balance of the body in which body fluids have a lower pH than normal.

**alkalosis** A disturbance in the body's acid–base balance in which the pH of the extracellular fluids is shifted toward the alkaline side of normal. See also *acidosis*.

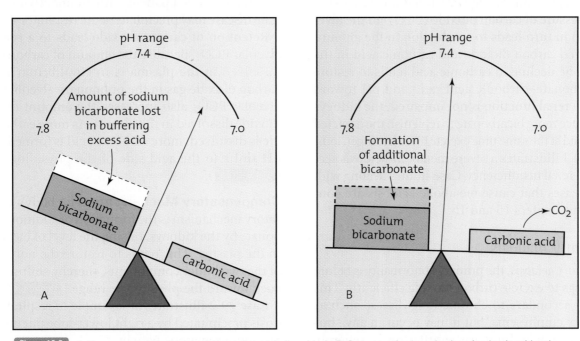

Figure 19-3    **A,** Derangement of acid–base balance in metabolic acidosis. **B,** Compensation by reduction of carbonic acid and formation of additional bicarbonate.

Ketosis commonly occurs in untreated type 1 diabetes because the body is unable to use carbohydrate efficiently and is forced to rely on fat as a major energy source (Chapter 16). Ketosis may also occur in any condition in which carbohydrate intake is inadequate, as in starvation, or if persistent vomiting prevents the retention of nutrients. In such cases, the body has to metabolize adipose tissue because carbohydrate is not available as an energy source. Some diets, called ketogenic diets, are actually designed to produce ketosis. They contain a large amount of fat, limited carbohydrates, and moderate protein. Ketogenic diets can be used to treat some types of epilepsy and have also been used to promote weight loss.

*Lactic acidosis* occurs in a number of different conditions, such as shock or severe heart failure, in which the tissues receive an inadequate supply of oxygen. The lactic acid is formed from the breakdown of glucose when there is not enough oxygen available to allow for the more efficient energy-generating aerobic (oxygen requiring) breakdown of glucose to its end products carbon dioxide and water. Instead, the body has to use a less efficient process (called anaerobic glycolysis) that produces lactic acid as its breakdown product, which leads to lactic acidosis.

## Compensatory Mechanisms

Compensation for metabolic acidosis is accomplished by both the lungs and the kidneys ( Figure 19-3B ). The acidosis stimulates the respiratory center in the brain stem, leading to an increase in both the rate and the depth of respiration. The hyperventilation reduces the partial pressure of carbon dioxide ($PCO_2$) in the alveoli, which in turn leads to a reduction in the amount of dissolved carbon dioxide and carbonic acid in the plasma. The decline in carbonic acid tends to restore the bicarbonate–carbonic acid ratio and pH toward normal. If renal function is not impaired, the kidneys also produce more bicarbonate to replenish the depleted supplies and at the same time excrete more hydrogen ions.

Case 19-1 illustrates a severe metabolic acidosis secondary to renal insufficiency. Case studies dealing with other diseases that cause metabolic acidosis are considered in Chapters 15 and 16.

## Respiratory Acidosis

In *respiratory acidosis*, the primary abnormality is failure of the lungs to excrete carbon dioxide efficiently. This is usually secondary to chronic lung disease such as pulmonary emphysema, but it may occur in any situation in which pulmonary ventilation is severely

**Case Study 19-1**

A 65-year-old woman consulted her physician because of discomfort in the lower back. Physical examination revealed moderate enlargement of both kidneys. Laboratory studies revealed a small amount of albumin in the urine and a moderate degree of anemia. Urea nitrogen was 57 mg/dL, a moderate elevation (normal range 10–20 mg/dL). A pyelogram revealed bilateral polycystic kidneys. The patient declined further treatment but was readmitted 6 months later because of further deterioration of her condition. She was more anemic, and the blood urea nitrogen had risen to 148 mg/dL. Blood pH was reduced to 7.2 (normal range 7.38–7.42). Plasma bicarbonate was also reduced to 10 mEq/L. The $PCO_2$ was 30 mm Hg, a slight decrease that was secondary to hyperventilation. The patient was considered to be in terminal renal failure with marked metabolic acidosis. Despite intensive therapy her condition did not improve, and she died in the hospital a few days later.

impaired (Chapter 12). In many instances, a respiratory infection in a patient with an underlying chronic lung disease may precipitate acute respiratory acidosis.

Retention of carbon dioxide leads to a rise in the alveolar $PCO_2$. Because the amount of carbon dioxide dissolved in the plasma is in equilibrium with the carbon dioxide gas in the pulmonary alveoli, a rise in alveolar $PCO_2$ also increases the amount of carbon dioxide dissolved in the plasma. As more carbon dioxide is dissolved, more carbonic acid is formed and the pH shifts to the acid side of the physiologic range ( Figure 19-4A ).

**Compensatory Mechanisms** The body's compensatory mechanism is the formation of additional bicarbonate by the kidneys, raising the level of bicarbonate in the plasma. This tends to restore the normal ratio of the two buffer components, thereby shifting the pH back toward the physiologic range ( Figure 19-4B ).

Case 19-2 illustrates an example of respiratory acidosis precipitated by a right lower-lobe pneumonia in an emphysematous patient.

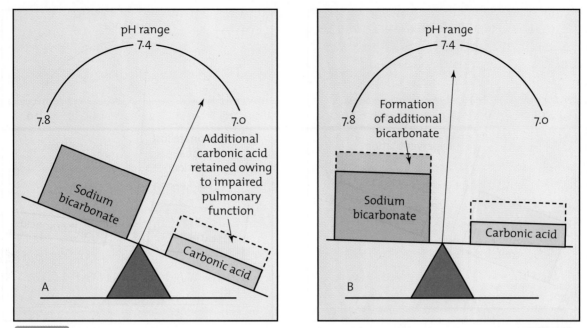

**Figure 19-4** **A,** Derangement of acid–base balance in respiratory acidosis. **B,** Compensation by formation of additional bicarbonate.

## Case Study 19-2

A 64-year-old man had noted progressive chronic cough and shortness of breath on exertion and repeated bouts of respiratory infection. He had become so short of breath that he was no longer able to climb stairs or do any kind of work around the house. Chest x-ray revealed hyperinflation of the lungs, compatible with pulmonary emphysema, and pulmonary function studies also showed marked impairment. Physical examination revealed a severely dyspneic (short of breath) man who was also slightly cyanotic. Scattered wheezes were heard throughout both lungs with a stethoscope. The temperature was slightly elevated. Chest x-ray revealed pulmonary emphysema and an area of consolidation in the right lower lobe of the lung representing a superimposed pneumonia. Arterial blood oxygen saturation was reduced; partial pressure of carbon dioxide was increased ($PCO_2$ 50 mm Hg), and blood pH was reduced (pH 7.30). The patient was treated with appropriate antibiotics and supplementary oxygen. He eventually recovered from the pneumonia and was able to leave the hospital.

## Metabolic Alkalosis

*Metabolic alkalosis* occurs less frequently than other acid–base disturbances and is caused by several different conditions that have in common an elevated sodium bicarbonate relative to the carbonic acid concentration, with an associated pH shift to the alkaline side of the physiologic normal range. The main causes include:

1. Loss of gastric juice resulting from vomiting or continuous aspiration of gastric contents
2. Excessive ingestion of sodium bicarbonate or other antacids to neutralize gastric juice
3. Blood chloride depletion
4. Adrenal corticosteroid excess

Compensation by raising carbonic acid to minimize the pH change induced by the high bicarbonate is not an option because shallow breathing to raise alveolar $PCO_2$ would only stimulate respirations and return $PCO_2$ to normal. The alkalosis can only be treated by correcting the patient's underlying disease or condition.

**Compensatory Mechanisms** Compensation is achieved by increased excretion of bicarbonate by the kidneys, which lowers the plasma bicarbonate and tends to restore the ratio of the buffer components toward normal.

## Respiratory Alkalosis

*Respiratory alkalosis* is a result of hyperventilation, which lowers the alveolar $PCO_2$. This in turn leads to a corresponding decrease in the amount of dissolved

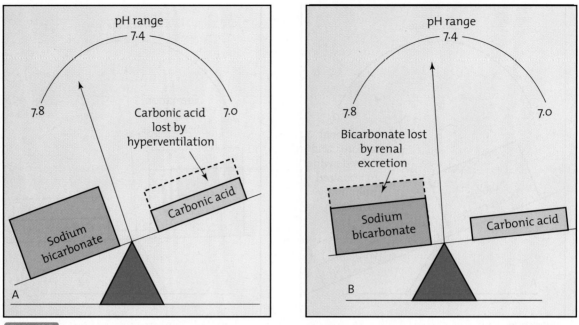

**Figure 19-5** **A,** Derangement of acid–base balance in respiratory alkalosis. **B,** Compensation by excretion of bicarbonate.

carbon dioxide and carbonic acid in the plasma. As a result, there is a relative excess of bicarbonate, and the blood pH tends to rise ( Figure 19-5A ). The hyperventilation that initiates this disturbance may result from stimulation of the respiratory center by drugs or may result from disease of the nervous system. Sometimes the hyperventilation is the result of an emotional disturbance such as severe anxiety. Compensation is archieved by excretion of bicarbonate by the kidneys to restore the normal ratio of the two buffer components ( Figure 19-5B ).

The temporary discomfort experienced by a vacationer traveling from sea level to a high altitude is caused in part by a mild respiratory alkalosis resulting from the hyperventilation induced by the lower $PO_2$

in the atmospheric air at high altitude. Fortunately, the body gradually learns to adapt and the initial discomfort gradually subsides.

## Diagnostic Evaluation of Acid–Base Balance

In evaluating the acid–base status of a patient, the clinician frequently determines the concentration of the bicarbonate in the plasma as an index of the patient's overall status. This is supplemented in many cases by the determination of the blood pH and the determination of the carbonic acid in the plasma. The clinical state of the patient, as evaluated by the clinician, together with these various laboratory tests, generally permits a determination of the patient's acid–base status and serves as a guide for effective treatment.

# CHAPTER REVIEW

## Summary

Most of the body consists of water containing dissolved mineral salts (electrolytes). Dehydration involves both body water and electrolytes, and usually results from inadequate intake, or excessive loss from vomiting or diarrhea. Overhydration usually results from excessive water intake, which also dilutes body fluids and may lead to serious life-threatening hyponatremia (low-serum sodium). Persons at risk include infants who are fed formula diluted with too much water, athletes consuming an excessive amount of water to prevent dehydration, and persons with kidney disease who are unable to excrete water efficiently.

Body fluids are slightly alkaline even though the body is an "acid-producing machine." Alkalinity is maintained by (1) the buffer systems of the blood as measured by the sodium bicarbonate–carbonic acid buffer system, (2) the lungs, which regulate carbonic acid by respiratory control of alveolar $PCO_2$, and (3) the kidneys, which regulate the bicarbonate concentration by either excreting or producing bicarbonate as required to maintain a normal blood pH. An acid–base balance disturbance that changes blood pH can be defined in terms of changes in bicarbonate or carbonic acid. In metabolic acidosis or alkalosis the primary disturbance is in the bicarbonate member of the buffer pair, which is regulated by the kidneys; in respiratory acidosis or alkalosis the primary disturbance is in the carbonic acid member of the pair, which is controlled by the lungs (regulating alveolar $PCO_2$). When the pH disturbance is caused by a change in one member of the buffer pair, the other member also changes (compensates) in an attempt to minimize the pH disturbance until the underlying disease or condition that caused the pH disturbance can be corrected. Metabolic acidosis results from a fall in bicarbonate resulting in accumulation of excess acids (kidney failure, ketosis, lactic acidosis), and the compensation is hyperventilation, which lowers carbonic acid by lowering alveolar $PCO_2$. Respiratory acidosis occurs in persons with inadequate pulmonary function, which raises alveolar $PCO_2$ and is accompanied by a corresponding rise in carbonic acid. Compensation is handled by the kidneys, which raise bicarbonate. Respiratory alkalosis is caused by hyperventilation, which lowers alveolar $PCO_2$ (and carbonic acid), and the compensation is excretion of bicarbonate by the kidneys. Metabolic alkalosis, which occurs less frequently than the other disturbances, is caused by conditions in which the pH change is associated with high blood bicarbonate, and there is no effective compensation.

## Questions for Review

1. What is the difference between intracellular fluid and extracellular fluid?
2. What is meant by the following terms: *milliequivalent*, *diuretic*, *carbonic anhydrase*, and *buffer*?
3. What is metabolic acidosis? How does it arise? What are the body's compensatory mechanisms?
4. What is respiratory acidosis? How does it arise? What are the body's compensatory mechanisms?
5. What is respiratory alkalosis? How does it arise? What are the body's compensatory mechanisms?

## Supplementary Reading

Almond, C. B. D., Shin, A. Y., Fortescue, E. B., et al. 2005. Hyponatremia among runners in the Boston marathon. *New England Journal of Medicine* 352: 1550–56.

> Four hundred eighty-eight participants in the Boston marathon provided a blood sample at the conclusion of the marathon and a completed questionnaire describing their fluid consumption and urine output during the race. Thirteen percent had a significant hyponatremia; three persons had a severe, potentially life-threatening hyponatremia of less than 120 mmol/L. Many runners drank more than 3 liters of fluid during the race, which diluted their body fluids and led to the hyponatremia. Excess fluid intake should be avoided during strenuous exercise because the kidneys may be unable to excrete the excess water efficiently.
>
> See also the accompanying editorial in the same issue: Levine, B. J., and Thompson, P. D. 2005.

Marathon maladies. *New England Journal of Medicine* 352:1516–17.

Beers, M. H., Fletcher, A. J., Jones, T. V., and Porter, R. 2003. *The Merck Manual of Medical Information. Second Home Edition.* New York: Pocket Books, a division of Simon & Schuster.

A very well-known medical reference based on the version produced for physicians. The material is very clearly written and concise.

Centers for Disease Control and Prevention. 1994. Hyponatremic seizures among infants fed commercial bottled drinking water. *Morbidity and Mortality Weekly Report* 43:641–43.

Several cases of severe water intoxication with hyponatremia are described in infants caused by supplementing infant formula with commercial bottled drinking water or when infant formula was diluted with water. Infants experienced irritability, drowsiness, and convulsions. Water should not be given to infants less than 6 months old.

Tierney, L. M., McPhee, S. J., and Papadakis, M. A. 2006. *Current Medical Diagnosis & Treatment*, 45th ed. New York: Lange Medical Books/McGraw-Hill.

Good section on fluids, electrolytes, and acid–base balance.

## Interactive Activities

### Fill-in-the-Blanks

1. Positively charged ions are called _____. and negatively charged ions are called _____.
2. The units of concentration of electrolytes are expressed as _____.
3. The two principal ions in intracellular fluids are _____ and _____.

### Matching

The numbered column lists several clinical conditions associated with acid–base balance disturbances. The lettered column lists the four types of acid–base disturbances. Match the letter with the clinical condition. There are six conditions but only four acid–base disturbances; thus, some letters are used more than once, and some may not be used at all.

| | |
|---|---|
| 1. Diabetes; excessive ketone bodies formed | A. Metabolic acidosis |
| 2. Hyperventilation; fall in alveolar $PCO_2$ | B. Respiratory acidosis |
| 3. Impaired lung function caused by chronic pulmonary disease | C. Metabolic alkalosis |
| 4. Kidney failure; retention of nonvolatile acids | D. Respiratory alkalosis |
| 5. Excess loss of gastric juice resulting from vomiting | |
| 6. Adrenal corticosteroid excess | |

### Critical Thinking

1. Eric Jones is a 57-year-old man with chronic kidney disease and was recently discharged from the hospital after being treated for kidney failure. He was told that his blood was "too acid." He asks you what this means, and why it developed. What would you tell him?
2. Mary Martin is a 28-year-old woman planning to enter the Boston marathon. She has been advised to drink lots of fluid during the marathon, but other people tell her not to drink too much fluid. She is confused about what to do. What would you tell her?

# The Endocrine Glands

## LEARNING OBJECTIVES

1. Explain the normal physiologic functions of the pituitary hormones. Name the common endocrine disturbances, and describe the methods of treating each disturbance.

2. Describe the major disturbances of thyroid function and their clinical manifestations, and explain the methods of treatment.

3. Explain the normal physiologic functions of the adrenal cortex and medulla. Name the common

endocrine disturbances resulting from dysfunction, and describe methods of treatment.

4. Define the causes and effects of parathyroid dysfunction, and describe the methods of treatment.

5. Understand the concept of ectopic hormone production by nonendocrine tumors.

6. Explain how stress affects the endocrine system.

## Endocrine Functions and Dysfunctions

Endocrine glands liberate their secretions directly into the bloodstream and exert a regulatory effect on various metabolic functions.

The major endocrine glands are the pituitary, thyroid, and parathyroid glands; the adrenal cortex and medulla; the pancreatic islets; and the ovaries and the testes. However, these glands are not the only sites of hormone

production. Many groups of specialized cells throughout the body also secrete hormones. Renin and erythropoietin are secreted by the kidneys; the hormones gastrin, secretin, and cholecystokinin are produced by the mucosa of the gastrointestinal tract. By convention, these hormones are considered along with the organs with which they are associated and are not generally regarded as part of the endocrine system.

The amount of hormone synthesized and released into the circulation by an endocrine gland may be regulated directly, by the level of hormone circulating in the blood, or indirectly, by the level of a substance under hormonal control, such as the concentration of glucose or sodium in the blood. Mechanisms of this type are called *feedback mechanisms*. Most commonly, an increase in the level of hormone or hormone-regulated substance suppresses further hormone output. This is called a *negative feedback mechanism* or *feedback inhibition* and is illustrated by the control mechanisms regulating output of pituitary hormones.

A disorder of an endocrine gland may consist of either hypersecretion of the gland, manifested as overactivity of the target organ regulated by the gland, or insufficient secretion, resulting in underactivity of the organ controlled by the gland.

The clinical effects of a disturbance of endocrine gland function are determined by the degree of dysfunction of the gland and by the age and sex of the affected individual. All degrees of glandular dysfunction may be encountered, ranging from barely detectable variations from normal to extreme hypofunction or hyperfunction.

The age of the person when the endocrine disturbance becomes manifest has a pronounced effect on the clinical features. Some endocrine glands, such as the thyroid gland, affect growth and development as well as metabolic processes; therefore, disturbed function in a child will produce a somewhat different clinical picture than will a similar disturbance in an adult.

The sex of the individual also influences the effect of disturbed endocrine function. Many hormones are concerned with the development and maintenance of sexual function and secondary sexual characteristics, and several endocrine glands produce sex hormones. Some endocrine disturbances cause alteration in sexual development in children, whereas the effects are much less pronounced in adults. Overproduction of an inappropriate sex hormone in some endocrine diseases causes masculinization (virilization) of the female or feminization of the male; conversely, overproduction of a sex hormone appropriate to the sex of the individual has little clinical effect.

# The Pituitary Gland

The *pituitary gland* is a small, pea-shaped gland suspended by a narrow stalk from the hypothalamus at the base of the brain. The gland is located within a small depression within the sphenoid bone called the *pituitary fossa* or *sella turcica* and is located just behind the optic chiasm. The gland is composed of an anterior lobe and a posterior lobe. Although many mammals also have an intermediate lobe located between the anterior and posterior lobes, in humans, it is no longer present as a distinct structure.

The *anterior lobe* is composed of cords of epithelial cells containing hormones that are synthesized and stored within this lobe. It has been conventional to classify anterior-lobe cells on the basis of the staining reaction of their cytoplasmic granules, using routine staining methods. Three cell types were recognized: eosinophils, which contain bright-red–staining cytoplasmic granules; basophils, which have abundant blue-staining granules in their cytoplasm; and chromophobe cells, which contain sparse, poorly stained granules. Newer, more specialized staining methods, however, have identified five different cell types, each producing its own specific hormones. Currently, these cells are more commonly designated by the hormones that they produce rather than by the staining reactions of their granules.

The anterior lobe is connected to the hypothalamus by a special system of blood vessels called a *portal system*, which begins as capillaries in the hypothalamus and extends down the pituitary stalk to terminate as capillaries around the cells of the anterior lobe. Release of the hormones stored within the cells of the anterior lobe is regulated by hormonal substances called *releasing hormones*, which are synthesized in the hypothalamus and carried to the cells of the anterior lobe in the blood flowing through the portal system.

The *posterior lobe* consists of a meshwork of nerve fibers intermixed with modified neuroglial cells. It is connected to the hypothalamus by bundles of nerve fibers extending through the pituitary stalk rather than by the portal circulation. The hormones in the posterior lobe are synthesized within the hypothalamus and are then transmitted down the nerve axons in the pituitary stalk to the posterior lobe, where they are stored. They are then released from the posterior lobe in response to nerve impulses transmitted from the hypothalamus down the pituitary stalk. Usually a hypothalamic-releasing hormone activates a single gland, but some releasing hormones exert an effect on more than one gland. Other hypothalamic hormones inhibit rather than stimulate specific glands, and the hormone response of the target gland reflects the net effect of the interaction between releasing and inhibiting hormones.

The **hypothalamus**, which controls release of hormones from both the anterior and posterior lobes, is in turn under the control of higher cortical centers; consequently, pituitary secretion is to some extent influenced by emotional stimuli such as anxiety, rage, and fear and is also influenced by sensory impulses that enter the nervous system and are in turn relayed to the hypothalamus.

## Pituitary Hormones

The pituitary gland secretes nine separate hormones that have multiple functions. Seven are produced by the anterior lobe. Four of these hormones, which regulate other endocrine glands as indicated by their names and abbreviations, are called *tropic hormones*.

1. Growth hormone
2. Prolactin
3. Thyroid-stimulating hormone (TSH)
4. Adrenocorticotrophic hormone (ACTH)
5. Melanin-stimulating hormone (MSH)
6. Follicle-stimulating hormone (FSH)
7. Luteinizing hormone (LH)

The posterior lobe produces two hormones: antidiuretic hormone (ADH) and oxytocin.

## Anterior Lobe Hormones

**Growth hormone** has multiple actions, all concerned with general tissue growth. **Prolactin** stimulates the secretion of milk by the breast that has been previously stimulated by estrogen and progesterone. **Thyroid-stimulating hormone (TSH)** stimulates the thyroid gland to secrete thyroid hormone. **Adrenocorticotrophic hormone (ACTH)** stimulates the adrenal cortex to manufacture and secrete adrenocortical hormones. It exerts its main effect on the adrenal hormones that control carbohydrate metabolism (glucocorticoids). ACTH is produced from a large precursor molecule that gives rise not only to ACTH but also to **melanin-stimulating hormone (MSH)** and some other products that also have MSH activity as a by-product of ACTH synthesis. MSH causes darkening of the skin by stimulating melanocytes but normally not enough is produced to have any significant effect when output of ACTH is normal. **Follicle-stimulating hormone (FSH)** and **luteinizing hormone (LH)** are called *gonadotropic hormones*. They regulate the growth and development of the gonads (ovaries and testes) and control the output of sex hormones that are responsible for the development of male and female secondary sex characteristics.

**Posterior Lobe Hormones** Antidiuretic hormone (ADH) causes the cells of the renal collecting tubules to become more permeable to water so that more water is absorbed and a concentrated urine is excreted. Secretion of ADH is regulated by receptors in the hypothalamus that respond to variations in the osmolarity of the extracellular fluid. If the osmolarity rises, the hypothalamic neurons send impulses to the posterior lobe to stimulate release of ADH. Water is retained instead of being excreted, which dilutes the extracellular fluid and lowers its osmolarity. Conversely, if the extracellular fluids become too dilute, the hypothalamus directs the pituitary to decrease its output of ADH. More water is excreted in the urine, which causes the osmolarity of the body fluids to rise.

**Oxytocin** stimulates the contraction of the pregnant uterus and causes ejection of milk from the lactating breast. Oxytocin is secreted in response to stimulation of the nipples during nursing. The sensory nerve impulses are transmitted to the hypothalamus, and the hypothalamic neurons in turn send impulses to the posterior lobe that cause the release of oxytocin.

## Physiologic Control of Pituitary Hormone Secretion

The level of the various tropic hormones elaborated by the pituitary is regulated by the level of circulating hormone produced by the target gland ( Figure 20-1 ). Cells in the hypothalamus measure the level of the various hormones in the blood and liberate various releasing and inhibiting hormones that control the release of pituitary hormones into the circulation. Generally hormones produced by the hypothalamus and pituitary gland are released in pulses, rather than as a continuous output. Many hormone levels may also vary over a 24-hour period, usually with the highest levels in the early morning followed by a gradual fall throughout the day. When the concentration of the hormone falls below a certain level, releasing hormones are elaborated. They travel by the portal venous system to the pituitary gland, causing release of the tropic hormone. This, in turn, affects the target organ. The level of the hormone elaborated by the target organ rises until it reaches the upper range of normal. At this point, the high level of circulating hormone "shuts off" further elaboration of tropic hormone. This mechanism maintains a relatively steady hormone output from the target organ

**hypothalamus** A portion of the brain stem that forms the floor of the third ventricle. It contains clusters of nerve cells that regulate various body functions.

**growth hormone** An anterior lobe pituitary hormone that stimulates growth of bone and other body tissues.

**prolactin** Hormone produced by the anterior lobe of the pituitary gland that stimulates milk secretion.

**thyroid-stimulating hormone (TSH)** Hormone secreted by the anterior lobe of the pituitary; regulates thyroid function.

**adrenocorticotrophic hormone (ACTH)** (ad-rēn´o-cor´tico-trō´fik) A hormone secreted by the anterior lobe of the pituitary that stimulates the adrenal cortex to manufacture and secrete adrenal cortical hormones.

**melanin-stimulating hormone (MSH)** One of the hormones produced by the pituitary. Causes darkening of the skin.

**follicle-stimulating hormone (FSH)** One of the gonadotropic hormones secreted by the anterior lobe of the pituitary, which regulates growth and function of the gonads (ovary and testis).

**luteinizing hormone (LH)** One of the gonadotropic hormones secreted by the anterior lobe of the pituitary that regulates growth and function of the gonads (ovary and testis).

**antidiuretic hormone (ADH)** (an-ti-dī-u-ret´tik) Posterior lobe pituitary hormone that regulates urine concentration by altering the permeability of the renal collecting tubules.

**oxytocin** (ox-i-to´sin) A hormone that is stored in the posterior lobe of the pituitary gland that causes uterine contractions during labor and ejection of milk from the breast lobules into the larger ducts.

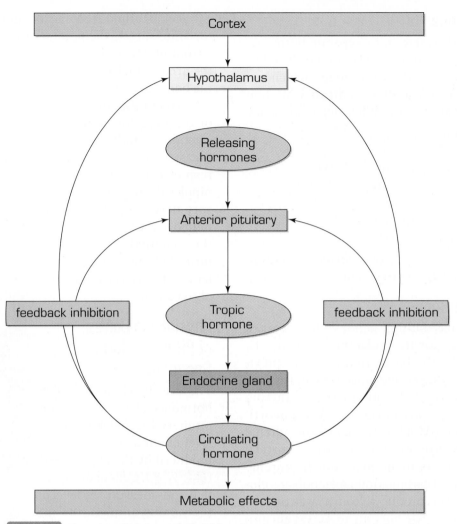

**Figure 20-1** Normal mechanisms controlling elaboration of tropic hormones by the pituitary gland.

and prevents wide fluctuations in hormonal level that might disrupt the smooth functioning of the body's hormone-regulated organ systems.

Prolactin secretion is regulated by a somewhat different mechanism from that of the other pituitary hormones. With other hormones, the main effect of hypothalamic releasing hormones is to stimulate secretion. For prolactin, however, the principal control is by an inhibitory hormone called prolactin inhibitory factor (PIF), which is a chemical mediator called **dopamine**. Secretion of prolactin would continue unabated if it were not continuously suppressed. If PIF output falls for any reason, prolactin secretion rises.

## Pituitary Hypofunction

Sometimes the anterior lobe of the pituitary gland is destroyed by a tumor or undergoes necrosis owing to a disturbance of its blood supply. In this condition, called **panhypopituitarism** (*pan* = multiple + *hypo* = decrease), the anterior lobe fails to secrete any hormones. The functions of the thyroid gland, adrenal glands, and gonads are impaired because tropic hormone stimulation is lost.

An isolated deficiency of growth hormone in a child leads to a condition called *pituitary dwarfism*, which is characterized by retarded growth and development. Normal growth and development can be restored by administering growth hormone produced by recombinant DNA technology (genetic engineering).

Diabetes insipidus is a rare disease that is usually caused by failure of the posterior lobe of the pituitary gland to secrete antidiuretic hormone (ADH) because of injury, tumor, or some other disease involving the posterior lobe. Because of the lack of ADH, the affected person is unable to absorb water from the renal collecting tubules and excretes a large volume of extremely dilute urine. Large amounts of water must be consumed to compensate for the excessive water loss and to prevent dehydration.

## Pituitary Tumors

Many conditions affecting the pituitary gland result from pituitary tumors involving the anterior lobe of the gland. Hormone-producing tumors are called *functional tumors*, and the clinical manifestations of a functioning tumor are determined by what hormone it makes, the size of the tumor, and the age of the subject. The two most common functional pituitary tumors are those that produce growth hormone and those that produce prolactin, and some tumors produce both hormones. Generally, each type of tumor produces a characteristic clinical syndrome. Tumors that do not produce hormones are called *nonfunctional tumors*. Although no hormones are produced, a nonfunctional tumor may cause problems because of its location, which is close to the optic chiasm, optic nerves, and other vital structures at the base of the brain. An enlarging tumor may erode the pituitary fossa, encroach on the optic chiasm, and may disrupt the hormone-producing functions of adjacent normal anterior lobe cells that are compressed by the expanding tumor.

Treatment of a pituitary tumor is determined by the type of tumor, the hormones that it produces, and the size of the tumor. A small prolactin-secreting adenoma may respond well to drugs that shrink the tumor, and some drugs can be used to suppress the secretion of growth hormone produced by a functional tumor. In most cases, however, the usual treatment of a pituitary tumor is surgical removal of the tumor, occasionally followed by radiation treatment in selected patients.

Because a pituitary tumor is so difficult to approach through the cranial cavity, it is usually resected through the nasal cavity and sphenoid sinus, a procedure called a transsphenoidal resection ( Figure 20-2 ). In this procedure the tumor is approached through the nose and through the sphenoid sinus. Then the anterior part of the pituitary fossa is resected to reach the tumor in the pituitary gland, followed by resection of the tumor.

## Overproduction of Growth Hormone

Overproduction of growth hormone in children and adolescents, whose epiphyses have not yet fused, causes excessive growth in the length of bones, and the subject becomes too tall. This condition is called pituitary gigantism. Some associated coarsening of the facial features usually occurs in response to the effect of growth hormone on the structure of the facial bones.

In adults, excessive growth hormone causes **acromegaly**. Because the epiphyses have fused, there can be no growth in height, but the growth hormone

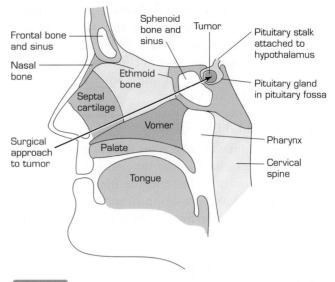

Figure 20-2    Transsphenoidal resection of a pituitary tumor as described in the text.

produces thickening and coarsening of bones and generalized enlargement of the viscera. Affected individuals have coarse facial features, large prominent jaws, and large spadelike hands, but they are no taller than normal ( Figure 20-3 ). The term *acromegaly* (*acron* = extremity + *megas* = large) describes one prominent feature of the disease.

**acromegaly** (ak′ro-meg′al-ē) A condition resulting from excessive secretion of growth hormone in the adult.

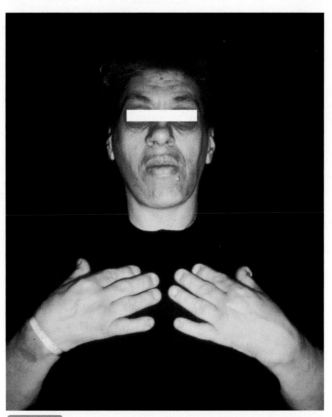

Figure 20-3    The appearance of a subject with advanced acromegaly.

In addition to the hormonal effects caused by a functional tumor, an enlarging tumor may also compress adjacent normal anterior lobe cells and disrupt their hormonal functions. Treatment consists of transsphenoidal resection of the tumor, sometimes supplemented by radiation therapy.

## Overproduction of Prolactin

In a nonpregnant woman, excess secretion of prolactin caused by a pituitary tumor may cause spontaneous secretion of milk from the breasts (**galactorrhea**) and cessation of menstrual periods (**amenorrhea**). Galactorrhea results from the effect of the hormone on breast tissue. Amenorrhea occurs because high prolactin also inhibits the secretion of pituitary gonadotropins FSH and LH, which in turn leads to cessation of ovulation and menstrual cycles. The manifestations of this condition are often called *the amenorrhea–galactorrhea syndrome*. Usually drugs can suppress growth of the tumor and its prolactin secretion.

**galactorrhea** (gā-lak-tō-rē′yuh) Secretion of milk by breast not associated with pregnancy or normal lactation.

**amenorrhea** (äh-men-ō-rē′äh) Absence of menses.

**colloid** An eosinophilic protein material present within the thyroid follicles.

# The Thyroid Gland

The thyroid gland consists of two lateral lobes connected by a narrow isthmus (Figure 20-4A). It is located in the neck overlying the upper part of the trachea and is regulated by pituitary thyroid-stimulating hormone (TSH). The four parathyroid glands are located on its posterior surface.

Histologically, the thyroid gland is composed of multiple minute spherical vesicles called thyroid follicles. Each follicle consists of a central mass of eosinophilic protein material called **colloid** containing a protein called *thyroglobulin* to which the thyroid hormone is attached. The colloid is surrounded by a layer of cuboidal epithelial cells called follicular cells (Figure 20-4B). Under the influence of TSH, the follicular cells synthesize two hormones called triiodothyronine ($T_3$) and thyroxin ($T_4$), which regulate the body's metabolic processes and are also required for the normal development of the nervous system. The term *thyroid hormone* is a general term referring to the two metabolic hormones $T_3$ and $T_4$, the numbers indicating the number of iodine atoms attached to the molecules. Most of the thyroid hormone circulates bound to a protein called thyroid-binding globulin and is biologically inactive. The small amount of hormone that circulates unbound to protein is the physiologically active form of the hormone.

Thyroid hormone controls the rate of metabolic processes; it is also required for normal growth and development. Sometimes the thyroid gland secretes an inappropriate amount of hormone. An excess of thyroid hormone, called *hyperthyroidism*, leads to an acceleration of all bodily metabolic functions. Conversely, a decrease in the level of thyroid hormone, called *hypothyroidism*, slows metabolic processes.

Clinically, some of the most pronounced effects of excess thyroid hormone are manifested in the cardiovascular and neuromuscular systems. The heart rate is accelerated. Reflexes are hyperactive, and frequently a fine tremor of the muscles is apparent. The hormone also has conspicuous effects on emotional and intellectual functions. Individuals with excess thyroid hormone are hyperactive, emotionally labile, and often quite irritable. They may have difficulty concentrating because mental processes are accelerated excessively.

**A**

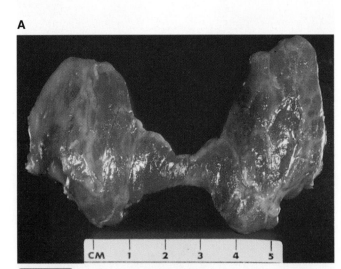

**B**

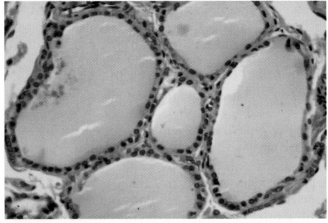

Figure 20-4 **A,** Normal thyroid gland, illustrating two lateral lobes connected by narrow isthmus. **B,** High-magnification photomicrograph of normal thyroid follicles, illustrating central masses of colloid surrounded by follicular epithelial cells (original magnification × 400).

## Table 20-1 — Comparison of Major Effects of Hyperthyroidism and Hypothyroidism

| | Hyperthyroidism | Hypothyroidism |
|---|---|---|
| Cardiovascular effects | Rapid pulse, increased cardiac output | Slow pulse, reduced cardiac output |
| Metabolic effects | Increased metabolism, skin hot and flushed, weight loss | Decreased metabolism, cold skin, weight gain |
| Neuromuscular effects | Tremor, hyperactive reflexes | Weakness, lassitude, sluggish reflexes |
| Mental, emotional effects | Restlessness, irritability, emotional lability | Mental processes sluggish and retarded, personality placid and phlegmatic |
| Gastrointestinal effects | Diarrhea | Constipation |
| General somatic effects | Warm, moist skin | Cold, dry skin |

The effects of thyroid hypofunction are the reverse of those in hyperthyroidism. The hypothyroid individual is slow and lethargic. Bodily metabolic functions are subnormal. Reflexes and speech are slow and sluggish. Table 20-1 summarizes the major clinical effects resulting from abnormal levels of thyroid hormone.

## Goiter

An enlargement of the thyroid gland is called a **goiter**. The gland may be uniformly enlarged, called a *diffuse goiter*, or multiple nodules of proliferating thyroid tissue may form a *nodular goiter*. An enlarged gland that produces an excessive amount of hormone and causes symptoms of hyperthyroidism is called a *toxic goiter*. A goiter that does not secrete excess thyroid hormone is called a *nontoxic goiter*.

**Nontoxic Goiter**  The basic cause of both nodular and diffuse nontoxic goiter is an inadequate secretion of thyroid hormone. The reduced hormone output causes the hypothalamus to elaborate releasing hormone, which in turn stimulates the pituitary to liberate more TSH ( Figure 20-5 ). As a result, the gland enlarges in order to produce more hormone.

Three major factors predispose to the development of a nontoxic goiter:

1. Iodine deficiency
2. Deficiency of enzymes required for synthesis of thyroid hormone or ingestion of substances that interfere with the function of these enzymes
3. Increased hormone requirements

**Iodine Deficiency**  If iodine is deficient in the diet, not enough will be available to produce adequate hormone for the needs of the individual. The enlargement of the gland in response to TSH stimulation is an attempt to extract the meager amount of iodine from the blood more efficiently to make enough hormone. Iodine deficiency is rarely a cause of goiter in the United States because table salt, bread, and many other foods are fortified with iodine. Consequently, the average American diet actually contains abundant iodine.

**Enzyme Deficiency or Impaired Enzyme Function**  Goiter more commonly results from a mild deficiency in a glandular enzyme that is required for hormone

**goiter**
(goy´ter) Any enlargement of the thyroid gland.

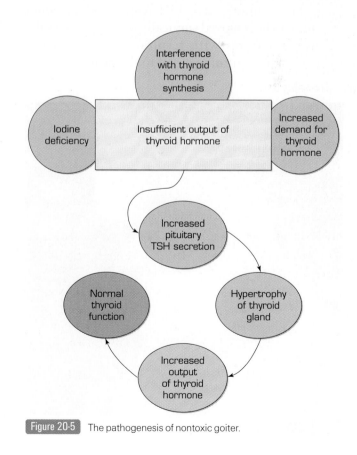

Figure 20-5   The pathogenesis of nontoxic goiter.

synthesis; the enzyme-deficient gland is unable to produce sufficient hormone without enlarging.

**Increased Hormone Requirements**  Normally, the need for thyroid hormone increases in puberty, during pregnancy, and under conditions of stress. In some individuals, the thyroid gland may be able to produce adequate hormone under normal circumstances but may be unable to increase its output in response to increased requirements without enlarging.

Whenever hormone output is inadequate, no matter what the cause, more TSH is released in order to step up hormone production. Because hormone requirements often fluctuate, a gland may undergo successive alternating periods of enlargement and reduction in size. At first, the gland enlarges uniformly in response to TSH stimulation, and it returns to its original size when increased hormone output is no longer required. Eventually, however, the gland may respond in an irregular manner to TSH stimulation. If this occurs, the enlargement of the gland is not uniform, and a nodular goiter results ( Figure 20-6 ).

**Treatment of Nontoxic Goiter**  Because a nontoxic goiter results from excessive stimulation of the thyroid gland by TSH, it is usually treated by administration of thyroid hormone, which suppresses TSH output by the negative feedback mechanism. Treatment usually causes the enlarged gland to shrink because it is no longer being stimulated by TSH. A large nodular goiter may have to be removed surgically if it compresses the trachea, interferes with respiration, or obstructs the neck veins returning blood to the heart.

## Hyperthyroidism

Many different conditions can cause an excess secretion of thyroid hormone, but usually hyperthyroidism is caused by an autoimmune disease in which autoantibodies target thyroid cells. This condition is usually called either Graves disease after the physician who described the condition, or exophthalmic (protruding eyes) goiter, which describes a common eye manifestation of the disease. The autoantibody combines with TSH receptors on thyroid cells, which drives the thyroid to secrete excess hormone unresponsive to the inhibitory feedback control mechanism that regulates normal thyroid activity. In most subjects, the thyroid gland is diffusely enlarged, but the degree of enlargement is not marked ( Figure 20-7 ).

The eye changes that occur in many subjects with Graves disease are also caused by the autoimmune disease. Activated T lymphocytes infiltrate the fat, connective tissue, and the muscles that move the eyes (extraocular muscles) located in the orbital cavities behind the eyes, which causes inflammation and swelling of the tissues and pushes the eyes forward.

**Treatment of Hyperthyroidism**  At present, no method is available to block the stimulation of the thyroid gland

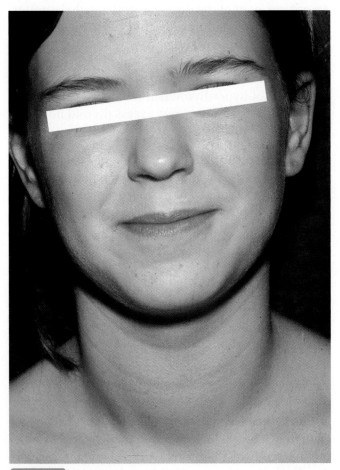

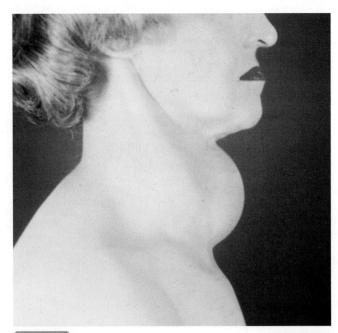

Figure 20-6  Large nodular goiter.

Figure 20-7  Small diffuse toxic goiter in young woman (Case 20-1).

by the autoantibodies that are causing the unregulated hypersecretion of thyroid hormone. It is possible, however, to control the hyperthyroidism. Three different methods of treatment can be used:

1. Antithyroid drugs can be administered to block the synthesis of hormone by the hyperactive gland.
2. A large portion of the gland can be removed surgically, reducing the source of the hormone.
3. A large dose of radioactive iodine can be administered to be taken up by the thyroid gland. The irradiation destroys part of the gland and reduces its hormone output.

The following case illustrates successful treatment of a diffuse toxic goiter by means of antithyroid drugs and thyroidectomy.

### Case Study 20-1

A 15-year-old girl was referred to her physician because of recent onset of hyperactivity, rapid speech, and some prominence of the eyes (see Figure 20-7). Examination revealed prominent eyes, a fine tremor, and hyperactive reflexes. Thyroid function studies indicated an elevated level of thyroid hormone in her blood, together with an increased uptake of iodine and increased synthesis of hormone as demonstrated by radioactive iodine tracer studies. The patient was considered to have a diffuse toxic goiter. She was treated initially by an antithyroid drug to control the hyperthyroidism, and a thyroidectomy was subsequently performed.

## Hypothyroidism

**Hypothyroidism in the Adult** Hypothyroidism in the adult is manifested by a general slowing of the body's metabolic processes. Hypothyroid individuals have low levels of circulating thyroid hormone and high levels of TSH that reflect stimulation of the gland in an unsuccessful attempt to increase hormone output. The condition is treated by supplying the deficient hormone, which results in clinical improvement, return of thyroid hormone level to normal, and a fall in TSH, as illustrated by Case 20-2.

**Neonatal Hypothyroidism** Hypothyroidism in the newborn infant is called congenital hypothyroidism. This condition may be caused by failure of the thyroid gland to develop or may result from a genetically determined deficiency of enzymes necessary for thyroid

### Case Study 20-2

A 25-year-old woman visited her physician because of recent weight gain and menstrual irregularities. On examination, she was moderately overweight, and her thyroid gland was slightly enlarged; however, there were no other abnormalities. The level of thyroid hormone in her blood was reduced to 2.1 micrograms/dL (normal range 4.5–11.0 micrograms/dL), and the thyroid-stimulating hormone (TSH) level was markedly increased to 310 microunits/mL (normal range 2–10 microunits/mL). She was considered to have hypothyroidism, probably the result of an autoimmune disease (often called chronic thyroiditis, which is described in a subsequent section). She was treated with a thyroid hormone preparation. The level of thyroid hormone rose, and the elevated TSH level gradually returned to normal. She felt much better and lost some weight. Her menstrual periods became normal.

hormone synthesis. If the condition remains undetected, the unfortunate infant will become permanently stunted in growth and mentally retarded. This condition is called **cretinism**. Fortunately, we have effective screening tests for neonatal hypothyroidism that are performed routinely on all newborn infants. Screening tests have ensured early recognition and prompt treatment of affected infants, thereby preventing cretinism, which is the unfortunate late manifestation of unrecognized and untreated neonatal hypothyroidism.

## Chronic Thyroiditis and Hashimoto Thyroiditis

Acute or chronic inflammation of the thyroid gland caused by a bacterial or viral infection is uncommon, and is usually called either acute or chronic thyroiditis, depending on its clinical manifestations and the type of inflammatory cells present within the gland. However, an autoimmune disease affecting the thyroid gland is also called **chronic thyroiditis**, or preferably Hashimoto thyroiditis to distinguish the condition from an infection of the thyroid gland. In Hashimoto thyroiditis, antithyroid autoantibodies and activated T lymphocytes attack and

**cretinism**
(krē′tin-izm)
Hypothyroidism in the infant.
**chronic thyroiditis**
An autoimmune disease in which an autoantibody directed against thyroid epithelial cells causes progressive destruction of the thyroid gland, leading to hypothyroidism. Also called *Hashimoto thyroiditis.*

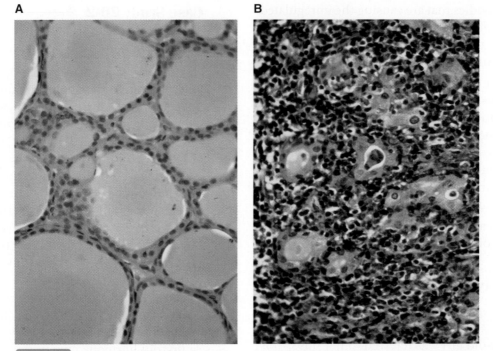

**Figure 20-8** Low-magnification photomicrographs comparing cellular structure of normal thyroid gland (**A**) with that in chronic thyroiditis (**B**). Gland is heavily infiltrated by lymphocytes. Follicles are small and lack colloid (original magnification x 100).

destroy the thyroid gland. This autoimmune disease is the most common cause of hypothyroidism in adults, which occurs predominantly in middle-aged women. The autoantibody is directed against TSH receptors on the thyroid cells, which destroys the receptors so that TSH is unable to attach to thyroid cells and stimulate the thyroid gland. Consequently, output of thyroid hormone falls as TSH receptor damage progresses. The normal feedback control system that regulates hormone output (Figure 20-1) responds to the low hormone level, and TSH rises as thyroid hormone falls.

The thyroid gland of a person with Hashimoto thyroiditis is usually enlarged by diffuse infiltration of activated T lymphocytes and plasma cells that are destroying the thyroid gland ( Figure 20-8 ). No specific treatment is available to arrest the relentless progression of the disease, but the hypothyroidism can be treated by administration of thyroid hormone.

## Tumors of the Thyroid

The thyroid gives rise to both benign and malignant tumors. Thyroid adenomas are well-circumscribed tumors composed of mature follicles that often contain large amounts of colloid ( Figure 20-9 ). There are two distinct types of thyroid cancer:

1. Well-differentiated carcinoma
2. Undifferentiated carcinoma

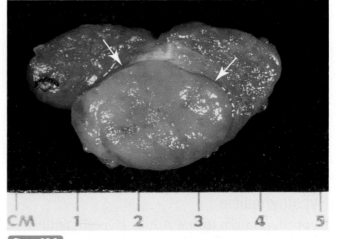

**Figure 20-9** A benign, well-circumscribed adenoma of the thyroid gland (*arrows*). The surrounding thyroid tissue appears normal.

Thyroid carcinomas usually are well-differentiated tumors that occur in young adults. The most common type, illustrated in Figure 20-10 , is called a papillary carcinoma because the tumor is composed of well-differentiated papillary processes covered by well-differentiated thyroid epithelial cells. A less common type of tumor is called a follicular carcinoma because the tumor cells form colloid-filled follicles, which resemble normal thyroid tissue. Treatment of both types is by surgical resection of the thyroid gland (thyroidectomy).

**A** **B**

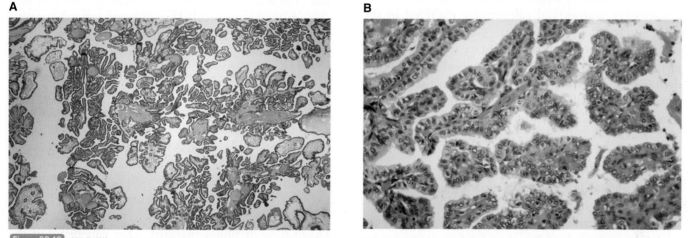

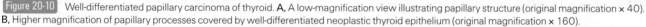

**Figure 20-10** Well-differentiated papillary carcinoma of thyroid. **A,** A low-magnification view illustrating papillary structure (original magnification × 40). **B,** Higher magnification of papillary processes covered by well-differentiated neoplastic thyroid epithelium (original magnification × 160).

*Undifferentiated carcinoma* develops in older persons, is composed of rapidly growing bizarre tumor cells, and has a poor prognosis. Treatment is by means of surgical resection combined with radiation and chemotherapy.

# The Parathyroid Glands and Calcium Metabolism

The blood calcium is in equilibrium with the calcium salts present in bone. Half the blood calcium is present as calcium ions ($Ca^{2+}$) and is the active form. The other half is bound to blood proteins and is biologically inactive. An adequate concentration of ionized calcium is required for normal cardiac and skeletal muscle contraction, for transmission of nerve impulses, and for coagulation of the blood. A subnormal level of ionized calcium causes increased excitability of nerve and muscle cells, leading to spasm of skeletal muscles, which is called **tetany**. Conversely, a high level of ionized calcium diminishes neuromuscular excitability and leads to generalized muscular weakness.

The level of ionized calcium in the blood is regulated primarily by parathyroid hormone, which is secreted by four small parathyroid glands located on the posterior surface of the lateral lobes of the thyroid gland. The parathyroid hormone regulates the level of calcium by regulating the release of calcium from bone, the absorption of calcium from the intestine, and the excretion of calcium by

**tetany**
(tet′an-ē) Spasm of skeletal muscles caused by subnormal level of ionized calcium in the blood.

the kidneys. The secretion of parathyroid hormone is regulated by the level of ionized calcium in the blood rather than by a tropic hormone elaborated by the pituitary gland. If the level of ionized calcium in the blood decreases, the parathyroid glands secrete more hormone. If the ionized calcium level rises, parathyroid hormone secretion declines. Any abnormality in the secretion of parathyroid hormone changes the concentration of ionized calcium in the blood and will eventually alter the amount of calcium deposited in bone.

**glucocorticoid** An adrenal cortical hormone that regulates carbohydrate metabolism.

## Hyperparathyroidism

Hyperparathyroidism is a relatively common problem and is usually the result of a hormone-secreting parathyroid adenoma. In response to increased output of hormone, the blood calcium rises (hypercalcemia), and excessive calcium is withdrawn from bone. The bones become excessively fragile and are easily broken.

Excessive amounts of calcium are excreted in the urine (hypercalciuria), sometimes leading to formation of calcium stones within the urinary tract. Occasionally, calcium precipitates from the blood and becomes deposited in the kidneys, lungs, and other tissues, producing tissue injury and functional impairment. Treatment consists of surgical removal of the tumor.

## Hypoparathyroidism

Hypoparathyroidism usually results from accidental removal of parathyroid glands during an operation for a diffuse toxic goiter or a nodular goiter in which most of the thyroid gland is removed. Blood calcium falls precipitously, which leads to increased neuromuscular excitability and tetany. Treatment consists of raising the level of blood calcium by the administration of a high-calcium diet and supplementary vitamin D, which promotes absorption of calcium from the intestinal tract.

# The Adrenal Glands

The adrenals are paired glands located above the kidneys. Each adrenal consists of two separate endocrine glands: an inner adrenal medulla surrounded by an outer adrenal cortex. The two glands secrete different hormones.

## The Adrenal Cortex

The adrenal cortex secretes three major classes of steroid hormones:

1. Glucocorticoids
2. Mineralocorticoids
3. Sex hormones

**Glucocorticoids** Glucocorticoids have three main actions:

1. They raise the blood glucose by decreasing glucose utilization in many tissues, except the brain, and promote fat breakdown with utilization of fatty acids rather than glucose as an energy source.
2. They inhibit protein synthesis and promote breakdown of body proteins, some of which are converted into glucose by the liver. The net effect is to deplete tissue proteins and raise blood glucose. (The adverse effect of glucocorticoids on wound healing and tissue repair is a result in part of their protein-depleting effects.)
3. They act as multiple sites to suppress the inflammatory reaction. (The use of adrenal corticosteroids to treat various types of inflammatory disease is related to the anti-inflammatory property of the glucocorticoids.)

Glucocorticoids are secreted in response to stimulation by adrenocorticotrophic hormone (ACTH), and their output is controlled by the same type of negative feedback mechanism that regulates secretion of thyroid hormone. The major glucocorticoid is **cortisol**.

**Mineralocorticoids** Mineralocorticoids regulate electrolyte and water balance by promoting absorption of sodium and water, and excretion of potassium by the renal tubules. The major mineralocorticoid is aldosterone, and its secretion is regulated by more than one mechanism. Although ACTH increases aldosterone secretion to some extent, the most potent stimulus for aldosterone secretion is the *renin–angiotensin system* (Chapter 15), which responds to a reduction in renal blood flow or blood pressure. One can think of the kidneys as "interpreting" the reduced blood flow and pressure to mean that blood volume is low; aldosterone secretion is then called for to promote retention of sodium and water, thus increasing blood volume.

**Sex Hormones** The adrenal cortex also produces weak androgenic (testosteronelike) steroid hormones in response to ACTH stimulation, which are further metabolized into testosterone and into estrogens by both males and females. In men, the estrogens have little effect because of the much greater testicular production of testosterone. In women, the testosterone is responsible for sex drive but otherwise has little physiologic effect because it is overshadowed by estrogen produced by the ovaries. The additional estrogens made from adrenal androgenic hormones do not add much to the large amount already made by the ovaries. However, in estrogen-deficient postmenopausal women, the estrogens produced from adrenal androgens may be very significant, as described in Chapter 13.

# Disturbances of Adrenal Cortical Function

Abnormal adrenal cortical function produces abnormalities in the metabolism of carbohydrates and protein as a result of abnormal glucocorticoid secretion, as well as disturbances of salt and water metabolism caused by disturbed mineralocorticoid secretion.

**Addison Disease**  Adrenal cortical hypofunction is called **Addison disease**. It results from atrophy or destruction of both adrenal glands, leading to a deficiency of all of the steroid hormones produced by these glands. In most cases the disease results from an autoimmune disorder in which destructive autoantibodies directed against adrenal cortical cells and invading cytotoxic lymphocytes destroy the cortex. Less commonly, the adrenal destruction is caused by tuberculosis, histoplasmosis, or metastatic carcinoma involving both adrenal glands.

As a result of a glucocorticoid (cortisol) deficiency, the blood glucose level is subnormal and may decline during fasting to such a low level that symptoms of hypoglycemia develop. The body's ability to regulate the content of sodium, potassium, and water in body fluids is disturbed as a result of the mineralocorticoid deficiency. Blood volume and blood pressure fall, as does the concentration of sodium in the blood, and blood potassium rises. The blood volume may become so reduced that the circulation can no longer be maintained efficiently.

The low corticosteroid hormone levels in Addison disease cause the pituitary gland to increase its output of ACTH, which is regulated by a negative feedback mechanism, in an unsuccessful attempt to stimulate the adrenal gland to produce more corticosteroid hormones. ACTH is produced from a precursor molecule

**A**

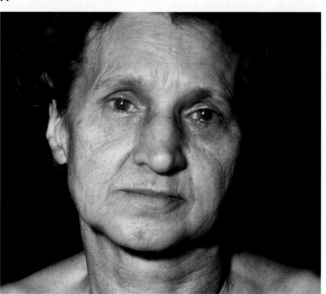

that also produces melanin-stimulating hormone (MSH) along with ACTH. When ACTH rises, so does MSH. Consequently many persons with Addison disease also frequently exhibit increased skin pigmentation resulting from the increased MSH that accompanies the rise in ACTH secretion. It is the MSH that simulates the melanin-producing cells in the skin and is responsible for the increased skin pigmentation characteristic of Addison disease ( Figure 20-11 ). Treatment of Addison disease consists of administering the deficient corticosteroids, as illustrated by Case 20-3.

**Cushing Disease and Cushing Syndrome**  Adrenal cortical hyperfunction causes a rather characteristic clinical syndrome, which results from excess production of adrenal corticosteroids. The glucocorticoid excess causes disturbances of carbohydrate, protein, and fat metabolism. The blood glucose rises. Protein synthesis is impaired, and body proteins are broken down, which leads to loss of sketetal muscle fibers and muscle weakness. Bones become weaker and more susceptible to fracture (osteoporosis) as the protein breakdown leads to loss of the connective tissue framework of the bones. The amount and distribution of body fat are altered. Fat tends to accumulate on the trunk, while the extremities appear thin and wasted because of muscle atrophy.

The skin becomes thin and bruises easily. Stretch marks (striae) often appear in the skin as fat deposits accumulate in the subcutaneous tissues of the trunk. The face appears full and rounded, which is sometimes called a "moon face." Salt and water are retained because of the increased output of mineralocorticoids, leading to an increase in blood volume and a rise in blood pressure. Excess adrenal androgens may lead to increased growth of facial and body hair in women.

**cortisol**
(kōr′ti-sol) The major glucocorticoid.
**Addison disease**  A disease caused by chronic adrenal cortical hypofunction.

**B**

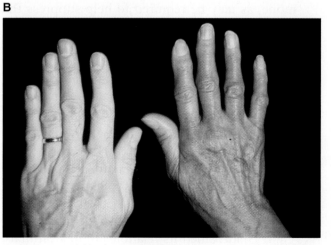

Figure 20-11  Patient with Addison disease (Case 20-3). **A,** Appearance of face illustrating increased skin pigmentation. **B,** Appearance of hand (*right side* of photograph) compared with hand of normal subject.

## Case Study 20-3

A 66-year-old woman had noted gradual loss of energy and some weight loss over the previous 2 or 3 years. Her skin had become darker. She was in the habit of working outdoors in the summer and becoming suntanned, but recently, her tan did not fade in the winter. Physical examination was unremarkable except for increased skin pigmentation. Pigmentation was also noted in the oral mucosa and in the skin creases. Laboratory studies revealed normal thyroid function. Plasma corticosteroid hormone level was reduced to 5 micrograms/dL (normal range 7–28 micrograms/dL). The plasma adrenocorticotrophic hormone (ACTH) level was markedly increased to more than 2000 pg/mL (normal level is less than 120 pg/mL). A diagnosis of Addison disease was made. The very high ACTH level represented a loss of feedback inhibition with stimulation of the adrenal by the pituitary in an attempt to increase hormone output. The patient was treated with cortisone and responded satisfactorily.

Four distinct conditions may give rise to this syndrome:

1. An ACTH-producing tumor of the pituitary gland, which stimulates the adrenal glands to enlarge and produce excess hormone
2. A corticosteroid–hormone-producing tumor of the adrenal cortex
3. Administration of large amounts of corticosteroid hormone to treat diseases that respond to the hormone, as may be required to help suppress the immune response in recipients of organ transplants or patients with autoimmune diseases, or to help induce remission in patients with leukemia
4. A malignant tumor, such as a lung tumor, that produces ACTH or a similar protein that resembles the "real" hormone, as described later in this chapter

The most common cause of a corticosteroid excess is a small ACTH-secreting pituitary adenoma (microadenoma), and this condition is called **Cushing disease** after the physician who described the clinical features of the disease and identified its relationship to a pituitary tumor. When this condition is caused by an

**Cushing disease**
A disease characterized by adrenal cortical hyperfunction caused by an ACTH-secreting tumor of the pituitary gland.

adrenal tumor, excess corticosteroid administration, or ACTH production by a non-endocrine tumor, the term *Cushing syndrome* is used.

The treatment of this condition depends on the cause. If it is Cushing disease caused by a pituitary microadenoma, the usual method of treatment is transsphenoidal resection of the tumor. Cushing syndrome caused by an adrenal cortical tumor is treated by resection of the adrenal tumor.

Successful treatment is followed by regression of the clinical manifestations of the disease. Figure 20-12 and Figure 20-13 illustrate the features of this condition and the favorable response to treatment.

# The Adrenal Medulla

The adrenal medulla produces two similar hormones called **norepinephrine** (noradrenaline) and **epinephrine** (adrenaline), which belong to a class of compounds called **catecholamines**. The hormone-producing cells of the medulla are arranged in small groups surrounded by a rich network of capillaries. The cell cytoplasm is filled with fine granules that become dark brown when treated with chromium salts, and the cells are termed chromaffin cells because of this staining affinity.

The catecholamines produced by the chromaffin cells are stored within the cells and are released in response to nerve impulses transmitted to the medulla by the sympathetic nervous system. Any emotional stress, such as anger, fear, or anxiety, activates the sympathetic nervous system and causes the adrenal medulla to release its hormones. The liberated catecholamines cause a rapid heart rate, rise in blood pressure, and other effects that prepare the individual to cope with the stress of an emergency.

## Tumors of the Adrenal Medulla

Rarely, a benign tumor called a **pheochromocytoma** arises from the chromaffin cells of the medulla. The tumor derives its unusual name from the staining reaction of the tumor cells to chromium salts, which gave the tumor its name (*pheo* = dark + *chromo* = color + *cyte* = cell + *oma* = tumor). A pheochromocytoma often secretes large amounts of catecholamines (such as epinephrine and related compounds) and produces severe effects on the heart and vascular system. The tumor may discharge catecholamines intermittently and induce periodic episodes of high blood pressure and increased heart rate. At times, the blood pressure may rise so high that a cerebral blood vessel ruptures, causing a cerebral hemorrhage. In other cases, the

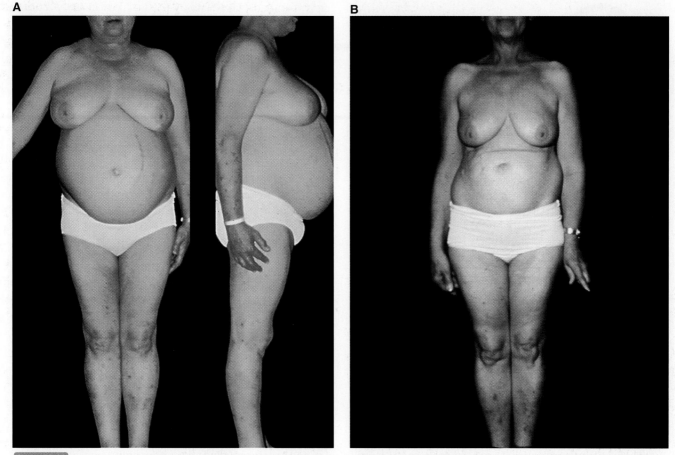

**Figure 20-12** Cushing disease before and after treatment. **A,** Before treatment, front and side views of subject illustrating trunk obesity with relatively thin extremities. **B,** After treatment, illustrating normal body configuration.

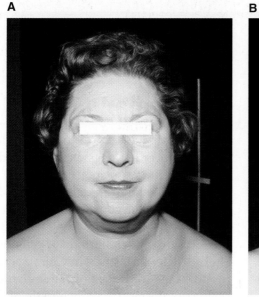 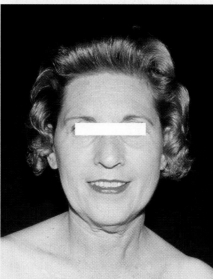

**Figure 20-13** Cushing disease before and after treatment. **A,** Full, rounded face ("moon face") prior to treatment. **B,** Normal facial appearance after treatment.

**norepinephrine**
(nor'ep-in-ef'rin)
One of the compounds (*catecholamines*) secreted by the adrenal medulla.

**epinephrine** (ep-in-ef'rin)
One of the compounds (*catecholamines*) secreted by the adrenal medulla.

**catecholamines**
(kat-eh-kōl'uh-mēnz) The adrenal medullary hormones *epinephrine* and *norepinephrine*.

**pheochromocytoma**
(fē'o-krō'mō-sī-tō'uh) Catecholamine-secreting tumor of the adrenal medulla.

*Harvey Cushing's accomplishments as a neurosurgeon are well known, but he also made a major contribution to blood pressure measurement, which is not as well known.*

You probably already have heard Harvey Cushing's name because of the disease named after him. He made a huge impact on the development of brain surgery. Born in 1869, he attended Harvard University Medical College, and later studied under eminent surgeons at Johns Hopkins Hospital in Baltimore, where in the early 1900s he developed many of the surgical methods for operating on the brain. He identified the cause of the disease named after him described in this chapter and he contributed to many other advances in neurosurgery.

Not nearly as well known is how Cushing introduced the measurement of the blood pressure into clinical medicine. Previously the only way to measure blood pressure was to actually insert a tube into an artery, which was a cumbersome procedure and not often done. This situation changed after he visited a colleague in Italy named Scipione Riva-Rocci. There he was introduced to a device developed and used by Riva-Rocci that determined the systolic pressure by measuring the pressure required to compress the brachial artery in the arm. The device consisted of a mercury-filled manometer (measuring device) attached to an inflatable cuff that could be wrapped around the upper arm. Then the cuff was inflated until the pressure was high enough to compress the brachial artery so that the pulse

in the radial artery at the wrist could no longer be felt. The pressure required to stop blood flow through the artery corresponded to the highest pressure in the artery, which is the systolic pressure. Harvey Cushing was amazed by the simplicity and applicability of the device, which could enable physicians to easily determine the blood pressure in their patients. When he returned to the United States he told American physicians about the device, and the news spread rapidly to physicians in the United States and soon to physicians throughout the world. The method was acclaimed as a major advance in the practice of medicine, and Harvey Cushing was also highly regarded for disseminating the information about the device and popularizing its use.

Initially the device was used only to measure the systolic pressure. Several years later a Russian physician named Nicolai Korotkov determined that the diastolic pressure also could be determined by listening with a stethoscope to changes in the sounds within a large artery near the bend of the elbow as the pressure in the cuff was lowered slowly. The sounds initially were loud as the cuff pressure was lowered gradually, which allowed progressively more blood to flow through the partially constricted artery. Finally the sound became muffled and disappeared when the pressure in the cuff no longer constricted the artery, which corresponded to the lowest pressure in the artery. This is the diastolic pressure. Even today, the sounds made as the cuff pressure is lowered are still called *the sounds of Korotkov*.

---

increased output of catecholamines by the tumor is continuous and causes a sustained high blood pressure. Treatment consists of surgical removal of the tumor.

## The Pancreatic Islets

In addition to manufacturing digestive enzymes, the pancreas functions as an endocrine gland. Scattered throughout the pancreas are more than a million small clusters of cells called the *pancreatic islets* or *islets of Langerhans*, which produce three different hormones: insulin, glucagon, and somatostatin. Diabetes mellitus, the most important disease affecting the pancreatic islets, was considered in conjunction with diseases of the pancreas (Chapter 16).

## The Gonads

The gonads have two functions: the production of germ cells, either eggs or sperm, and the production of sex hormones responsible for the development of secondary sexual characteristics. (This function is controlled by the gonadotrophic hormones of the pituitary gland.)

Occasionally, sex-hormone–secreting tumors develop in the ovary or testis. They may secrete sex hormone appropriate to the sex of the individual or, paradoxically, sex hormone characteristic of the opposite sex. No endocrine symptoms result from a tumor that produces the "proper" sex hormone; however, elaboration of the inappropriate sex hormone by the tumor causes masculinization in the female or feminization in the male. Sex-hormone–secreting tumors of the gonads are usually benign, and the disorder can be cured by surgical excision.

# Hormone Production by Nonendocrine Tumors

Sometimes nonendocrine tumors secrete hormones that produce the same clinical manifestations as those of tumors arising from endocrine glands. Such hormones are called *ectopic hormones* (*ecto* = outside) because they are formed outside the endocrine glands, which are the normal sites of hormone production. An ectopic hormone is a protein that is either identical with the true hormone produced by the endocrine gland or has such a close resemblance that it mimics the action of the true hormone. Many different ectopic hormones have been identified, including ACTH, TSH, gonadotropins, parathyroid hormone, and insulin. Most hormone-producing nonendocrine tumors are malignant, and most are produced by carcinomas of lung, pancreas, or kidneys, or by malignant connective-tissue tumors.

# Stress and the Endocrine System

The body is an integrated collection of cells organized into complex organ systems and regulated by a wide variety of control mechanisms, all designed to maintain a stable internal environment in which the cells can function efficiently. The maintenance of a steady state by the body's internal control systems is called *homeostasis*, and anything that disturbs the body's well-ordered internal environment brings into play regulatory mechanisms that attempt to reestablish the steady state under which the body functions most effectively. In a general sense, stress is any event that disturbs this stable internal environment. The event may be physical trauma, such as an injury or surgical operation, prolonged exposure to cold, vigorous exercise, pain, or a strong emotional stimulus such as anxiety or fear. Any of these events call forth a response that helps the body cope with the stress. There are two distinct but overlapping responses to stress, and the type of response generated depends on both the intensity and the duration of the stress. The acute, short-term response is mediated by the sympathetic nervous system and the adrenal medulla. The chronic, longer-term response

includes the participation of several endocrine glands, with the adrenal cortex playing the major role. Both the acute and the chronic responses are initiated in the hypothalamus, which directs both the autonomic nervous system and many endocrine glands, and the hypothalamus in turn receives input from higher cortical centers.

## Acute Stress Response

The acute stress response is the well-known fear–fight–flight reaction triggered by the sympathetic nervous system. Norepinephrine released from sympathetic nerve endings, supplemented by norepinephrine and epinephrine released from the adrenal medulla in response to sympathetic nerve impulses, prepares the body to deal with the acute situation. Blood glucose rises as liver glycogen is broken down into glucose and released into the bloodstream. Peripheral vessels constrict, diverting more blood to the brain, heart, and skeletal muscles. The blood pressure rises, and the heart beats more forcefully. All of these systemic effects are of short duration and gradually subside when the stressful event is no longer present.

## Chronic Stress Response

In contrast, long-term stress of any type, either physical or emotional, initiates a slower but more complex chain of events. Hypothalamic-releasing hormones, acting through the pituitary gland, cause the adrenal cortex to increase its output of cortical hormones; they also increase the output of growth hormone and thyroid hormone while suppressing the output of gonadotropic hormones. Excess cortisol production has pronounced effects on glucose, protein, and fat metabolism, as described earlier in connection with Cushing disease. The cortisol excess also dampens the inflammatory response and reduces the responsiveness of the immune system. In addition, cortisol excess tends to raise blood pressure by making the peripheral arterioles more responsive to the vasoconstrictor effect of norepinephrine released from sympathetic nerve endings. Increased aldosterone output promotes retention of salt and water, which also tends to raise blood pressure by increasing intravascular fluid volume.

The stress-related fall in gonadotropin output impairs gonadal function, which has widespread physiologic effects, and in women may lead to stress-related cessation of menstrual periods. Stress-related amenorrhea has well-defined adverse effects on the skeletal system, as described in Chapter 22.

The increased output of thyroid hormone speeds up metabolic processes in order to allow the body to deal more effectively with the stress, as does increased output of growth hormone, which also stimulates the body's metabolic processes.

Unfortunately, chronic stress takes its toll on the body and, over the long term, may predispose to illness. Excessive demands are placed on the cardiovascular system, which may contribute to heart disease, and the chronic corticosteroid excess places undue demand on the vascular system, as well as on other organ systems. Perhaps even more important, the chronic corticosteroid excess may increase our susceptibility to many types of illnesses by reducing our ability to generate an effective inflammatory reaction and by reducing the responsiveness of our immune system.

Stress initiates many physiologic responses that are designed to help protect us from harm, but chronic, unrelieved stress can cause us harm, and stress-relieving activities can help protect us from its long-term injurious effects.

# CHAPTER REVIEW

## Summary

The endocrine glands discharge their secretions into the bloodstream and various mechanisms regulate hormone production. The pituitary produces nine separate hormones under hypothalamic control. Several pituitary hormones target other endocrine glands, such as the thyroid (via TSH), the adrenal (via ACTH), and the gonads (via gonadotropic hormones). Complete failure of pituitary function impairs the functions of all the endocrine glands under pituitary control. An isolated deficiency of growth hormone leads to pituitary dwarfism, which can be corrected by providing growth hormone. Functioning pituitary tumors can produce excess growth hormone (causing gigantism or acromegaly) or prolactin (causing the amenorrhea–galactorrhea syndrome), and some tumors produce both hormones. Nonfunctioning pituitary tumors don't produce hormones, but their growth may damage the optic nerves and other structures at the base of the brain, and may disrupt the functions of the normal pituitary cells adjacent to the tumor. Some pituitary tumors can be treated by drugs to shrink the tumor, but many require surgical treatment by transsphenoidal resection.

The thyroid gland produces two hormones designated $T_3$ and $T_4$ (based on their iodine content) which regulate metabolic processes. An enlarged thyroid gland is called a goiter, and if it produces excess thyroid hormone, it is called a toxic goiter. Graves disease is the most common cause of hyperthyroidism, which is caused by an autoantibody that stimulates thyroid hormone output. Hashimoto thyroiditis is also an autoimmune disease in which the autoantibody slowly destroys the gland function by damaging the TSH receptors on the cell, which leads to hypothyroidism. The parathyroid glands, located on the posterior surface of the thyroid gland, control the level of ionized calcium in the bloodstream. Functioning parathyroid tumors occur frequently, lead to hypercalcemia, and are treated by resection of the tumor.

The adrenal cortex produces three classes of steroid hormones: glucocorticoid, mineralocorticoid, and sex hormones. Adrenal hyperfunction causes Cushing disease and Cushing syndrome. Adrenal cortical hypofunction causes Addison disease, which is an autoimmune disease in which the autoantibody destroys the adrenal cortex and causes manifestations related to reduced output of adrenal corticosteroid hormones. The skin pigmentation results from high MSH that is formed as a by-product when ACTH is elevated. The disease is treated by supplying the missing hormones. The adrenal medulla is part of the sympathetic nervous system. A tumor of the adrenal medulla secretes excess epinephrine and norepinephrine, leading to severe and sometimes life-threatening hypertension (high blood pressure), which can cause a cerebral hemorrhage. The gonads may also give rise to functioning tumors that produce excess male or female hormones.

The endocrine system also responds to stress, which causes many physiologic responses to protect us from harm, but chronic unrelieved stress can be both mentally and physically harmful and should be avoided.

## Questions for Review

1. What are the major hormones produced by the pituitary gland? What factors regulate secretion of pituitary hormones?
2. What is the effect of overproduction of growth hormone?
3. What factors regulate the rate of production of thyroid hormone? What are the major effects of an abnormal output of thyroid hormone?
4. Why does the thyroid gland become enlarged as a result of iodine deficiency?
5. What is the difference between thyrotoxicosis and thyroiditis?
6. What are the main classes of hormones elaborated by the adrenal cortex? What diseases result from adrenal cortical dysfunction?
7. What factors regulate the output of parathyroid hormone? What are the possible effects of parathyroid dysfunction?
8. What are the clinical effects of hyperprolactinemia? What are the causes of hyperprolactinemia?
9. What is Addison disease? What is the cause of the skin pigmentation?

## Supplementary Reading

Beers, M. H., et al. 2006. *The Merck Manual of Diagnosis and Therapy, 18th edition.* Whitehouse Station, NJ: Merck Research Laboratories.

> An excellent source of current information relating to diagnosis and management of disease. Contains a very comprehensive discussion of endocrine diseases.

Eisenbarth, G. S., and Gottlieb, P. A. 2004. Autoimmune polyendocrine syndromes. *New England Journal of Medicine* 350:2068–79.

> Autoantibodies may target more than one endocrine gland leading to complex endocrine deficiencies, such as Addison disease coexisting with Graves disease, which must be managed carefully to avoid serious problems.

Melmed, S. 2008. Acromegaly. *New England Journal of Medicine* 355:2558–73.

> Pituitary tumors account for 15 percent of intracranial tumors and produce a variety of hormones. Recent advances in diagnosis and treatment are reviewed.

Schlechte, J. A. 2003. Prolactinomas. *New England Journal of Medicine* 349:2035–41.

> Describes the clinical manifestations of prolactin-secreting pituitary tumors and associated amenorrhea–galactorrhea syndrome. Primary treatment is a dopamine agonist drug. Surgery is recommended as a last resort if medical treatment is ineffective.

## Interactive Activities

### Matching
Match the abnormalities in the right column with the diseases in the left column.

1. Acromegaly
2. Amenorrhea–galactorrhea syndrome
3. Exophthalmic goiter
4. Addison disease
5. Cushing disease
6. Cushing syndrome
7. Cretinism
8. Chronic thyroiditis (Hashimoto disease)
9. Hyperparathyroidism
10. Episodes of severe hypertension

A. Neonatal hypothyroidism
B. ACTH-producing tumor
C. Growth–hormone-producing tumor
D. Administration of excess corticosteroids
E. Autoantibody-induced thyroid hyperfunction
F. Autoantibody-induced destruction of adrenal cortex
G. Autoantibody-induced destruction of thyroid gland
H. Prolactin-secreting pituitary tumor
I. Hormone-secreting parathyroid tumor
J. Catecholamine-secreting adrenal tumor

## True or False

Indicate whether a statement is true or false by writing T or F at the end of the statement.

1. A person with Hashimoto disease has a higher than normal level of thyroid hormones._____

2. Cushing disease is caused by an ACTH-secreting tumor of the pituitary gland._____

3. A catecholamine-producing tumor of the adrenal medulla is a **common cause** of hypertension._____

4. Untreated neonatal hypothyroidism leads to impaired growth and mental development._____

5. A functional parathyroid tumor leads to increased blood calcium._____

6. Most persons with diabetes fail to secrete enough insulin to maintain a normal blood glucose._____

7. An excess of growth hormone usually leads to calcium loss and loss of bone density._____

## Critical Thinking

1. Mary Jones has just delivered a baby girl and a sample of the baby's blood (umbilical cord blood) was sent to the laboratory to have thyroid function tests performed. She asks you why this was done, and what it means if the results are not normal. What would you tell her?

2. George Harrison, a 52-year-old man, hasn't been feeling well lately, and he says that his skin is darkening, like a suntan, although it is winter and he doesn't go outside very often. He doesn't understand why this is happening. What should he do, and what would you tell him?

3. Mary Martin is a 37-year-old woman who has recently started to gain weight and is about 30 pounds heavier than she was 6 months ago. She doesn't think that she has been overeating and wonders if her endocrine glands are responsible. What would you tell her, and what should she do?

# The Nervous System

## LEARNING OBJECTIVES

1. Describe the normal structure and basic functions of the brain, meninges, and cerebrospinal fluid as they relate to neurologic disease.

2. Define muscle tone and voluntary motor activity, and relate these concepts to the two forms of muscle paralysis.

3. Explain the pathogenesis and clinical manifestations of closure defect of the central nervous system. Name the techniques used for prenatal diagnosis.

4. Describe the pathogenesis and manifestations of hydrocephalus, and relate them to treatment measures.

5. Name the causes, manifestations, and treatment of transient ischemic attacks.

6. Differentiate between the two principal types of stroke in regard to pathogenesis, prognosis, and treatment.

7. Describe the pathogenesis, manifestations, and treatment of congenital cerebral aneurysms.

8. Name the types of tumors that affect the central nervous system, and explain their origin, pathogenesis, clinical manifestations, and treatment.

9. Explain the pathogenesis, major clinical manifestations, and general principles of treatment of Parkinson disease, meningitis, and multiple sclerosis.

# Structure and Function

The central nervous system (CNS) consists of the brain and spinal cord, surrounded by several membranes called **meninges**. The firm, fibrous outer membrane is called the **dura**. The thin inner membrane, which adheres to the surface of the brain and spinal cord, is called the **pia**. The middle membrane, interposed between the pia and the dura, is called the **arachnoid**. The space between the arachnoid and the underlying pia is called the **subarachnoid space**. It contains cerebrospinal fluid (CSF) together with fine strands of arachnoidal connective tissue that extend through the space and attach to the tips of the gyri.

The *brain* is divided into the *cerebrum*, *brain stem*, and *cerebellum*. The brain is hollow, containing four interconnected cavities called ventricles. Arterial blood is supplied to the brain by large blood vessels entering the base of the skull. These arteries join to form a circle of vessels (*the circle of Willis*) at the base of the brain. Branches from the circle extend outward to supply all parts of the brain. Venous blood is returned from the brain into large venous sinuses in the dura, which eventually drain into the jugular veins.

The brain and spinal cord are surrounded by cerebrospinal fluid and are encased within protective bony structures: the *cranium* and the *vertebral column*. The bony case protects the soft and rather fragile nervous tissue, and the cerebrospinal fluid acts as a hydrostatic cushion to insulate the brain from shocks and blows.

The nerve tissue of the brain and spinal cord is composed of nerve cells called neurons and supporting cells called neuroglia (Chapter 2). Each individual neuron has a central body and one or more long processes extending from the cell body to transmit the impulses. Processes carrying impulses into the nerve cell are called dendrites, and those carrying impulses out of the nerve cell are called axons. Sometimes the general term *nerve fiber* is used when referring to either type. Neurons are frequently arranged in chains; the neurons interconnect with other neurons to transmit impulses, but they are not in direct contact with one another. They are separated by minute gaps called *synapses*. The transmission of a nerve impulse across a synapse is by means of a chemical called a *neurotransmitter* that is released from the end of an axon and activates receptors on the dendrite or cell body of the adjacent neuron. There are several types of neurotransmitters, and each type of neuron has its own specific type. When a nerve fiber leaves the central nervous system, it becomes invested by cells called *Schwann cells* that wrap around the fiber. These cells produce the myelin that insulates the fiber. The myelin surrounding nerve fibers within the central nervous system is produced by glial cells called **oligodendroglia**.

A nerve that transmits impulses into the nervous system is called a *sensory nerve* or *afferent nerve* (*ad* = to + *ferre* = carry). A *motor nerve* or *efferent nerve* (*e* = away) conducts impulses from brain or spinal cord to muscle. The gray matter of the brain and cord is composed primarily of nerve cells and their processes. The *white matter* consists mostly of bundles of nerve fibers covered by fatty myelin sheaths.

The nervous system may be regarded as a giant switchboard, receiving sensory impulses and relaying this information to brain and spinal cord centers concerned with perception of sensation and with motor activity. The cerebral cortex receives sensory input and initiates voluntary motor activity. In the depths of each cerebral hemisphere are masses of gray matter: the thalami and the basal ganglia (basal nuclei). The paired thalami function as relay stations that receive sensory impulses from lower levels and transmit them to the cortex. The basal ganglia in each hemisphere are part of a complex neuron system that is concerned with control of automatic functions that do not require constant attention, such as walking. The brain stem also contains neurons that are involved in multiple functions not under direct cortical control, and also carries the bundles of nerve fibers that pass to higher and lower levels within the CNS. The cerebellum regulates muscle tone, coordination, posture, and balance.

The spinal cord is the continuation of the brain stem. Its central gray matter receives sensory input from spinal nerves entering the cord, and motor neurons exit from the cord to innervate muscles. Spinal sensory and motor neurons are involved in many reflex functions not under cortical control, and are also activated by motor impulses originating from cortical neurons. The spinal motor neurons in turn discharge impulses to the skeletal muscles that they supply, causing them to contract.

The fiber tracts conveying sensory impulses to the cortex and those conveying motor impulses from the cortex cross within the brain stem to the opposite side as they transmit impulses to their destination. Consequently, the right hemisphere registers sensation from the left half of the body and innervates the muscles on the left side. Conversely, the left hemisphere receives

**meninges**
(men-in´jēz)
The membranes covering the brain and spinal cord.

**dura** (dū´rä) The outer covering of the brain and spinal cord.

**pia** (pē´yuh) The innermost of the three membranes covering the brain and spinal cord.

**arachnoid** (ar-ak´noyd) The middle of the three meninges that cover the brain and spinal cord.

**subarachnoid space** (sub-är-ak´noyd) The space between the arachnoid and the pia, containing large blood vessels supplying the brain.

**oligodendroglia** (ol´ig-ō-den-drog´li-ah) One type of neuroglia that surrounds nerve fibers within the central nervous system.

sensation from the right side of the body and activates muscles on the right side.

# Development of the Nervous System

In the embryo, the CNS first appears as a thickened band of surface cells (ectoderm) called the neural plate. Its lateral margins become elevated to form neural folds, and the two folds then fuse to form a hollow tube called the neural tube. Fusion begins in the middle of the developing tube and progresses toward both ends until a completely closed tube is formed by the end of the fourth week of embryonic development. Three expansions, called the forebrain, midbrain, and hindbrain, develop from one end of the neural tube ( Figure 21-1 ). The other end remains narrow and becomes the spinal cord.

The *cerebral hemispheres* develop as lateral outgrowths from the forebrain and soon overgrow the remaining parts of the brain. The remainder of the forebrain becomes the *diencephalon*, which is located between the cerebral hemispheres (*dia* = between + *encephalon* = brain). The

*midbrain* persists as a small area connecting the forebrain and the hindbrain. The hindbrain gives rise to parts of the brain called the *pons*, *medulla*, and *cerebellum*. The diencephalon, midbrain, pons, and medulla together form the *brain stem*. The central cavity within the neural tube develops into the *ventricular system* of the adult brain. The embryonic cells (mesoderm) surrounding the developing neural tube give rise to the cranial cavity, vertebral bodies, and adjacent tissues.

# Muscle Tone and Voluntary Muscle Contraction

A skeletal muscle contracts in response to impulses discharged from motor neurons in the spinal cord or from corresponding neurons of the cranial nerves in the brain stem. Voluntary motor activity is controlled by two separate motor systems. One system, called the *pyramidal system*, controls voluntary motor functions, and the other system, called the *extrapyramidal system*, regulates muscle groups concerned primarily with balance, posture, and coordination.

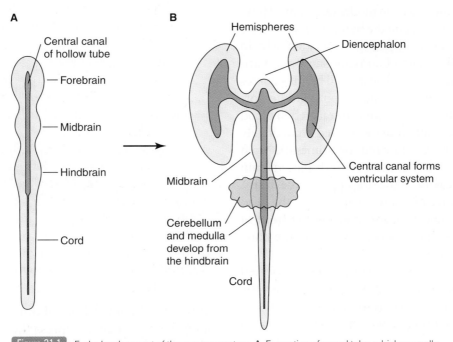

**A**

Central canal of hollow tube

— Forebrain

— Midbrain

— Hindbrain

— Cord

**B**

Hemispheres

Diencephalon

Central canal forms ventricular system

Midbrain

Cerebellum and medulla develop from the hindbrain

Cord

Figure 21-1 Early development of the nervous system. **A**, Formation of neural tube, which normally closes at both ends. Central canal in tube is the precursor of the ventricular system. **B**, Cerebral hemispheres grow from the forebrain and the central region becomes the diencephalon. The hindbrain forms the medulla and cerebellum. The tube becomes the ventricular system. The two lateral ventricles follow the contours of the developing hemispheres, which communicate with the third ventricle in the diencephalon by channels called interventricular foramina. The channel in the midbrain becomes the cerebral aqueduct, which expands into the fourth ventricle in the medulla. Each ventricle develops a choroid plexus to make the cerebrospinal fluid that flows through the ventricular system, exits through openings in the fourth ventricle, and circulates around the brain and spinal cord.

The pyramidal system and the extrapyramidal system function together as a single system under cortical control to produce the smooth integrated functions of muscle groups involved in voluntary motor activity. Malfunction of the extrapyramidal system leads to loss of coordinated motor functions. The muscles do not function smoothly, and the malfunction also gives rise to abnormal uncontrollable muscular movements.

# Muscle Paralysis

A muscle that is no longer subject to voluntary control is said to be paralyzed. There are two different types of paralysis:

1. *Flaccid paralysis* results when the spinal motor neurons are destroyed by disease, as in poliomyelitis.
2. *Spastic paralysis* results from disease affecting the cortical motor neurons or their fibers, as occurs when a person has a stroke.

Spastic paralysis occurs more frequently than flaccid paralysis because cortical neurons are more often damaged by disease than are spinal motor neurons.

# Cerebral Injury

The brain is well protected from moderate trauma. However, a severe blow may injure the brain, and sometimes the skull also is fractured ( Figure 21-2 ). Injury to the brain may be manifested by loss of consciousness and various neurologic disturbances. The injured brain becomes swollen and often shows evidence of pinpoint hemorrhages caused by disruption of small intracerebral blood vessels. Usually the brain injury is located immediately adjacent to the site of the blow, but sometimes the brain injury is caused by violent contact of the displaced brain against the cranial cavity on the side opposite the injury. For example, the force of a blow to the back of the head may displace the brain forward, injuring the front of the brain where it strikes against the front of the bony cranial cavity ( Figure 21-3 ).

Sometimes a head injury tears blood vessels located between the cranial bones and the dura or under the dura. The escaping blood may accumulate in any of several locations, depending on which vessels have been damaged:

1. Between the outer layer of dura and the cranial bones (*epidural hemorrhage*)
2. Between the dura and the arachnoid (*subdural hemorrhage*)
3. Between the arachnoid and the pia (*subarachnoid hemorrhage*)

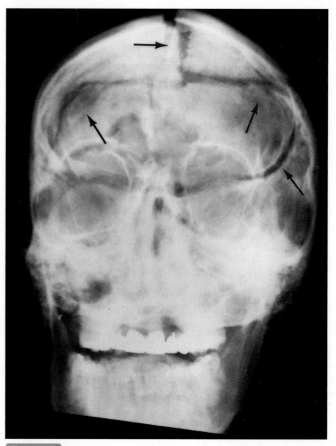

Figure 21-2 Skull x-ray illustrating large skull fracture (*arrows*) associated with extensive injury to underlying brain.

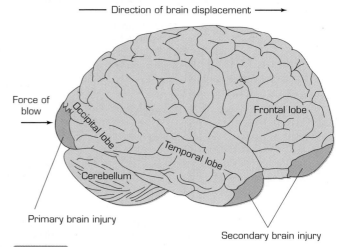

Figure 21-3 Mechanism of injury to frontal and temporal poles of brain caused by a blow to the back of the head.

A localized epidural or subdural collection of blood (a *hematoma*) may compress the brain and impair its function. In a subarachnoid hemorrhage, the blood often mixes with the cerebrospinal fluid and spreads diffusely through the subarachnoid space.

Unfortunately, the rigid cranial cavity, which normally serves a protective function, is a disadvantage if the brain is seriously injured. The brain often swells at the site of injury, and the unyielding cranial cavity restricts the swelling and compresses the swollen brain, leading to high intracranial pressure. The elevated pressure adversely affects cerebral function and may also interfere with the blood supply to the brain by compressing cerebral blood vessels.

# Neural Tube Defects

Failure of either end of the neural tube to close properly leads to serious congenital malformations called *neural tube defects*, which involve not only the nervous system but the surrounding tissues as well. A closure defect involving the end of the tube destined to form the cerebral hemispheres (called the *cephalic end*) leads to a condition called **anencephaly** (*ana* = without + *encephalon* = brain). **Spina bifida** results if the opposite end of the tube (the *caudal* end) fails to close normally. These are the two most common congenital malformations of the nervous system. The combined incidence of these malformations is about 2 per 1000 births in the United States and even higher in some other countries. The malformations follow a multifactorial pattern of inheritance (Chapter 7) and tend to recur in subsequent pregnancies. If parents have already given birth to an offspring with a neural tube defect, the risk of recurrence in a subsequent pregnancy is approximately 1 in 20. The risk is 1 in 10 when the parents have had two affected infants.

A deficiency of folic acid during the early part of pregnancy when the neural tube is forming plays an important role in causing neural tube defects. Intake of 0.4–0.8 mg of folic acid daily beginning one month before conception and during the early part of pregnancy (first trimester) can reduce by one-half the frequency of neural tube defects. However, these defects follow a multifactorial inheritance pattern, and the folic acid deficiency functions along with genetic factors to cause the neural tube defect.

## Anencephaly

Anencephaly occurs most commonly in female infants and is incompatible with postnatal life. Because the cephalic end of the neural tube fails to close, the exposed neural tissue undergoes secondary degenerative changes that convert it into a mass of vascular connective tissue intermixed with masses of degenerated brain and choroid plexus. The anencephalic infant has a striking appearance ( Figure 21-4 ). The brain is absent, as are the soft tissues of the scalp and the bones making up the vertex of the skull. The exposed base of the skull is covered only by a vascular membrane. The base of the cranial cavity is abnormally formed, and the orbits are

**anencephaly**
(an-en-seff′uh-lē) A congenital malformation: absence of brain, cranial vault, and scalp as a result of defective closure of the neural tube.

**spina bifida**
(spī′-nuh bif′fid-duh) Incomplete closure of vertebral arches over the spinal cord, sometimes associated with protrusion of meninges and neural tissue through the defect (*cystic spina bifida*).

A

B

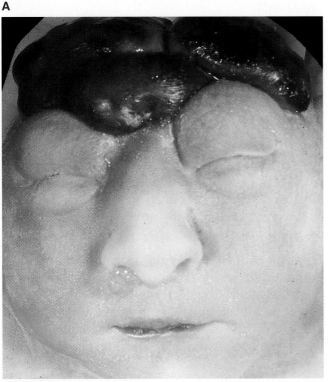

Figure 21-4    Characteristic appearance of anencephalic infant. Most of brain, top of skull, and scalp are absent. Maldevelopment of skull causes protrusion of eyes. **A,** Frontal view. **B,** Lateral view.

shallow, causing the eyes to bulge outward. The trunk is short, the shoulders are broad, and the neck is not normal; the head arises directly from the trunk and cannot be flexed.

The following case illustrates some of the obstetric problems associated with anencephaly.

## Case Study 21-1

A female anencephalic infant was born to a 28-year-old woman who was pregnant for the first time. The fetal heartbeat could be heard by the obstetrician throughout the last part of the pregnancy. When the patient's abdomen was examined near term, the obstetrician became concerned about the possibility of anencephaly because of the inability to feel the fetal head. An x-ray film taken of the patient's abdomen confirmed the clinical impression because only the base of the fetal skull could be seen in the x-ray film. The bones of the cranial vault were absent. The rest of the fetal skeleton appeared normally formed. The patient was delivered at term with some difficulty because the anencephalic head was unable to flex normally as it passed through the mother's pelvis, and the infant was delivered face first. The infant survived for several hours after delivery. The autopsy revealed complete absence of the cerebral hemispheres, the cerebellum, and most of the brain stem.

## Spina Bifida

**meningocele** (men-in′go-sēl) A protrusion of meninges through a defect in the spinal vertebral arches.

**meningomyelocele** (men-ing-gō-mī′el-ō-sēl) A type of spina bifida characterized by protrusion of meninges and cord through the defect in the vertebral arches.

Malformations of the opposite (caudal) end of the neural tube and related vertebral arches are generally considered together under the term *spina bifida*. This term means literally *split spine* and refers to the characteristic failure of fusion of the vertebral arches common to all types of spina bifida ( Figure 21-5 ). Failure of fusion of vertebral arches in the lower lumbar region occurring as an isolated abnormality is called *occult spina bifida* (Figure 21-5A); this type produces no clinical symptoms. The more severe types of spina bifida, sometimes called collectively *cystic spina bifida*, are characterized by a saclike

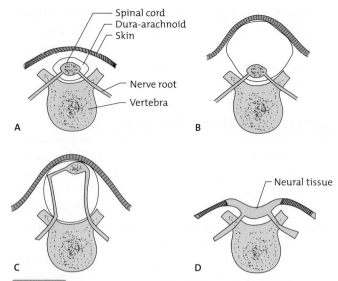

**Figure 21-5** Various types of spina bifida. **A,** Occult spina bifida. Failure of formation of vertebral arches. No protrusion of meninges. **B,** Meningocele. Meninges protrude through defect in the vertebral arches. Cord and nerve trunks are not present in the sac. **C,** Meningomyelocele. Protrusion of both meninges and nerve tissue. The spinal cord and nerve trunks are frequently incorporated into the wall of the sac. **D,** Failure of the neural tube to form and separate from the surface ectoderm. The neural tissue is continuous with the adjacent skin.

protrusion of meninges or meninges and nerve tissue through the defect in the vertebral arches. The malformation is called a **meningocele** if the protrusion consists only of meninges (Figure 21-5B) and is called a **meningomyelocele** (*myelo* = cord) if parts of the spinal cord or nerve roots also are included in the sac (Figure 21-5C).

In meningomyelocele, there is often a severe neurologic deficit below the level of the sac because the nerve tissue is actually incorporated into the wall of the sac and is disorganized so that the conduction of nerve impulses is impaired or completely interrupted. In the most severe (and fortunately rare) form of spina bifida, the caudal end of the neural tube completely fails to close. The distal end of the spinal cord is represented by a flattened mass of nerve tissue that is continuous with the adjacent skin (Figure 21-5D). The larger meningomyelocele sacs often are covered not by skin but merely by a thin, easily ruptured membrane composed only of meninges ( Figure 21-6 ).

**Treatment of Spina Bifida** Occult spina bifida is asymptomatic, and no treatment is required. A meningocele usually can be repaired without difficulty by excising the sac and closing the spinal dura, and the results are usually very satisfactory. Unfortunately, a large meningomyelocele is much more difficult to treat, and results are much less satisfactory. Because spinal cord and nerve roots are often incorporated in the sac, there is frequently some loss of sensation and motor power

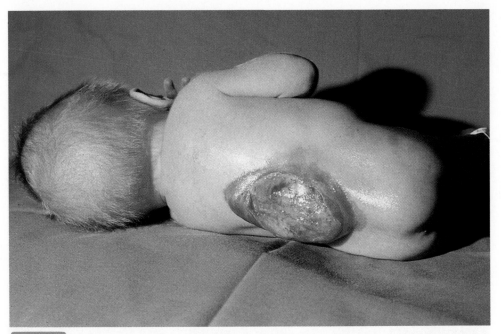

Large thoracic meningomyelocele covered only by a thin membrane. This condition is associated with neurologic disturbances resulting from incorporation of neural tissue into the wall of the sac.

in the lower extremities. Bowel and bladder function also may be impaired, leading to stasis of urine in the bladder and predisposing to urinary tract infections. These individuals are managed best by a team of specialists in a medical center specializing in the care of patients with severe disabilities of this type. Many patients can be treated successfully and are able to lead happy and productive lives despite their disability.

## Prenatal Detection of Neural Tube Defects

It is usually possible to identify a fetus with a neural tube defect prior to birth. An elevated concentration of **alpha fetoprotein (AFP)** detected on a routine screening test of maternal blood may suggest the possibility of a neural tube defect, and the defect can be confirmed by an ultrasound examination of the fetus performed at about 16-weeks' gestation, as described in Chapter 7.

Alpha fetoprotein is produced in the fetal liver beginning early in pregnancy and can be readily detected in the fetal blood. The concentration in fetal blood is highest at about 13 weeks and then gradually declines. A small amount of AFP normally diffuses from the fetal blood into the amnionic fluid and also into the mother's blood. High amnionic fluid AFP levels are encountered when the fetus is anencephalic or has a cystic spina bifida in which the defect is covered only by a thin membrane. Consequently, AFP can more easily diffuse from the fetal blood and cerebrospinal fluid into the amnionic fluid, and AFP levels are much higher than in a normal pregnancy.

# Hydrocephalus

Cerebrospinal fluid serves as a protective cushion around the brain and spinal cord. The fluid is secreted by the choroid plexuses of the ventricles. It flows from the lateral ventricles into the third ventricle, through the cerebral aqueduct (*aqueduct of Sylvius*) into the fourth ventricle and then out into the subarachnoid space through three small openings in the roof and lateral walls of the fourth ventricle. The fluid circulates around the cord and over the convexity of the brain and is resorbed into the large venous sinuses in the dura. Secretion of cerebrospinal fluid continues even if the flow of fluid through the ventricular system is blocked. Obstruction to the normal circulation of spinal fluid distends the ventricles proximal to the site of obstruction, with associated compression atrophy of brain tissue around the dilated ventricles. This condition, which is called **hydrocephalus**, may be either congenital or acquired ( Figure 21-7 ).

**Congenital Hydrocephalus** *Congenital hydrocephalus* is usually caused by a congenital abnormality in the ventricular system, either a congenital obstruction or abnormal formation of the cerebral aqueduct, a narrow channel connecting the third and fourth ventricles, or failure of the openings in the roof and lateral walls of the fourth

**alpha fetoprotein (AFP)** (al'fuh fē'tō-prō'tēn) Protein produced by fetal liver early in gestation. Sometimes produced by tumor cells. Level is elevated in amnionic fluid when fetus has neural tube defect.

**hydrocephalus** Dilatation of the ventricular system caused by pressure arising from accumulation of cerebrospinal fluid within the ventricles.

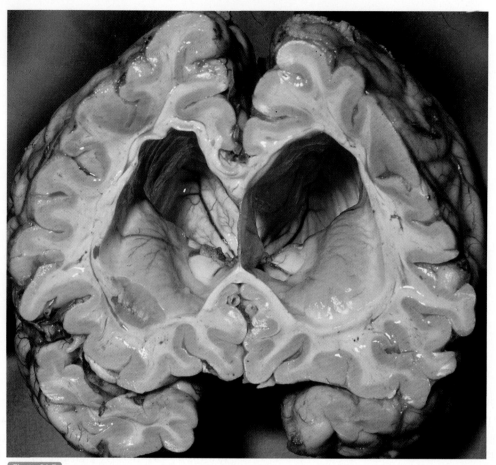

**Figure 21-7** Coronal section of brain revealing marked dilatation of ventricles in patient with congenital hydrocephalus.

ventricle to form normally, which blocks escape of cerebrospinal fluid into the subarachnoid space. An aqueduct obstruction leads to distention of the lateral and third ventricles. An obstruction of the outlet channels in the fourth ventricle leads to distention of all four ventricles. Because the distention develops before the skull bones have fused, the head enlarges greatly and the brain undergoes pronounced atrophy secondary to compression by the dilated ventricles. Hydrocephalus may occur in the fetus prior to birth, and the head may become so large that it is unable to enter the maternal pelvis during labor. More often, the hydrocephalus develops insidiously after birth.

**Acquired Hydrocephalus** *Acquired hydrocephalus* is most commonly caused by obstruction of the circulation of the cerebrospinal fluid in the region of the fourth ventricle by fibrous adhesions, which sometimes form after a bacterial infection of the meninges (meningitis) and block the outflow of fluid from the fourth ventricle, or by blockage of the ventricular system secondary to a brain tumor. Acquired hydrocephalus develops after the skull bones fuse, and the

skull cannot enlarge as in the congenital form of hydrocephalus.

**Treatment of Hydrocephalus** Hydrocephalus can often be treated successfully by inserting a plastic tube into one of the dilated ventricles and rerouting (*shunting*) the fluid into another part of the body where it can be absorbed. The fluid can be shunted into the right atrium (*ventriculoatrial shunt*) or into the peritoneal cavity (*ventriculoperitoneal shunt*). A small opening is made in the skull to allow insertion of a plastic drainage tube through cerebral hemisphere into one of the dilated lateral ventricles. The other end of the tube is passed through the subcutaneous tissues behind the ear. In a ventriculoatrial shunt, the tube is inserted into the jugular vein and threaded down the vein so that the tip is positioned in the right atrium. In the more commonly used ventriculoperitoneal shunt the tube is passed through the subcutaneous tissues of the neck, chest, and upper abdomen and introduced into the abdominal cavity through a small incision in the peritoneum. Whatever type of shunt is used, a one-way valve is incorporated in the tube to prevent any reflux of blood or peritoneal fluid into the ventricles ( Figure 21-8 ).

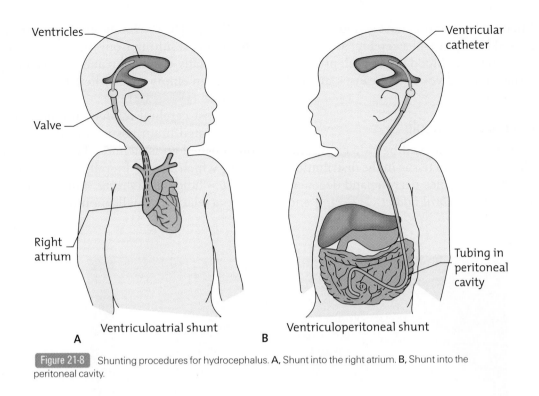

Ventricles

Valve

Right
atrium

Ventriculoatrial shunt

**A**

Ventricular
catheter

Tubing in
peritoneal
cavity

Ventriculoperitoneal shunt

**B**

**Figure 21-8** Shunting procedures for hydrocephalus. **A,** Shunt into the right atrium. **B,** Shunt into the peritoneal cavity.

Case 21-2 illustrates some of the obstetric and pediatric problems encountered when hydrocephalus occurs in the fetus before delivery.

**Case Study 21-2**

A 24-year-old woman who was pregnant for the first time noted marked enlargement of her abdomen during the last part of pregnancy. X-ray examination of the abdomen revealed a hydrocephalic infant having a head diameter that was larger than the diameter of the mother's pelvis, indicating that delivery could not be accomplished vaginally. At term, an elective cesarean section was performed, and the infant was evaluated soon after delivery by a neurosurgeon. A shunt was performed in order to control the progressing hydrocephalus. The shunt prevented further enlargement of the head, and the infant did reasonably well after this operation.

# Stroke

The term **stroke**, also called a **cerebrovascular accident** or simply **CVA**, is used to designate any injury to brain tissue resulting from disturbance of blood supply to the brain and encompasses three conditions: (1) cerebral

thrombosis, (2) cerebral embolism, and (3) cerebral hemorrhage.

A **cerebral thrombosis**, as indicated by the name, results from thrombosis of a cerebral artery narrowed by arteriosclerosis and is the cause of most strokes.

A **cerebral embolus**, which occurs less frequently than a cerebral thrombosis, is caused by blockage of a cerebral artery by a fragment of a blood clot dislodged from the surface of an ulcerated arteriosclerotic plaque in the carotid artery and carried to the brain, or from a blood clot that formed within the heart. Three cardiac conditions predispose to cerebral emboli:

1. A mural thrombus that formed on the wall of the left ventricle adjacent to a healing myocardial infarct.
2. A thrombus that formed on the rough surface of a diseased mitral or aortic valve.
3. A small thrombus in the left atrial appendage (auricle) of a person with atrial fibrillation. Atrial thrombi tend to develop because the atria are not contracting normally. Consequently, the blood pools in the atrial appendages instead of being ejected normally, which predisposes to formation of blood clots in the stagnant atrial appendage blood.

**stroke**
Any injury to the brain caused by disturbance of its blood supply.

**cerebrovascular accident (CVA)** An injury to the brain resulting in a disturbance of cerebral blood flow caused by a cerebral thrombosis, cerebral embolism, or cerebral hemorrhage.

**cerebral thrombosis**
A stroke caused by thrombosis of an arteriosclerotic cerebral artery.

**cerebral embolus**
A stroke caused by blockage of a cerebral artery by a blood clot that had formed elsewhere in the circulatory system and was transported in the bloodstream to the brain.

A **cerebral hemorrhage** is the most serious type of stroke. It is caused by rupture of a cerebral artery in a person with hypertension. Blood under high pressure escapes from the ruptured vessel and causes marked damage to the brain.

## Cerebral Thrombi and Emboli

When a cerebral artery is blocked by either a thrombus on an embolus, the brain tissue in the distribution of the blocked vessel becomes necrotic and degenerates, which is called a *cerebral infarct* (Figure 21-9 and Figure 21-10). The myelin sheath material breaks down and the debris resulting from the necrosis of brain tissue is eventually cleaned up and removed by phagocytes, leaving an empty space where the necrotic tissue was removed (Figure 21-11).

In most cerebral infarcts, no blood leaks into the degenerated brain tissue, and this type of infarct is often called an ischemic infarct (pronounced *is-key-mik*), which means literally that blood is held back (*ischo* = hold back + *heme* = blood). However, sometimes a relatively small amount of blood leaks into the

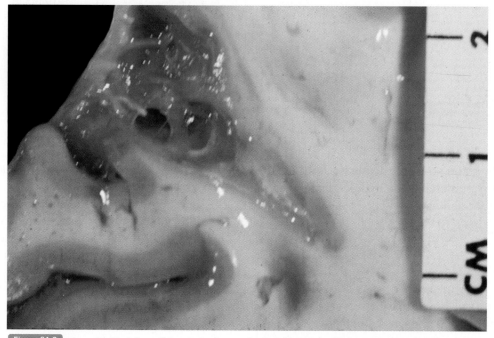

Figure 21-9    A small, older infarct of the cerebral cortex that is undergoing cystic breakdown (encephalomalacia).

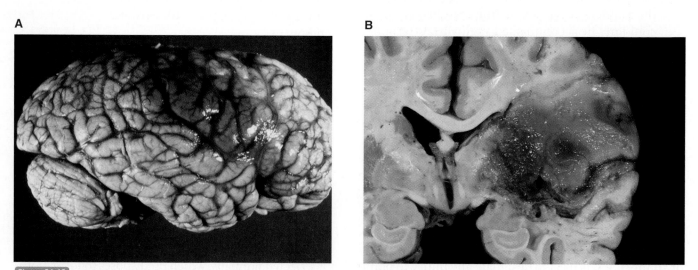

Figure 21-10    Large recent infarct of right cerebral hemisphere caused by thrombosis of middle cerebral artery. **A**, External surface of brain illustrating the swollen, dark, infarcted area in the right hemisphere. **B**, Coronal section through hemispheres at level of basal ganglia. Cerebral tissue is necrotic and discolored and involves a large part of the hemisphere.

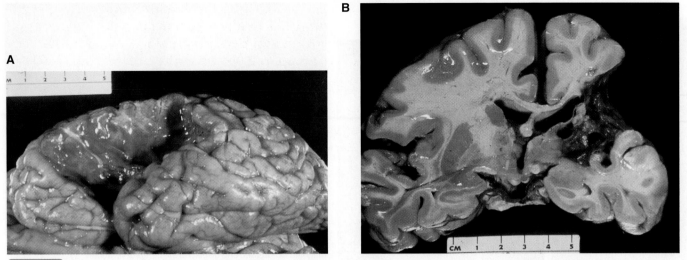

**Figure 21-11** A large, old infarct in the left hemisphere sustained several years previously, which caused paralysis of right side of body and loss of speech. A, External surface of the brain, illustrating the large defect in the left hemisphere at the site of the old infarct. B, Coronal section through the hemisphere revealing complete loss of cerebral tissue at the site of the old infarct, leaving only a few strands of glial tissue.

degenerated brain tissue from adjacent damaged cerebral blood vessels, as illustrated in Figure 21-10.

Some patients who have had a stroke caused by thrombosis of a cerebral artery may benefit from the same type of thrombolytic drugs used to dissolve blood clots in coronary arteries (Chapter 10). Unfortunately, there is very little time available to restore flow through a blocked cerebral artery before permanent brain damage occurs, and sometimes the thrombolytic drug treatment may be complicated by hemorrhage within the damaged brain tissue.

## Stroke Caused by Arteriosclerosis of Extracranial Arteries

A stroke may also be caused by atherosclerosis of one of the major arteries arising from the aorta to supply the brain, before the vessel enters the cranial cavity. A commonly affected site is at the origin of the internal carotid artery in the neck, where atheromatous plaques may narrow the lumen and reduce cerebral blood flow. The plaques may also become ulcerated, and thrombi may form on the roughened surfaces. Bits of arteriosclerotic debris or thrombus material may break loose from the plaque and be carried into the blood vessels in the brain, where they may block small cerebral arteries. Rarely, the internal carotid artery may become completely blocked by a thrombus that has formed on the roughened surface of the artery, leading to a large cerebral infarction. Figure 21-12 illustrates the possible effects of arteriosclerosis of the internal carotid artery in the neck.

**Diagnosis of Extracranial Vascular Disease** Cerebral blood flow can be studied by injecting a radiopaque dye into the carotid and vertebral arteries that arise

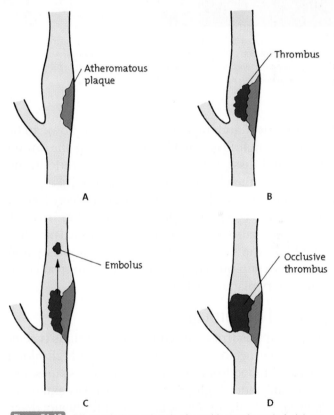

**Figure 21-12** Effects of atherosclerosis of carotid artery in neck. A, Atherosclerotic plaque narrows lumen, and surface frequently becomes ulcerated. B, Formation of thrombus on ulcerated surface of plaque, further narrowing vessel. C, Thrombus material dislodged from plaque to form emboli, which are carried to brain. D, Complete occlusion of artery by thrombus. (Escourolle and Poirier. *Manuel élémentaire de neuropathology*. Masson S. A., Paris, 1977. English translation: W. B. Saunders. Philadelphia, 1978.)

from the arch of the aorta to supply the brain. In this procedure, called a *cerebral angiogram*, the course of the dye is followed by serial x-ray studies, using methods similar to those used to visualize the coronary arteries. Arteriosclerotic plaques that occlude the

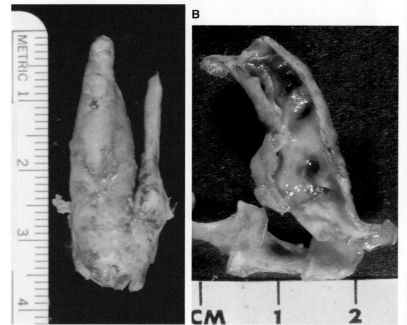

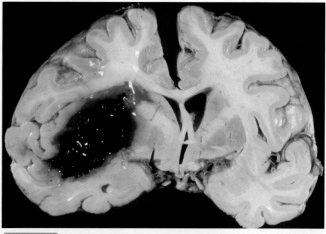

Figure 21-14 Coronal section of brain illustrating large cerebral hemorrhage that has compressed and displaced the cerebral ventricles.

Figure 21-13 Carotid endarterectomy. **A,** Resected atherosclerotic plaque material has the contour of the common carotid artery and its two major branches, where it formed. **B,** An opened endarterectomy specimen revealing rough internal surface with areas of ulceration and hemorrhage in the atheromatous plaque.

carotid artery and impede cerebral blood flow can be removed surgically by making an incision in the carotid artery and dissecting out the arteriosclerotic lining and plaque, thereby opening up the artery ( Figure 21-13 ). The procedure is called a *carotid endarterectomy* (*endo* = within + artery + *tome* = incision). Other less invasive methods are also being investigated in selected patients, including the same type of balloon angioplasty and stent insertion procedures that are used to treat coronary artery plaques (Chapter 10).

## Cerebral Hemorrhage

A *cerebral hemorrhage* is a much more serious type of stroke that occurs in persons who have high blood pressure. Blood from the ruptured vessel escapes into the brain under high pressure and causes extensive damage to brain tissue. A large cerebral hemorrhage is frequently fatal ( Figure 21-14 ).

It is possible to distinguish a cerebral infarct from a cerebral hemorrhage by a specialized x-ray study called a computed tomographic (CT) scan (Chapter 1). A CT scan can localize abnormal areas in the brain and determine their density. A cerebral hemorrhage appears as a dense area within the brain because blood is denser than normal brain tissue ( Figure 21-15 ). In contrast, an infarct is often swollen by edema and appears less dense than normal brain tissue. Magnetic resonance imaging (MRI) provides similar information and is equally effective.

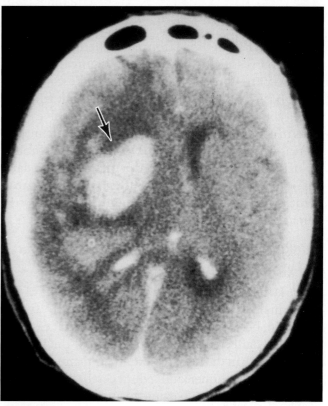

Figure 21-15 A computed tomographic (CT) scan of a patient with cerebral hemorrhage (*arrow*), which appears white because blood is denser than brain tissue.

## Manifestations of Stroke

The clinical effects of a stroke depend on the location of the brain damage and the amount of brain tissue injured. Small infarcts may cause little functional disturbance and are usually followed by prompt recovery with little or no residual disability. Unfortunately, many strokes result from occlusions of the middle cerebral artery or one of its major branches or from a hemorrhage in a part of the brain supplied by the artery.

Frequently the injury is extensive and causes partial paralysis by disrupting the nerve fibers that carry impulses to the spinal motor neurons and motor neurons of the cranial nerves. Nerve fibers carrying sensory impulses to the cortex are often damaged as well, leading to various sensory disturbances.

As mentioned earlier, sensory and motor fiber tracts cross in the brain stem as they ascend or descend; so the motor neurons from the right cerebral hemisphere supply the left side of the body, and sensory impulses received by this hemisphere come from the left side of the body. Conversely, the left hemisphere controls the right half of the body and receives sensory input from the right side. Consequently, a stroke involving one cerebral hemisphere often leads to weakness or paralysis on the opposite side, called **hemiplegia** (*hemi* = half + *plege* = stroke) or *hemiparesis* (*paresis* = weakness) and often to some sensory impairment on the paralyzed side as well. Speech also may be affected, but usually the affected individual does not lose consciousness.

### Rehabilitation of the Stroke Patient

Many patients who suffer a major stroke are partially paralyzed, and some may have speech impairment as well. Rehabilitation, which is begun as soon as possible, helps the patient achieve several goals:

1. To regain the ability to walk
2. To relearn self-care activities, such as washing, combing the hair, and eating, which may have been impaired by the stroke
3. To prevent stiffness and limitation of motion in the joints of the paralyzed limbs
4. To make an emotional adjustment to the disability

These goals are achieved primarily by a program of exercises and relearning. If speech is impaired, speech therapy also is started. Many patients can learn to walk again, although in some cases a leg brace and cane may be required. It is more difficult to regain useful function in a paralyzed upper limb.

# Transient Ischemic Attack

The term **transient ischemic attack**, often abbreviated **TIA**, refers to brief episodes of neurologic dysfunction such as temporary paralysis of an arm or leg, loss of speech, or disturbances of vision. The episodes, which tend to occur in older persons, last from a few minutes to a few hours and clear completely. They are usually caused by bits of thrombus or arteriosclerotic debris that break loose from an ulcerated plaque in the internal carotid artery and obstruct a small cerebral artery. The episodes are brief because the obstructing debris or small clot becomes fragmented and dissolved, and the circulation through the blocked vessel is restored before permanent damage to brain tissue occurs.

About one-third of patients with transient ischemic attacks eventually suffer a major stroke, but most have no further difficulties. Treatment consists either of surgical resection of the ulcerated plaque in the carotid artery by means of a *carotid endarterectomy* or administration of drugs that decrease the likelihood that thrombi will form on the ulcerated plaques. A narrowing of the carotid artery is significant if the lumen of the artery is reduced by 50 percent. This degree of narrowing corresponds to a 75 percent reduction in the cross-section area of the lumen and is associated with a large reduction in flow rate through the artery.

**hemiplegia** (hem-ē-plē´-jē-uh) Paralysis of one side of the body.

**transient ischemic attack (TIA)** (isskē´mik) Temporary cerebral dysfunction as a result of transient obstruction of a cerebral vessel by a bit of atheromatous debris or blood clot usually embolized from an arteriosclerotic plaque in the carotid artery.

# Cerebral Aneurysm

Occasionally, aneurysms occur in the large cerebral arteries at the base of the brain. The most common type, a *congenital cerebral aneurysm*, results from a congenital defect in the elastic and muscular tissue of the vessel wall, usually at the point where the artery branches. Because of the congenital weakness, the lining of the arterial wall (*intima*) eventually protrudes through the defect at the point of branching, leading to the formation of a saclike outpouching ( Figure 21-16 ).

Although the weakness of the vessel wall is congenital, the actual aneurysm does not develop until young adulthood or middle age. Persons with congenital

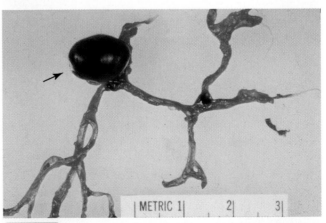

| METRIC 1| | 2| | 3|

Figure 21-16   Dissection of vessels from the brain of a person with large congenital cerebral aneurysm (*arrow*).

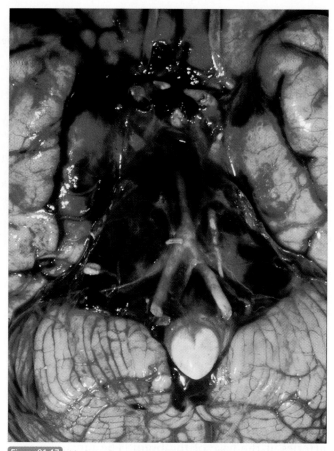

Figure 21-17 Undersurface of brain, illustrating subarachnoid hemorrhage secondary to ruptured cerebral aneurysm.

polycystic kidney disease (Chapter 15) are prone to develop aneurysms of this type. Congenital aneurysms are hazardous because they may rupture, producing severe and sometimes fatal subarachnoid hemorrhage within the cranial cavity ( Figure 21-17 ). Persons with high blood pressure are especially prone to this complication. The initial symptoms of a ruptured aneurysm are severe headache and a stiff neck. The headache results from the increased intracranial pressure caused by the sudden escape of blood into the subarachnoid space. The stiff neck occurs because the escaping blood irritates the meninges, setting off reflex contraction of the neck muscles.

The location of the aneurysm can be determined by a *cerebral angiogram*. Radiopaque material (contrast medium) is injected into the arteries supplying the brain and fills the aneurysm sac, defining both its size and position ( Figure 21-18 ). Treatment usually consists of occluding (closing off) the aneurysm. Often this can be accomplished by applying a small metal clip to the narrow neck of the sac at its attachment to the arterial wall, but other procedures may be used depending on the size and location of the aneurysm.

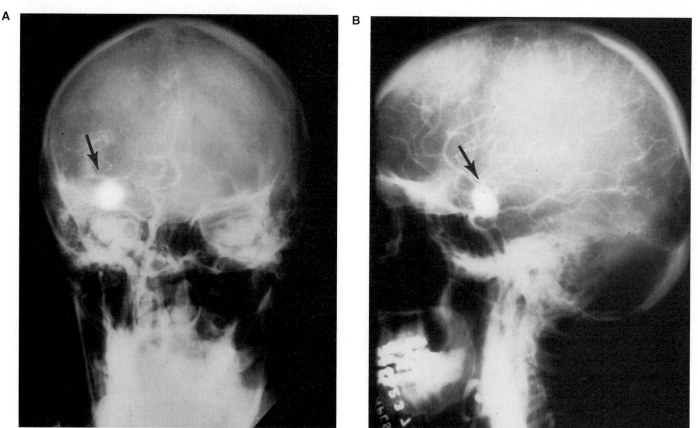

Figure 21-18 A cerebral aneurysm (*arrow*) demonstrated by an angiogram. A, Front view. B, Side view.

# Infections of the Nervous System

Many different organisms can infect the nervous system, including bacteria, viruses, and fungi. An infection that predominantly affects the meninges surrounding the brain and spinal cord is called a **meningitis**. An infection of the brain tissue is called an **encephalitis**. If both brain and meninges are affected, the term *meningoencephalitis* is often used. An infection of the spinal cord is called a **myelitis**.

The manifestations of an infection of the CNS are those of any systemic infection: elevated temperature and other nonspecific symptoms. In addition, there are manifestations of meningeal irritation, consisting of a headache and a stiff neck. Involvement of brain tissue is associated with alteration of consciousness and neurologic symptoms resulting from dysfunction of localized areas within the brain.

Diagnosis of a CNS infection is established by examination of the spinal fluid, which contains a large number of leukocytes and an elevated protein concentration if infection is present. In bacterial infections, the leukocytes are primarily neutrophils, whereas lymphocytes predominate in viral infections. In bacterial and fungus infections, the organism responsible for the infection can often be identified in stained smears prepared from the spinal fluid and by culture of the spinal fluid.

## Meningitis Caused by Bacteria and Fungi

Two organisms are responsible for most cases of bacterial meningitis: the meningococcus (*Neisseria meningitides*) and the pneumococcus (*Streptococcus pneumoniae*) as illustrated in Figure 21-19. Until recently, a third organism, *Hemophilus influenzae*, was a common cause of meningitis in children. Now infants and children are routinely immunized against this organism, and *Hemophilus influenzae* meningitis, as well as other infections caused by this organism, occurs much less frequently than in the past.

Meningococcal infections occur primarily in young adults and often become epidemic where people live in close quarters, such as college dormitories and army camps. If an individual develops meningococcal meningitis, persons who have had close contact with the infected individual are treated with prophylactic antibiotics. If several cases occur in a community, college dormitory, or army camp, mass immunizations are undertaken to prevent an epidemic of meningococcal meningitis. In contrast, pneumococcal meningitis occurs sporadically in older adults, but it is not transmitted from person to person as is meningococcal meningitis.

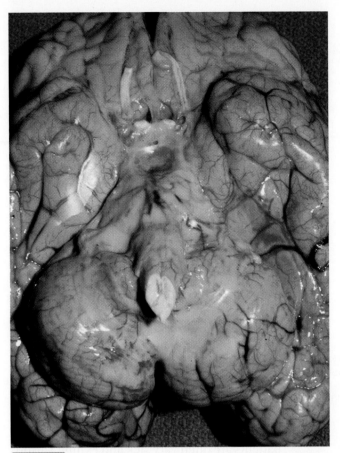

**Figure 21-19** Bacterial meningitis, illustrating purulent exudate in the meninges. Exudate is most noticeable over the pons (*middle* of photograph) and cerebellum.

Consequently, persons who have had contact with an individual who develops pneumococcal meningitis do not require antibiotic prophylaxis, and communitywide immunizations are not required. Other bacteria may occasionally cause meningitis, especially in persons whose immunologic defenses have been weakened by disease or immunosuppressive therapy, or under conditions in which bacteria are introduced directly into the nervous system.

Bacterial meningitis is often preceded by a mild upper-respiratory infection, during which small numbers of bacteria gain access to the bloodstream. The bacteria are carried to the meninges, where they localize and initiate an acute infection. Occasionally, the pathogens may spread directly to the meninges from a sinus or middle-ear infection, or they may be introduced into the nervous system directly from a serious head injury such as a gunshot wound or other severe injury in which the scalp is lacerated and the skull is fractured.

Meningitis caused by the tubercle bacillus or a pathogenic fungus is uncommon and tends to be chronic rather than acute. *Tuberculous meningitis* results from

**meningitis** (men-in-jī′tis) Inflammation of the meninges.

**encephalitis** (en-sef-äl-ī′tis) An inflammation of the brain.

**myelitis** (mī-el-ī′tis) An inflammation of the spinal cord.

spread of bacteria from a primary infection in the lung (Chapter 12). *Fungus meningitis* also is usually secondary to a fungal infection of the lung, and many of the cases develop in immunocompromised persons. Bacterial and fungal infections are treated with appropriate antibiotics.

## Viral Infections

Many viruses can infect the nervous system, including the measles and mumps viruses, various intestinal and respiratory viruses, the herpes simplex virus, cytomegalovirus, poliomyelitis virus, and an important group of viruses called *arboviruses*.

## Manifestations of Nervous System Virus Infection

A viral infection may affect either the meninges (meningitis) or the brain tissue (encephalitis). A viral infection restricted to the meninges is often called *aseptic meningitis* to distinguish it from *suppurative* (pus-producing) *meningitis* caused by pathogenic bacteria. The affected individual has an elevated temperature, headache, and a stiff neck but does not usually appear seriously ill and recovers completely. *Viral encephalitis* is a much more serious infection. Affected patients are often very sick and exhibit various neurologic disturbances, such as confusion, disorientation, coma, cranial nerve dysfunction, weakness, and paralysis. Some cases are fatal, and patients who recover may be left with some permanent neurologic disability. Unfortunately, there is no specific treatment for most cases of viral encephalitis. However, some antiviral drugs may be effective if administered early in the course of the disease.

**poliomyelitis**
(pō′lē-yo-mī-e-lī′tis) An inflammation of the gray matter of the spinal cord, caused by a virus.

## Arbovirus Infections

This important group of viruses is responsible for many cases of meningitis and encephalitis. The viruses infect birds and animals as well as humans and are transmitted by mosquitoes. The term *arbovirus* is a contraction of the term *arthropod–borne-virus*. Several different types of arboviral encephalitis are recognized. In the United States, *western equine encephalitis* occurs primarily in the West, and *eastern equine encephalitis* in the eastern part of the country. Two other types of encephalitis, called *St. Louis encephalitis* and *California encephalitis*, are not limited to the area implied by their names but are quite widely distributed.

**West Nile Virus Infections** The West Nile virus was first identified in 1937 in an infected woman living in the West Nile province of Uganda in Africa. From there the virus soon spread to Europe, where it became established and eventually spread to the United States in 1999, where the first case was identified in a person living in the New York City area.

Soon afterwards the virus spread rapidly through the United States, as well as into Canada and Mexico, where it caused the largest outbreak of arbovirus infections ever recorded in the Western Hemisphere. The West Nile virus infects many species of wild birds, horses, and other animals, as well as people, and many species of mosquitoes can transmit the virus. The virus can also be transmitted across the placenta from a pregnant virus-infected mother to her infant and in breast milk from an infected mother to a nursing infant.

Most persons infected with West Nile virus have no symptoms of infection, but about 20 percent of infected persons develop a fever and neurologic manifestations that can vary from mild aseptic meningitis to severe and sometimes fatal encephalitis. Some affected persons have developed a poliomyelitislike flaccid paralysis. No vaccine is available to immunize against the virus, and no antiviral therapy is available to treat the disease.

**Poliomyelitis** Poliomyelitis was formerly a very important and serious disease that caused much disability and many deaths. The virus enters the body through the gastrointestinal tract, localizing in the gray matter of the spinal cord and sometimes also in the cell bodies of cranial nerves in the brain stem. Destruction of motor neurons leads to paralysis of the muscles supplied by the affected neurons. The name of the disease refers to the affinity of the virus for the gray matter of the spinal cord (*polios* = gray). Fortunately, widespread immunization has eliminated this disease in the developed countries of the world, and an extensive immunization effort directed toward persons at risk in third world countries may soon lead to worldwide elimination of poliomyelitis. Hopefully, poliomyelitis will soon join smallpox as another disease that has been completely eradicated by an effective immunization program.

**The Postpolio Syndrome** About half the persons who survived paralytic poliomyelitis have begun to experience slowly progressive muscular atrophy, weakness, and muscle fatigue, and the onset of these manifestations began many years after the original episode of acute poliomyelitis from which they had recovered. The weakness usually involves muscles or muscle groups that had been affected during the original bout of poliomyelitis and from which the individual had made a partial or apparent complete recovery. This late-onset muscle weakness and muscle atrophy have been called the *postpolio syndrome*.

The exact cause of the postpolio syndrome is unknown. One likely explanation is that the surviving spinal motor neurons that were not damaged by poliomyelitis took over the function of the spinal neurons destroyed by poliomyelitis. These neurons established new axon connections with the muscle fibers that had lost their nerve supply, thereby reestablishing function in the previously paralyzed muscles. Overuse of the muscles with their reestablished nerve supply eventually caused the overworked neurons to fail many years later, which led to weakness and atrophy of the involved muscles as they gradually lost their nerve supply. Unfortunately, there is no specific treatment that can restore function to the muscles that have become weak and atrophic.

# Creutzfeldt–Jakob Disease

Named after the physicians who described it, Creutzfeldt–Jakob (CJ) disease is a very unusual disease caused by a very unusual infectious agent. The disease occurs sporadically but can also be transmitted like an infectious disease, from contact with the infected tissues of a person with the disease.

The infectious agent is unusually resistant to inactivation by heat, by many disinfectants, and by ultraviolet light, but it can be destroyed by autoclaving or by household bleach. CJ is caused by an abnormal form of a specific protein called a **prion**, which is a contracted term for *proteinaceous infectious particle*. The normal form of the protein (the "good prion") is found in the cell membranes of neurons and in some other tissues. The abnormal form of the protein (the "bad prion") is identical except for the way the protein is folded, which causes the protein to have a different configuration (conformation) when viewed in three dimensions. The abnormal prion is able to function as an infectious agent because of its ability to convert normal prions into abnormal forms. As progressively more prion proteins are converted into abnormal forms, a self-perpetuating chain reaction follows as the newly formed abnormal prions convert more normal prions. As the abnormal prion proteins continue to accumulate, they disrupt the functions of the brain cells, which leads to the characteristic clinical and histologic manifestations of CJ disease.

The sporadic cases of CJ disease, which occur in older adults (as does Alzheimer disease described in the next section), are caused by a spontaneous mutation of a normal gene, and the mutated gene codes for the abnormal prion protein responsible for CJ disease.

Clinically, CJ disease is characterized by rapidly progressive mental deterioration (*dementia*) associated with neurologic disturbances. The disease is usually fatal within 6 months after the onset of symptoms.

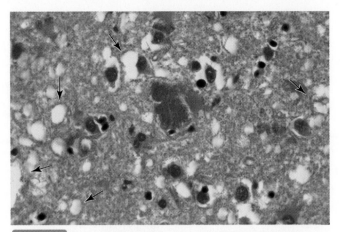

**Figure 21-20** A photomicrograph of cerebral tissue from patient with Creutzfeldt–Jakob disease, illustrating multiple small vacuoles throughout the cortex (*arrows*) with loss of neurons and proliferation of astrocytes but no inflammatory reaction. The clump of eosinophilic material in the center of the photomicrograph is an aggregate of abnormal prion protein (original magnification × 400).

Histologically, the brains of affected persons contain a large number of vacuoles within the neurons, which causes the affected brain tissue to have a spongy appearance. The affected neurons degenerate, and astrocytes proliferate in response to the neuron loss; however, there is no inflammatory reaction (Figure 21-20). Unfortunately, no treatment is available for this devastating disease.

The cases of CJ disease caused by contact with infected tissues have been traced to biologic products or tissue contaminated with abnormal prions, such as cornea and organ transplants obtained from persons with unsuspected CJ disease.

**prion**
(pri′-on) A protein infectious particle responsible for Creutzfeldt-Jakob disease and some other degenerative diseases of the nervous system.

# Mad Cow Disease

Somewhat similar prion diseases occur in animals, which can be transmitted between animals of the same or different species by feeding animal tissues from infected animals to healthy animals. One such prion-related disease occurs in cattle and has raised concerns that it may cause CJ disease in humans. The cattle disease was recognized in 1985 when several dairy cows in the United Kingdom developed bovine spongiform encephalopathy, a prion disease that is usually called by the more familiar term *mad cow disease* because of the bizarre behavior of infected animals. During subsequent years, the number of infected cows increased to over 170,000. This epidemic was traced to cattle feed that had been mixed with protein-rich tissues obtained from sheep that had been infected with a similar prion disease. This feeding practice was discontinued, and the frequency of the cattle disease

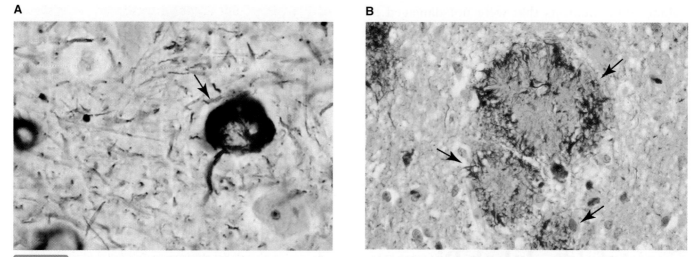

**Figure 21-21** Alzheimer disease. **A,** Thickened neurofilaments encircle and obscure nucleus of nerve cells (*arrow*) forming neurofibrillary tangle (silver stain, original magnification × 400). **B,** Three neuritic plaques (*arrows*), composed of broken masses of thickened neurofilaments (silver stain, original magnification × 100).

declined. Now use of animal tissues in animal feed is banned in both Britain and the United States.

The disease in cattle was followed several years later by cases of CJ disease, which had clinical features that were somewhat different from the usual manifestations of CJ disease, and has been called *new variant Creutzfeldt–Jakob disease.* This variant disease was contracted from eating meat from infected cows, and many people were concerned that more cases would occur since there was a lag time between consumption of infected beef and onset of clinical manifestations, but a great increase in new cases has not materialized.

# Alzheimer Disease

**Alzheimer disease** is a chronic progressive disease that affects primarily middle-aged and older persons. The disease is characterized by progressive failure of recent memory and difficulties in thinking, reasoning, and judgment; it is often associated with emotional disturbances such as depression, anxiety, and irritability.

The brains of affected patients exhibit progressive loss of neurons with atrophy of cerebral cortex and two rather characteristic histologic changes: *neurofibrillary tangles* and *neuritic plaques.* Neurofibrillary tangles result from degenerative changes affecting the thin, delicate, wirelike neurofilaments, which are located within the cytoplasm of the neurons. They become converted into thick, tangled, ropy masses encircling or displacing the nuclei of nerve

cells and are demonstrated by special stains containing silver compounds ( Figure 21-21A ). Neuritic plaques are masses of broken, thickened nerve filaments that stain intensely with silver-containing stains and that surround a core of acellular protein material, called *amyloid protein,* with distinct staining properties ( Figure 21-21B ). In general, there is a correlation between the degree of intellectual deterioration and the severity of the histopathologic changes. The brains of patients with advanced Alzheimer disease contain large numbers of neuritic plaques and neurofibrillary tangles, whereas those with mild disease have less-striking changes.

The diagnosis of Alzheimer disease is made by excluding other conditions that can impair brain function, such as chronic infections of the nervous system or multiple strokes. Unfortunately, there is no specific treatment that can arrest the relentless progression of the disease, although some drugs may be useful to improve cerebral function temporarily.

# Multiple Sclerosis

**Multiple sclerosis** is a chronic disease characterized by focal randomly distributed degeneration of the myelin sheaths covering groups of nerve fibers in the brain and spinal cord. The areas of demyelination disrupt the conduction of nerve impulses, and the damaged areas eventually heal by proliferation of fibers made by neuroglial cells called **astrocytes** ( Figure 21-22 ). The disease is named from the multiple areas of demyelination, and the term sclerosis refers to the proliferation of fibers made by astrocytes, although the fiber proliferation is not the same as a fibrous tissue scar made by connective tissue cells. The discrete areas of myelin

**Alzheimer disease**
(ahls′-hīm-er) A degenerative disease of the nervous system with characteristic structural abnormalities within neurons.

**multiple sclerosis**
Chronic disease characterized by focal areas of demyelination in the central nervous system, followed by glial scarring.

**astrocyte** A large stellate cell having highly branched processes. Forms the structural framework of the nervous system. One of the neuroglial cells.

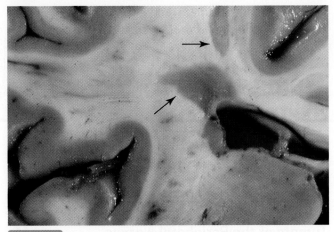

**Figure 21-22** Coronal section of brain illustrating areas of glial scarring (*arrows*) adjacent to ventricle in multiple sclerosis. The demyelinated areas appear much darker than the adjacent normal white matter because of loss of myelin.

loss with glial scarring are called multiple sclerosis plaques. They are readily demonstrated within the nervous systems of affected persons by means of magnetic resonance imaging (MRI; described in Chapter 1). This diagnostic procedure is extremely useful for evaluating patients with neurologic disease in whom multiple sclerosis is suspected ( Figure 21-23 ).

Multiple sclerosis is a disease of young adults. The onset of symptoms before the age of 15 or after the age

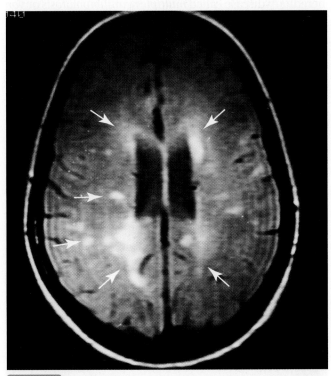

**Figure 21-23** Multiple sclerosis demonstrated by MRI. The ventricular system is well demonstrated in the *center* of the photograph. Dense white areas adjacent to posterior horns of the ventricles and scattered throughout the brain lateral to the ventricles (*arrows*) are multiple sclerosis plaques.

of 40 is rare. Clinically, the disease is characterized by periodic episodes of acute neurologic disturbances, the nature depending on the location of the demyelination. Each episode is followed by a period of recovery and remission. The course of the disease is prolonged and quite unpredictable, with repeated acute episodes followed by remissions extending over many years. Eventually, the neurologic disabilities become permanent as a consequence of multiple areas of glial scarring, which impair conduction of nerve impulses in the brain and spinal cord. There is no specific treatment that can arrest the progression of the disease. A number of measures, however, are available to relieve symptoms, shorten the recovery from an acute episode, and minimize the neurologic disabilities. Much evidence indicates that multiple sclerosis is an autoimmune disease, possibly initiated by a viral infection in a genetically predisposed person that stimulates an abnormal immune response manifested by focal demyelination of nerve tissue.

# Parkinson Disease

**Parkinson disease** is a chronic disabling disease characterized by rigidity of voluntary muscles and tremor of fingers and extremities. The disease results from a progressive loss of neurons in a part of the midbrain called the substantia nigra. The axons of these neurons synapse with neurons in the basal ganglia, where they release the neurotransmitter dopamine, and this is one of the important connections of the extrapyramidal motor system. As a result of the progressive neuron loss in the substantia nigra, fewer fibers are available to release dopamine in the basal ganglia, and the concentration of dopamine in the basal ganglia falls. The muscular rigidity, increased muscle tone, and abnormal repetitive involuntary movements, which are common manifestations of the disease, result from the deranged function of the extrapyramidal system.

**Parkinson disease** A chronic disease of the central nervous system characterized by rigidity and tremor, caused by decreased concentration of dopamine in the central nervous system.

The manifestations of the disease can be relieved by a drug called L-*dopa*, which is converted within the brain into dopamine. The drug therapy alleviates symptoms because it raises the concentration of dopamine in the basal ganglia, thereby supplying the neurotransmitter that is deficient. Various other drugs also have been used successfully to control the manifestations of Parkinson disease. Treatment, however, does not arrest the progressive neuron loss in the substantia nigra, nor does it stop the progression of the disease.

# Huntington Disease

This is an uncommon but relatively well-known hereditary autosomal dominant disease that is characterized by progressive mental deterioration associated with abnormal jerky and writhing movements. The first manifestations in affected persons occur between ages 30 to 50 years. The disease progresses slowly and is usually fatal within about 15 to 20 years. Huntington disease causes progressive atrophy of groups of neurons called basal ganglia that are located deep within the cerebral hemispheres. These structures are part of the extrapyramidal motor system, which regulates smooth and coordinated muscle movements, and damage to the system gives rise to the abnormal movements characteristic of the disease. The cerebral cortex is also affected, which eventually leads to dementia as the disease progresses. CT scans of affected subjects demonstrate the cortical and basal ganglia atrophy characteristic of the disease.

Unfortunately, there is no way to arrest the progression of the disease, but drugs are available to help control some of its manifestations. Children of persons with Huntington disease should be offered genetic counseling and should be advised that they can be tested to determine whether they carry the abnormal gene. However, not all of the children of affected persons want this information. Some prefer living with an uncertain future rather than being tested and possibly learning that they carry the abnormal gene and are destined to acquire the disease.

# Degenerative Diseases of Motor Neurons

A group of diseases of unknown cause affecting middle-aged and older adults is characterized by degeneration of motor neurons in the cortex, of cranial nerve neurons in the brain stem, and of spinal motor neurons. Most cases occur sporadically, and no hereditary background can be identified. Many of these diseases receive specific names, depending on which neuron groups are affected most severely, and the clinical manifestations of the neuron degeneration depend on which part of the nervous system suffers the greatest degenerative changes. In general, the symptoms are rapidly progressive muscular weakness leading to severe incapacitation and breathing difficulties resulting from weakness or paralysis of respiratory muscles. Death usually results from respiratory failure, often complicated by superimposed pulmonary infections. Unfortunately, there is no way to arrest the relentless progression of these devastating diseases. One of the best known of these neuronal degenerative diseases is called *amyotrophic lateral sclerosis*, better known as Lou Gehrig disease.

# Tumors of the Nervous System

Tumors of the nervous system may arise from three sites:

1. The peripheral nerves
2. The meninges
3. Cells within the brain or spinal cord

## Tumors of the Peripheral Nerves

Tumors of peripheral nerves arise from the Schwann cells that surround the nerve fibers. Such tumors may be solitary or multiple, benign or malignant.

Most solitary Schwann cell tumors are benign. They form discrete, well-circumscribed nodules attached to larger nerve trunks and usually can be dissected easily from the adjacent nerve (see Chapter 8, Figure 8-1). This type of tumor is often called a *neuroma*, although the terms *schwannoma* or *neurofibroma* also are used. Sometimes a neuroma arises from one of the cranial nerves at the base of the brain or from one of the spinal nerves within the spinal canal. A tumor in either of these locations is much more difficult to remove.

Multiple tumors of the peripheral nerves occur in a hereditary disease called *multiple neurofibromatosis* or *von Recklinghausen* disease, an uncommon condition transmitted as a Mendelian dominant trait. In this condition, the skin is disfigured by multiple tumors that grow from the cutaneous nerves and appear as variously sized nodules covering the entire body (Figure 21-24). The nodules are usually associated with localized light-brown patches

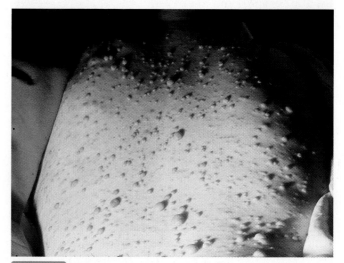

**Figure 21-24** Multiple skin tumors in a patient with multiple neurofibromatosis.

of hyperpigmented skin. Multiple tumors also arise from the more deeply placed nerves supplying the internal organs. There is no specific treatment for this disease. Large tumors that encroach on vital organs or are cosmetically disfiguring can be removed surgically.

## Tumors of the Brain

Malignant tumors arising in the breast, colon, lung, or other sites frequently metastasize to the brain. *Primary brain tumors* are less common than metastatic tumors. They may arise from the meninges, from the glial-supporting tissues of the brain, from the cells lining the ventricular system, or rarely from other tissues such as the blood vessels within the brain. Neuromas may also arise from the cranial nerves, as described in the foregoing section. Tumors do not develop from neurons because adult nerve cells are no longer capable of cell division.

A tumor of meninges is called a **meningioma**. This is a well-circumscribed benign tumor arising from arachnoid cells and is firmly adherent to the dura. The tumor causes symptoms as a result of compression of the underlying brain and can be removed successfully if it is located in an accessible location.

Any tumor of neuroglial origin is called a **glioma**. These tumors are further classified according to the type of glial-supporting cell from which the neoplasm arises. The most common type arises from astrocytes and is called an *astrocytoma*. A special name, *glioblastoma multiforme*, is applied to a highly undifferentiated, rapidly growing astrocytoma. The name describes the primitive appearance of the neoplastic astrocytes (*blast* = primitive cell) and their great variability in shape and appearance (*multiform* = having many shapes). Gliomas arise less frequently from other supporting cells. Lymphomas also may arise within the CNS and they are relatively common tumors in patients with AIDS.

Primary CNS tumors do not normally spread outside the nervous system, but many carry a poor prognosis because they often lie deep within the brain. Treatment consists of surgical resection of as much of the tumor as possible. In selected cases, surgery is followed by radiation and sometimes by anticancer chemotherapy as well. Primary lymphomas respond poorly to treatment, although radiotherapy may control the tumor for a time.

The symptoms of a brain tumor depend on the size and location of the neoplasm. Headache is a common initial manifestation because the increased volume within the cranial cavity caused by the tumor raises the intracranial pressure. Growth of the tumor also disrupts nerve cells and fiber tracts within the brain, leading to various neurologic disturbances.

## Tumors of the Spinal Cord

The types of tumors that affect the brain may also occur in the spinal cord. In addition, metastatic tumors within the vertebral bodies or **multiple myeloma**, a tumor of plasma cells within the bone marrow (Chapter 8), may extend from the vertebrae to compress or invade the adjacent spinal cord. If this occurs, sensation and motor function below the level of cord injury may be partially or completely lost.

# Peripheral Nerve Disorders

Peripheral nerves and nerve roots may undergo demyelination and varying degrees of axon degeneration, and the condition is usually called peripheral neuritis. Clinical manifestations depend on the degree of nerve degeneration and on which nerves are affected. Involvement of a single nerve is usually secondary to injury or external compression. A frequently compressed nerve is the median nerve as it travels into the hand accompanied by the flexor tendons that attach to the thumb and fingers. These structures all travel through a narrow channel called the carpal tunnel that is interposed between the carpal bones posteriorly and a dense fibrous tissue ligament anteriorly. The nerve compression causes pain and **paresthesias** (abnormal sensations such as burning, numbness, and tingling) in the index and middle fingers, together with decreased sensation in the part of the hand supplied by the nerve. The small muscles of the hand at the base of the thumb, which are supplied by the nerve, may also undergo atrophy. Sometimes symptoms can be relieved by conservative measures such as injecting a corticosteroid mixed with a local anesthetic into the confined space (called the *carpal tunnel*) in which the nerve is compressed. In many cases, however, it may be necessary to cut the ligament that forms the anterior boundary of the carpal tunnel, thereby enlarging the tunnel to relieve the median nerve compression.

**meningioma** (men-in-jē-ō′muh) A benign tumor arising from the meninges.

**glioma** (glē-ō′muh) Any brain tumor arising from glial (supporting) cells of the brain.

**multiple myeloma** (my-el-ō′muh) A malignant neoplasm of plasma cells.

**paresthesia** (par-es-thē′ze-ah) An abnormal sensation, such as burning, prickling, or numbness.

**polyneuritis** (päl-ē-nū-rī′tis) An inflammation of multiple nerves.

## Polyneuritis (Peripheral Neuritis)

**Polyneuritis**, also called *peripheral neuritis*, is characterized by progressive muscular weakness, numbness and tingling, tenderness, and pain in the parts of the body supplied by the peripheral nerves (called the *distribution* of the nerves). Often the muscles supplied by the involved nerves also exhibit some degree of atrophy. Usually the weakness and sensory disturbances affect the distal parts of the limbs, whereas strength and sensation remain relatively normal in the proximal parts of the extremities. This "glove-and-stocking" pattern of sensory and motor dysfunction is quite characteristic of polyneuritis. Most cases result from systemic diseases such as long-standing diabetes or various autoimmune diseases, or from occupational exposure to toxic drugs, heavy metals, or industrial compounds. Alcoholism is another common cause of peripheral neuritis, which is probably related to a coexisting vitamin B deficiency, as described in Chapter 18. Treatment of the alcoholism and its associated vitamin and nutrient deficiencies may improve the peripheral neuritis.

# Neurologic Manifestations of Human Immunodeficiency Virus Infections

The nervous system is often involved in persons infected with the human immunodeficiency virus (AIDS virus; described in Chapter 8). Neurologic manifestations of AIDS virus infections fall into three large categories:

1. Infections of the nervous system directly caused by the AIDS virus
2. Infections of the nervous system caused by opportunistic pathogens
3. AIDS-related tumors of the nervous system

## HIV Infections of the Nervous System

Although HIV causes its major damage by infecting and destroying helper T lymphocytes, the virus also infects monocytes that can transport the virus into the brain, where it can injure the nervous system. In some patients, the infection may be manifested as acute viral meningitis occurring soon after the initial infection with the virus. In others, the infection causes a more chronic progressive degeneration of the brain with symptoms similar to those of Alzheimer disease, which is called *AIDS-related dementia* or *AIDS encephalopathy* (*encephalon* = brain + *pathy* = disease).

## Opportunistic Infections of the Nervous System

Many of the opportunistic viruses, bacteria, fungi, and parasites that afflict AIDS patients can cause a primary infection of the nervous system. The clinical manifestations depend on the location of the infection within the nervous system and the amount of neurologic damage caused by the pathogen. Some of the more common opportunistic infections of the nervous system are those caused by the herpesvirus, cytomegalovirus, the fungus *Cryptococcus neoformans* and the protozoan parasite *Toxoplasma gondii* (Chapter 5). Some of these infections respond to appropriate antibiotics and chemotherapeutic agents.

## AIDS-Related Tumors

Persons with AIDS are at risk of various malignant tumors, especially Kaposi sarcoma and lymphoma, and these tumors may metastasize to the nervous system as well as to other sites within the body. AIDS patients may also develop primary lymphomas of the nervous system. These tumors carry a very poor prognosis and do not respond well to treatment.

# CHAPTER REVIEW

## Summary

This chapter begins with an overview of the structure and function of the nervous system, which can be regarded as a giant switchboard receiving nerve impulses and relaying them to their proper destination. The pyramidal and extrapyramidal motor systems function together to facilitate both voluntary motor activity and motor functions concerned with maintaining posture, balance, and coordination of activities such as walking, running, or swimming. Muscle paralysis results when its connection with the nervous system is lost. Flaccid paralysis results when spinal motor neurons are destroyed by disease, such as poliomyelitis, and the affected muscles become atrophic. Spastic paralysis results from damage to cortical neurons or their axons that connect with spinal neurons, as after a stroke. Control of the affected muscles is lost but the muscles do not become atrophic.

The brain is well protected within the cranial cavity but may be damaged by a severe blow, and the skull may fracture. Intracerebral bleeding may follow. If the neural tube does not form normally, the brain or spinal cord may be affected. Anencephaly is incompatible with postnatal life. Spina bifida may vary from only defective formation of the bony arch overlying the spinal cord to a profound developmental disturbance called a meningomyelocele. Results of treatment depend on the severity of the malformation. Hydrocephalus is a distention of the ventricular system caused by an obstruction of cerebrospinal fluid (CSF) movement through the ventricular system. In infants the head enlarges because the cranial bones have not fused, which does not occur in an affected adult. Treatment involves shunting the fluid through a tube extending from the dilated ventricular system into the peritoneal cavity, where the CSF is reabsorbed into the circulation by blood vessels within the peritoneal cavity.

A stroke, also called a cerebrovascular accident or CVA, may result from a thrombosis of a cerebral blood vessel, an embolus from a thrombus within the heart or overlying an atheromatous plaque in the internal carotid artery, or from rupture of an intracerebral blood vessel in a person with severe hypertension; a cerebral hemorrhage follows, which is a life-threatening catastrophe. A transient ischemic attack, often called a TIA, is a brief episode of neurologic dysfunction that subsides in a short time, and is usually caused by short-duration blockage of a cerebral artery by atheromatous plaque material or a bit of thrombus material extruded from a plaque within the internal carotid artery. A cerebral aneurysm results from a congenital defect in the muscle or elastic tissue in the wall of an artery at the base of the brain; the protrusion usually occurs where the artery branches. The lining of the artery (intima) projects as a saclike extension from the artery, which may rupture and cause a subarachnoid hemorrhage. Various methods are available to prevent rupture of a known aneurysm, or to deal with the results of a ruptured aneurysm.

Infections of the nervous system may be caused by bacteria, such as the meningococcus or pneumococcus, or by viruses such as the West Nile virus. Less commonly the mycobacterium causing tuberculosis may infect the meninges, and various fungi may infect immunocompromised persons. Appropriate antibiotics are available to treat many of these infections. An entirely different problem results from an infection caused by the abnormal prion that causes sporadic Creutzfeldt–Jakob (CJ) disease, and the new variant CJ disease caused by ingestion of meat from cows infected with mad cow disease (bovine spongiform encephalopathy).

A number of other diseases affect the nervous system and impair CNS function including (1) Alzheimer disease, caused by progressive neuron loss and nephritic plaques; (2) Parkinson disease, caused by degeneration of dopamine-producing cells in the midbrain; (3) multiple sclerosis, an autoimmune disease affecting the white matter of the nervous system; and (4) Huntington disease, a progressive hereditary disease affecting the basal ganglia that disrupts the functions of the extrapyramidal system.

There are also several degenerative diseases of unknown cause affecting middle-aged and older adults. The diseases are characterized by progressive nerve cell degeneration, leading to progressive muscular weakness, eventually affecting respiratory muscles and leading to death from respiratory failure. The best known of these is a condition called amyotrophic lateral sclerosis, better known as Lou Gehrig disease.

Various primary tumors also affect the nervous system, arising from peripheral nerves (neuromas and neurofibromas), and from neuroglial cells (various gliomas including astrocytomas and the highly malignant glioblastoma multiforme). One relatively common hereditary disease is characterized by the formation of multiple neurofibromas in the skin and deeper tissues, which is called multiple neurofibromatosis. Metastatic tumors may also involve the nervous system.

Peripheral nerve degeneration is called peripheral neuritis, and many cases are caused by harmful drugs or other agents, or as a result of nutritional deficiencies in persons with chronic alcoholism. Isolated nerve degeneration may also follow nerve compression, as in the carpal tunnel syndrome where the nerve is compressed within the carpal tunnel as it passes through the wrist. Some cases of polyneuritis appear to be a manifestation of an autoimmune disease. An HIV infection may also affect the nervous system, presenting as a meningitislike syndrome during the initial infection, as an infection by various opportunist pathogens in persons with AIDS, or occasionally as a malignant lymphoma related to failure of the immune defense system in an AIDS patient.

## Questions for Review

1. Briefly describe the organization of the central nervous system. Describe the function and circulation of cerebrospinal fluid.
2. What are some of the possible effects of a severe blow to the head?
3. What is a stroke? What are the common causes of a stroke? What is a congenital aneurysm of the circle of Willis?
4. What are the common causes of hydrocephalus? How does a brain tumor cause hydrocephalus?
5. What is a neural tube defect? How can it be recognized before birth?
6. What is meant by the following terms: *arachnoid, subdural hemorrhage, anencephaly,* and *meningioma*?
7. What is a transient ischemic attack? How is it treated?
8. Describe the common tumors of the nervous system. What are their clinical manifestations?
9. What is the difference between a polyneuritis (peripheral neuritis) and an isolated nerve compression, as in the carpal tunnel syndrome?
10. Compare Creutzfeldt–Jakob disease and Alzheimer disease.
11. Describe the role of magnetic resonance imaging in the diagnosis of multiple sclerosis.
12. Describe the effects of human immunodeficiency virus infections on the nervous system.

## Supplementary Reading

Brown, P. 1997. The risk of spongiform encephalopathy ("mad cow disease") to human health. *Journal of the American Medical Association* 278:1008–11.

A review of the variant form of Creutzfeldt–Jakob disease transmitted from infected cattle to humans.

Caplan, L. R. 1998. Stroke treatment: Promising but still struggling [Editorial]. *Journal of the American Medical Association* 279:1304–6.

Many technical advances have improved the management of affected patients. Thrombolytic therapy may be helpful in selected cases, but carries a risk of causing a brain hemorrhage and must be used within a few hours after the onset of stroke symptoms.

Centers for Disease Control and Prevention. 1993. Recommendations for use of folic acid to reduce the number of spina bifida cases and other neural tube defects. *Journal of the American Medical Association* 269:1233–38.

All women of childbearing age should consume 0.4 mg of folic acid per day to reduce their risk of having a pregnancy affected with a neural tube defect.

DeAngelis, L. M. 2001. Brain tumors. *New England Journal of Medicine* 344:114–23.

A comprehensive review article dealing with the clinical features, classification, diagnosis, prognosis, and management of the various types of glial and meningeal tumors.

Hollander, H., Schaefer, P. W., and Hedley-Whyte, E. T. 2005. Case 22-2005: An 81-year-old man with cough, fever, and altered mental status. *New England Journal of Medicine* 353:287–95.

A clinical and pathological case study of an older man with the fatal West Nile virus infection. Autopsy revealed encephalomyelitis with the most marked damage in spinal cord anterior horn cells and in motor nuclei of the brain stem, changes similar to those encountered in poliomyelitis. Less marked changes were also detected in the thalamus, cerebellum, and cerebral cortex.

JAMA Patient Page. 1998. How do you know when someone is having a stroke? *Journal of the American Medical Association* 279:1324.

A review for the lay person of risk factors, manifestations, and what to do when someone is having a stroke.

Johnson, R. T., and Gibbs, C. J., Jr., 1998. Creutzfeldt–Jakob disease and related transmissible spongiform encephalopathies. *New England Journal of Medicine* 339:1994–2004.

This review article discusses the relationship of mad cow disease to Creutzfeldt–Jakob disease.

Jubelt, B., and Agre, J. C. 2000. Characteristics and management of postpolio syndrome. *Journal of the American Medical Association* 284:412–14.

A discussion of clinical manifestations and management of postpolio syndrome, which affects about half the persons who developed paralytic poliomyelitis many years previously.

Noseworthy, J. H., Lucchinetti, C., Rodriguez, M., and Weinshenker, B. G. 2000. Multiple sclerosis. *New England Journal of Medicine* 343:938–52.

A comprehensive review of clinical manifestations, epidemiologic features, genetic factors, and treatment.

Ojemann, R. G. 1981. Management of unruptured intracranial aneurysm [Editorial]. *New England Journal of Medicine* 304:725–26.

From approximately 3 to 4 percent of patients each year with an asymptomatic aneurysm will experience cerebral hemorrhage as the result of rupture. The larger the aneurysm, the greater the likelihood of rupture. Aneurysm larger than 7 mm should be treated surgically.

Sacco, R. L. 2001. Extracranial carotid stenosis. *New England Journal of Medicine* 345:1113–18.

A review of methods of treatment, risk of strokes and other complications under various conditions, and guidelines for treatment. Patients with symptoms who have severe carotid artery stenosis should be treated surgically.

Tyler, K. L. 2003. Creutzfeldt–Jakob disease [Perspective]. *New England Journal of Medicine* 348:681–82.

Current status of new variant Creutzfeldt–Jakob disease and tests available for diagnosis. The number of new cases in the United Kingdom is decreasing.

# Interactive Activities

## Matching

Match the disease or condition in the left column with its characteristic features or manifestations in the right column.

| Disease or Condition | Features or Manifestations |
| --- | --- |
| 1. Alzheimer disease | A. Demyelinating disease |
| 2. Glioblastoma | B. Brain degeneration caused by abnormal prions |
| 3. Transient ischemic attack | C. Neuritic plaques and neurofibrillary change in cerebral neurons |
| 4. Neurofibroma | D. Nerve compression |
| 5. Mad cow disease | E. Progressive nerve cell degeneration in older adult |
| 6. Lou Gehrig disease | F. Malignant brain tumor |
| 7. Carpal tunnel syndrome | G. Protrusion of meninges through defect in spine |
| 8. Multiple sclerosis | H. Enlarged ventricles |
| 9. Cystic spina bifida | I. Benign tumor of nerve |
| 10. Hydrocephalus | J. Short episode of neurologic dysfunction. |

## True or False

Mark the answer true (T) or false (F) in the space provided.

1. Lou Gehrig disease is caused by abnormal prions that destroy brain tissue._____
2. Multiple neurofibromatosis is a hereditary disease resulting in formation of multiple benign tumors in skin and deeper tissues._____
3. Anencephaly results from failure of the neural tube to close normally._____
4. A saclike protrusion of the lining of a cerebral artery through a defect in the arterial wall is called a cystic spina bifida._____
5. The frequency of neural tube defects can be reduced significantly by ingestion of folic acid before conception and during pregnancy._____
6. Most glioblastomas in older adults respond well to treatment and have a good prognosis._____
7. Persons who had poliomyelitis many years ago with muscle paralysis who have recovered muscle function may have a recurrence of their paralysis many years later._____

8. Mad cow disease is a type of rabies that causes the cows to become aggressive and hostile._____

9. New variant Creutzfeldt–Jakob disease is acquired from eating meat from cows infected with abnormal prions._____

10. The West Nile virus usually causes a measleslike skin rash._____

## Critical Thinking

1. Jane Anderson said that her 62-year-old father was drinking coffee in a restaurant and he had a brief episode when he lost the strength in his hand and dropped the cup, spilling his coffee. The hand weakness persisted for about 30 minutes and then his muscle strength returned. She asks you what this means and should she be concerned about it. What would you tell her?

2. Susan Smith is a 25-year-old computer operator who has begun to experience pain in the right wrist and hand especially after she has been working at the computer for a long period of time. She also has developed some weakness on some of her thumb muscles. She asks you what to do about this. What would you tell her?

# The Musculoskeletal System

1. Name the common congenital abnormalities of the skeletal system.

2. List the three major types of arthritis. Describe their pathogenesis and clinical manifestations, and explain the methods of treatment.

3. Describe the causes and effects of osteoporosis, and name the methods of treatment.

4. Describe the structure of the intervertebral disks, and explain their function. Describe the clinical manifestations of a herniated disk.

5. Compare the pathogenesis and clinical manifestations of muscular atrophy and muscular dystrophy. Name and describe the common types of each.

6. Describe the pathogenesis, manifestations, and treatment of myasthenia gravis.

7. Describe the manifestations, complications, and treatment of scoliosis.

# Structure and Function of the Skeletal System

The skeleton is the rigid supporting structure of the body. All bones have the same basic structure. They are composed of an outer layer of *compact bone*, the cortex, and an inner, spongy layer in which the bone is arranged in a loose meshed latticework of thin strands called *bone trabeculae*. The spaces between the trabeculae contain the bone marrow, which consists of fat and blood-forming tissue.

Individual bones vary in size and appearance. They may be long, short, flat, or irregular in shape. The typical long bone, such as is found in the upper and lower limbs, has a tubular shape with expanded ends. The *shaft* is the long cylindrical part, and the expanded ends of the shaft are called the *epiphyses*. The center of the shaft is hollowed out to form the marrow cavity, which is filled with fat and bone marrow. This type of construction provides considerable strength without excessive weight.

Bone is a specialized type of connective tissue. It is composed of a dense connective-tissue framework (called osteoid before it is calcified) which soon becomes impregnated with calcium phosphate salts along with smaller amounts of calcium carbonate and other minerals. Three different types of cells are found in bone: osteoblasts, osteocytes, and osteoclasts. *Osteoblasts* are the active bone-forming cells that produce the collagenous bone matrix. They secrete an enzyme, *alkaline phosphatase*, that promotes deposition of calcium phosphate salts in the bone matrix to calcify the bone. As the bone matrix is formed and calcified, the osteoblasts become incorporated within the bone and become transformed into relatively inactive mature bone cells called *osteocytes*. Osteoclasts are multinucleated cells concerned with bone resorption. They remove the bone matrix by phagocytosis, dissolve the bone salts, and release the calcium and phosphate ions into the circulation. Bone is not a static structure. It is continually being broken down and reformed, and calcium salts in bone and calcium ions in the blood and body fluid are continuously interchanged.

In general, the strength and thickness of the bones depend on the activities of the individual. A person accustomed to strenuous physical labor has thicker, heavier bones than one who is normally engaged in light, sedentary activities. If an extremity is immobilized and is not allowed to bear weight, as after a fracture, the immobilized bone undergoes significant thinning and decalcification, called disuse atrophy.

The bones of the skeleton are connected by *joints*. There are three types: fibrous joints, cartilaginous joints, and synovial joints. In a *fibrous joint*, such as occurs between the bones of the skull, the bones are firmly joined by fibrous tissue to form a firm union called a *suture line*. In a *cartilaginous joint*, such as occurs between adjacent vertebral bodies in the spine and between the pubic bones of the pelvis (symphysis pubis), the ends of the bones are joined by fibrocartilage. Joints of this type have very little mobility. A *synovial joint* is a movable joint. The ends of the bones that move against one another are covered by smooth hyaline cartilage, which is called the *articular cartilage* (*articulare* = to connect). The ends of the bones are held together by dense fibrous bands (ligaments). The joint capsule is lined by a thin synovial membrane (the *synovium*), which secretes a small amount of mucinous fluid to lubricate the joint. Figure 22-1 illustrates

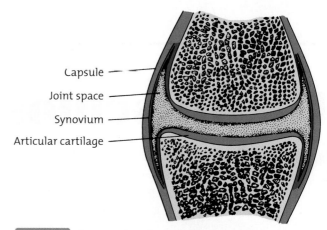

Labels: Capsule, Joint space, Synovium, Articular cartilage

**Figure 22-1** Structure of a typical movable joint.

the structure of a typical movable joint. Figure 22-2 illustrates the histologic appearance of the articular cartilage and underlying bone, and the appearance of a normal synovium. In joint disease, the structures are altered by inflammation and degeneration, leading to derangement in the functions of the joints.

## Bone Formation

There are two types of bone formation, and they are fundamentally similar. In one type, called **intramembranous bone formation**, the embryonic connective-tissue cells (mesodermal cells) are transformed directly into bone-forming cells (osteoblasts). The osteoblasts secrete a collagenous material called *osteoid*, which then becomes calcified to form bone. The bones of the vertex of the skull, the facial bones, and a few other bones are formed in this manner. Most of the skeletal system, however, is formed by a process called **endochondral bone formation** (*endo* = within + *chondral* = cartilage). In endochondral bone formation, the mesodermal cells differentiate first into cartilage cells, and the bones are formed initially as cartilage models. The cartilage is then absorbed and replaced by bone. Conversion of cartilage into bone is accomplished by vascular bone-forming mesoderm, which invades the cartilage. The areas of active bone formation are termed *centers of ossification*.

Bones that have been preformed in cartilage undergo ossification at specific times throughout fetal and postnatal life. The time of appearance of the various centers of ossification is characteristic for each bone. In the long bones, ossification begins first in the shaft; later, centers of ossification form at the ends (epiphyses) of the bone. The actively growing zone of cartilage between the shaft and the epiphysis of a long bone is called the epiphyseal plate.

**intramembranous bone formation** Direct formation of bone by osteoblasts without prior formation of a cartilage model.

**endochondral bone formation** (en-dō-kon'drul) Formation of bone as, first, a cartilage model that is then reabsorbed and converted into bone.

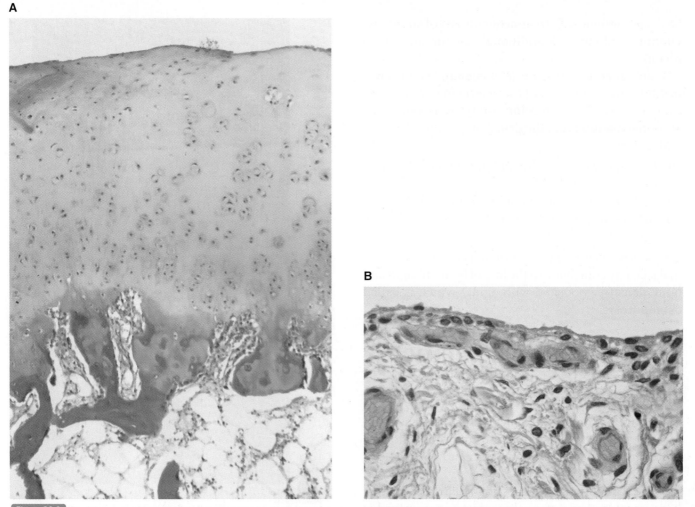

**A** **B**

**Figure 22-2** **A,** A low-magnification photomicrograph of cellular structure of normal articular surface, illustrating articular cartilage at *top* of photograph, junction of bone and cartilage in *middle* of photograph, and normal bone with fatty bone marrow at *bottom* of photograph (original magnification × 40). **B,** Normal synovium composed of synovial cells (*top* of photograph) covering loose connective tissue.

## Bone Growth

Bone grows in both length and thickness and is continually remodeled as it grows by absorption of bone in some areas and formation of new bone in others. Bone grows thicker by adding to its external surface newly formed bone that is produced by the periosteum, a layer of specialized connective-tissue cells surrounding the bone. The periosteal cells differentiate into osteoblasts, which in turn produce bone. Growth in the length of bone is the result of proliferation of cartilage at the epiphyseal plate, which is converted into bone. Growth in bone length continues into adolescence. Eventually, epiphyseal growth ceases, and the cartilagenous epiphyseal plate becomes converted into bone—called closure of the epiphyses. Thereafter, no further growth in length of bone is possible.

Normal bone growth and maturation require a normal amount of vitamin D, which can be obtained by exposure of the skin to sunlight, or obtained from the diet in vitamin D-fortified milk and other foods. Normal amounts of calcium and phosphate are also needed to calcify the bone as it is formed, and the parathyroid glands, which regulate the level of blood calcium, must function normally.

**Bone Growth Disturbances Caused by Vitamin D Deficiency** As described in Chapter 18, children lacking adequate vitamin D develop rickets, which is an uncommon disease because most children receive vitamin D supplements. However, if vitamin D is insufficient, calcium is not absorbed normally from the intestinal tract and the blood calcium tends to fall. The parathyroid glands respond to the low calcium by increasing the secretion of parathyroid hormone, which raises blood calcium but also causes the level of phosphate in the blood to fall. As a result, the deposition of calcium phosphate in the bone matrix is impaired because there is not enough phosphate available to combine with calcium, and the bone matrix is not adequately calcified. Osteoid is formed in excess at the epiphyseal ends of the growing bones, but it lacks strength because it is so poorly calcified. Consequently, the weakened bones tend to become bowed when weight bearing is attempted. Treatment consists of supplying vitamin D along with additional calcium and phosphate.

A similar condition caused by vitamin D deficiency in adults is called *osteomalacia*, a term that means *softening of bone*. The condition occurs in middle-aged and elderly adults, and the deficiency is caused by several factors:

1. Inadequate exposure to sunlight, which is required to produce vitamin D
2. Reduced intake of vitamin D-fortified foods
3. Increased vitamin D requirements associated with aging

The poorly calcified bone formed in persons with osteomalacia may contribute to the loss of bone strength and bone density associated with aging, which is called **osteoporosis**.

# Congenital Malformations

## Abnormal Bone Formation

The two most important genetically determined diseases of the skeletal system that result from abnormal bone formation are achondroplasia and osteogenesis imperfecta.

In **achondroplasia**, endochondral bone formation is faulty. The abnormality, which is transmitted as a Mendelian dominant trait, is characterized by disturbed endochondral bone formation at the epiphyseal plates (growth centers) of the long bones. The disturbance impairs growth of the extremities, causing a type of dwarfism in which the limbs are disproportionately short in relation to the trunk (*achondroplastic dwarfism*). The head is also abnormally formed because of disturbed endochondral ossification of the bones forming the base of the skull, and there is usually also an exaggerated curvature (lordosis) of the lumbar spine ( Figure 22-3 ).

**Osteogenesis imperfecta** (meaning literally "imperfect bone formation") is characterized by the formation of very thin and delicate bones that are easily broken under very minimal stress. In the most severe cases, the infant is born with multiple fractures. Some fractures occur before birth, having been sustained as a result of the very minor stresses resulting from the movements of the fetus within the uterus; other fractures occur

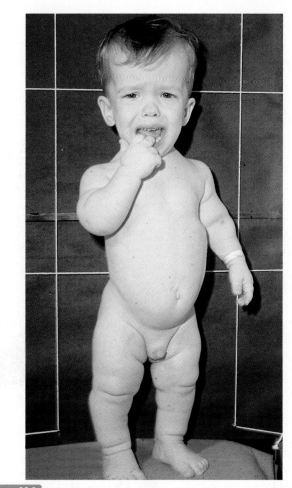

Figure 22-3    Characteristic appearance of child with achondroplasia, illustrating the relatively large head and disproportionate shortening of the extremities.

during delivery. The intrauterine fractures of the extremities usually heal in poor alignment, causing the limbs to appear bent and disproportionately short ( Figure 22-4 ). In milder forms of the disease, the abnormal fragility of the bone may not become apparent until childhood or adolescence.

## Congenital Clubfoot (Talipes)

**Clubfoot** is a relatively common congenital abnormality, having an incidence of about 1 in 1000 infants. The malformation is characterized by an abnormal position of the foot that prevents normal weight-bearing, and the affected individual tends to walk on the ankle rather than on the sole of the foot (*talus* = ankle + *pes* = foot). Figure 22-5 illustrates the most common type of clubfoot deformity called *talipes equinovarus*, in which the foot is turned inward at the ankle (varus position) and fixed in tiptoe (equinus) position. Often the malposition can be corrected by application of casts or splints. Surgical correction may be required if more conservative treatment is not successful.

**osteoporosis** (ă′stē-ō-por-ō′sis) Generalized thinning and demineralization of bone that tends to occur in post-menopausal women.

**achondroplasia** (a-kon-dro-pla′zi-yuh) A congenital disturbance of endochondral bone formation that causes a type of dwarfism.

**osteogenesis imperfecta** A congenital disturbance of bone formation characterized by excessively thin and delicate bones that are easily broken.

**clubfoot** Congenital malposition of foot. In most common type, foot is turned inward at ankle and heel is elevated.

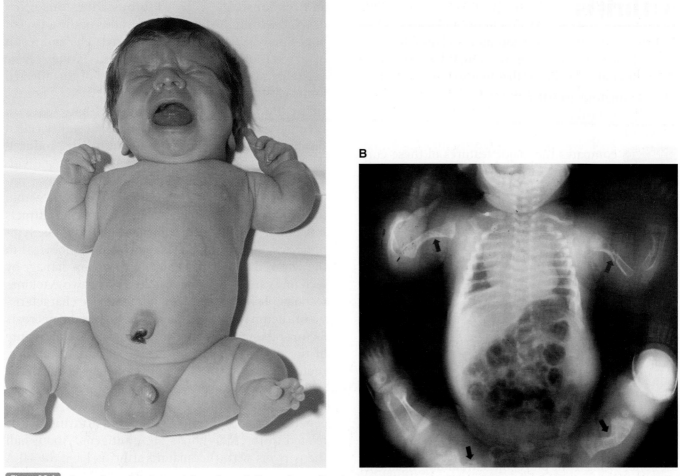

Figure 22-4   Severe form of osteogenesis imperfecta. **A,** Shortening and bowing of the limbs resulting from multiple intrauterine fractures that have healed in poor alignment. **B,** X-ray film showing multiple fractures of ribs and limb bones, some showing poor alignment and evidence of healing. *Arrows* indicate the location of four fractures.

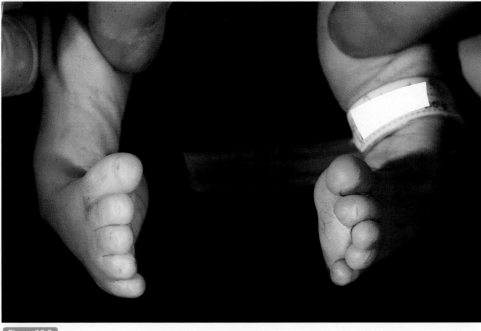

Figure 22-5   Common type of congenital clubfoot (*talipes equinovarus*) in newborn infant.

# Arthritis

Arthritis is one of the most common and disabling diseases of the skeletal system. Although there are many different kinds of arthritis, the three most common are

1. Rheumatoid arthritis
2. Osteoarthritis
3. Gout

Table 22-1 compares the major features of these conditions.

## Rheumatoid Arthritis

**Rheumatoid arthritis** is a systemic disease affecting the connective tissues throughout the body, but the most pronounced clinical manifestations are in the joints. Clinically, the disease is seen as a chronic, disabling, and often deforming arthritis affecting several joints. Rheumatoid arthritis is encountered most frequently in young and middle-aged women; it usually affects the small joints of the hands and feet. In the joints, the arthritis produces a chronic inflammation and thickening of the synovial membrane. The inflammatory tissue extends over the surface of the articular cartilage, destroying the cartilage (Figure 22-6). The severe damage to the articular surfaces makes the joint unstable; this in turn leads to deviation or displacement of the bones owing to the pull of the surrounding ligaments and tendons (Figure 22-7). Fibrous adhesions often develop within the joint, and the ends of the adjacent bones may become completely fused. The end result of these various structural derangements is often severe disability and conspicuous deformity of the affected joints (Figure 22-8).

The blood and synovial tissues of patients with rheumatoid arthritis often contain a substance called *rheumatoid factor*, which is an autoantibody produced by B lymphocytes that is directed against the individual's own gamma globulin. Immune complexes composed of gamma globulin and autoantibody form within the joints, which activates complement and attracts inflammatory cells that damage the joints. The lymphocytes and macrophages (activated monocytes) in the synovial tissues also contribute to joint damage by secreting various injurious cytokines. The two cytokines responsible for much of the joint damage characteristic of rheumatoid arthritis are called **tumor necrosis factor** and **interleukin-1**. Because of the systemic nature of the disease and the presence of autoantibodies, rheumatoid arthritis is usually classified as one of the autoimmune diseases (Chapter 4).

As with some other autoimmune diseases, there is a genetic susceptibility to rheumatoid arthritis that is related to the individual's HLA antigens. About half the persons with rheumatoid arthritis have the HLA

## Table 22-1 | Comparison of Major Features of Common Types of Arthritis

|  | Rheumatoid Arthritis | Osteoarthritis | Gout |
|---|---|---|---|
| Age and sex of usual patient | Young and middle-aged, female | Adult, older persons, both sexes | Middle-aged, male |
| Major characteristic | Systemic disease with major effects in joints; causes chronic synovitis | "Wear-and-tear" degeneration of articular cartilage | Disturbance of purine metabolism; acute episodes caused by crystals of uric acid in joints |
| Secondary effects of disease | Ingrowth of inflammatory tissue over cartilage destroys cartilage, leads to destruction of joint space; deformities common | Overgrowth of bone; thickening of periarticular soft tissues | Deposits of uric acid in joints with damage to joints (gouty arthritis); soft tissue tophi |
| Joints usually affected | Small joints of hands and feet | Major weight-bearing joints | Small joints; joint at base of great toe often affected |
| Special features | Autoantibody against gamma globulin (rheumatoid factor) | No systemic symptoms or biochemical abnormalities | High blood level of uric acid |

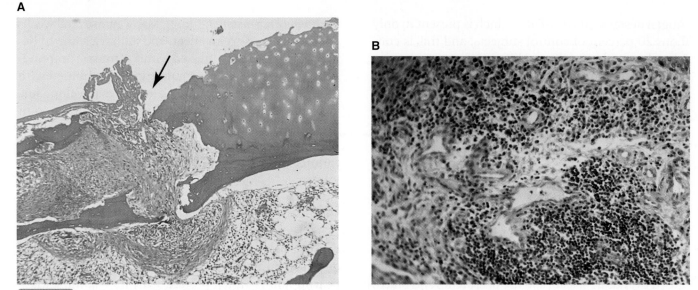

Figure 22-6    Rheumatoid arthritis. **A,** Low-magnification photomicrograph illustrating destruction of articular cartilage by inflammatory reaction (*arrow*) extending from synovial surface (original magnification × 25). **B,** Photomicrograph of chronic inflammatory reaction in synovium (original magnification × 100).

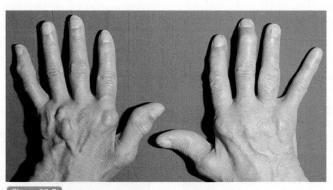

Figure 22-7    Rheumatoid arthritis. Early manifestations, illustrating swelling of knuckle joints (metacarpophalangeal joints) as a result of inflammation.

**rheumatoid arthritis** (rōōm´uh-toyd) A systemic disease primarily affecting the synovium with major manifestations in the small joints.

**tumor necrosis factor** A cytokine that can destroy foreign or abnormal cells.

**interleukin-1** (in-ter-loo´-kin) A cvytokine that promotes lymphocyte proliferation and maturation and also produces mediators of inflammation that causes inflammation, which may lead to tissue damage.

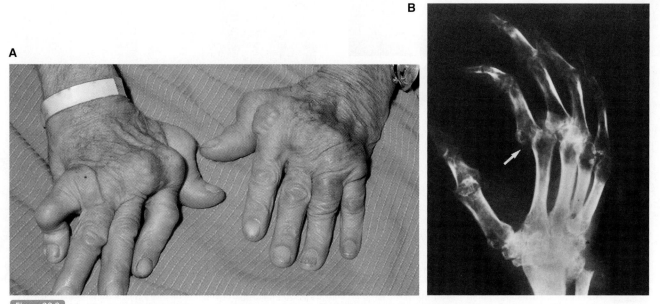

Figure 22-8    **A,** Advanced joint deformities caused by rheumatoid arthritis. **B,** Radiograph illustrating destruction of articular surfaces and anterior dislocation of base of index finger (*arrow*) as a result of joint instability.

antigen designated HLA-DR4, which is present in only about 20 percent of control subjects, and this is considered a highly significant difference.

Rheumatoid arthritis tends to fluctuate in severity. Periods in which the disease is active may alternate with periods in which it is inactive. Although there is no cure for rheumatoid arthritis, a number of measures can be used to control the disease and minimize its attending disability and deformity.

The primary objectives of treatment are reduction of joint inflammation and pain, maximal preservation of joint function, and prevention of joint deformity if possible. Treatment consists of rest periods for several hours every day while the disease is active, use of splints to support inflamed joints and reduce deformities caused by muscle spasm, and use of crutches and braces to aid weight-bearing. The affected joints are exercised gently in order to preserve joint mobility and muscle strength. Anti-inflammatory drugs such as aspirin are prescribed to reduce inflammation within the joints. In selected cases, corticosteroids are administered orally or injected into the affected joints. Often other measures are used to slow the progression of the disease, which are grouped under the general term of *disease-modifying anti-rheumatic drugs*. Many take several weeks or months to exert an effect, and all have some toxicity. Many patients are treated with a cytotoxic immunosuppressive drug called methotrexate combined with other drugs. If severe joint deformities develop, surgical procedures can be performed to improve joint function. These measures include excision of thickened inflamed synovium, surgical correction of joint dislocations, or even complete reconstruction of damaged joints.

## Osteoarthritis

In contrast to rheumatoid arthritis, which is a systemic disease, **osteoarthritis** is a result of "wear-and-tear" degeneration of one or more of the major weight-bearing joints (*osteo* = bone + *arthro* = joint + *itis* = inflammation). The disease is seen in older adults. The primary change in osteoarthritis is degeneration of the articular cartilage, leading to roughening of the articular surfaces of the bones ( Figure 22-9 ). As a consequence, the bones grate against one another when the joint moves, instead of gliding smoothly. Degeneration of the cartilage sometimes leaves large areas of underlying bone exposed. Secondary overgrowth of

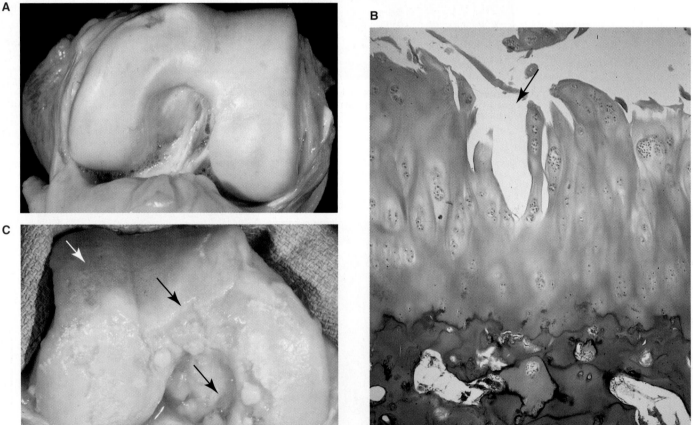

Figure 22-9    **A,** Knee joint, illustrating smooth articular surface of femoral condyles. **B,** Early histologic changes of osteoarthritis, illustrating splitting and fragmentation of articular cartilage (*arrow*) (original magnification × 160). Compare with normal articular cartilage in Figure 22-2A. **C,** Advanced osteoarthritis, illustrating loss of articular cartilage (*left arrow*) and nodular overgrowth of bone (*right arrows*).

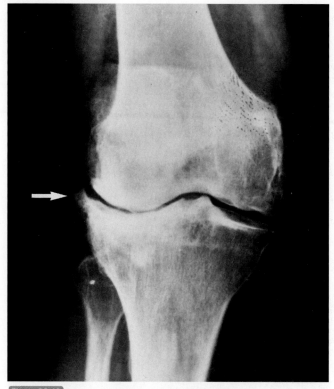

Osteoarthritis. Radiograph illustrates increased bone density of femoral condyle (*left side* of photograph) and adjacent tibia, with overgrowth of bone at margin of tibia (*arrow*).

bone frequently occurs in response to the trauma of weight-bearing (Figure 22-10), and some thickening of the synovium and adjacent soft tissues is also common.

Clinically, persons with osteoarthritis experience stiffness, creaking, and some pain on motion of the joints, but disability is usually not severe, and the joints are not destroyed. However, occasional patients may experience considerable pain and disability from advanced arthritis affecting one or both hip joints. In such cases, it is possible to remove the affected femoral head and articular surface of the hip bone surgically and to replace them with an artificial hip joint. Similar types of joint replacement procedures have been performed on the knee joint and some other joints as well. Joint replacement operations can provide excellent pain relief and greatly improved joint function in many patients.

## Gout

**Gout** is a clinical syndrome associated with an elevated level of uric acid in the blood and body fluids (hyperuricemia), leading to precipitation of uric acid as sodium urate crystals in joints and other tissues. In most patients, the condition is caused by a metabolic disorder of purine metabolism, which leads to an overproduction of uric acid, an inadequate excretion of uric acid, or a combination of both. This condition is called **primary gout** to distinguish it from the much less common **secondary gout** in which the elevated uric acid is secondary to some other disease or condition.

**Primary Gout** Purines are double-ring nitrogen compounds that are used to form the nucleotides adenine and guanine. Along with the pyrimidine nucleotides, they make up the large DNA molecules within the nuclei of our cells. Although our body can produce purines from nonpurine precursor substances, most of the purines that we use to make nucleoproteins for new cells are salvaged (recycled) from our own worn-out cells when the cells are broken down. The purines that are not salvaged and recycled are converted into the end-product uric acid, which is excreted in the urine. Because uric acid is not very soluble in body fluids, any significant elevation may lead to precipitation of the uric acid in joints and other tissues.

Clinically, the person afflicted with gout experiences periodic episodes of extremely painful acute arthritis usually involving initially only a single joint, often the joint at the base of the great toe (Figure 22-11A). The acute episodes are caused by crystallization of uric acid within the joint, which incites an intense inflammatory reaction. Gradually the symptoms of an acute attack subside, and joint function returns to normal until the next attack. If the disease is not treated, however, the attacks last longer, occur more frequently, and may involve several joints. Eventually, lumpy masses called gouty tophi are deposited in the soft tissues around the joints (Figure 22-11B) and in other locations. The tophi consist of large masses of urate surrounded by macrophages, multinucleated giant cells, and fibrous tissue. When viewed under polarized light, the needlelike urate crystals have a characteristic appearance diagnostic of gout (Figure 22-12). In untreated patients, masses of urate crystals deposited in and around the articular surfaces of the joints damage the joint surfaces and adjacent bone; this is called *gouty arthritis* (Figure 22-13).

In many persons with gout, the disease also targets the kidneys and urinary tract. Many develop uric acid kidney stones. The uric acid also may precipitate from the tubular filtrate within the kidney tubules, which blocks the tubules, damages the kidneys,

**osteoarthritis** (ă′stē-ō) A "wear and tear" degeneration of the major weight-bearing joints.

**gout** A disorder of nucleoprotein metabolism characterized by elevated uric acid and deposition of uric acid in and around joints.

**primary gout** A metabolic disease caused by overproduction of uric acid, reduced excretion of uric acid, or a combination of both factors. Clinical manifestations are related to precipitation of uric acid in joints, kidneys, and other sites.

**secondary gout** Elevated uric acid and clinical manifestations of gout not caused by the metabolic disease, primary gout, but instead caused by some other disease that raises the blood uric acid excessively, such as kidney failure or excessive breakdown of white blood cells in patients with leukemia.

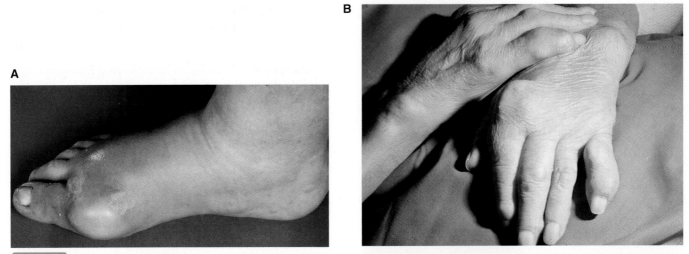

**Figure 22-11** **A,** Acute gout affecting right great toe (photograph courtesy of Dr. Jeffrey Felt). **B,** Deformities of hands caused by accumulation of uric acid crystals (tophi) in and around finger joints.

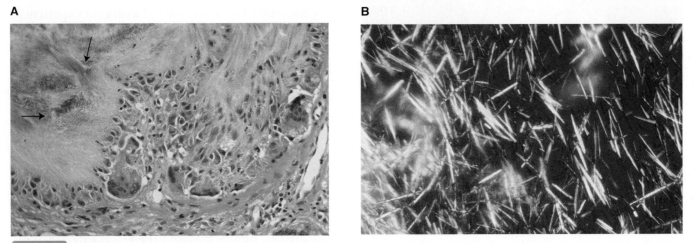

**Figure 22-12** **A,** Margin of tophus illustrating mass of urate crystals (*arrows*) and adjacent zone of macrophages, multinucleated giant cells, and fibrous tissue formed in response to crystal deposits (original magnification × 250). **B,** Characteristic histologic appearance of needlelike sodium urate crystals from tophus viewed under polarized light (original magnification × 400).

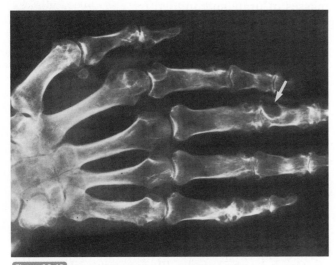

**Figure 22-13** Radiograph of right hand of patient with gouty arthritis illustrating area of bone destruction (*arrow*) caused by masses of uric acid crystals.

and impairs renal function. This condition is called *urate nephropathy*, as described in Chapter 15.

Gout is treated by administering drugs that reduce the concentration of uric acid in the blood by interfering with the formation of uric acid within the body, or by promoting the excretion of uric acid by the kidneys.

**Secondary Gout** Other conditions may also raise blood uric acid, caused either by inadequate excretion of uric acid or excessive breakdown of nucleoprotein. Sometimes the uric acid level may be so high that the uric acid precipitates from the blood and produces the same manifestations as gout caused by the metabolic disorder of purine metabolism. This condition is often called *secondary gout* because the elevated uric acid is secondary to some other disease, either a kidney-related problem in which uric acid excretion is impaired or a blood disease characterized by a marked overproduction of white blood cells. For example, patients with kidney failure may have high blood uric acid because the diseased kidneys are unable to excrete the uric acid efficiently, and some diuretics also may impair renal uric acid excretion. Hyperuricemia may be a problem in patients with leukemia who have a greatly increased number of white blood cells, especially after treatment with drugs that destroy the leukemic cells and release large amounts of nucleoprotein from the disrupted cells. The breakdown of the nucleoprotein yields a large amount of uric acid derived from the purine-containing nucleotides in the nucleoprotein. In these conditions, there is no underlying metabolic defect of purine metabolism.

# Fracture

A **fracture** is a break in bone. In a *simple fracture*, the bone is broken into only two pieces. The term *comminuted fracture* is used when the bone is shattered into several pieces. A *compound fracture* is one in which the overlying skin has been broken. A compound fracture is more serious than the other types because of the possibility that bacteria may invade the fracture site and cause secondary infection of bone (*osteomyelitis*).

After a fracture, the ends of the broken bone may remain aligned, or they may be displaced out of position. The term *reduction of a fracture* refers to realigning the ends of the broken bone so that the bone will heal in its normal anatomic position. Sometimes a bone may become so weakened by disease such as metastatic tumor that it breaks after minimal stress (for example, coughing or sneezing). A fracture of this type through a diseased area in bone is called a *pathologic fracture*.

# Osteomyelitis

Osteomyelitis is an infection of bone and adjacent marrow cavity (*osteo* = bone + *myelos* = marrow + *itis* = inflammation) that is usually the result of staphylococci or various gram-negative bacteria. The infecting organisms gain access to bone in two ways:

1. They may be transported to bone from a distant site by way of the bloodstream, which is called *hematogenous osteomyelitis*.
2. Bacteria may be implanted directly in the bone from various causes.

## Hematogenous Osteomyelitis

Hematogenous osteomyelitis is more common in children than in adults. The bacteria are usually carried to the bone from a skin infection, such as a boil, from a kidney infection, or from some other distant site.

In children, the organisms tend to lodge in the growing end of the bone on the diaphyseal (shaft) side of the epiphyseal plate, where they proliferate and incite an acute inflammation. Local injury to bone near its very vascular growing end seems to favor localization of bacteria in the bone, probably because a small hemorrhage forms secondary to the injury, and the collection of blood provides conditions favorable for the growth of bacteria.

Hematogenous osteomyelitis sometimes occurs in adults. Although hematogenous osteomyelitis may affect any bone, the infection frequently localizes in the vertebral bodies rather than in the long bones. Probably the stresses and trauma associated with weight-bearing predispose to localization in the spine.

**fracture** (frak-tūr) A broken bone.

## Osteomyelitis as a Result of Direct Implantation of Bacteria

Various conditions may expose bone to direct infection, including compound fractures, gunshot wounds, or other severe injuries affecting bone. Various surgical procedures performed on bone, such as open reduction and internal fixation of fractures or total joint replacement, may also be complicated by osteomyelitis. Chronic ulcers of the feet, which sometimes develop in diabetic patients, may expose the small bones of the feet to chronic infection.

## Clinical Manifestations and Treatment

Usually, osteomyelitis is manifested as an acute febrile illness associated with localized pain, tenderness, and swelling over the affected bone.

Osteomyelitis is treated by a prolonged course of antibiotic therapy. In some patients, the infection may become chronic and may recur periodically. Chronic osteomyelitis is much more difficult to treat. In addition to intensive antibiotic treatment, surgical procedures may be required to remove infected degenerated bone and drain collections of pus in the bone.

Pathogenic fungi, tubercle bacilli, and various unusual opportunistic organisms may at times cause osteomyelitis, especially in immunocompromised adults. The infections are treated by appropriate antibiotics supplemented by various surgical procedures, if needed.

# Tumors of Bone

Bone is often affected by metastatic tumors. Carcinoma of breast or prostate, as well as many other tumors, frequently metastasize to bone ( Figure 22-14 ). Occasionally, the skeletal system may be so heavily infiltrated by

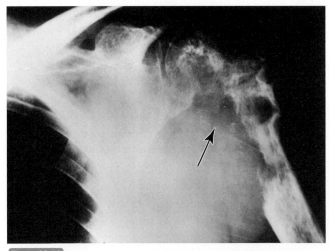

Figure 22-14 Metastatic carcinoma in the humerus. The primary tumor was in the kidney. Bone destruction by metastatic carcinoma is indicated by marked irregularity in the contour of the head and neck of the humerus (*arrow*).

# Osteoporosis

Osteoporosis, literally meaning "porous bones," is a generalized thinning and demineralization of the entire skeletal system. Most cases are found in postmenopausal women, beginning in their 50s, and a significant degree of osteoporosis is said to be present in approximately one-fourth of all women in their 60s. Osteoporosis develops whenever bone resorption exceeds bone production. The incidence is high in postmenopausal women because the loss of ovarian function results in estrogen deficiency. Estrogen inhibits bone resorption, and loss of estrogen accelerates the rate of bone resorption, which results in slowly progressive thinning of the bones. Osteoporosis also develops in older men, but it occurs at a much later age and is usually less severe than in women.

The osteoporotic bones are quite fragile and susceptible to fracture. Fractures of vertebral bodies are frequent, either from the stress of weight-bearing or after minor exertion ( Figure 22-15 ). Such fractures produce back pain and tenderness and are often characterized by collapse of the anterior portions of the vertebral bodies (*compression fractures*). Collapse of vertebral bodies may compress the spinal nerve roots passing through the intervertebral foramina, causing pain to radiate along the course of the compressed nerve.

Maximum bone density is attained in young adults, and then it slowly but steadily declines as they get

tumor that hematopoietic cells within the marrow are crowded out, leading to anemia, leukopenia, and thrombocytopenia (Chapter 11). Nodular deposits of neoplastic plasma cells are frequently present throughout the skeletal system in multiple myeloma (Chapter 8). Benign cysts and benign tumors of bone are encountered occasionally, but primary malignant tumors of bone are unusual. A malignant tumor of cartilage is called a *chondrosarcoma*. One arising from bone-forming cells is called an *osteosarcoma*.

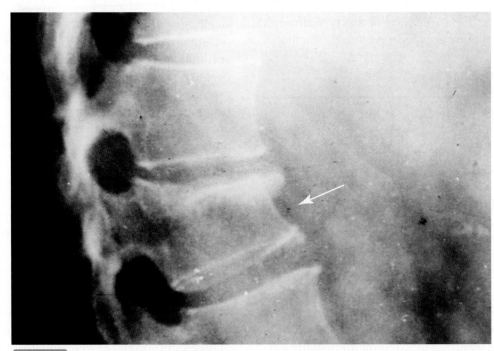

Figure 22-15 Osteoporosis with a compression fracture of vertebral body. Vertebral bodies are less dense than normal, and the front of one vertebral body has collapsed (*arrow*). Compare the compression fracture in this vertebral body with the vertebra above in which the anterior and posterior surfaces are the same height.

older. The greater the bone density one has as a young adult, the longer it will take before there is enough bone loss to increase the risk of fractures. To use an analogy, bone density is like a savings account at a bank where money is deposited for retirement. The more money one has accumulated, the longer it takes before the savings account is depleted.

Bone loss can be retarded by regular weight-bearing exercises, which help maintain bone density, by a high-calcium diet and calcium supplements if necessary to ensure an adequate calcium intake, and by an adequate intake of vitamin D, which is required to promote calcium absorption from the intestine and incorporation into bone. Estrogens are no longer recommended to retard bone loss in postmenopausal women because of the long-term risks associated with estrogen use.

Once marked osteoporosis has developed and fractures occur, it is difficult to restore bone density. A number of drugs are available that may be helpful. Each has advantages and disadvantages.

Significant loss of bone density may also occur in women athletes who engage in prolonged, intense physical activity, such as runners and gymnasts. The high level of physical activity triggers the hypothalamus and pituitary gland to increase adrenal corticosteroid output as an adaptation to the exercise-induced stress. This event, however, is also associated with a fall in the pituitary gonadotropic hormones that stimulate ovarian function. The ovaries, no longer adequately stimulated by pituitary gonadotropins, fail to produce adequate estrogen, which leads to cessation of menses called *exercise-induced amenorrhea*. In addition, the estrogen-deficient athlete is also at risk of the same type of estrogen-deficiency osteoporosis that develops in postmenopausal women and is subject to the same osteoporosis-related complications.

Osteoporosis related to exercise-induced amenorrhea can be prevented by reducing the level of physical activity enough to reestablish normal menstrual cycles. Alternatively, the athlete who elects to continue the same level of exercise can reduce her risk of osteoporosis by taking supplementary estrogen and progesterone hormones to replace the missing ovarian hormones and by taking calcium supplements.

X-ray and radioisotope methods are now available that make a quantitative assessment of a patient's bone density and compare the results with normal ranges established for persons of the same age and sex. Those patients whose bones are losing mineral content to a greater extent or more rapidly than normal are at high risk of fractures and other complications related to osteoporosis. They should be treated vigorously in an attempt to retard further bone demineralization.

# Structure and Function of the Spine

The vertebral column forms the central axis of the body. It consists of a series of vertebrae joined by intervertebral disks and fibrous ligaments. The vertebral column has four curves. The *cervical* and *lumbar curves* arch forward. Those in the thoracic and sacral regions bend in the opposite direction ( Figure 22-16A ).

A typical vertebra has a large cylindrical *body* and a *bony arch* that encloses the spinal canal and protects the spinal cord. The parts of the arch that extend posteriorly from the body are called the *pedicles*, and the parts that roof the spinal canal are called the *laminae* (singular, *lamina*). A single midline spinous process projects posteriorly from the bony arch, and paired *transverse processes* extend laterally ( Figure 22-16B ).

When the vertebrae are viewed from the side, the superior and inferior margins of the vertebral pedicles appear concave. Small disklike articular surfaces called *articular processes* are present on the upper and lower surfaces of each vertebral arch, and the vertebral bodies articulate with each other by means of small *synovial joints*. The spaces between the concave surfaces of the pedicles of adjacent vertebrae form oval openings called

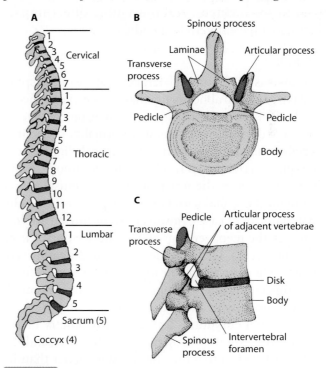

**Figure 22-16** **A,** Side view of vertebral column illustrating normal curves. Vertebrae are numbered. **B,** Structure of typical vertebra viewed from above. The vertebral arch extends posteriorly from the vertebral body. The spinous process projects posteriorly from the arch, and the transverse processes project laterally. The articular processes of adjacent vertebrae articulate with each other by means of small synovial joints. **C,** Side view of two vertebrae, illustrating the intervertebral disk, articular processes, and intervertebral foramen.

intervertebral foramina (singular, foramen), through which the spinal nerves leave the spinal canal ( Figure 22-16C ).

The **intervertebral disks**, interposed between adjacent vertebral bodies, consist of a peripheral fibrous ring, the annulus fibrosus, and a soft central *nucleus pulposus*. The **annulus fibrosus** ("fibrous ring") is structured as a ring of interlacing connective-tissue bundles firmly adherent to adjacent vertebral bodies. Longitudinal bands of connective tissue called the *anterior* and *posterior longitudinal ligaments* run the entire length of the vertebral column to reinforce the annulus. The **nucleus pulposus** ("pulpy nucleus") consists of a gelatinous material containing a carbohydrate substance called a mucopolysaccharide that contains about 80 percent water. Because of its very high water content, it is relatively incompressible.

The intervertebral disks function somewhat like shock absorbers. Pressure applied to the disks is distributed evenly around the annulus by the soft nucleus pulposus, absorbing the forces of compression to some extent, and preventing direct impact between adjacent vertebral bodies.

## Scoliosis

**Scoliosis** is an abnormal lateral curvature of the spine and is a common abnormality that is estimated to occur in about 4 percent of people. A small percentage of cases result from a congenital abnormality of a spinal vertebra that disturbs the normal vertical alignment of the spinal vertebrae, or results from a neurologic problem that disturbs the innervation of the muscles that maintain the spinal vertebrae in proper position. The vast majority of cases, however, occur during adolescence as the teenager is growing, and we don't know why this occurs. This condition is called **idiopathic scoliosis**. (The term *idiopathic* means that we don't know why this condition develops.) Scoliosis occurs much more frequently in adolescent girls than in boys.

The spinal curvatures lead to an asymmetry of the trunk so one shoulder is higher than the other, and the pelvis is tilted so that one iliac crest is higher than its counterpart on the opposite side. Some degree of rotation of the vertebrae accompanies the curvatures, which may lead to some asymmetry of the ribs that attach to the thoracic vertebrae ( Figure 22-17A ). Posterior protrusion of the ribs on one side of the thorax may cause a noticeable humplike deformity.

If scoliosis is identified, x-rays are taken to measure the extent of the curvature. A small curvature may not require treatment, but the adolescent needs to be checked periodically because some curves may get worse as the adolescent grows. Usually a curvature doesn't progress after the teenager stops growing, but a marked curvature may continue to get worse even after growth stops. Severe degrees of scoliosis may cause significant disability. A marked thoracic curvature greatly reduces the size of the thorax, which interferes with lung function ( Figure 22-17B ).

Treatment depends on the degree of curvature. Slight curves may not require treatment but should be watched because the curve may get worse. A growing teenager with a curvature that is getting worse is treated by means of a spinal brace to help maintain the normal position of the spine and stop the progression of the curvature. A marked scoliosis may require surgical treatment, and various surgical procedures are used to stabilize the spine and correct the curvature.

# Intervertebral Disk Disease

With age, the intervertebral disks undergo a progressive wear-and-tear degeneration of both the nucleus and the annulus. The nucleus becomes denser because its water content is reduced, and the annulus becomes weakened and thinned. When marked compression force is applied to the anterior part of the disk during flexion of the spine, the nucleus is forced posteriorly against the weakened annulus, and part of the nucleus may be forced into the spinal canal through a weak area or tear in the annulus ( Figure 22-18 ). Generally, a disk protrusion occurs in the lumbosacral region because this is the part of the vertebral column where the disks are subject to the greatest mechanical compression during lifting. The disk usually protrudes in a posterolateral direction because the dense posterior longitudinal ligament reinforces the annulus in the midline, preventing a direct posterior protrusion.

Symptoms of disk protrusion, sometimes called a "slipped disk," consist of sudden onset of acute back pain after an episode of lifting. Frequently, the pain is also felt in the leg and thigh on the side of the protrusion. This occurs because the extruded disk material often impinges on lumbosacral nerve roots, causing pain to radiate along the course of the nerve compressed by the protruded nucleus pulposus. Treatment consists of bed rest and measures to minimize pain and disability, such as administration of aspirin or other pain-relieving medications, local application of heat, and use

**intervertebral disk** A fibrocartilaginous joint between adjacent vertebral bodies.

**annulus fibrosus** (an´ū-lus) The dense peripheral ring of fibrocartilage making up the intervertebral disk.

**nucleus pulposus** (nū´klē-us) The soft elastic center of the intervertebral disk.

**scoliosis** (sko-lee-oh´-sis) An abnormal lateral curvature of the spine.

**idiopathic scoliosis** (id´-ē-opath´-ik skō-lē-ō´-sis) Lateral curvature of the spine. Idiopathic means cause of condition is unknown.

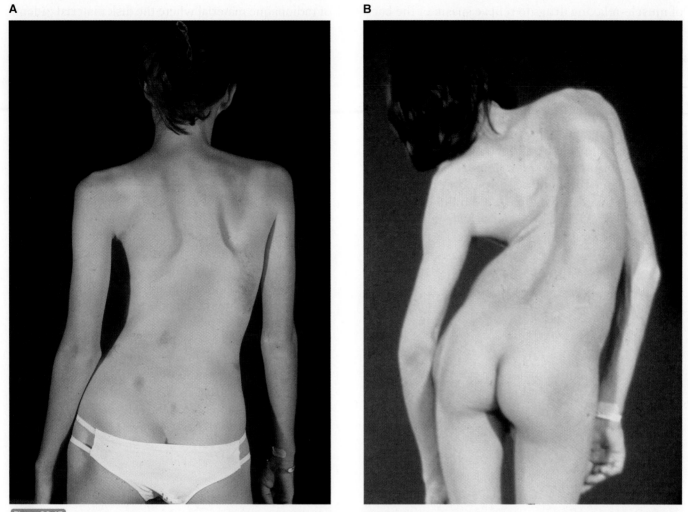

**Figure 22-17** Scoliosis. **A,** Moderate scoliosis. **B,** Severe scoliosis that caused marked asymmetry of trunk and greatly reduced the size of the thoracic cavities, interfering with pulmonary function.

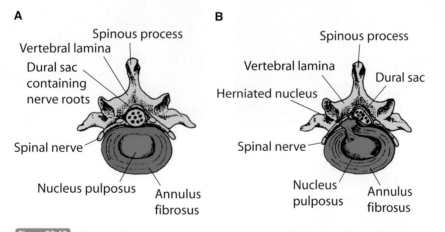

**Figure 22-18** Cross section through the lumbar spine at the level of the intervertebral disk. **A,** Normal relationships of intervertebral disk to spinal canal, dura, and spinal nerves. **B,** Posterior protrusion of nucleus pulposus, impinging on dural sac and spinal nerve exiting through intervertebral foramen.

of muscle-relaxing drugs to relieve spasm of the back muscles that occurs after a disk protrusion and contributes to the disability. Protruded disk material may be resorbed, and the tear in the annulus may be repaired by fibrous tissue. Sometimes, however, surgical removal of the protruded disk material may be required.

The protrusion of the disk material into the spinal canal can be demonstrated by means of a special radiologic procedure called a myelogram, which is used less often than in previous years. Radiopaque material is introduced into the dural sac surrounding the cord and nerve roots in order to outline the contour of the dural sac ( Figure 22-19A ). The extruded disk material can be recognized in the x-ray film as a filling defect in the column of radiopaque material where the disk material indents the dural sac. CT and MRI scans, noninvasive radiologic examinations described in Chapter 1, have largely replaced myelograms for identifying disk protrusions, but myelograms still have some limited use in special circumstances ( Figure 22-19B  and  Figure 22-19C ).

# Structure and Function of Skeletal Muscle

Muscle cells are highly specialized contractile cells. Three different types of muscle are recognized: smooth muscle, skeletal muscle, and cardiac muscle. Smooth muscle is found in the walls of the gastrointestinal tract, biliary tract, urogenital system, respiratory tract, and blood vessels. Skeletal muscle is attached to the skeleton by tendons and ligaments; it functions in voluntary muscular activity. Cardiac muscle closely resembles skeletal muscle but has certain special features related to its function of producing rhythmic contractions of the heart. Lesions of smooth muscles are rare, and disorders of cardiac muscle are considered in Chapter 10. A discussion of skeletal muscle, the great bulk of muscle within the body, follows.

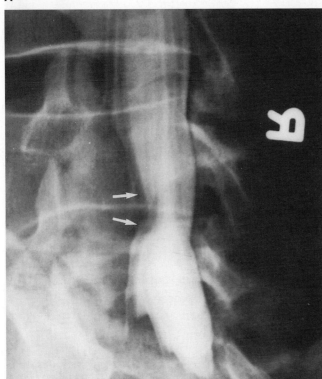

A

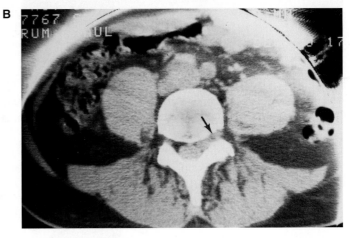

B

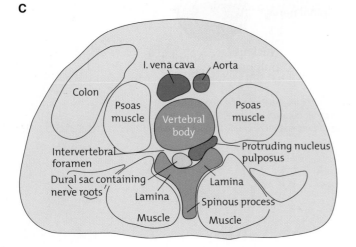

C

Figure 22-19  Demonstration of herniated nucleus pulposus ("slipped disk"). A, X-ray examination obtained after radiopaque contrast material was instilled into dural sac (myelogram). Indentation of dural sac (*arrows*) results from herniated nucleus pulposus impinging on spinal dura.
B, CT scan of lumbar region. Protruding nucleus pulposus (*arrow*) is located adjacent to dural sac and fills intervertebral foramen (*arrow*). Compare with appearance of normal intervertebral foramen on opposite side.
C, Schematic of anatomic structures and lesion as demonstrated on CT scan.

## Contraction of Skeletal Muscle

Skeletal muscles are long, straplike fibers that measure as much as 30 centimeters in length. The cytoplasm (sarcoplasm) contains multiple nuclei located just beneath the cell membrane (sarcolemma). Filling the cytoplasm are long threadlike myofibrils composed of the contractile myofilaments actin and myosin. The cytoplasm also contains many energy-rich organic compounds, ions, and enzymes required for the metabolic activity of the muscle cell.

Muscle cells contract in response to motor nerve impulses conveyed to the muscle. The area of communication between the nerve endings and the muscle cell is called the *myoneural junction*. The actual stimulation of the muscle cell is the result of a chemical called **acetylcholine**, which is released from the nerve endings at the myoneural junction and interacts with acetylcholine receptors on the surface of the muscle fibers. The chemical mediator acetylcholine initiates the biochemical chain of events that causes the actin and myosin filaments to slide together, which leads to shortening of the muscle fiber. The duration of the chemical mediator is quite brief because this substance is rapidly broken down by the enzyme *cholinesterase*, which is present at the myoneural junction.

## Factors Affecting Muscular Structure and Function

The normal structural and functional integrity of skeletal muscle depends on an intact nerve supply, normal transmission of impulses across the myoneural junction, and normal metabolic processes within the muscle cell.

As considered in Chapter 21, skeletal muscles that are not used or muscles deprived of their nerve supply undergo marked atrophy. Conversely, when additional work is required of the muscles, they undergo hypertrophy in response to the increased demands.

Diseases of skeletal muscle are uncommon. The principal disorders consist of inflammatory lesions, muscular atrophy, degeneration (dystrophy) of muscle, and disturbance of impulse conduction at the myoneural junction.

# Inflammation of Muscle (Myositis)

## Localized Myositis

Small areas of inflammation in skeletal muscle are encountered in many systemic diseases. Inflammation of muscle may also follow injury or muscular overexertion. The inflammation is secondary to necrosis and disruption of muscle cells and is associated with swelling and tenderness of the affected muscle. The inflammation gradually subsides as the muscle injury heals.

## Generalized Myositis

Generalized inflammation of skeletal muscle (polymyositis) is an uncommon but serious systemic disease of unknown etiology, characterized by widespread degeneration and inflammation of skeletal muscle. One type of polymyositis, associated with swelling and inflammation of the skin, is called *dermatomyositis*. These disorders are often classified as autoimmune connective tissue (collagen) diseases (Chapter 4) because of the necrosis of connective tissue fibers in the affected muscles and because these diseases are presumed to have an immunologic basis.

# Muscular Atrophy and Muscular Dystrophy

A group of relatively rare diseases is characterized by progressive atrophy or degeneration of skeletal muscle. Many are hereditary. Various clinical syndromes are recognized, depending on the muscle groups affected, the patterns of inheritance, and the rate of progression of the disease. In general, the diseases are characterized by progressive muscular weakness and gradually increasing disability, eventually terminating in death from paralysis of the respiratory muscles or superimposed respiratory infection.

**acetylcholine**
(as-et-il-kō´lēn) A chemical secreted by nerve endings that activates neurons or muscle cells.

It is customary to classify these diseases into two large categories: the *muscular atrophy group* and the *muscular dystrophy group*.

In the progressive muscular atrophy group of diseases, the muscular weakness and atrophy are secondary to progressive degeneration of motor nerve cells in the cerebral cortex, brain stem, and spinal cord, described in Chapter 21, "Degenerative Diseases of Motor Neurons." The clinical manifestations are related to the location of the degenerating nerve cells within the CNS and the rate at which the neuronal degeneration progresses.

In the muscular dystrophy group, the nerve supply to the muscles is unaffected. The basic disturbance is an abnormality in the muscle fibers that causes them to degenerate. The most common and severe type is called *Duchenne muscular dystrophy*, and a milder form of muscular dystrophy is called *Becker muscular dystrophy*. Both forms result from the mutation of a large gene on the X chromosome, and the disease is transmitted as an X-linked trait to male children of women who carry the defective gene. The normal gene codes for a muscle protein called *dystrophin*, which is located on the inner surface of the sarcolemma, where it plays a role in maintaining the structure and functions of the muscle fibers.

As a result of the gene mutation, dystrophin is absent in the muscle fibers of persons afflicted with Duchenne muscular dystrophy and is apparently responsible for the manifestations of the disease, which appear first during early childhood and progress rapidly, leading to death in late adolescence or early adulthood. The muscles primarily affected are those of the lower extremities, trunk, hips, and shoulder girdle. Often the extent of atrophy is masked because the muscles are infiltrated by fat and fibrous tissue as they atrophy. The fat infiltration may at times be so extreme that the affected muscles appear hypertrophied, leading to the paradox of profound muscular weakness in an individual whose muscles appear very well developed. The apparent hypertrophy is an illusion, which is why the term *pseudohypertrophic* is applied to this type of muscular dystrophy.

The less-severe Becker muscular dystrophy also is caused by a mutation of the same dystrophin-producing gene that causes Duchenne muscular dystrophy. Dystrophin is produced by the mutated gene but is either abnormal or produced in insufficient amounts. In both diseases, the muscle enzyme creatine kinase (CK) leaks from the abnormal muscle fibers, and very high enzyme levels can be detected in the blood of affected persons. (This is the same enzyme that leaks from heart muscle when the muscle is damaged, as described in Chapter 10.) The diagnosis of muscular dystrophy is made on the basis of the clinical features together with the very high CK blood concentration. Genetic testing reveals the gene mutation, and muscle biopsies reveal absence of dystrophin in Duchenne dystrophy and an abnormal or reduced amount of dystrophin in Becker dystrophy. Although the various types of muscular atrophy and muscular dystrophy are uncommon, they are of major concern not only to the patient, but to the family because of the hereditary nature of many of these illnesses. Unfortunately, there is no way at present to arrest the relentless progression of the disease.

Gene therapy to eventually allow insertion of replacement genes in muscle fibers to code for the synthesis of the missing or defective dystrophin is being actively investigated but has not yet been successful.

# Myasthenia Gravis

**Myasthenia gravis** is a chronic disease characterized by abnormal fatigability of the voluntary muscles as a result of an abnormality at the myoneural junction. Fatigue develops rapidly when the muscles are used and subsides when they are rested. Often, the dysfunction is most conspicuous in the small muscles of the face and in the muscles concerned with eye movement (extraocular muscles). Myasthenia gravis appears to be an autoimmune disease. The blood of affected patients contains an autoantibody directed against acetylcholine receptors on the surface of the muscle fibers at the myoneural junction. The manifestations of the disease occur because the antibody damages and greatly reduces the number of receptors available to interact with the acetylcholine liberated from motor nerve endings.

Symptoms can be relieved by drugs that inhibit the action of the enzyme cholinesterase. This prolongs the action of the chemical mediator acetylcholine so that it can continue to stimulate the reduced numbers of receptors for a longer time. Many patients with myasthenia gravis have either a tumor or a benign hyperplasia of the thymus gland, which is probably also related to a disturbance of the immune system. Patients with hyperplasia or a tumor of the thymus gland sometimes are improved by removal of the thymus.

# CHAPTER REVIEW

## Summary

Our skeleton is our rigid supporting framework composed of dense connective tissue impregnated with calcium salts. Normal bone structure depends on a normal amount of calcium in our diet, normal amounts of vitamin D, and normal parathyroid gland function. Achondroplasia and osteogenesis imperfecta are genetically determined abnormalities affecting bone formation and clubfoot (talipes) results from abnormal positioning of the limb skeleton.

The three principal types of arthritis are osteoarthritis, rheumatoid arthritis, and gout. Osteoarthritis is a "wear-and-tear" degeneration of the articular cartilage of a weight-bearing joint that exposes the underlying bone, followed by reactive proliferation of the exposed bone. Rheumatoid arthritis is an autoimmune disease that targets the synovium and leads to secondary destruction of joint surfaces; joint instability follows, often association with misalignment or dislocation of affected bones, and associated disability. Treatment is directed toward controlling the autoimmune-mediated joint damage. Gout is a disorder of purine metabolism that leads to elevated uric acid (as sodium urate) in blood and body fluids. Because urate is not very soluble, it is prone to precipitate from solution in and around joints when its concentration is higher than normal, leading to episodes of acute joint pain as well as progressive joint damage resulting from the urate deposits. Urate may also precipitate from the tubular fluid within the kidney tubules, plugging the tubules and leading to kidney damage as well as joint damage caused by gout.

Bones are sturdy, but they may break, and fractures are classified based on the characteristics of the fracture. The most serious type is a compound fracture in which the overlying skin is broken, exposing the fracture site to infection. A bone may also break if it has been weakened by disease, such as by a deposit of metastatic carcinoma. Such a disease-associated fracture is called a pathologic fracture.

An infection in a bone is called osteomyelitis, which is usually caused by a pathogenic bacteria carried to the bone in the bloodstream from an infection elsewhere in the body (hematogenous spread), or introduced directly into the bone, as may occur following a compound fracture or as a complication of a surgical procedure, such as a hip replacement operation. Treatment consists of antibiotics, sometimes supplemented by surgical procedures.

Malignant tumors may involve bone. Primary bone tumors such as osteosarcoma or chondrosarcoma are uncommon. Most are metastatic tumors spreading from other sites, such as colon, breast, prostate, or lung. Myeloma, a neoplasm of plasma cells, is also relatively common, and may cause multiple areas of bone destruction.

Loss of bone density (osteoporosis) predisposes to fracture, and the condition occurs most frequently in postmenopausal women. It is easier to prevent excessive bone loss by adequate calcium intake, vitamin D, and weight-bearing exercise than it is to restore bone density after it has been lost. However, various treatments are available and are effective.

The spine that supports us may cause problems, such as scoliosis. Early detection and treatment prevent severe disability. Another common problem is a herniated intervertebral disk impinging on a nerve root and causing back pain radiating down the leg. Treatment may require surgical removal of the herniated disk tissue.

Myositis is an inflammation of skeletal muscle. Mild localized myositis may follow injury from overexertion. Generalized myositis is a systemic autoimmune disease and is more difficult to treat. Progressive muscular atrophy results from degeneration of nerve cells supplying the affected muscles for which there is no treatment. Muscular dystrophy is a hereditary X-linked disease affecting the muscle protein dystrophin, which leads to progressive muscle degeneration. Myasthenia gravis is an autoimmune disease in which the antibody targets acetylcholine receptors at the muscle–nerve junction, which impairs transmission of nerve impulses from nerve to muscle. Symptoms are relieved by drugs that prolong the action of acetylcholine. Some affected patients have a tumor of the thymus (thymoma) and can be improved by removing the thymic tumor.

## Questions for Review

1. Describe the structure of the typical movable joint (see Figure 22-1).
2. What are the three most common types of arthritis? What are their distinguishing features (see Table 22-1)?
3. What is the difference between a simple fracture and a compound fracture? What are the complications of a compound fracture? What is a comminuted fracture? A pathologic fracture?
4. What is osteoporosis? Why does it develop? What symptoms and complications result from osteoporosis?
5. What is a "slipped disk"? Why does it occur? Why does it sometimes produce pain radiating down the leg? How is it treated?
6. What is meant by the following terms: *osteoporosis*, *multiple myeloma*, *nucleus pulposus*, *rheumatoid factor*?
7. What are the types of muscle cells?
8. What is meant by the following terms: *myoneural junction*, *acetylcholine*, and *myositis*?
9. What is the difference between muscular atrophy and muscular dystrophy? What are the most common types of atrophic disease of the muscles? Of dystrophic disease?
10. What is myasthenia gravis? What is its relationship to the immune system? How is it treated?

## Supplementary Reading

Brender, E. 2005. Vitamin D. *Journal of the American Medical Association* 394:2386.

A short one-page article designed for patient education describing the amount of sunlight exposure required to ensure adequate vitamin D (10–15 minutes twice per week), the diseases resulting from the deficiency (rickets and osteomalacia), the persons at risk of deficiency (breastfed infants receiving less than 2 cups a day of vitamin D-fortified formula or milk, persons with dark pigmented skin, persons with very limited sun exposure, persons with fat malabsorption diseases, persons with liver or kidney disease, persons in the northern hemisphere during winter).

Cauley, J., Lui, L. Y., Ensrud, K. E., et al. 2005. Bone mineral density and the risk of incident nonspinal fracture in black and white women. *Journal of the American Medical Association* 293:2102–8.

Age, female sex, slender body configuration, and white race are well-known risk factors for osteoporosis. Although many factors affect bone mineral density (BMD), middle-aged and older black men and women have higher BMD and lower fracture rates than whites. Decreased total hip and femoral neck BMD is associated with increased fracture risk in both black and white women. At any level of BMD, fracture rates in black women were 30 to 40 percent lower than in white women. Separate race-specific databases may be appropriate to define osteoporosis and fracture risk in black and white women.

Drinkwater, B. L., Nilson, K., Ott, S., and Chesnut, C. H. 1986. Bone mineral density after resumption of menses in amenorrheic athletes. *Journal of the American Medical Association* 256:380–82.

Bone mass may not be completely restored.

Felson, D. T. 2006. Osteoarthritis of the knee. *New England Journal of Medicine* 354:841–48.

Describes risk factors, manifestations, and principle of treatment.

Holick, M. F. 2007. Vitamin D deficiency. *New England Journal of Medicine* 357:266–81.

Vitamin D deficiency is still a problem despite fortification of foods with supplements. In adults the deficiency may increase the risk of bone fractures by contributing to the development of osteoporosis, and may also cause osteomalacia. Without vitamin D only about 10–15 percent of dietary calcium and about 60 percent of phosphorous is absorbed. Most cells and tissues in the body have vitamin D receptors, and vitamin D has many effects unrelated to the skeletal system. Vitamin D inhibits cell proliferation of both normal cells and cancer cells, and promotes normal differentiation of cells. Vitamin D is required for normal immune system function, which may explain why black Americans, who are often vitamin D deficient, are more prone to tuberculosis than are whites, and tend to have more aggressive disease. People living at higher or lower latitudes (farther away from the equator where sunlight is most intense and prolonged) have a greater risk of a number of diseases than are persons living closer to the equator. Current recommendations for vitamin D supplements are too low, and many persons are vitamin D deficient.

Johnson, R. J., and Rideout, B. A. 2004. Uric acid and diet—Insights in the epidemic of cardiovascular disease. *New England Journal of Medicine* 350:1071–73.

Neither the total protein intake nor the intake of purine-rich vegetables was correlated with the development of gout. Gout is most common among persons whose diet is high in meat and low in dairy products. Genetic and other factors also modulate the uric acid levels. Many persons with chronic gout and persisting high uric acid develop urate nephropathy. Diets that contain abundant fruits, vegetables, and low-fat dairy foods not only reduce the frequency of hypertension but also the frequency of gout.

LeBoff, M. S., Kohlmeier, L., Hurwitz, S., et al. 1999. Occult vitamin D deficiency in postmenopausal U.S. women with acute hip fracture. *Journal of the American Medical Association* 281:1505–11.

Many postmenopausal women with hip fractures have occult vitamin D deficiency, which impairs absorption of calcium and mineralization of bone and also stimulates compensatory increase in parathyroid hormone secretion. These factors predispose to fractures. Older people need 600 IU of vitamin D daily, which should be increased to 800 IU in winter.

Loucks, A. B., Mortola, J. F., and Girton, S. S. C. 1990. Alterations in the hypothalamic–pituitary–ovarian and the hypothalamic–pituitary–adrenal axis in athletic women. *Journal of Clinical Endocrinology and Metabolism* 68: 402–11.

Describes pathophysiology of exercise-induced amenorrhea.

O'Dell, J. R. 2004. Therapeutic strategies for rheumatoid arthritis. *New England Journal of Medicine* 350:2591–602.

Irreversible joint damage occurs early in rheumatoid arthritis. Early diagnosis and prompt treatment with disease-modifying antirheumatic drugs (DMARD) are essential to minimize joint damage. Nonsteroidal anti-inflammatory drugs improve symptoms but do not slow the progression of the disease. Corticosteroid drugs suppress inflammation and slow disease progression but have significant side effects. DMARD vary in effectiveness and toxicity. Methotrexate is the most widely used, and many patients are treated with methotrexate combined with two other DMARD agents. Tumor necrosis factor inhibitor drugs are generally reserved for patients whose disease cannot be controlled by a combined therapy with DMARD.

Raisz, L. G. 2005. Screening for osteoporosis. *New England Journal of Medicine* 353:164–71.

Measurement of bone mineral density at the lumbar spine and proximal femur is a reliable and safe way to assess the risk of fracture. Screening should provide an estimate of fracture risk during the subsequent 5 or 20 years.

Rott, K. T., and Agudelo, C. A. 2003. Gout. *Journal of the American Medical Association* 289:2857–60.

Current concepts on pathogenesis, factors raising uric acid, clinical manifestations, drugs available for treating gout, and new treatment methods being investigated.

Shahinian, V. B., Kuo, Y. F., Freeman, J. L., and Goodwin, J. S. 2005. Risk of fracture after androgen deprivation for prostate cancer. *New England Journal of Medicine* 532:154–64.

Orchiectomy or drug-induced suppression of testicular function in men with prostate cancer significantly increases their risk of fractures by promoting more rapid decline in bone density resulting from loss of androgens.

## Interactive Activities

### Matching

Match the type of arthritis on the right with the disease characteristic on the left.

1. Affects primarily small bones of the hands and feet

2. Autoantibodies formed    A. Osteoarthritis

3. Disturbed purine    B. Rheumatoid
   metabolism          arthritis

4. Major weight-bearing    C. Gout
   joints involved

5. Fragmentation and degeneration of articular cartilage

6. Destructive cytokines produced by inflammatory cells

7. Uric acid deposits in and around joints

8. May lead to kidney damage

## True or False

Indicate whether each statement is true or false by writing T or F at the end of the statement.

1. Most patients with gout have autoantibodies directed against articular cartilage that damage the joints._____
2. Myasthenia gravis is an autoimmune disease in which the autoantibody targets acetylcholine receptors at the myoneural junction._____
3. Muscular dystrophy results from degeneration of motor neurons in the spinal cord._____
4. Rheumatoid arthritis is caused by degeneration of the articular cartilage in weight-bearing joints._____

## Critical Thinking

1. Mary Jones is a college student who has heard that the risk of osteoporosis developing later in life can be minimized by measures that promote strong bones. What should she do to promote strong bones and minimize her osteoporosis risk?

2. John Cunningham is a middle-aged man who had an acute episode of pain and swelling at the base of his great toe. What conditions could account for the pain and swelling? What measures would help establish the cause of the condition?

# General References

## Anatomy and Physiology

Ganong, W. F. 2003. *Review of Medical Physiology,* 21st ed. New York. Lange Medical Books/McGraw-Hill.

Guyton, A. C., and Hall, J. E. 1997. *Human Physiology and Mechanisms of Disease,* 6th ed. Philadelphia: W.B. Saunders Company.

Martini, F. H., Timmons, M. J., and Tallitsch, R. B. 2006. *Human Anatomy,* 5th ed. San Francisco: Pearson/Benjamin Cummings.

Martini, F. H. 2006. *Fundamentals of Anatomy and Physiology,* 7th ed. San Francisco: Pearson/Benjamin Cummings.

## Medicine

Andrioli, T. E., Carpenter, C. C. J., Griggs, R. C., and Loscalzo, J. 2006. *Cecil Essentials of Medicine,* 6th ed. Philadelphia: W.B. Saunders Company.

Beers, M. H., Fletcher, A. J., Jones, T. V., et al. 2003. *The Merck Manual of Medical Information; Home Edition,* 2nd ed. New York: Pocket Books/Simon and Schuster, Inc.

Greenspan, F. S., and Gardner, D. G. eds. 2004. *Basic and Clinical Endocrinology,* 7th ed. New York: Lange Medical Books/McGraw-Hill.

Tierney, L. M., McPhee, S. J., and Papadakis, M. A. eds. 2006. *Current Medical Diagnosis and Treatment 2006,* 45th ed. New York: Lange Medical Books/McGraw-Hill.

## Microbiology

Murray, P. R., Rosenthal, K. S., and Pfaller, M. A. 2005. *Medical Microbiology,* 5th ed. Philadelphia: Mosby.

## Obstetrics and Gynecology

Boston Women's Health Book. 1998. *Our Bodies, Ourselves for the New Century: A Book for and by Women.* New York: Simon and Schuster, Inc.

Decherney, A. H, Nathan, L., and Goodwin, T. M. 2006. *Current Obstetric & Gynecologic Diagnosis and Treatment,* 10th ed. New York. Lange Medical Books/McGraw-Hill.

## Pathology

Kumar, V., Abbas, A. K., and Fausto, N. 2005. *Robbins and Cotran Pathologic Basis of Disease,* 7th ed. Philadelphia: Elsevier Saunders.

## Pediatrics

Hay, W. W., Levin, M. J., Sondheimer, J. M., and Deterling, R. R. 2005. *Current Pediatric Diagnosis and Treatment,* 17th ed. New York: Lange Medical Books/McGraw-Hill.

## Surgery

Doherty, G. M. 2006. *Current Surgical Diagnosis and Treatment,* 12th ed. New York: Lange Medical Books/McGraw-Hill.

Sabiston, D. C., and Lyerly, H. K. 2005 *Textbook of Surgery: The Biological Basis of Modern Surgical Practice,* 16th ed. Philadelphia: W.B. Saunders Company.

## Urology

Schrier, R. W. 2003. *Renal and Electrolyte Disorders,* 6th ed. Baltimore: Lippincott Williams & Wilkins.

# Answers to Interactive Activities

## Chapter 1

**Multiple Choice:** 1A; 3D; 5B

**Critical Thinking:**

1. It is a good idea to be screened because you both will know whether you carry the sickle cell gene. If only one of you has the gene, it may be passed to the child and could lead to sickle cell trait, which would not be a problem. If you both carry the sickle cell gene, there is a possibility that a child will acquire both S genes and have sickle cell anemia, which is a serious disease. Prenatal diagnosis is available so you will know the genes carried by the fetus. If the fetus has two sickle cell genes, you will know that the fetus will have the disease. Then you will have to decide whether to continue the pregnancy.

## Chapter 2

**Matching:** 1G; 3E; 5C; 7A

**True or False:** 1T; 3T; 5T

**Critical Thinking:**

1. The increased muscle mass results from hypertrophy of individual muscle fibers resulting from weight lifting; Charles' high-protein diet is supplying the necessary protein to cause the muscle fibers to become larger, but intake of more protein is unlikely to be beneficial.

3. Sally's brother has hemophilia because he received the X chromosome containing the mutant gene. Since he is a male, there is no second X chromosome to offset the effect of the mutant gene on the X chromosome that he received. Sally could have received from her mother the normal X chromosome, or the chromosome containing the mutant gene. In the latter situation, she would be a carrier of the abnormal gene that she could transmit to a male child. Further studies to determine the amount of antihemophilic globulin (AHG) she produces could provide information as to whether Sally has two normal X chromosomes and produces a normal amount of AHG, or is a carrier of an abnormal X, and has a reduced amount of AHG. Other more specialized tests are available in specialized centers dealing with hemophilia.

## Chapter 3

**Matching:** 1H; 3C; 5A; 7B; 9I

**True or False:** 1F; 3T; 5T

**Critical Thinking:**

1. Ambrose has an infection with lymphangitis and lymphadenitis and should be on antibiotic treatment. It would be helpful to obtain a culture from the wound to identify the responsible organism and its sensitivity to the antibiotic he is receiving to be sure that the organism will respond to the antibiotic. He probably has been immunized against tetanus, but this should be checked. He may also require a booster dose of tetanus toxoid or antitoxin, depending on his immunization status.

## Chapter 4

**Matching:** 1E; 3H; 5A; 7B; 9K; 11F; 13G

**True or False:** 1F; 3T; 5T

**Critical Thinking:**

1. The exposure to pig brain tissue may have caused John to form anti-pig brain antibodies. Pig tissue contains many antigens similar to those in human tissue, and an anti-pig brain antibody may have cross-reacted with similar antigens in human nervous system, tissues, which may have caused the neurologic symptoms.

## Chapter 5

**Matching 1:** 1I; 3H; 5D; 7B; 9C

**Matching 2:** 1A; 3G; 5E; 7H; 9F

**Matching 3:** 1B; 3E; 5D

**True or False:** 1F; 3F; 5T; 7F; 9T

**Critical Thinking:**

1. The oral herpes is caused by the herpes simplex virus, but has nothing to do with herpes zoster that is caused by a different virus called the varicella zoster virus. This organism causes chickenpox, but after the infection subsides the virus "hides out," usually in spinal sympathetic ganglia. Then years later, in some people, the virus may become active again. When this occurs, the virus travels down the sympathetic nerve to cause a vesicular skin eruption in the distribution of the nerve attached to the ganglion where the virus had been previously dormant.

3. This may be the only worm in Michael's intestinal tract, but there could be others. An examination of Michael's stool for eggs may be helpful, followed by treatment to eliminate the worms if eggs are identified.

## Chapter 6

**True or False:** 1T; 3T; 5T; 7T; 9F

**Critical Thinking:**

1. Chlamydia may spread from the cervix to infect the fallopian tubes, and the infection may lead to scarring that may block or partially obstruct one or both tubes, putting her at risk of sterility (if both tubes are obstructed) or ectopic pregnancy (if the scarring delays transport of a fertilized egg through the tube). The infection can be transmitted to a partner during intercourse. The infection responds well to antibiotic therapy, and she should be treated to prevent complications.

3. Gonorrhea is not a benign disease, and it may not remain confined to the genital tract. It may spread in the bloodstream to infect other tissues, such as the joints as in the present case, or infect heart valves. Gonococcal skin lesions may also occur. Casual sex with a new partner is always risky.

# Chapter 7

**Multiple Choice:** 1D; 3B

**True or False:** 1T; 3F; 5T

**Matching:** 1B; 3D

**Critical Thinking:**

1. Hemophilia is transmitted on the X chromosome from Mary's mother, who is a carrier of the abnormal X chromosome. If Mary received the normal X chromosome, then both X chromosomes are normal. If she received the abnormal X, she is a carrier but will not have hemophilia because the normal X chromosome can function to produce enough antihemophilic globulin (AHG) so that she will not have any bleeding problems. On the other hand, her brother has only one X chromosome, which happens to carry the abnormal gene, so he has hemophilia. Mary could have received from her mother the normal X chromosome or the abnormal X chromosome. If she receives the abnormal X, she will not have hemophilia because the normal X chromosome will produce enough antihemophilic globulin (AHG) so that she will not have any difficulties, although she may produce a reduced amount of AHG. If she carries the abnormal X chromosome, she could transmit the chromosome to her infant, should she become pregnant. A male infant would have hemophilia; a female would be a carrier like the mother. Mary could obtain information about whether she is a carrier by a blood test to determine the amount of AHG she produces, which is subnormal in a carrier. More sophisticated studies are also available at medical centers dealing with hemophilia. Specialized chromosome studies can determine whether the genes on both of her X chromosomes that are responsible for producing AHG are normal, or whether one is abnormal, which makes her a carrier of the abnormal gene.

3. The urinary tract infection should be treated with an antibiotic. The Food and Drug Administration places all drugs into one of five categories according to the degree of possible risk to the fetus, and her physician would select one that poses no risk to the fetus (category A).

# Chapter 8

**True or False:** 1F; 3T; 5T; 7T; 9F

**Matching:** 1E; 3F; 5A

**Critical Thinking:**

1. This is a screening test looking for disturbances of cell maturation (dysplasia) usually caused by a carcinogenic strain of papillomavirus that may progress to cervical carcinoma. If abnormalities are found, additional treatment can eradicate the abnormal erpithelium and prevent cervical cancer.

3. Peter heard correctly that a person whose immune system doesn't function properly has an increased risk of cancer. The immune system recognizes abnormal cells that may arise during cell division and eliminates the abnormal cells before they proliferate excessively and possibly form a tumor.

# Chapter 9

**True or False:** 1F; 3T; 5T; 7T; 9T

**Matching:** 1C; 3B

**Select the Proper Answer:** 1B; 3A

**Critical Thinking:**

1. Mary may not be a good contraceptive pill candidate. Even low-dose contraceptive pills can increase the concentration of coagulation factors, which may slightly increase her risk of developing a blood clot. However, her blood pressure is slightly elevated, which is not normal for a woman her age, and she smokes, which also significantly increases her risk of developing a thrombus. She has several factors that suggest she should consider another contraceptive method, such as condoms for her partner, or a diaphragm for her. An intrauterine contraceptive device could be considered but may occasionally be complicated by a uterine infection that could spread and involve the fallopian tubes, which could jeopardize her fertility and may not be a good choice.

# Chapter 10

**Matching:** 1B; 3D; 5C

**Multiple Choice:** 1B; 3D; 5C

**Critical Thinking:**

1. Such marked elevation in a young person is unusual and probably is not primary hypertension. Other possibilities are an adrenal tumor producing excess epinephrine, possibly a corticosteroid-producing adrenal tumor, an aldosterone-producing tumor, or hyperthyroidism. These less likely conditions could be excluded by appropriate clinical and laboratory tests. The most likely possibility is an aortic coarctation, which is characterized by significant blood pressure differences between upper and lower limbs and characteristic changes in a chest x-ray that show regularities in the ribs caused by the vigorous pulsations of the intercostal arteries carrying blood to the aorta distal to the coarctation. Additional studies could identify the site of the coarctation, and resection of the narrowed area with reconnection of the aorta should cure the hypertension.

3. Weight control, treatment of hypertension and diabetes if present, an anti-coronary diet, and mild exercise. Often drugs to reduce myocardial irritability are also recommended along with statin drugs.

# Chapter 11

**Multiple Choice:** 1D; 3C

**Critical Thinking:**

1. Mary's white cells and platelets are normal, which suggests that the anemia is not caused by leukemia or some other disease that destroys or replaces the bone marrow with abnormal cells. She probably has an iron-deficiency anemia, possibly from excessive menstrual bleeding leading to iron deficiency. This can be confirmed by examination of a blood smear to see whether she has a hypochromic microcytic anemia, and laboratory tests to confirm an iron deficiency.

# Chapter 12

**Multiple Choice:** 1B; 3B; 5D; 7A; 9C

**Fill-in-the-Blanks:**

1. ventilation; gas exchange
3. tension (positive pressure) pneumothorax; insert chest tube to evacuate the air
5. surfactant deficiency
7. multinucleated giant cell
9. neonatal acute respiratory distress syndrome
11. silicosis
13. carcinoma; mesothelioma
15. cigarette smoking

**Critical Thinking:**

1. Peter probably has chronic obstructive pulmonary disease (COPD) from long-time cigarette smoking. He may also have a lung carcinoma for the same reason. Peter needs further studies including a chest x-ray, and possibly also a bronchoscopic examination and lung biopsy if the chest x-ray suggests a tumor in addition to COPD. He should stop smoking. Although he will not be able to repair the lung damage, he may be able to slow further lung damage by stopping smoking.

# Chapter 13

**Fill-in-the-Blanks:**

1. ovary
3. gynecomastia
5. sentinel node

**True or False:** 1T; 3F; 5F; 7F; 9F; 11T; 13F; 15F

**Critical Thinking:**

1. Breast cancer would be unlikely in such a young woman. It is more likely to be a benign cyst or a fibroadenoma but further study is needed to confirm this. Her physician might want to insert a needle into the lump and try to aspirate fluid, confirming that it is a benign cyst. If no fluid is obtained, smears of any aspirated material can be examined histologically, which would confirm that the lump is a fibroadenoma that could be removed under local anesthesia. Alternatively, the physician may prefer to have a mammogram to obtain further information about the lump before attempting to aspirate or biopsy the lump.

3. The atypical cells may be secondary to a mild inflammation or possibly a papillomavirus infection. The Pap smear should be repeated in 6 months, along with a HPV test. If the repeat Pap test and HPV test are negative, no further examinations other than routine gynecologic care are needed. If the Pap smear is still atypical and the HPV test is positive, cervical biopsies are indicated and further treatment will depend on the biopsy results.

# Chapter 14

**Multiple Choice:** 1C; 3A; 5C

**True or False:** 1T; 3F; 5F; 7F; 9T

**Critical Thinking:**

1. Rh hemolytic disease is no longer a major problem because we know how to prevent it. Because Maria is Rh negative, she could have an Rh-positive fetus if her spouse is Rh positive and passes the Rh (D) gene to the fetus. However, many Rh-positive men are heterozygous Rh positive (genotype Dd) and may not pass the Rh-positive (D) gene to the fetus. If the fetus were Rh-positive, sensitization probably would occur when Rh-positive fetal cells were transferred into the maternal circulation as the placenta separated from the uterus after delivery of the infant. Administration of Rh-immune globulin to the mother during pregnancy and postpartum would eliminate any Rh-positive fetal cells entering the mother's circulation so that the mother would not become sensitized to the Rh antigen. Consequently, her next Rh-positive pregnancy would not be affected.

3. Contraceptive pills work by providing estrogen and progestin, which suppresses gonadotropin hormone output from the pituitary gland. Since there are no gonadotropic hormones to stimulate follicle maturation and ovulation, the woman can't become pregnant because she doesn't ovulate. The postcoital contraceptive pills ("the morning-after pill") act primarily by changing the character of the endometrium so that a fertilized ovum (which takes about 7 days from ovulation to implantation) is unable to implant. The pills may also have effects on ovulation and tubal transport that also work against a successful implantation.

# Chapter 15

**Matching 1:** 1B; 3A; 5C

**Matching 2:** 1D; 3A; 5C

**Fill-in-the-Blanks:**

1. gonococcus-chlamydia; antibiotics
3. prostatic specific antigen (PSA); prostatic carcinoma
5. malignant teratoma
7. gubernaculum

**True or False:** 1F; 3F

**Critical Thinking:**

1. The swelling of the legs and abdomen is caused by accumulation of fluid in the tissues. The marked protein loss in the urine lowers serum albumin and reduces its osmotic effect, which tends to pull fluid back into the bloodstream (discussed in Chapter 9). Usually in a child the cause is a minimal change in the permeability of the glomerular filter, and the child will probably recover without any long-term aftereffects.

3. Urinary tract infections are more common in women than in men, because the short female urethra allows bacteria easier access to the bladder. Sexual intercourse may also predispose to bladder infections, as does infrequent urination, which allows bacteria to multiply.

5. Martin's right testis is in the scrotum and spermatogenesis presumably is normal, so his fertility is not in jeopardy even though the abdominal testis is sterile. However, the incidence of testicular carcinoma is significantly higher in an abdominal testis than in a scrotal testis, and he would not be able to recognize the tumor until it was far advanced and had already metastasized. Removing the abdominal testis should be recommended.

# Chapter 16

**Matching 1:** 1E; 3B; 5C; 7F

**Matching 2:** 1E; 3F; 5H; 7G

**True or False:** 1F; 3T; 5T; 7F; 9T; 11F; 13T; 15T; 17F

**Critical Thinking:**

1. Hepatitis A can be transmitted by oral–genital contact if John's partner has hepatitis A or is recovering from a recent infection. Virus excreted in the stool may contaminate the perianal and genital region, and any oral contact may lead to an infection. Intestinal parasites and intestinal pathogens also can be transmitted this way as well. He can reduce his risk by avoiding promiscuous sexual contacts, avoiding oral–genital contacts and anal–genital contacts without a condom, which will reduce his risk of hepatitis B and HIV.

3. Naomi has three problems. She is overweight, her blood pressure is higher than it should be, and her blood glucose is slightly elevated. She should lose weight, which may bring her blood pressure and glucose back to normal. We don't know her cardiovascular status, but she has risk factors that suggest a metabolic syndrome, which is usually associated with abnormal blood lipids.

# Chapter 17

**Matching:** 1E; 3L; 5G; 7F; 9A; 11K

**True or False:** 1F; 3T; 5T; 7F; 9F

**Critical Thinking:**

1. The combination of obesity, diabetes, and hypertension is consistent with the metabolic syndrome. Susan needs to get her weight under control, which may lower her blood glucose and get her diabetes under control, which may also lower her blood pressure. Medical treatment is available, but she lacks the commitment to follow through so surgical treatment can be considered. A Roux-Y gastric bypass would lower her weight and probably improve her diabetes, but she needs to be committed to a lifelong change in her eating habits. Many surgeons will not perform a surgical procedure unless the patient has made this commitment.

# Chapter 18

**Matching:** 1D; 3A; 5B

**Critical Thinking:**

1. He undoubtedly has a nutritional deficiency, because he is not eating and has chronic diarrhea, either caused by his disease or a coexisting chronic bacterial or parasitic intestinal infection. The treatment should be to improve his appetite and stop the diarrhea. He needs a medical evaluation of his HIV status and perhaps a change in treatment, and

stool studies to see whether there is a treatable bacterial or parasitic intestinal infection. Initial treatment should be followed by gradually increasing his food intake to restore his nutritional status to normal.

3. This unfortunate man has two common alcohol-related problems resulting from a thiamin deficiency. The tingling pain and muscle weakness results from peripheral nerve degeneration, called peripheral neuritis, which may improve with intensive thiamin treatment. Unfortunately, the memory problems indicate a thiamin deficiency-related brain degeneration and may not improve. However, thiamin treatment and stopping heavy drinking may prevent the brain problem from becoming worse by developing into the more advanced disease called the Wernicke–Korsakoff syndrome.

## Chapter 19

**Fill-in-the-Blanks:**

1. cations; anions
3. potassium; phosphate

**Matching:** 1A; 3B; 5C

**Critical Thinking:**

1. "Acid blood" refers to metabolic acidosis caused by retention of waste products normally excreted by the kidneys that have accumulated in the blood and have been buffered by sodium bicarbonate, which lowers Eric's blood bicarbonate. The ratio of bicarbonate to carbonic acid is disturbed, which lowers his blood pH.

## Chapter 20

**Matching:** 1C; 3E; 5B; 7A; 9I

**True or False:** 1F; 3F; 5T; 7F

**Critical Thinking:**

1. The test on cord blood is to detect hypothyroidism, which could lead to impaired growth and mental development if untreated. The test is required on all infants so that treatment can be started promptly if indicated.

3. Although overweight may occasionally be related to endocrine gland disturbances, in most cases it is related to overeating. Thyroid function tests can check for hypothyroidism, and tests can detect Cushing disease or syndrome. If these tests are negative, then Mary's eating and exercise activities should be evaluated to see whether overeating with reduced exercise may be the problem.

## Chapter 21

**Matching:** 1C; 3J; 5B; 7D; 9G

**True or False:** 1F; 3T; 5T; 7T; 9T

**Critical Thinking:**

1. Jane's dad had a transient ischemic attack (TIA) probably caused by temporary plugging of an artery in the brain by arteriosclerotic plaque material or a bit of thrombus material on the surface of a plaque in his carotid artery that soon was removed by the body's protective mechanisms, and blood flow returned. The TIA is a manifestation of vascular disease and he should have a further investigation to evaluate his cardiovascular system and see whether the carotid artery is the source.

## Chapter 22

**Matching:** 1B; 3C; 5A; 7C

**True or False:** 1F; 3F

**Critical Thinking:**

1. Mary should consume an adequate diet containing sufficient calcium, phosphate, and vitamin D. Moderate exercise, but not excessive, which leads to exercise-induced amenorrhea.

# Glossary

## Common Prefixes and Suffixes

### Prefixes

**a, an**—without

**ab**—from, away from

**ad**—toward

**ante**—before

**bi**—twice, two

**circum**—around

**co**—together

**contra**—against, opposed

**de**—down, from, away

**dis**—apart

**dys**—abnormal, difficult

**endo**—within

**epi**—upon

**exo**—outside

**extra**—outside

**hemi**—half

**hetero**—different

**homo**—same

**hyper**—above, beyond, excessive

**hypo**—below, under, deficient

**infra**—beneath

**inter**—between

**intra**—within

**meta**—after, beyond

**para**—beside

**peri**—around

**post**—behind, after

**pre**—before

**pro**—before

**sub**—beneath

**supra**—above

**syn**—together

### Suffixes

**—blast**, applied to formative cells
(e.g., osteoblast)

**—cyte**, applied to adult cells
(e.g., osteocyte)

**—itis**, inflammation of

**—oid**, like

**—ology**, study of

**—oma**, a swelling or tumor

### An Approximate Guide to Pronunciation

**a:** as in lad

**ā:** as in late

**ä:** as in calm

**e:** as in met

**ē:** as in meet

**i:** as in pill

**ī:** as in pile

**o:** as in rob

**ō:** as in robe

**u:** as in shut

**ü:** as in chute

**oi:** as in joy

**ōō:** as in fool

**ou:** as in loud

# A

**ABO hemolytic disease** A mild hemolytic disease in group A or B infants or group O mothers, as a result of maternal anti-A and anti-B antibodies.

**abscess** (ab´sess) A localized accumulation of pus in tissues.

**acetone** (as´e-tōn) An organic compound (ketone) derived from the ketone bodies acetoacetic acid and beta-hydroxybutyric acid.

**acetylcholine** (as-et-il-kō´lēn) A chemical secreted by nerve endings that activates neurons or muscle cells.

**acetyl coenzyme A** (acetyl-CoA) A combination of a two-carbon acetate fragment with a complex organic compound called coenzyme A.

**achondroplasia** (a-kon-dro-pla´zi-yuh) A congenital disturbance of endochondral bone formation that causes a type of dwarfism.

**acidosis** A disturbance in the acid–base balance of the body in which body fluids have a lower pH than normal.

**acquired immune deficiency syndrome (AIDS)** An infection caused by the human immunodeficiency virus. The virus attacks and destroys helper T lymphocytes, which compromises cell-mediated immunity, leading to increased susceptibility to infection and some tumors.

**acromegaly** (ak´ro-meg´al-ē) A condition resulting from excessive secretion of growth hormone in the adult.

**ACTH** See *adrenocorticotrophic hormone*.

**actinic keratosis** (ak-ti´-nik ke-rä-tō´sis) A precancerous warty proliferation of squamous epithelial cells in sun-damaged skin of older persons.

**acute coronary syndrome** A general term for the three most serious manifestations of coronary artery disease: unstable angina, non-ST-segment elevation myocardial infarction, and ST-segment elevation myocardial infarction.

**Addison disease** A disease caused by chronic adrenal cortical hypofunction.

**adenoma** (ad-en-ō´muh) A benign tumor arising from glands.

**ADH** See *antidiuretic hormone*.

**adhesions** (ad-hē´shuns) Bands of fibrous tissue that form subsequent to an inflammation, and bind adjacent tissues together.

**adjustable gastric banding** A method for treating obesity by applying an adjustable gastric band to the stomach in order to reduce its capacity, thereby promoting weight loss.

**adrenocorticotrophic hormone (ACTH)** (ad-rēn´o-cor´tico-trō´fik) A hormone secreted by the anterior lobe of the pituitary that stimulates the adrenal cortex to manufacture and secrete adrenal cortical hormones.

**aldosterone** A steroid hormone produced by the adrenal cortex that regulates the rate of sodium absorption from the renal tubules.

**alkalosis** A disturbance in the body's acid–base balance in which the pH of the extracellular fluids is shifted toward the alkaline side of normal. See also *acidosis*.

**allele** (äh´lēl) One of several related genes that may occupy the same locus on a homologous chromosome.

**alpha cells** (al´fuh) Glucagon-secreting cells of the pancreatic islets.

**alpha fetoprotein (AFP)** (al´fuh fē´tō-prō´tēn) Protein produced by fetal liver early in gestation. Sometimes produced by tumor cells. Level is elevated in amnionic fluid when fetus has neural tube defect.

**Alzheimer disease** (ahls´-hīm-er) A degenerative disease of the nervous system with characteristic structural abnormalities within neurons.

**amenorrhea** (äh-men-ō-rē´äh) Absence of menses.

**amnionic sac** (am-nē-on´ik) The fluid-filled sac surrounding the embryo. One of the fetal membranes.

**anaphylactoid reaction** (a-na-fil-ack´-toyd) A hypersensitivity reaction resembling anaphylaxis but not caused by IgE antibodies.

**anaphylaxis** (a-nä-fil-aks´is) A severe generalized IgE-mediated hypersensitivity reaction characterized by marked respiratory distress and fall in blood pressure.

**anastomosis** (ä-nas-ta-mō´sis) A communication between two blood vessels or other tubular structures. Also refers to a surgical connection of two hollow tubular structures, such as the divided ends of the intestine or a blood vessel (*surgical anastomosis*).

**anemia** (an-ē´mē-uh) A decrease in hemoglobin or red cells or both.

**anencephaly** (an-en-seff´uh-lē) A congenital malformation: absence of brain, cranial vault, and scalp as a result of defective closure of the neural tube.

**aneurysm** (an´ūr-izm) A dilatation of a structure, such as the aorta, a cerebral artery, or a part of the ventricular wall.

**angina pectoris** (an-jī´nuh pek´tōr-is) Precordial pain experienced on exertion owing to inadequate blood supply to the heart muscle.

**angiogram** (an´jē-ō-gram) Same as *arteriogram*.

**angiotensin-converting enzyme** An enzyme that converts angiotensin I to angiotensin II.

**angiotensinogen** (an-jē-o-ten-sin´o-gen) A blood protein converted to angiotensin I by renin secreted by the kidneys. Part of the renin-angiotensin-aldosterone system.

**anion** (an´ī-on) An ion carrying a negative charge.

**anorexia nervosa** Excessive self-induced weight loss because of a false perception of being fat.

**annulus fibrosus** (an´ū-lus) The dense peripheral ring of fibrocartilage making up the intervertebral disk.

**antidiuretic hormone (ADH)** (an-ti-dī-u-ret´tik) Posterior lobe pituitary hormone that regulates urine concentration by altering the permeability of the renal collecting tubules.

**aplastic anemia** (ā-plas´tik) An anemia caused by bone marrow failure.

**arachnoid** (ar-ak´noyd) The middle of the three meninges that cover the brain and spinal cord.

**aromatase inhibitor** (air-ō´-muh-tase) A drug that inhibits the conversion of adrenal androgenic steroids to estrogens, used as post-resection adjuvant therapy to treat postmenopausal women with estrogen-positive breast carcinoma.

**arteriogram** (är-tēr´ē-ō-gram) An x-ray technique for studying the caliber of blood vessels by injection of radiopaque material into the vessel.

**arteriolosclerosis** (är-tēr-ē-ólo-skler-ō´-sis) One type of arteriosclerosis characterized by thickening and degeneration of small arterioles.

**asbestos body** (as-bes´tus) An asbestos fiber coated with protein and iron that is found in lungs and sputum of patients with asbestosis.

**asbestosis** (as-bes-tō´sis) A type of pneumoconiosis caused by inhalation of asbestos fibers.

**ascites** (a-si´tēz) Accumulation of fluid in the abdominal cavity.

**astrocyte** A large stellate cell having highly branched processes. Forms the structural framework of the nervous system. One of the neuroglial cells.

**atelectasis** (ah-tel-ek′tuh-sis) Collapse of the lung, either caused by bronchial obstruction (*obstructive atelectasis*) or external compression (*compression atelectasis*).

**atheroma** (ah-ther-ō′muh) A mass of lipids and debris that accumulates in the intima lining of an artery and narrows its lumen.

**atherosclerosis** A thickening of the lining (*intima*) of blood vessels caused by accumulation of lipids, with secondary scarring and calcification.

**atopic** (ā-top′ik) Having a genetic predisposition to certain allergic conditions such as hay fever and asthma.

**atrioventricular (AV) valve** (a′trē-o-ven-trik′ū-lar) The flaplike heart valve located between the atrium and ventricle.

**autoantibody** (aw′tō-an′ti-bod-ē) An antibody formed against one's own cells or tissue components.

**autoimmune disease** A disease associated with formation of cell-mediated or humoral immunity against the subject's own cells or tissue components.

**autosome** (aw′tō-sōm) A chromosome other than a sex chromosome.

# B

**Barr body** The inactivated X chromosome that is applied to the nuclear membrane in the female. Sex chromatin body.

**Barrett esophagus** A condition in which the epithelial lining of the esophagus changes from squamous to columnar type, usually as a result of reflux esophagitis.

**basophil** A cell that contains numerous variable-sized granules that stain intensely purple with basic dyes. See also *eosinophil*.

**beta cells** (bā′tuh) Insulin-secreting cells of the pancreatic islets.

**bile** A secretion of the liver containing bile salts, cholesterol, and other substances.

**bile canaliculus** (kan-al-ik′u-lus) Small terminal bile channel located between liver cords.

**bile salts** Derivatives of bile acids present in bile that act as emulsifiers to promote fat digestion and absorption.

**biliary cirrhosis** Diffuse liver cell damage and scarring with distortion of liver cell structure and function (cirrhosis) caused by obstruction of bile ducts.

**biliary colic** Abdominal pain that results when a gallstone enters the biliary duct system.

**bilirubin** (bil-i-rū′bin) One of the bile pigments derived from breakdown of hemoglobin.

**biopsy** (bī′op-sē) Removal of a small sample of tissue for examination and diagnosis by a pathologist.

**blastocyst** A stage of development of the fertilized ovum (*zygote*) in which a central cavity accumulates within the cluster of developing cells.

**B lymphocyte** A lymphocyte that differentiates into plasma cells and is associated with humoral immunity.

**body stalk** The structure connecting the embryo to the chorion. Eventually develops into the umbilical cord.

**Bowman's capsule** The cuplike expanded end of the nephron that surrounds the tuft of glomerular capillaries.

**bradykinin** (brā-dē-kī′nin) A chemical mediator of inflammation derived from components in the blood plasma.

**bronchiectasis** (bron-kē-ek′tuh-sis) Dilatation of bronchi caused by weakening of their walls as a result of infection.

**bronchiole** (bron′ke-ōl) One of the small terminal subdivisions of the branched bronchial tree.

**bronchus** One of the large subdivisions of the trachea.

**bulimia nervosa** Weight control by compulsive overeating followed by self-induced vomiting and other methods in order to prevent weight gain.

**buffer** A substance that minimizes change in pH of a solution when an acid or base is added.

# C

**calculus** A stone formed within the body, as in the kidney or gallbladder.

**carcinoma** (kär-sin-ō′-mah) A malignant tumor derived from epithelial cells.

**cardiac catheterization** A specialized technique to determine the blood flow through the chambers of the heart, and to detect abnormal communications between cardiac chambers.

**cardiac cycle** The sequence of events during a single contraction and relaxation of the atria and ventricles.

**cardiac output** The amount of blood ejected from a single ventricle in one minute, calculated by multiplying the cardiac stroke volume by the heart rate in beats per minute.

**cardiospasm** (kär′-dē-o-spazm) Spasm of the lower gastroesophageal (cardiac) sphincter.

**caries** (ka′rēz) Tooth decay.

**catecholamines** (kat-eh-kōl′uh-mēnz) The adrenal medullary hormones *epinephrine* and *norepinephrine*.

**cation** (kat′ ī-on) An ion that carries a positive charge.

**cell-mediated immunity** Immunity associated with population of sensitized lymphocytes.

**cellulitis** (sell-ū-līē′-tis) An acute spreading inflammation affecting the skin or deeper tissues.

**cerebral embolus** A stroke caused by blockage of a cerebral artery by a blood clot that had formed elsewhere in the circulatory system and was transported in the bloodstream to the brain.

**cerebral hemorrhage** A stroke caused by rupture of a cerebral artery, usually in a person with hypertension, which allows blood to escape under high pressure into the brain.

**cerebral thrombosis** A stroke caused by thrombosis of an arteriosclerotic cerebral artery.

**cerebrovascular accident (CVA)** An injury to the brain resulting in a disturbance of cerebral blood flow caused by a cerebral thrombosis, cerebral embolism, or cerebral hemorrhage.

**cholelithiasis** (kō′lē-lith-ī′uh-sis) Formation of gallstones.

**cholesterol** (kō-les′ter-ol) A complex compound (*sterol*) containing several ring structures.

**chordae tendineae** (kor′dā ten-din′ē-ā) Fibrous cords that extend from the free margins of the atrioventricular valves to attach to the papillary muscles.

**choriocarcinoma** (kōr′rē-ō-kär-sin-ō′muh) A malignant proliferation of trophoblastic tissue.

**chorion** (kō′ri-on) The layer of trophoblast and associated mesoderm that surrounds the developing embryo.

**chorionic vesicle** The chorion with its villi and enclosed amnion, yolk sac, and developing embryo.

**chorionic villi** Fingerlike columns of cells extending from the chorion that anchor the chorionic vesicle in the endometrium.

**chromatid** (krō′mä-tid) One of two newly formed chromosomes held together by the centromere.

**chronic obstructive pulmonary disease (COPD)** A chronic pulmonary disease characterized by emphysema and coexisting chronic bronchitis.

**chronic thyroiditis** An autoimmune disease in which an autoantibody directed against thyroid epithelial cells causes progressive destruction of the thyroid gland, leading to hypothyroidism. Also called *Hashimoto thyroiditis*.

**cirrhosis of the liver** (si-rō′sis) A disease characterized by diffuse intrahepatic scarring and liver cell degeneration.

**clearance test** (klēr′ans) A test of renal function that measures the ability of kidneys to remove (clear) a substance from the blood and excrete it in the urine.

**cleft lip** Defect in the upper lip of variable degree, as a result of a developmental disturbance.

**cleft palate** Defect in hard palate allowing communication between oral cavity and nasal cavity, as a result of a developmental disturbance.

***Clostridium*** (klä-strid′ē-yum) Anaerobic gram-positive spore-forming rod-shaped bacterium.

**clubfoot** Congenital malposition of foot. In most common type, foot is turned inward at ankle and heel is elevated.

**colitis** (kō-lī′tis) Inflammation of the colon, such as chronic ulcerative colitis.

**collateral circulation** An accessory circulation capable of delivering blood to a tissue when the main circulation is blocked, as by a thrombus or embolus.

**colloid** An eosinophilic protein material present within the thyroid follicles.

**colposcope** (kol′po-skōp) A binocular magnifying instrument used to view the cervix and endocervical canal.

**communicable disease** A disease transmitted from person to person.

**complement** A group of blood proteins that are activated by antigen–antibody interaction and a few other conditions, leading to release of components that "complements" the body's response to infection.

**computed tomographic (CT) scan** (tō-mo-graf′ik) An x-ray technique producing detailed cross-sectional images of the body by means of x-ray tube and detectors connected to a computer. Sometimes called a CAT scan.

**condyloma** (kon-di-lō′ma) A warty tumorlike overgrowth in the squamous epithelium of the anorectal or genital tract, caused by a virus that is spread by sexual contact.

**congenital** Present at birth.

**conjugated bilirubin** A more soluble form of bilirubin produced by the addition of two molecules of glucuronic acid to the bilirubin molecule.

**cortisol** (kōr′ti-sol) The major glucocorticoid.

***Corynebacterium*** (kōr-rī′nē-bak-te′rī-yum) An aerobic nonspore-forming gram-positive rod-shaped bacterium.

**cotyledon** (co-ti-lē′don) A unit of the placenta visible grossly on the maternal surface as an irregularly shaped lobe circumscribed by a depressed area.

**creatinine** (krē-at′in-ēn) A waste product derived from the breakdown of a compound present in muscle (phosphocreatine) that is excreted in the urine.

**cretinism** (krē′tin-izm) Hypothyroidism in the infant.

**Crohn disease** (krō′-n) A chronic autoimmune disease characterized by segmental areas of inflammation and scarring within the intestine, often involving primarily the distal ileum. Also called *regional ileitis*.

**crossover** Interchange of genetic material between homologous chromosomes during synapse and meiosis.

**Cushing disease** A disease characterized by adrenal cortical hyperfunction caused by an ACTH-secreting tumor of the pituitary gland.

**cyanosis** A blue tinge of the skin and mucous membranes that results from an excessively large amount of reduced hemoglobin in the blood when blood oxygenation is insufficient.

**cystitis** (sis-tī′tis) Inflammation of the bladder.

**cytokine** A general term for any protein secreted by cells that functions as an intercellular messenger and influences cells of the immune system. Cytokines are secreted by macrophages and monocytes (monokines), lymphocytes (lymphokines), and other cells.

# D

**daughter cell** A cell resulting from division of a single cell (called the *parent cell*).

**decidua** (de-sid′ū-ah) The endometrium of pregnancy.

**delta cells** (del′tuh) Somatostatin-secreting cells of the pancreatic islets.

**dental plaque** Masses of bacteria, bacterial products, and salivary proteins adherent to teeth, which predisposes to tooth decay.

**dentine** (den′tēn) Bony structure of the tooth.

**deoxyribonucleic acid (DNA)** The nucleic acid present in the chromosomes of the nuclei of cells that carries genetic information.

**dermatophyte** (der-mat′o-fīt) A fungus that causes a superficial infection of the skin.

**desensitization** A method of inducing a diminished response to allergens by inducing the formation of specific IgG and IgA antibodies.

**diabetes mellitus** (dī-u-bē′tēz mel′lit-is) A metabolic disease characterized by hyperglycemia and caused by insufficient insulin secretion or inefficient utilization of insulin.

**diabetic ketosis** A disturbance of the body's acid–base balance (acidosis) caused by an inability to utilize glucose, which requires the body to use fat as an energy source. Fat metabolism generates excessive amounts of acid ketone bodies, which disrupts the normal alkalinity of body fluids.

**diagnosis** The determination of the nature and cause of a patient's illness.

**disease** Any disturbance of the structure or function of the body.

**dissecting aneurysm of the aorta** (an′ūr-izm) A dissection of blood into the wall of the aorta secondary to degeneration of the arterial wall with an associated tear of the lining (*intima*) of the artery.

**disseminated intravascular coagulation syndrome** A disturbance of blood coagulation as a result of activation of the coagulation mechanism and simultaneous clot lysis.

**diverticulitis** (dī-vur-tik-u-lī′tis) An inflammation of a diverticulum.

**diverticulosis** (dī-vur-tik-u-lō'sis) A condition characterized by an outpouching of the colonic mucosa through weak areas in the muscular wall.

**diverticulum** (dī-vur-tik'u-lum) An outpouching from an organ, as from the mucosa of the colon, which projects through the muscular wall.

**DNA repair genes** Genes that monitor and correct errors in DNA replication during cell division.

**dominant gene** A gene that expresses a trait in the heterozygous state.

**dopamine** (dō'puh-mēn) Chemical mediator released by hypothalamic neurons.

**dura** (dū'rä) The outer covering of the brain and spinal cord.

**dysfunctional uterine bleeding (DUB)** Irregular uterine bleeding caused by disturbance of the normal cyclic interaction of estrogen and progesterone on the endometrium.

**dysmenorrhea** (dis-men-ō-rhē'uh) Painful menstruation.

**dysplasia** (dis-plā'sē-yuh) Abnormal maturation of cells.

# E

**eclampsia** (ek-lamp'-sē-ā) One or more convulsions in a pregnant woman with preeclampsia.

**ejection fraction** The volume of blood ejected from a ventricle in systole (stroke volume) expressed as a percentage of the total volume of blood within the ventricle in diastole (end-diastolic volume).

**electrocardiogram** (ē lek-trō-kär'dē-ō-gram) A technique for measuring the serial changes in the electrical activity of the heart during the various phases of the cardiac cycle. (Often called ECG or EKG.)

**electrolyte** (ē-lek'trō-līt) A compound that in solution dissociates into positive and negative ions.

**embolism** (em'bō-lizm) A condition in which a plug composed of a detached clot, mass of bacteria, or other foreign material (*embolus*) occludes a blood vessel.

**embryo** (em'brē-ō) The developing human organism from the third through the seventh weeks of gestation.

**embryonal carcinoma** A malignant testicular tumor in which the malignant cells have features resembling rapidly growing trophoblastic tissue.

**enamel** Dense outer covering of the exposed surface of the tooth.

**encephalitis** (en-sef-äl-ī'tis) An inflammation of the brain.

**end-diastolic volume** (die-e-stahl'-ik) The volume of blood in the ventricle just before the beginning of ventricular systole.

**endemic disease** (en-dem'ik) A communicable disease in which small numbers of cases are continually present in a population.

**endochondral bone formation** (en-dō-kon'drul) Formation of bone as, first, a cartilage model that is then reabsorbed and converted into bone.

**endometrial cyst** (en-dō-mē'trē-ul) An ovarian cyst lined by endometrium and filled with old blood and debris. A manifestation of endometriosis.

**endometriosis** (en-dō-mē trē-ō'sis) Presence of endometrial tissue in abnormal locations, such as in the ovary or pelvis.

**endoscopy** (en-däs'kō-pē) An examination of the interior of the body by means of various lighted tubular instruments.

**endothelium** (en-dō-thē'lē-um) The internal lining of blood vessels and interior of heart.

**enteritis** (en-ter-ī'tis) Inflammation of the intestine.

**eosinophil** (ē-ō-sin'o-fil) A cell whose cytoplasm is filled with large, uniform granules that stain intensely red with acid dyes. See also *basophil*.

**epidemic disease** (ep-i-dem'ik) A communicable disease affecting concurrently large numbers of persons in a population.

**epinephrine** (ep-in-ef'rin) One of the compounds (catecholamines) secreted by the adrenal medulla.

**Epstein-Barr virus** A virus that causes infectious mononucleosis.

**erythroblast** (e-rith'rō-blast) A precursor cell in the bone marrow that gives rise to red blood cells.

**erythropoietin** (er-ith-rō-poy'e-tin) A humoral substance made by the kidneys that regulates hematopoiesis.

**esophageal varices** (var'i-sēz) Dilated (varicose) veins of the esophagus, which are often present in patients with cirrhosis of the liver.

**etiology** (ē-tē-ol'ō-jē) The cause, especially the cause of a disease.

**exchange transfusion** Partial replacement of blood of infant with hemolytic disease by blood lacking the antigen responsible for hemolytic disease, as when transfusing Rh-negative blood to an Rh-positive infant. Performed to reduce intensity of hemolytic jaundice.

**exudate** (ex'yū-dāt) The fluid, leukocytes, and debris that accumulate as a result of an inflammation.

# F

**fetal hemoglobin** A type of hemoglobin containing two alpha and two gamma chains, which is able to take up and release oxygen at much lower $PO_2$ (oxygen partial pressures) than in adult hemoglobin.

**fetus** The unborn offspring after eight weeks' gestation.

**fibrillation** (fi-bril-lā'shun) Uncoordinated quivering of cardiac muscle that prevents normal contraction of the heart muscle.

**fibrin monomer** (mä'nō-mer) A derivative of fibrinogen that polymerizes to form the fibrin clot during blood coagulation.

**follicle-stimulating hormone (FSH)** One of the gonadotropic hormones secreted by the anterior lobe of the pituitary, which regulates growth and function of the gonads (ovary and testis).

**fracture** (frak-tūr) A broken bone.

# G

**galactorrhea** (gā-lak-tō-rē'yuh) Secretion of milk by breast not associated with pregnancy or normal lactation.

**gametes** Reproductive cells, eggs, and sperm, each containing 23 chromosomes, which unite during fertilization to form a zygote containing 46 chromosomes.

**gametogenesis** (gam-ē'-toe-genesis) The development of mature eggs and sperm from precursor cells.

**gangrene** (gang-grēn') Term has two different meanings. Refers to (1) infection caused by gas-forming anaerobic bacteria (*gas gangrene*) or (2) necrosis of an extremity caused by interruption of its blood supply (*ischemic gangrene*).

**gastroenteritis** Inflammation of the stomach and intestine.

**gene product** A protein or enzyme specified (coded) by a gene.

**genetic code** (jen-et'ik kōd) The information carried by the codons of DNA molecules in chromosomes.

**genome** (jee′nōm) The total of all the genes contained in a cell's chromosomes.

**germ cell** A precursor cell capable of developing in a mature sperm or ovum.

**germ disk** A three-layered cluster of cells that will eventually give rise to an embryo.

**gestational diabetes** Elevated blood glucose caused by insulin resistance resulting from elevated hormones related to the pregnancy. Blood glucose returns to normal postpartum, but woman has increased risk of diabetes later in life.

**gestational trophoblast disease** (jes-tay′-shun-ul tro′-fo-blast) A general term for all diseases characterized by abnormal trophoblast proliferation. Includes both hydatidiform mole and choriocarcinoma.

**glioma** (glē-ō′muh) Any brain tumor arising from glial (supporting) cells of the brain.

**glomerulonephritis** (glo-mär′ū-lō-nef-rī′tis) An inflammation of the glomeruli caused by either antigen-antibody complexes trapped in the glomeruli, or by antiglomerular basement membrane antibodies.

**glucocorticoid** An adrenal cortical hormone that regulates carbohydrate metabolism.

**glycosylated hemoglobin** (gli-ko′-sil-ay-ted) Hemoglobin to which glucose molecules have become permanently attached. Concentration is related to concentration of glucose in the blood.

**goiter** (goy′ter) Any enlargement of the thyroid gland.

**gonad** (gō′nad) A general term referring to either the ovary or the testis.

**gout** A disorder of nucleoprotein metabolism characterized by elevated uric acid and deposition of uric acid in and around joints.

**granulosa cells** (gran-u-lō′suh) Cells lining the ovarian follicles.

**growth hormone** An anterior lobe pituitary hormone that stimulates growth of bone and other body tissues.

**gubernaculum** (goo′-ber-nak′-ū-lum) A band of fibrous tissue extending from the fetal testis into the scrotum that promotes descent of the testis.

# H

**Hashimoto thyroiditis** Another name for chronic thyroiditis.

**heart block** Delay or complete interruption of impulse transmission from the atria to the ventricles.

**hemiplegia** (hem-ē-plē′-jē-uh) Paralysis of one side of the body.

**hemizygous** A term applied to genes located on the X chromosome in the male.

**hemochromatosis** (hemo-crow-mah-toe′-sis) A genetic disease characterized by excessive iron absorption, leading to accumulation of excessive amounts of iron in the body, causing organ damage.

**hemodialysis** (hēm-ō-dī-al′i-sis) A dialysis procedure by which waste products are removed from the blood of patients in chronic renal failure, usually by means of an artificial kidney machine.

**hemoglobin** An oxygen transport protein within red cells composed of an iron-porphyrin complex (heme) combined with a protein chain (globin).

**hemolytic anemia** An anemia caused by increased blood destruction.

**hemorrhoids** (hem′or-oyds) Varicosities of anal and rectal veins.

**hepatitis B core antigen** The antigen contained in the core of the hepatitis B virus.

**hepatitis B surface antigen** The coating of the hepatitis B virus that is also found in great excess in the blood of infected patients.

**hereditary spherocytosis** A hereditary anemia caused by a defect affecting the red cell membrane that causes the biconcave disk-shaped red cells to change into small spherical cells that do not survive normally in the circulation.

**hernia** (her′nē-yuh) A protrusion of a loop of bowel through a narrow opening, usually in the abdominal wall.

**Hodgkin's disease** One type of lymphoma.

**homologous chromosomes** A matched pair of chromosomes, one derived from each parent.

**host** Individual infected with a disease-producing organism.

**human chorionic gonadotropin (HCG)** (kōr-ē-on′ik gō-na-dō-trō′pin) A hormone made by the placenta in pregnancy having actions similar to pituitary gonadotropins. Same hormone is made by neoplastic cells in some types of malignant testicular tumors.

**human leukocyte antigens** Unique histocompatibility antigens (self-antigens) on the surface of cells. Also called major histocompatibility complex (MHC) antigens.

**human placental lactogen (HPL)** (lak′tō-jen) One of the hormones produced by the placenta that has properties similar to pituitary growth hormone.

**humoral immunity** Immunity associated with formation of antibodies produced by plasma cells.

**hydatidiform mole** (hī-da-tid′i-form mōl) A neoplastic proliferation of trophoblast associated with formation of large cystic villi.

**hydrocele** (hī′-drō-cēl) An accumulation of excess fluid within the tunica vaginalis of the testis.

**hydroceph′alus** Dilatation of the ventricular system caused by pressure arising from accumulation of cerebrospinal fluid within the ventricles.

**hydronephrosis** (hydro-nef-rō′sis) A dilatation of the urinary drainage tract proximal to the site of an obstruction.

**hydrothorax** (hī-drō-thor′ax) Accumulation of fluid in the pleural cavity.

**hydroureter** A dilatation of the ureter secondary to obstruction of the urinary drainage system, often associated with coexisting dilatation of the renal pelvis and calyces (*hydronephrosis*).

**hyperglycemia** (hī-per-glī-sē′mi-uh) Excessively high blood glucose concentration.

**hyperosmolar coma** (hī-per-oz-mō′lär) Coma resulting from neurologic dysfunction caused by hyperosmolarity of body fluids as a consequence of severe hyperglycemia.

**hyperplasia** (hī-per-plā′sēē-uh) An increase in the number of cells.

**hypersensitivity** A state of abnormal reactivity to a foreign material.

**hypertension** High blood pressure.

**hypothalamus** A portion of the brain stem that forms the floor of the third ventricle. It contains clusters of nerve cells that regulate various body functions.

# I

**idiopathic scoliosis** (id′-ē-opath′-ik skō-lē-ō′-sis) Lateral curvature of the spine. Idiopathic means cause of condition is unknown.

**immune complex** An aggregate consisting of an antigen combined with a specific antibody to which complement may also be fixed, which is often associated with autoimmune diseases.

**immune-response genes** Genes on chromosome 6 that control the immune response to specific antigens.

**immunity** Resistance to disease.

**immunoglobulin** (im'mū-nō-glob'u-lin) An antibody protein.

**immunotherapy** (im'mū-nō-ther'uh-pē) Treatment given to retard growth of a disseminated malignant tumor by stimulating the body's own immune defenses.

**impotence** Inability of the male to achieve an erection.

**inclusion bodies** Spherical structures in the nucleus or cytoplasm of virus-infected cells.

**infection** Inflammation caused by a disease-producing organism.

**inner cell mass** A group of cells that are derived from the fertilized ovum and are destined to form the embryo.

**interferon** (in-tur-fēr'on) A broad-spectrum antiviral agent manufactured by various cells in the body.

**interleukin** A general term for a cytokine liberated by lymphocytes that causes a response in other cells.

**interleukin-1** (in-ter-loo'-kin) A cytokine that promotes lymphocyte proliferation and maturation and also produces mediators of inflammation that cause inflammation, which may lead to tissue damage.

**intervertebral disk** A fibrocartilaginous joint between adjacent vertebral bodies.

**intramembranous bone formation** Direct formation of bone by osteoblasts without prior formation of a cartilage model.

**intussusception** (in'tus-us-cep'shun) A telescoping of one segment of bowel into an adjacent segment.

**invasive mole** An aggressive hydatidiform mole that invades the uterine wall.

**islets of Langerhans** (län'ger-hänz) Cluster of endocrine cells in the pancreas.

# J

**jaundice** (jawn'dis) Yellow color of the skin that results from accumulation of bile pigment within the blood.

**juxtaglomerular apparatus** (jux'tu-glo-mār'u-lär) A specialized group of cells at the vascular pole of the glomerulus that regulates blood flow through the glomerulus of the kidneys.

# K

**karyotype** (kār'-ē-ō-type) An arrangement of chromosomes from a single cell arrangement in pairs in descending order according to size of the chromosomes and the positions of the centromeres.

**keratinocyte** (ker-u-tin'ō-cyte) A keratin-forming cell in the epidermis.

**ketosis** (kē-tō'sis) An excess of ketone bodies (acetoacetic acid, beta-hydroxybutyric acid, and acetone) in the blood resulting from utilization of fat as the primary source of energy.

# L

**laparoscope** (lap'-ā-rō-skōp) A long tubular telescopelike instrument passed through the abdominal wall to examine structures within the peritoneal cavity.

**lecithin** (les'ith-in) A phosphorus-containing lipid (*phospholipid*) having detergent properties similar to bile salts.

**Legionnaires disease** A type of pneumonia caused by an airborne bacterium called *Legionella pneumophila.*

**lentigo maligna** A precancerous, pigmented skin lesion arising from proliferation of atypical melanin-producing epithelial cells (melanocytes).

**lesion** (lē'shun) Any structural abnormality or pathologic change.

**leukemia** (lōō-kē'mē-yuh) A neoplastic proliferation of leukocytes.

**leukopenia** (lōō-kō-pē'ni-uh) An abnormally small number of leukocytes in the peripheral blood.

**leukoplakia** A white patch of hyperplastic and usually atypical squamous epithelium on the oral mucosa or genital tract mucosa.

**leukotriene** (lōō-kō-try'-ēn) A prostaglandinlike mediator of inflammation.

**LH** Luteinizing hormone, one of the gonadotrophic hormones.

**liver lobule** A histologic subdivision of the liver in which columns of liver cells converge toward a central vein and portal tracts are located at the periphery.

**lithotripsy** (lith-o-trip'sē) A method for removing stones from the urinary tract by breaking them into small bits that can be excreted in the urine.

**locus** The position of a gene on a chromosome. Different forms (*alleles*) of the same gene are always found at the same locus on a chromosome.

**luteinizing hormone (LH)** One of the gonadotropic hormones secreted by the anterior lobe of the pituitary that regulates growth and function of the gonads (ovary and testis).

**lymphadenitis** (limf-a-den-ī'tis) An inflammation of lymph nodes draining a site of infection.

**lymphangitis** (limf'an-jī'tis) An inflammation of lymph vessels draining a site of infection.

**lymphokine** (limf'ō-kīn) A soluble substance liberated by lymphocytes.

**lymphoma** (limf-ō'muh) A neoplasm of lymphoid cells.

# M

**major histocompatibility complex** (his-tō'com-pat-i-bil'i-tē) A group of genes on chromosome 6 that determine the antigens on the surface of cells.

**Mallory body** An irregular red-staining structure in the cytoplasm of injured liver cells, usually resulting from alcohol-induced liver injury.

**mammogram** (mam'ō-gram) An x-ray of the breast, used to detect tumors and other abnormalities within the breast.

**mast cell** A specialized connective-tissue cell containing granules filled with histamine and other chemical mediators.

**matrix** (mā'trix) Material in which connective-tissue cells are embedded.

**Meckel diverticulum** (dī-vur-tik'kū-lum) A tubular outpouching from the distal ileum; remnant of the vitelline duct.

**megakaryocyte** (mega-carry'-o-site) A very large bone marrow cell having abundant granular cytoplasm and multilobed nucleus that forms the platelets circulating in the bloodstream.

**megaloblast** (meg'al-ō-blast) An abnormal red cell precursor resulting from vitamin $B_{12}$ or folic acid deficiency.

**meiosis** (mī-o'sis) A special type of cell division occurring in *gametes* (ova and sperm), in which the number of chromosomes is reduced by one-half in the ovum and sperm.

**melanin** Dark pigment found in the skin, in the middle coat of the eye, and in some other regions.

**melanin-stimulating hormone (MSH)** One of the hormones produced by the pituitary. Causes darkening of the skin.

**melanocyte** (mc lan´o-cyte) Melanin-producing cell in the epidermis.

**meninges** (men-in´jēz) The membranes covering the brain and spinal cord.

**meningioma** (men-in-jē-ō´muh) A benign tumor arising from the meninges.

**meningitis** (men-in-jī´tis) Inflammation of the meninges.

**meningocele** (men-in´go-sēl) A protrusion of meninges through a defect in the spinal vertebral arches.

**meningomyelocele** (men-ing-gō-mī´el-ō-sēl) A type of spina bifida characterized by protrusion of meninges and cord through the defect in the vertebral arches.

**mesangial cell** (mes-an´jē-yul) Modified connective-tissue cells at the vascular pole of the glomerulus that hold the capillary tuft together.

**mesothelium** (me-sō-thē´li-um) A layer of flat squamous epithelial cells that covers the surfaces of the pleural, pericardial, and peritoneal cavities.

**metabolic syndrome** A group of conditions consisting of obesity, hypertension, elevated blood glucose, and blood lipids, which predisposes to cardiovascular disease and diabetes.

**metaplasia** (met-uh-plā´sē-yuh) A change from one type of cell to a more resistant cell type.

**metastasis** The spread of cancer cells from the primary site of origin to a distant site within the body.

**micelle** (mi-sell´) An aggregate of bile salt and lecithin molecules by which cholesterol is brought into solution in bile.

**mitosis** The type of cell division of most cells in which chromosomes are duplicated in the daughter cells and are identical with those in the parent cell. The characteristic cell division found in all cells in the body except for the gametes.

**monocyte** (mon´ō-sīt) A leukocyte having a kidney-shaped nucleus and light blue cytoplasm; a phagocytic cell that forms part of the reticuloendothelial system.

**monokine** A cytokine secreted by monocytes and macrophages.

**monosomy** A condition of a cell in which one chromosome of a homologous pair is missing.

**morula** A mulberry-shaped solid cluster of cells formed by division of the fertilized ovum.

**MSH** See *melanin-stimulating hormone.*

**multiple myeloma** (my-el-ō´muh) A malignant neoplasm of plasma cells.

**multiple sclerosis** Chronic disease characterized by focal areas of demyelination in the central nervous system, followed by glial scarring.

**myasthenia gravis** (mī-as-thē´nē-uh grä´vis) An autoimmune disease characterized by abnormal fatigability of muscle and caused by an autoantibody that damages the acetylcholine receptors at the myoneural junction.

**myelitis** (mī-el-ī´tis) An inflammation of the spinal cord.

**myelodysplastic syndrome** (my´elo-dis-plas´tik) A disturbance of bone marrow function that is characterized by anemia, leukopenia, and thrombocytopenia and that may be a precursor to leukemia in some patients.

**myocardial infarction** (mī-o-kar´dī-ul in-färk´shun) Necrosis of heart muscle as a result of interruption of its blood supply. May affect full thickness of muscle wall (*transmural infarct*) or only part of the wall (*subendocardial infarct*).

**myoma** (mī-ō´muh) A benign smooth muscle tumor such as commonly develops in the uterus.

# N

**natural killer cells** Lymphocytes capable of destroying foreign or abnormal cells, although they have not had any prior antigenic contact with the cells.

**necrosis** (nek-rō´sis) Structural changes associated with cell death.

**neoplasia** (nē-ō-plā´se-yuh) The pathologic process that results in the formation and growth of a tumor.

**nephron** (nef´rän) The glomerulus and renal tubule.

**nephrosclerosis** Thickening and narrowing of the afferent glomerular arterioles as a result of disease.

**nephrotic syndrome** (nef-rä´tik sin´drōm) A generalized edema resulting from excessive protein loss in the urine, caused by various types of renal disease.

**neuroglia** (noo-rog´-lē-ah) Supporting cells of tissue of the nervous system.

**neuron** (nū´ron) A nerve cell, including the nerve cell body and its processes.

**NK cells** An abbreviation for natural killer cells.

**norepinephrine** (nor´ep-in-ef´rin) One of the compounds (*catecholamines*) secreted by the adrenal medulla.

**nucleus pulposus** (nū´klē-us) The soft elastic center of the intervertebral disk.

# O

**oligodendroglia** (ol´ig-ō-den-drog´li-ah) One type of neuroglia that surrounds nerve fibers within the central nervous system.

**oligohydramnios** (ol-ig-ō-hī-dram´nē-yus) An insufficient quantity of amnionic fluid.

**one-second forced expiratory volume (FEV$_1$)** The maximum volume of air that can be expelled from the lungs in one second.

**opportunistic infection** (op-por-too-nis´tik) An infection in an immunocompromised person caused by an organism that is normally nonpathogenic or of limited pathogenicity.

**organelle** A small structure present in the cytoplasm of the cell, such as a mitochondrion.

**organic disease** A disease associated with structural changes in the affected tissue or organ.

**osteoarthritis** (ä´stē-ō) A "wear and tear" degeneration of the major weight-bearing joints.

**osteogenesis imperfecta** A congenital disturbance of bone formation characterized by excessively thin and delicate bones that are easily broken.

**osteomalacia** (ä´stē-ō-māh-lāy´see-yāh) Impaired calcification of bone in an adult caused by vitamin D deficiency, which also contributes to bone loss caused by osteoporosis.

**osteoporosis** (ä´stē-ō-por-ō´sis) Generalized thinning and demineralization of bone that tends to occur in postmenopausal women.

**oxytocin** (ox-i-to'sin) A hormone that is stored in the posterior lobe of the pituitary gland that causes uterine contractions during labor and ejection of milk from the breast lobules into the larger ducts.

# P

**panhypopituitarism** Failure of secretion of all anterior lobe pituitary hormones.

**papilloma** (pap-pil-ō'muh) A descriptive term for a benign tumor projecting from an epithelial surface.

**Pap smear** A study of cells from various sources, commonly used as a screening test for cancer.

**parenchyma** (par-en'ki-muh) The functional cells of an organ, as contrasted with the connective and supporting tissue that forms its framework.

**parenchymal cell** (par-en'ki-mul) The functional cell of an organ or tissue.

**paresthesia** (par-es-thē'ze-ah) An abnormal sensation, such as burning, prickling, or numbness.

**Parkinson disease** A chronic disease of the central nervous system characterized by rigidity and tremor, caused by decreased concentration of dopamine in the central nervous system.

**partial thromboplastin time (PTT) test** (throm-bō-plas'tin) A test that measures the overall efficiency of the blood coagulation process.

**pathogen** A disease-causing bacterium or other harmful organism.

**pathogenesis** (path-ō-jen'e-sis) Manner in which a disease develops.

**pathogenic** (path-ō-jen'ik) Capable of producing disease.

**pathology** The study of the structural and functional changes in the body caused by disease.

**percutaneous coronary intervention** (per'cue-tāy'ne-yus) An angioplasty procedure in which a balloon catheter covered by a stent is inserted into the site of a severely narrowed or blocked coronary artery, followed by expansion of the balloon, which enlarges the lumen of the artery and simultaneously expands the stent to keep the artery open.

**periodontal disease** (per-i-ō-don'tal) An inflammation of the gums around the roots of the teeth.

**petechia** (pe-tē'kēy-uh) A small pinpoint hemorrhage caused by decreased platelets, abnormal platelet function, or capillary defect.

**pheochromocytoma** (fē'o-krō'mō-sī-tō'muh) Catecholamine-secreting tumor of the adrenal medulla.

**phosphodiesterase** (fahs-foh-di-ester'-ase) An enzyme that breaks down cyclic guanosine monophosphate (cGMP) into a substance that dilates penile blood vessels to promote erection of the penis. A drug that inhibits phosphodiesterase inhibits cGMP breakdown, which prolongs its action, thereby facilitating penile erection in men with erectile dysfunction.

**phototherapy** Fluorescent light treatment of jaundiced babies to reduce the concentration of unconjugated bilirubin in their blood.

**pia** (pē'yuh) The innermost of the three membranes covering the brain and spinal cord.

**placenta previa** (prē'vē-yuh) Attachment of the placenta in the uterus such that it partially or completely covers the cervix.

**pleura** (plōōr'äh) The mesothelial covering of the lung (*visceral pleura*) and chest wall (*parietal pleura*).

**pneumoconiosis** (nōō'mō-kō-nēēiō'sis) An occupational lung disease caused by inhalation of injurious substances such as rock dust.

*Pneumocystis carinii* (new-mō-cis'tis cär-in'-ē-ī) (now called *Pneumocystis jiroveci* [jir-o-vek-key]) A protozoan parasite that causes severe pulmonary infections in immunocompromised persons.

**polar body** Structure extruded during the meiosis of the oocyte. Contains discarded chromosomes and a small amount of cytoplasm.

**poliomyelitis** (pō'lē-yo-mī-e-lī'tis) An inflammation of the gray matter of the spinal cord, caused by a virus.

**polycythemia** (päl-ē-sī-thē'mē-yuh) Increased number of red cells. May be caused by some types of chronic heart or lung disease (*secondary polycythemia*) or by marrow erythroid hyperplasia of unknown causes (*primary polycythemia*).

**polyhydramnios** (päl-ē-hī-dram'nē-yus) An excess of amnionic fluid.

**polyneuritis** (päl-ē-nū-rī'tis) An inflammation of multiple nerves.

**polyp** A descriptive term for a benign tumor projecting from an epithelial surface.

**portacaval shunt** (por'tuh-kay'vul) Surgically created anastomosis between the portal vein and the vena cava, performed to lower portal pressure in the treatment of esophageal varices.

**portal tract** Branch of hepatic artery, portal vein, and bile duct located at periphery of liver lobule.

**preeclampsia** (pre'ek-lamp'-sē-ă) A pregnancy-related complication characterized by hypertension and proteinuria, which usually occurs after the twentieth week of gestation, thought to be caused by placental dysfunction.

**primary gout** A metabolic disease caused by overproduction of uric acid, reduced excretion of uric acid, or a combination of both factors. Clinical manifestations are related to precipitation of uric acid in joints, kidneys, and other sites.

**prion** (prī'-on) A protein infectious particle responsible for Creutzfeldt-Jakob disease and some other degenerative diseases of the nervous system.

**prognosis** The probable outcome of a disease or a disorder; the outlook for recovery.

**prolactin** Hormone produced by the anterior lobe of the pituitary gland that stimulates milk secretion.

**prostaglandin** (pros-ta-glan'din) A complex derivative of a fatty acid (prostanoic acid) that has widespread physiologic effects.

**prothrombin time test** A test that measures that phase of the coagulation mechanism after the formation of thromboplastin.

**proto-oncogene** (pro-to-on'-koh-jēn) A normal gene that regulates some aspect of cell growth, maturation, or division.

**purpura** (pur'pura) A condition characterized by hemorrhage in the skin and mucous membranes (petechiae and ecchymoses).

**pyelonephritis** (pī'el-ō-nef-rī'tis) A bacterial infection of the kidney and renal pelvis.

# R

**recessive gene** A gene that expresses a trait only when present in the homozygous state.

**reflux esophagitis** Inflammation of the lining of the esophagus caused by reflux of acidic gastric secretions through an incompetent lower gastroesophageal sphincter.

**renin** (ren'in) A humoral substance secreted by the kidneys in response to fall in blood pressure, blood volume, or sodium concentration.

**respiratory unit** A functional unit of the lung consisting of a cluster of respiratory bronchioles, alveolar ducts, and alveoli derived from a single terminal bronchiole.

**reticulocyte** (rē-tik´ū-lō-sīt) A young red cell that can be identified by special staining procedures.

**Reye syndrome** (Rī) A disease characterized by a fatty liver and neurologic disturbances, probably related to aspirin administration in association with a viral infection.

**rheumatoid arthritis** (rōōm´uh-toyd) A systemic disease primarily affecting the synovium with major manifestations in the small joints.

**ribonucleic acid (RNA)** A type of nucleic acid contained in the nucleoli of cells. A component of messenger, transfer, and ribosomal RNA.

**rickets** Impaired calcification of bone in a growing child, caused by vitamin D deficiency, which leads to bowing of leg bones when weight bearing is attempted.

**roentgenogram** (rent´gen-ō-gram) A photograph taken with x-rays.

# S

**sarcoma** (sar-kō´muh) A malignant tumor arising from connective and supporting tissues.

**scoliosis** (sko-lee-oh´-sis) An abnormal lateral curvature of the spine.

**secondary gout** Elevated uric acid and clinical manifestations of gout not caused by the metabolic disease, primary gout, but instead caused by some other disease that raises the blood uric acid excessively, such as kidney failure or excessive breakdown of white blood cells in patients with leukemia.

**self-antigen** A group of unique genetically determined antigens on the cells of an individual.

**seminoma** (sem-in-ō´ma) One type of malignant tumor of testis.

**sentinel node** The lymph node in a group of lymph nodes that is located closest to a malignant tumor, which is examined to determine whether the tumor has spread to the node. If the sentinel node is not involved, additional lymph node dissection is not required.

**septicemia** (sep-ti-sē´mē-yuh) An infection in which large numbers of pathogenic bacteria are present in the bloodstream.

**serotonin** (sēr-o-tō´-nin) A vasoconstrictor mediator of inflammation released from platelets.

**sex-linked gene** Gene present on the X chromosome.

**sickle cell anemia** A hereditary anemia characterized by formation of an abnormal hemoglobin that causes the red cells to become sickle shaped when the oxygen content of the blood is reduced.

**silicosis** (sil-ik-ō´sis) A type of occupational lung disease caused by inhalation of rock dust.

**sinoatrial (SA) node** (sign-o-atrial´) The part of the cardiac conduction system that depolarizes at the fastest rate, thereby functioning as the cardiac pacemaker to regulate the heart rate; also called *sinus node*.

**spermatids** Germ cells in a late stage of sperm development just before complete maturation to mature sperm.

**spermatogenesis** Formation of mature sperm from precursor cells.

**spherocytosis** See *hereditary spherocytosis*.

**spina bifida** (spī´-nuh bif´fid-duh) Incomplete closure of vertebral arches over the spinal cord, sometimes associated with protrusion of meninges and neural tissue through the defect (*cystic spina bifida*).

**splenorenal shunt** (splē´no-rē´nul) Surgically created anastomosis between splenic vein and renal vein, performed to lower portal pressure in the treatment of esophageal varices.

**spores** Spherical structures formed within some bacteria that are extremely resistant to heat, disinfectants, and other agents that destroy bacteria. Spores form when conditions are unfavorable for the bacteria, and they can germinate to form actively growing bacteria when conditions are more favorable.

**stent** An expandable metal hollow tubular device placed within the lumen of a structure such as a blood vessel, often used to expand the lumen of the vessel, where it functions as a support to prevent narrowing of the dilated vessel.

**stroke** Any injury to the brain caused by disturbance of its blood supply.

**stroke volume** The amount of blood ejected from a ventricle by a single ventricular contraction.

**stroma** (strō´muh) The tissue that forms the framework of an organ.

**subarachnoid space** (sub-är-ak´noyd) The space between the arachnoid and the pia, containing large blood vessels supplying the brain.

**surfactant** (sur-fak´tant) A lipid material secreted by alveolar lining cells that facilitates respiration by decreasing the surface tension of the fluid lining the pulmonary alveoli.

**synapse** (sin´aps) Pairing of homologous chromosomes in meiosis.

# T

**teratoma** (tār-uh-tō´muh) A tumor of mixed cell components.

**tetany** (tet´an-ē) Spasm of skeletal muscles caused by subnormal level of ionized calcium in the blood.

**thalassemia** (thal-uh-seem´-mia) A hereditary anemia characterized by defective production of globin chains required to produce normal hemoglobin, leading to a hypochronic microcytic anemia.

**thrombin time** A laboratory test measurement that determines the concentration of fibrinogen in the blood by determining the clotting time of the blood plasma after addition of thrombin.

**thrombocytopenia** (throm´bō-sī-tō-pē´ny-yuh) A deficiency of platelets.

**thrombolytic therapy** (throm-bo-lit´-tik) Intravenous administration of clot-dissolving drugs to dissolve a blood clot in an artery blocked by a thrombus in an attempt to reestablish blood flow through the artery.

**thrombosis** A blood clot formed within the vascular system.

**thyroid-stimulating hormone (TSH)** Hormone secreted by the anterior lobe of the pituitary; regulates thyroid function.

**tissue** A group of similar cells joined to perform a specific function.

**T lymphocyte** A type of lymphocyte associated with cell-mediated immunity.

**transient ischemic attack (TIA)** (isskē´mik) Temporary cerebral dysfunction as a result of transient obstruction of a cerebral vessel by a bit of atheromatous debris or blood clot usually embolized from an arteriosclerotic plaque in the carotid artery.

**transjugular intrahepatic portosystemic shunt** A nonsurgical method used to lower portal vein pressure in a person with cirrhosis by connecting an intrahepatic branch of the portal vein to a hepatic vein branch.

**trisomy** The presence of an extra chromosome within a cell; having three of a given chromosome instead of the usual pair.

**trophoblast** Cell derived from the fertilized ovum that gives rise to the fetal membranes and contributes to the formation of the placenta.

**TSH** Thyroid-stimulating hormone.

**tumor necrosis factor** A cytokine that can destroy foreign or abnormal cells.

**tumor suppressor gene** A gene that suppresses cell proliferation.

# U

**urate nephropathy** (nĕf-rop´-uh-thē) Kidney damage caused by precipitation of urate crystals within the kidney tubules of a person with gout.

**urea** (ū-rē´yuh) The nitrogen waste product derived from protein metabolism and excreted in the urine.

**uremia** (ur-ē´mi-yuh) An excess of urea and other waste products in the blood, resulting from renal failure.

**urinalysis** (ur-in-al´i-sis) A commonly performed chemical and microscopic analysis of the urine.

# V

**valve stenosis** (sten-ō´sis) Impaired flow of blood through a heart valve that does not open properly.

**varicocele** (var´-ik-kō-sēl) Varicose veins within the spermatic cord that drain blood from the testis.

**vasodilator** A substance that dilates blood vessels.

**vesicoureteral reflux** (ves´i-kō-ūr-ēt´er-al) Retrograde flow of urine from the bladder into the ureter during voiding.

**virulence** (vir´u-lenz) The ability of an organism to cause disease.

**vital capacity** The maximum volume of air that can be forcefully expelled after a maximum inspiration.

**volvulus** (vol´vū-lus) A rotary twisting of the intestine on its mesentery, with obstruction of the blood supply to the twisted segment.

# W

**Wilms tumor** A malignant renal tumor of infants and children.

# Y

**yolk sac** A sac that is formed adjacent to the germ disk and that will form the gastrointestinal tract and other important structures in the embryo.

# Z

**zygote** (zī´gōt) The fertilized ovum.

# Index

## M

Macleod, J.J.R., 387
Macroglobulin, 53
Macrophages, 49
Mad cow disease, 481–482
Magnetic resonance imaging (MRI),
    11, 420
Major histocompatibility complex (MHC),
    34, 50, 52
Malaria, 82, 83, 86
Malignant tumors, 132–135
Mallory bodies, 374
Malnutrition
    in adults, 427–428
    alcohol, role of, 428
    causes of, 426–427
    in children, 427
Mammary ridges, 270–271
Mammograms, 8, 269–270
Mantoux test, 254
Marasmus, 427
Mast cells, 41, 42
Mastectomies, 276
Matrix, 19
Meckel diverticulum, 409
Mediators, inflammation
    blood plasma, 42
    cell-derived, 41–42
Megakaryocytes, 156, 225
Megaloblasts, 230
Meiosis, 28–29, 30
Melanin, 137
Melanin-stimulating hormone (MSH),
    447, 457
Melanocytes, 137
Meninges, 466, 485
Meningioma, 485
Meningitis, 70, 71, 82, 479–480
Meningocele, 470
Meningomyelocele, 470
Mesangial cells, 326
Mesenteric thrombosis, 418–419
Mesothelium, 18
Metabolic acidosis, 438, 439–440
Metabolic alkalosis, 438, 441–442
Metabolic diseases, 2
Metabolic syndrome, 388
Metaphase, 29, 30
Metaplasia, 24
Metastasis, 132, 134
Metazoal infections, 82, 82–89, 90
Micelles, 380
Microcephaly, 124
Microorganisms
    bacteria, 66–74
    chlamydiae, 75
    fungi, 80–82

mycoplasmas, 75
    rickettsiae and ehrlichiae, 75
    types of harmful, 65–66
    viruses, 75–80
Miliary tuberculosis, 254
Mineralocorticoids, 456
Minerals, importance of, 426, 431
Miscarriages, 305–306
Mitochondria, 17, 18
Mitosis, 28, 29–30, 113
Mitral valve prolapse, 191–192
Monocytes, 224, 225
Monokines, 48
Mononuclear cells, 39
Mononucleosis, 237–238
Monosomy, 112
Morulae, 75, 298
Mosaic, 113
Mother-to-infant transmission of HIV, 106
Multifactorial inheritance, 125
Multiple myeloma, 149–150, 485
Multiple neurofibromatosis, 119, 120
Multiple sclerosis, 482–483
Muscle
    paralysis, 468
    skeletal, 506–507
    tissue, 19–20
    tone and voluntary contraction,
        467–468
Muscular atrophy and dystrophy,
    507–508
Musculoskeletal system
    arthritis, 496–499
    bone formation, 492
    bone formation, abnormal, 494
    bone growth, 493–494
    bone tumors, 501–502
    clubfoot, congenital, 494
    fractures, 501
    gout, 499–501
    intervertebral disk disease, 504, 506
    muscular atrophy and dystrophy,
        507–508
    myasthenia gravis, 60, 508
    myositis, 507
    osteomyelitis, 501
    osteoporosis, 494, 502–503
    skeletal muscle, structure of, 506–507
    spine, structure and function of,
        503–504
    structure and function of, 491–494
Mutation, 140
Myasthenia gravis, 60, 508
*Mycobacterium avium* complex,
    72, 104
*Mycobacterium tuberculosis*, 72
Mycoplasmas, 75